THE 2003 Credentialing AND Privileging
DESK REFERENCE

CONTRIBUTING EDITOR:
Kathy Matzka, CMSC, CPCS

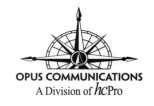

OPUS COMMUNICATIONS
A Division of *hc*Pro

The 2003 Credentialing and Privileging Desk Reference is published by Opus Communications, Inc., a subsidiary of HCPro Corp.

Copyright 2003 by Opus Communications, Inc., a subsidiary of HCPro Corp.

All rights reserved. Printed in the United States of America.   5   4   3   2   1

ISBN 1–57839–227-6

The information provided in this Book is for your personal use only and not for commercial exploitation. You may not rent, lease, loan, sell, sublicense, or create derivative works from this Book or its Contents. You may not copy, modify, reproduce, republish, distribute, display, or transmit for commercial, nonprofit or public purposes all or any portion of this Book, except to the extent permitted above. Any unauthorized use of this Book or its Contents is prohibited.

Except as expressly provided above, nothing contained herein shall be construed as conferring any license or right, by implication, estoppel or otherwise, under copyright or other intellectual property rights. You further agree that the Book and its Contents are protected by copyrights, trademarks or other proprietary rights and laws. If you do not agree to these terms, return this book immediately for a refund. The right to return and refund does not extend to your transferee.

No part of this publication may be reproduced, in any form or by any means, without prior written consent of Opus Communications or the Copyright Clearance Center (978/750-8400). Please notify us immediately if you have received an unauthorized copy.

Opus Communications provides information resources for the health care industry. Neither HCPro Corp. nor Opus Communications, Inc. is affiliated in any way with the Joint Commission on Accreditation of Healthcare Organizations, which owns the JCAHO trademark.

Kathy Matzka, CMSC, CPCS, Contributing Editor
Dale Seamans, Executive Editor
Elaine Koritsas, Senior Copy Editor
Rena Cutchin, Senior Managing Editor
Erin E. Callahan, Managing Editor
Tracy Gieske, Editorial Assistant
Michele L. Wilson, Editorial Assistant
Jean St. Pierre, Creative Director
Mike Mirabello, Senior Graphic Artist
Suzanne Perney, Publisher

Advice given is general. Readers should consult professional counsel for specific legal, ethical, or clinical questions. Arrangements can be made for quantity discounts.

For more information, contact:

Opus Communications
PO Box 1168
Marblehead, MA 01945
Telephone: 800/650-6787 or 781/639-1872
Fax: 781/639-2982
E-mail: customerservice@hcpro.com

Visit Opus Communications at its World Wide Web sites:
www.hcmarketplace.com, www.hcpro.com, **and** *www.credentialinfo.com*

Table of Contents

About the Contributing Editor vii

Preface viii

Chapter 1: Areas of Credentialing 1

Chapter 2: Areas of Privileging 11

Chapter 3: Roles and Responsibilities in Credentialing 27

Chapter 4: Managed Care Credentialing 33

Chapter 5: Schools, Colleges, and Educational Programs 47

    Medical School Degrees, Residencies, Internships, and Fellowships. 55
    Osteopathic Medical Schools. 139
    Canadian Medical Schools 147
    Dental Schools 159
    Podiatry Schools 179
    Chiropractic Schools 183
    Physician Assistant Programs 193
    Nursing Schools 221
    Nurse Anesthesia (CRNA) Programs 227
    Nurse-Midwifery Programs 257

Chapter 6: Licensing Agencies 275

    Medical Licensing Agencies. 287
    Canadian College of Physicians and Surgeons Provincial Offices. 331
    Dental Licensing Agencies. 341
    Podiatric Licensing Agencies 375
    Chiropractic Licensing Agencies. 395
    Physician Assistant Licensing Agencies 415
    Nursing Licensing Agencies 435
    Psychology Licensing Agencies 455

Chapter 7: Board Certification 477

    American Board of Medical Specialties (ABMS) Boards. 485
    American Osteopathic Association (AOA) Boards 498
    American Dental Association (ADA) Boards 505
    American Podiatric Medical Association (APMA) Boards 510
    Nursing Boards 511
    Psychology Boards 513
    Other Boards 514

Table of Contents

Chapter 8: How to Use Practitioner Data Banks 517

    National Practitioner Data Bank (NPDB) 519
    Healthcare Integrity and Protection Data Bank 526
    Federation of State Medical Boards 527
    Federation Credentials Verification Service 530
    American Medical Association Physician Masterfile 530
    National Register of Health Service Providers in Psychology 533
    Chiropractic Information Network/Board Action Databank 533
    American Osteopathic Association
        Official Osteopathic Physician Profile Report 534
    Quick Checklist Guide to the NPDB 537

Chapter 9: Specialty Associations, Societies, Colleges, and Academies .539

    Addictionology 543
    Allergy, asthma, and immunology 544
    Allied health-general 545
    Anesthesiology 547
    Cardiology 549
    Chiropractic 549
    Colon and rectal surgery 550
    Counseling 550
    Critical care/trauma medicine 550
    Dentistry 551
    Dermatology 553
    Emergency medicine 554
    Endocrinology 555
    Endoscopy 555
    Environmental medicine 556
    Family medicine 556
    Gastroenterology 557
    General medicine 558
    Geriatric medicine 562
    Head and neck surgery 562
    Hematology 563
    Hospice care 563
    Hospital-related organizations 564
    Internal medicine 567
    Laser medicine 568
    Managed care 568
    Maxillofacial surgery 568
    Nephrology 569
    Neurological surgery 569
    Neurology 570
    Nuclear medicine 570
    Nursing 571
    Obstetrics and gynecology 583

Occupational medicine...584
Occupational therapy..584
Oncology...585
Ophthalmology..585
Optometry..587
Oral surgery..587
Orthopedic surgery...587
Osteopathic medicine...587
Otolaryngology..592
Otology..593
Pain management..593
Pathology..594
Pediatrics..595
Pharmacology/Pharmacy...597
Physiatry/Rehabilitative medicine.....................................598
Physical therapy...599
Physician and medical assistants......................................599
Plastic surgery...600
Podiatry..600
Preventive medicine..601
Psychiatry..602
Psychology...603
Public health...604
Radiology..605
Respiratory care...607
Rheumatology..608
Social work...608
Speech, language, hearing...609
Surgery..609
Thoracic medicine..611
Thyroid medicine..612
Urology..612
Video data transmission...613
Wound care..613

Chapter 10: Credentialing and Privileging Resources 615

Professional Associations..617
Accreditors...618
National Credentials Verification Organizations (CVOs).................626
Regional Credentials Verification Organizations (CVOs)................631
Software Vendors..636
Books, Periodicals, and Multimedia..................................639

Appendix: Table of Board Certification Time Limits 647

Index 653

About the Contributing Editor

Kathy Matzka, CMSC, CPCS, is a writer and speaker on medical and professional staff issues with more than 15 years' experience in medical and professional staff services. Having been a member of the National Association of Medical Staff Services since 1991, she is well known within the field. She currently serves as President of the Missouri Association of Medical Staff Services.

Matzka has served on NAMSS' *OverView* editorial board, strategic planning, and nominating committees. She currently serves on the editorial advisory board for Opus Communications' *Briefings On Credentialing* and C&R Publications' *The Advisor for Medical & Professional Staff*. Matzka is the author of the professional development book, *MSSPs Take Charge: Practical Tips to Promote Yourself and Get the Respect You Deserve*. She developed and edited Unit III, *Meeting Management, Documentation, and Management of Information* of NAMSS' *Core Curriculum for Persons Responsible for Medical Staff Management and Provider Services,* and is the contributing editor of Module III of NAMSS' Independent Study Program, *Principles of Medical Staff Organization and Healthcare Finance*. She is also a contributing editor for NAMSS' Certification Preparatory Courses for Certified Provider Credentialing Specialist and Certified Medical Staff Coordinator.

Preface

When I began my career in medical staff services more than 15 years ago, I went into it with no training or experience. In addition to needing to know why physicians are credentialed, I also needed to know where and how to contact the primary sources needed to accomplish this function. I would have been so grateful for a resource like this book.

Often, getting the information we need is as simple as knowing whom to ask. This book not only tells you whom to contact, but gives you names, addresses, phone and fax numbers, e-mail and Web site addresses and the cost for verification. This comprehensive resource provides information on medical and allied health professional schools, licensing agencies, specialty boards and associations, and data banks all organized in easy-to-read chapters. The book begins with a chart that provides quick reference to key credentialing and privileging issues. In addition, a listing of additional credentialing and privileging resources that can provide further helpful information is included.

All this in one publication makes *The 2003 Credentialing and Privileging Desk Reference* the premier credentialing resource for both new and "seasoned" medical and professional staff services professionals.

Kathy Matzka, CMSC, CPCS

CHAPTER 1
Areas of Credentialing

Chapter 1
Areas of Credentialing

Credentialing is the process of collecting and verifying data that will serve as the basis for decisions regarding appointments and reappointments to the medical staff and delineation of clinical privileges for medical staff applicants and others with privileges. The JCAHO requires the medical staff to consider information concerning the applicant's licensure, training/experience, current competence, and the ability to perform the privileges requested. Although individual state laws may have some requirements dealing with credentialing, any additional information an organization decides to use in making credentialing decisions is up to the organization.

In a number of legal cases, the hospital's governing body has been held responsible for adopting corporate and medical staff bylaws that hold the medical staff accountable to the board for ensuring the adequacy of the credentials review process. Failure of the hospital to do so may lead to a finding of negligent credentialing.

The following chart includes basic credentialing issues with current JCAHO standards referenced. The chart is not meant to be all-inclusive. State and federal regulations may contain additional requirements. We suggest that you use this chart as a basis for understanding, and strongly encourage you to review the appropriate standards in the relevant accreditor manuals for more details.

Chapter 1

Credentialing Area	Associated *CAMH* Standard No.	Allowed	Req'd	Rec'd	Explanation
Closed and difficult-to-reach facilities and military credentials	MS.5.4.3.1.	√		√	It may not always be feasible to obtain information from the primary source. Hospitals may not no longer exist or the applicant's records may have been lost or destroyed. Applicants may have received education, training, in a foreign country and verification information is not accessible. In these cases, JCAHO allows use of designated equivalent sources or other reliable secondary sources. This may include written statements from individuals who were in a leadership positions in the closed organization, or statements from a successor organization. In this case, you must document the attempt to contact the primary source. Usually, if a hospital has closed, the medical staff records will have been transferred to another facility. If the hospital is part of a healthcare system, the system's main office or another system hospital can provide information as to the location of files. Also the medical staff office of other hospitals in the same city will often have information concerning the location of these records. If a military applicant was recently discharged, the last place the practitioner was stationed may still have all records. Since the record follows the person from assignment to assignment, personnel at the last assignment should have all information in the file to verify dates of military affiliation and training. If a base is closed and documentation is needed for verification of current competency or training, ask the applicant to provide the current location of his/her training program director or physician supervisor. For verification of prior military service, you can write to the Military Records Center, 9700 Page Boulevard, St. Louis, MO 63132-5100.
Core criteria	MS.5.4 through MS.5.4.3		√		Each hospital should have professional criteria as the basis for medical staff appointment and granting initial or renewed or revised clinical privileges. These criteria must pertain to, at the very least, evidence of current licensure, relevant training and experience, current competency, and ability to perform privileges requested. This includes health status as it relates to the privileges requested. Criteria must be applied consistently to all applicants.
Credentialing AHPs	MS.1.1.1 through MS.1.1.3 HR.2		√	√	AHPs are usually designated as "dependent" or "independent". Independent AHPs are licensed practitioners who are allowed by the hospital and state law to function without physician supervision. Under JCAHO standards, these AHPs are considered licensed independent practitioners and are granted appointment and privileges through the same credentialing and privileging process as a physician. Dependent AHPs often are employees of a medical staff appointee. These individuals usually function under a job description, but are not granted medical staff appointment or privileges. Typically, the physician employer is granted privileges to utilize the services of the AHP in the hospital

Areas of Credentialing

Credentialing Area	Associated *CAMH* Standard No.	Allowed	Req'd	Rec'd	Explanation
					setting. JCAHO's Medical Staff standards do not address dependent AHP's.

Your hospital or medical staff policies should detail the best method for credentialing applicants classified as dependent AHPs and complementary, integrative, or alternative practitioners (CIAs). You should also make sure that your hospital's classifications of LIPs, AHPs, and CIAs match your state's classifications.

You should evaluate a dependent AHP's education, training, and current competency just as you would for a physician. This evaluation may be done in either the medical staff office or the human resources department. Generally, if an AHP is a physician employee, credentialing occurs in the medical staff office.

Although the JCAHO does not specifically require primary source verification of AHP credentials, most hospitals do whenever feasible to avoid liability.

The JCAHO also does not require recredentialing every two years for dependent AHPs, but again it is suggested to do so to avoid liability. At the minimum, this evaluation should include current licensure or certification, an annual evaluation by the physician employer, and any other medical staff requirements.

If the AHP is practicing through a contractual arrangement between the hospital and the AHP, the JCAHO HR standards apply to this contracted individual, meaning the hospital must manage the contracted personnel just as it manages direct employees. This includes maintaining a written job description and a completed competence assessment, evaluation, or appraisal tool for each individual and confirmation of the applicants' credentials, qualifications, experience, education, and ability. The hospital must define, either in the contract or in policy, criteria for performance of the contracted service; or it must, review and adopt the contract organization's policies and practices. The contract should specify that the contracted organization will provide only staff who are qualified in relation to their education, training, licensure, and competence as defined by the organization.

Further, the medical staff may privilege hospital-contracted AHPs. In some hospitals, certain AHPs—such as psychologists, social workers, and nurse clinicians— are offered appointment to a medical staff category separate from physicians, in addition to being privileged. Any of these options is acceptable to the JCAHO. |
| Credentialing using data banks | MS.5.4.3.2 | | | √ | The JCAHO standards encourage hospitals to research medical staff applicants using additional resources. The standards specifically cite the Federation of State Medical Boards Physician Disciplinary Data Bank. The reasoning is that by using additional sources, you may learn more about the applicant or see "red flags" such as an inconsistency. |

CVO use/ Delegated credentialing	MS.5.4.3.2					Delegated credentialing may refer to: • A hospital assigning portions of the credentialing process to another organization such as a CVO, • Multiple hospitals centralizing the credentialing process at a central office, or • A managed care organization assigning credentialing responsibility to a physician group, and then overseeing the process. JCAHO allows hospitals to use an external agency (or CVO) to collect information from primary sources. The agency must furnish the hospital with any information from the primary source(s). The hospital then evaluates the individual's credentials by comparing the information in his or her application with the information provided by the primary source to the external agency. Any hospital using a CVO should have confidence in the completeness, accuracy, and timeliness of that information.
Current competence	MS.5.4.3.–MS.5.4.3.1.1 MS.5.6 MS.5.12 through 5.12.3 MS.5.13 Intent Statement MS.5.15		√			The professional criteria considered at appointment and reappointment must include current competence. For applicants in fields doing operative and other procedure(s), evaluation should include the types of operative procedures performed, including information on appropriateness and outcomes. For applicants in nonsurgical fields, the evaluation should include types and outcomes of medical conditions managed. At the time of reappointment, current competence is determined by the results of performance-improvement activities. Relevant practitioner-specific information from organization performance improvement activities should be considered and compared to aggregate information. If a physician has not had a level of activity at your hospital in the period since his/her last reappointment that would allow an evaluation of current competence, additional information should be solicited from other hospitals where the physician has been working. See the Intent Statement for MS.5.4.3.1 for addition requirements for using CVOs.
Disclosing credentialing information			√			Medical staff offices are limited by hospital and medical staff policy as to what information about a practitioner they can make available on request from the public or from another healthcare organization. Every medical staff office should consult with both legal counsel and the medical staff and develop a policy regarding the release of information. Here are some examples of information hospitals might routinely disclose: • Practitioners' specialties, general areas of privileges, foreign language capabilities, and office locations • Medical staff appointment status and length of appointment • General details about a practitioner's practice record, such as number of admissions and number of procedures completed (but only to other healthcare organizations and only if they have a practitioner's signed consent and release) Prior to releasing information that contains disciplinary

Areas of Credentialing

					actions, the medical staff office should consult with administration and legal counsel. Many state licensure boards have databanks that provide information about adverse actions. Most of these databanks are open to the public.
Fast-track credentialing	MS.5.1.1	√			The JCAHO allows expedited credentialing by enabling the governing body to delegate membership-privilege decisions to a committee consisting of at least two governing body members. The standards require this committee to "be consistent with the governing body bylaws as they relate to forming a governing body committee ", which means that this committee should be allowed by and defined in the policies or bylaws of the board. The governing body 's bylaws must specify the criteria for delegation. The standard does list conditions under which expedited credentialing may not be used, e.g., the applicant's application is incomplete. Review the standard for more details.
Locum tenens physicians	5.14.4	√		√	Locum tenens physicians are employed for a short-term, specific purpose, usually through an employment agency. These physicians typically complete an abbreviated application process or all or part of the primary source verification may be delegated to the locum tenens company. All requirements for granting temporary privileges as specified in JCAHO's standards must be met prior to granting temporary privileges. (See Temporary Privileges section.) Locum tenens physicians may also qualify for "emergency privileges." See privileging section for more information.
Peer recommendation	MS.5.4 Intent Statement MS.5.7		√		A peer recommendation is a statement provided in support of an applicant's request for appointment/reappointment and/or privileges by a practitioner in the same professional discipline as the applicant. A physician must provide the peer recommendation for a physician, dentist for dentist, podiatrist for podiatrist, nurse for nurse, etc. In situations where there is no peer available for a specific category or LIP, a physician with essentially equal qualifications, who is familiar with the LIPs performance, can provide the reference. For example, a pediatrician could provide a reference for a pediatric nurse practitioner, or an internist could provide a reference for an adult nurse practitioner. The recommendation should come from someone in the same clinical specialty. For new applicants, peer recommendations are usually letters of reference. For reappointments, JCAHO standards allow statements from an applicant's colleagues who are members of the same department, members of the credentials committee, or medical executive committee to serve as the peer recommendation on reappointment.
Peer review	MS.8-MS.8.4 And MS.5.12-MS.5.12.3		√	√	Peer Review is defined as the evaluation or review of the performance of colleagues by professionals with similar types and degrees of clinical expertise. The peer should come from the same medical discipline and specialty. JCAHO standards require a properly designed peer review process to evaluate LIPs. Further, the JCAHO does state that

					peer review results are important and should be measured, aggregated, and trended over time; and that medical staffs should be using them in a constructive way to make credentialing and privileging decisions.
Photographs				√	Requiring applicants to provide photographs may guard against imposters with falsified credentials. Prior to requiring this, make sure to consult with your hospital's attorneys to be sure you are in compliance with the law.
Primary-source verification	MS.5.4.3 and MS.5.4.3.1 through MS.5.4.3.2		√		This is verifying important credentials with the primary source, that is, the person or organization able to attest directly to their validity. The JCAHO requires primary-source verification for professional school education, licensure, postgraduate or specialty training, and current competence. There are some acceptable designated equivalent sources for specific credentials.

The JCAHO allows hospitals to use an external agency (or CVO) to collect information from primary sources. The agency must furnish the hospital with any information from the primary source(s). The hospital then evaluates the individual's credentials by comparing the information in his or her application with the information provided by the primary source to the external agency. Any hospital using a CVO should have confidence in the completeness, accuracy, and timeliness of that information.

You may verify by means other than a traditional written document, (such as the Internet) but the source must be adequately documented and must be a primary source of the information. For example, a state licensing agency's Web site would be an acceptable primary source for current license verification.

According to the JCAHO, a documented telephone conversation can be utilized as primary-source verification for all information including licensure, education, training, experience, competence, and peer references. When verifying information via telephone, the following documented should include the date of the conversation, the name and title of the person providing the information, the name of the organization when appropriate, e.g., the school, certifying board, employing organization, etc., the specific information provided, and the date and signature of the person receiving the information. |
| Supplemental credentialing criteria | MS.5.5-MS.5.5.3.1 | | √ | √ | Medical staff bylaws and rules may provide for applicants for medical staff appointment or reappointment (or for initial, revised, or renewed clinical privileges) to provide information that is supplemental to the core criteria (current licensure, relevant training or experience, current competence, and ability to perform requested privileges). Examples of supplemental information include: challenges to any licensure or regulation, relinquishment of licensure or registration, voluntary or involuntary termina-tion of medical staff privileges/appoint ment, malpractice suits or settlements, etc. |
| Temporary privileges | MS. 5.14.4 | √ | | | The JCAHO standards allow the CEO (or his or her designee) to grant temporary privileges based on the recommendation of the department chair or the president of the medical staff. For new applicants, these privileges cannot exceed 120 days. Temporary privileges are not to be routinely used for admin-istrative purposes such as when an LIP fails to provide all |

Areas of Credentialing

						information necessary to the processing of his/her reappointment in a timely manner and failure of the organization staff to verify performance data and information in a timely manner. JCAHO standards lists two circumstances for which the granting of temporary privileges to an LIP would be acceptable – to fulfill an important patient care need and when an applicant with a complete, "clean" application is awaiting review and approval of the medical staff executive committee and board. The following examples of a "patient care need" are given: • A physician becomes ill or takes a leave of absence and an LIP would need to cover his/her practice until he/she returns • A specific LIP has the necessary skills to provide care to a patient that an LIP currently privileged does not possess In order for an application to be considered "complete and clean" there must be verification of current licensure, relevant training or experience, current competence, ability to perform the privileges requested, and any other criteria required by the organization's medical staff bylaws. The National Practitioner Data Bank query results must have been obtained and evaluated. It is also required that the new applicant has a complete application with no current or previously successful challenge to licensure or registration, has not been subject to involuntary termination of medical staff appointment at another organization, and has not been subject to involuntary limitation, reduction, denial, or loss of clinical privileges. Medical staff bylaws, rules and regulations, or policies must describe the mechanism used for granting temporary privileges and must stipulate that, in an emergency, any medical staff member who has clinical privileges is permitted to provide any type of patient care necessary as a life-saving measure or to prevent serious harm—regardless of his or her medical staff status or clinical privileges—provided that the care provided is within the scope of the individual's license. The temporary status may also be granted to locum tenens physicians. These physicians are employed for a short-term, specific purpose, usually through an employment agency. These physicians typically complete an abbreviated application process or all or part of the primary-source verification may be delegated to the locum tenens company. All requirements for granting temporary privileges must be met prior to granting temporary privileges
Emergency privileges	MS. 5.14.4.1	√			√	JCAHO allows emergency privileges to be granted case-by-case basis when the hospital's emergency management plan has been activated, and the organization is unable to handle the immediate patient needs. The medical staff must • identify in writing the individual(s) responsible for granting emergency privileges. • describe in writing the responsibilities of the individual(s) responsible for granting emergency privileges.

- describe in writing a mechanism to manage the activities of individuals who receive emergency privileges. There is a mechanism to allow staff to readily identify these individuals.
- addresses the verification process as a high priority.

The verification process for the credentials and privileges of those granted emergency privileges must begin as soon as the immediate situation is under control. This privileging process must be identical to the process for granting temporary privileges to fulfill an important patient care need.

The chief executive officer or president of the medical staff or his or her designee(s) *may* grant emergency privileges upon presentation of any of the following:

- A current picture hospital ID card
- A current license to practice and a valid picture ID issued by a state, federal, or regulatory agency
- Identification indicating that the individual is a member of a Disaster Medical Assistance Team
- Identification indicating that the individual has been granted authority by a federal, state or municipal entity to render patient care in emergency circumstances
- Presentation by current hospital or medical staff member(s) with personal knowledge regarding practitioner's identity

CHAPTER 2
Areas of Privileging

Chapter 2
Areas of Privileging

Determining the procedures that each medical staff appointee may perform and conditions that he or she may treat—commonly known as delineation of clinical privileges—is one of the most difficult jobs that department chairs and other medical staff leaders face. Delineation of clinical privileges requires fairly and consistently analyzing whether each appointee's education, training, experience, and clinical competence match the particular procedures the appointee wishes to perform and the conditions he or she seeks to treat.

The JCAHO requires privileges delineation, but does not specify how to organize privileges or the level of detail in which privileges must be described. In fact, the JCAHO requires that a hospital's privilege delineation be "hospital specific"—tailored to take into account the hospital's technical and staff capability of supporting the procedures.

The following chart includes basic privileging issues with current JCAHO standards referenced. The chart is not meant to be all-inclusive. State and federal regulations may contain additional requirements. We suggest that you use this chart as a basis for understanding and strongly encourage you to review the appropriate standards in the relevant accreditor manuals for more details.

Privileging Area	Associated *CAMH* Standard No.	Allowed	Req'd	Rec'd	Explanation
Classifying clinical privileges	MS.5.14 Intent Statement through MS5.15.4		√		The JCAHO does not specify the exact method a medical staff must use to categorize privileges, but it does require an accurate, detailed, and specific description of the clinical privileges granted. Many hospitals categorize privileges by specialty areas—for example, surgery, internal medicine, or pediatrics or into subspecialties—for example, orthopedics, neurosurgery, thoracic surgery, or cardiology. Other hospitals, or departments, categorize privileges by severity of illness or intensity of service—for example, Level I privileges encompass procedures and treatments that do not involve threat to life or long-term health, whereas Level II privileges include procedures and treatments that require hospital admission to a general care unit, but do not involve threat to life or long-term health. Privileges can also be delineated by disease and disease classes (for example, tuberculosis, AIDS, or oncology), or by body area (for example, hand surgery, thoracic surgery, or neurology). Medical staffs may delineate privileges using core privileges (see Core Privileging below), laundry lists (which includes every procedure or treatment a LIP may perform), or a combination of both.
Clinical data and references	MS.5.4.3		√	√	Prior to reviewing or granting clinical privileges, clinical data and references should be acquired. Clinical data may include information such as numbers and types of procedures. Your hospital's policy should specify requirements for clinical data from those requesting privileges. The data collected should include outcomes. According to the JCAHO, for applicants in fields doing operative and other procedures, evaluation should include the types of operative procedures performed, including information on appropriateness and outcomes. For applicants in nonsurgical fields, the evaluation should include types and outcomes of medical conditions managed. At the time of reappointment, current competence is determined by the results of performance-improvement activities. If a physician has not had a level of activity at your hospital in the period since his/her

Areas of Privileging

Privileging Area	Associated *CAMH* Standard No.	Allowed	Req'd	Rec'd	Explanation
					last reappointment that would allow an evaluation of current competence, additional information should be solicited from other hospitals where the physician has been working.
Complying with the ADA and documentation of health status	MS.5.4.3 Intent Statement		√		JCAHO does require that evaluating current competence for privileges include consideration of health status. However, the ADA restricts employer access to employee health information. In consideration of this, the current JCAHO standards require only that applicants be asked to describe their ability to perform requested privileges. This covers relevant aspects of health status and avoids requesting information about an applicant's general health or potential disabilities. The JCAHO does also require that an individual familiar with the applicant's work confirm the applicant's health status, as it relates to ability to perform requested privileges. As of yet, there are few formal legal decisions that have clarified how the courts view medical staff appointment and privileges in regard to the ADA. Therefore, each hospital should work with its attorneys to develop policies that comply with the ADA.
Core privileging				√	Core privileging is a common alternative to the traditional "laundry list" approach to credentialing. Core privileging is considered more effective because it uses predefined criteria in conjunction with clinically realistic, well-defined descriptions of core privileges for each specific clinical specialty or subspecialty treatment area. A successful core privileging system should include the following for each specialty ("core set"): • Predefined criteria for each privilege that outlines specific education, training, and experience requirements • Descriptions of clinical privileges that are accurate, detailed, comprehensive, and specific • A system that is designed to avoid denials by clearly stating the minimum education, training, and experience needed to apply for specific clinical privileges In addition to defining this "core set," the medical staff should outline privilege

Chapter 2

Privileging Area	Associated *CAMH* Standard No.	Allowed	Req'd	Rec'd	Explanation
					requests that require individual applications. Such special requests nearly always reflect new advances in technology, volume-sensitive privileges not automatically incorporated within the core, and issues that occasionally cross specialty lines.
Delineation of clinical privileges	MS.5.4 through 5.4.5, MS.5 through 5.16, and MS.6.8		√		The JCAHO requires all individuals who are permitted by law and the hospital to care for patients independently (LIPs) have delineated clinical privileges, whether or not they are medical staff members. Further, the JCAHO requires that the hospital have in place a mechanism that ensures the quality of patient care by all individuals with delineated clinical privileges, whether or not they are medical staff appointees. Delineating clinical privileges means determining the procedures that each medical staff appointee may perform and conditions that he or she may treat. This includes an accurate, detailed, and specific description of the clinical privileges granted. This requires fair and consistent analysis of whether each appointee's education, training, experience, and clinical competence match the particular procedures the appointee wishes to perform and the conditions he or she seeks to treat. The underlying structure of the privilege categories—or delineation—should be common sets of skills required to carry out procedures. Whenever two or more procedures require the same set of skills, those procedures should be covered by a single privilege. It is not necessary to designate those procedures as separate privileges. A hospital with an effective privilege delineation system fulfills the following objectives: • It decides which procedures and treatments the hospital should offer to patients. This involves examining the hospital's ability to meet the requirements that each procedure and treatment area demands, from equipment to support staff. • It organizes the procedures and treatments it offers into specific privilege categories. For each privilege category, a hospital must define:

Areas of Privileging

Privileging Area	Associated *CAMH* Standard No.	Allowed	Req'd	Rec'd	Explanation
					– the scope of the privilege—that is, exactly which procedures the privilege includes. – the training and experience requirements a practitioner must demonstrate to be awarded the privilege. – the requirements for automatic renewal of the privilege upon expiration. This might include, for example, the minimum number of times the privilege was used in the past two years without significant negative outcomes. • It evaluates each practitioner's qualifications against the established criteria for each specific procedure or treatment area in which the practitioner wishes to be privileged. • Once it grants a practitioner privileges, it continually monitors the practitioner's activities to ensure that the practitioner is always competent and practicing within his or her privileged area(s). The JCAHO allows hospitals a lot of leeway regarding privilege categories; it requires privileges delineation, but does not specify how to organize privileges or the level of detail in which privileges must be described. In fact, the JCAHO requires that a hospital's privilege delineation system be tailored to the hospital in that it must take into account the hospital's technical and staff capability of supporting the procedures.
Peer recommendation	MS.5.4 Intent Statement, and MS.5.7		√		A peer recommendation is a statement provided in support of an applicant's request for appointment, reappointment, or privileges by a practitioner in the same professional discipline as the applicant. A physician must provide the peer recommendation for a physician, dentist for dentist, podiatrist for podiatrist, nurse for nurse, etc. In situations where there is no peer available for a specific category or LIP, a physician with essentially equal qualifications, who is familiar with the LIPs performance, can provide the

Privileging Area	Associated *CAMH* Standard No.	Allowed	Req'd	Rec'd	Explanation
					reference. For example, a pediatrician could provide a reference for a pediatric nurse practitioner, or an internist could provide a reference for an adult nurse practitioner. The recommendation should come from someone in the same clinical specialty. For new applicants, peer recommendations are usually letters of reference. For reappointments, JCAHO standards allow statements from an applicant's colleagues who are members of the same department, members of the credentials committee, or medical executive committee to serve as the peer recommendation on reappointment.
Peer review	MS.8-MS.8.4 And MS.5.12-MS.5.12.3		√		Peer review is the evaluation or review of the performance of colleagues by professionals with similar types and degrees of clinical expertise. The peer should come from the same medical discipline and specialty. The JCAHO standards require a properly designed peer review process to evaluate medical staff. Further, the JCAHO does state that peer review results are important and should be measured, aggregated, and trended over time; and that medical staffs should be using them in a constructive way to make credentialing and privileging decisions.
Privileges for admitting patients to a hospital	MS.5.14.1 through MS.5.14.3, and MS.6 through 6.5.2		√		The JCAHO's requirements for privileging practitioners to admit patients to a hospital state that healthcare organizations must privilege medical staff members to admit patients, and only those with these privileges may admit patients to inpatient services. Furthermore, the admitting privilege must comply with both state law and the criteria for standards of medical care that the medical staff established. Standards MS.6.2 through MS.6.3, which detail the H&P requirements for patients who are admitted, requires that each admitted patient have a medical history taken and receive a physical examination. The standards state that the onus for the quality of medical histories and patient examinations rests with the medical staff. In order to ensure this quality, only a qualified physician or LIP who is credentialed and privileged should oversee this. For non-inpatient admissions, MS.6.3 defines the JCAHO's expectation that the medical staff will determine which patients

Areas of Privileging

Privileging Area	Associated *CAMH* Standard No.	Allowed	Req'd	Rec'd	Explanation
					need a history and physical examination. The intent statement for these standards assigns practitioner-specific responsibilities for completion of H&P. The standards are very specific about what a hospital's policy should contain. When a hospital allows non-physicians to admit patients, make sure to follow state law and the following JCAHO standards that deal with coordinating responsibility between physicians and other professionals: MS.6.1, MS.6.2, MS.6.2.1, MS.6.2.2, MS.6.2.2.1, MS.6.2.2.2, MS.6.2.2.3, and MS.6.5 through MS.6.5.2. JCAHO standards require the medical staff to ensure an appropriately qualified practitioner who is competent to deliver the required clinical treatment to each patient. The medical staff must define criteria that determine which clinical procedures or treatments or medical, surgical, or psychiatric conditions require consultation with, or management by, a physician or other licensed independent practitioner.
Privileging (See Delineation of Clinical Privileges above)	MS.5.4 through 5.4.5, MS.5 through 5.16, and MS.6.8		√		JCAHO defines privileging as the process whereby a specific scope and content of patient care services (that is, clinical privileges) are authorized for a health care practitioner by a health care organization based on evaluation of the individual's credentials and performance. Privileging should ensure that all practitioners practicing within or under the auspices of a hospital or other health care organization are competent to carry out any and all clinical procedures they undertake. The JCAHO does not specify the exact way a hospital must delineate privileges, but it does require all medical staff appointees and others with clinical privileges to have an accurate, detailed, and specific description of the clinical privileges granted.
Privileging AHPs	MS. Privileging Standards apply to AHPs granted clinical privileges. HR standards apply to contracted AHPs	√	√	√	AHPs are non-physician practitioners who have patient contact. Generally, AHPs are dependent practitioners; in other words, most do practice with medical direction or supervision. There are some exceptions. AHPs are usually designated as "dependent" or "independent". Independent AHPs are licensed practitioners who are allowed by the hospital and state law to function without physician supervision. Under JCAHO

The 2003 Credentialing and Privileging Desk Reference

Privileging Area	Associated *CAMH* Standard No.	Allowed	Req'd	Rec'd	Explanation
					standards, these AHPs are considered licensed independent practitioners and are granted appointment and privileges through the same credentialing and privileging process as a physician.
					Some dependent AHPs are employees of a medical staff appointee. These individuals usually function under a job description, but are not granted medical staff appointment or privileges. Typically, the physician employer is granted privileges to utilize the services of the AHP in the hospital setting. JCAHO's Medical Staff standards do not address dependent AHPs.
					Although the JCAHO does not require it, you should evaluate a dependent AHPs education, training, and current competency just as you would for a physician. This evaluation may be done in either the medical staff office or the human resources department. Generally, if an AHP is a physician employee, credentialing occurs in the medical staff office.
					Your hospital or medical staff policies should detail the best method for credentialing applicants classified as dependent AHPs and complementary, integrative, or alternative practitioners (CIAs). You should also make sure that your hospital's classifications of LIPs, AHPs, and CIAs match your state's classifications.
Privileging for outpatient services for non-privileged physicians		√			Hospitals may perform outpatient services, such as lab work, filling prescriptions, or a service such as physical therapy, for the patient of a physician who does not have a relationship with the hospital.
					JCAHO requires that, if state law and regulation requires an order from a licensed independent practitioner to perform a laboratory test or radiology procedure, or to provide outpatient care such as physical, occupational or speech therapy, then the organization needs to determine that the person ordering the tests, procedures or care is in fact licensed by the state, prior to performing such test, procedures or care. In this type of situation, the hospital need only establish that the physician (or for that matter, any other type of practitioner) has a current, valid license and is practicing within the scope of that license in ordering the lab test, medication, or therapy.

Areas of Privileging

Privileging Area	Associated *CAMH* Standard No.	Allowed	Req'd	Rec'd	Explanation
					Orders or prescriptions from out-of-state practitioners can be recognized as state law permits, but the hospital is well advised to check for a current, valid license, controlled substance license, and DEA in the practitioner's home state.
Privileging in clinics and physician offices					JCAHO privileging requirements for clinics and physician offices depend upon the ownership of the facilities. When a clinic or office is not part of an accredited hospital or network and is itself not a candidate for accreditation, there are no privileging requirements. As long as practitioners and clinic owners practice within the scope of their licenses, they are free to carry out whatever clinical procedures they and their patients agree upon. By contrast, when a clinic or physician office is owned or controlled by an accredited hospital, the JCAHO treats it as part of the hospital, so it is subject to survey when the rest of the hospital is surveyed and is surveyed under the same set of standards. This means that all LIPs involved must be privileged. Their privileges may be the same ones they exercise within the hospital—if the hospital privilege descriptions are written so that they encompass these outpatient settings—or they may be a different set of privileges, written to match the outpatient settings. If a practitioner does not have privileges in the hospital, he or she must have a set of outpatient privileges. In short, all doctors working in private offices that are owned by a hospital must have privileges to work there.
Privileging in the case of a merger or acquisition	MS.1 through 1.3	√			The JCAHO recognizes that, if two or more hospitals merge, the medical staffs may also merge. The intent of MS.1 states that a single medical staff may operate in more than one accredited hospital. In such a case, make sure that practitioners' privileges are tailored to fit the facility in which they are working. If a practitioner works in only one of the facilities, he or she should have privileges applicable only to that facility. If there are separate medical staffs in the healthcare organization, a physician working at both hospitals would presumably go through two credentialing processes and be evaluated twice for privileges.

			√		
Privileging LIPs (See Privileging and Delineation of Privileges Sections above)			√		The JCAHO requires that all LIPs be privileged. According to the JCAHO, an LIP is someone who is permitted by state law and the hospital to practice without medical direction or supervision. This covers both employees and contracted practitioners if granted privileges through the medical staff function. A physician is an example of an LIP.
Privileging house staff	MS.2.5 and MS.6.9	√		√	The JCAHO requires hospitals with house staffs (such as residents, interns, or employed doctors who work in some sort of restricted or supervised status) to have a means of specifying what house staff can do and how house staffs are supervised. The medical staff must have a defined process for supervision by a licensed independent practitioner with appropriate clinical privileges for each house staff physician and a mechanism for effective communication between the committee(s) responsible for residency program and the medical staff and governing body. Written descriptions of the roles, responsibilities, and patient care activities or residents must be provided to the medical staff by the residency program. Medical staff rules and regulations and policies must delineate those residents who may write orders, the circumstances under which they may do so, and what entries, must be countersigned by a supervising LIP. If a house staff physician works as an LIP outside of the residency program, such as when covering the emergency room, he or she must be credentialed and privileged.
Privileging trainees				√	Although there are no JCAHO standards dealing with trainees such as medical students, nursing students, pharmacy interns, and psychology interns, principles of risk management suggest that all trainees who have patient contact should have some sort of credentials review, specific statements regarding the limits of what they can do, and documented supervision. The hospital may also have employee health requirements, such as TB testing, that these trainees must meet.
Sedation, anesthesia, and privileging	TX.2 through TX.2.4.1		√		Anesthesiology is a highly specialized, high-risk discipline that involves rendering a patient insensible to pain and emotional stress during surgical, obstetrical, and certain medical procedures and to which hospitals must pay close attention. The JCAHO recognizes that special care is required for sedation and anesthesia administration; its specific standards

Areas of Privileging

					require pre-sedation, pre-anesthesia, intra-anesthesia, and post-sedation and post-anesthesia procedures and documentation. The JCAHO standards require moderate or deep sedation and anesthesia are provided by qualified individuals and that individuals administering moderate or deep sedation and anesthesia are qualified and have the appropriate credentials to manage patients at whatever level of sedation or anesthesia is achieved, either intentionally or unintentionally. A practitioner credentialed to perform moderate sedation needs to have the ability to • evaluate patients prior to moderate or deep sedation and anesthesia • rescue patients who slip into a "deeper-than-desired" level of sedation or anesthesia • manage a compromised airway during a procedure • provide adequate oxygenation and ventilation In addition to the abilities noted above, a physician credentialed to perform deep sedation must be able to handle a compromised cardiovascular system during a procedure. Usually these privileges are restricted to those trained in anesthesia.
Telemedicine	MS.5.16	√			JCAHO standards require the medical staff to recommend any clinical services to be provided by telemedicine and to credential and privilege physicians who prescribe, diagnose or treat patients via telemedicine the same as other medical staff appointees.
Temporary Privileges	MS. 5.14.4	√			The JCAHO standards allow the CEO (or his or her designee) to grant temporary privileges based on the recommendation of the department chair or the president of the medical staff. For new applicants, these privileges cannot exceed 120 days. Temporary privileges are not to be routinely used for administrative purposes such as when an LIP fails to provide all information necessary to the processing of his/her reappointment in a timely manner and failure of the organization staff to verify performance data and information in a timely manner. JCAHO standards lists two circumstances for which the granting of temporary privileges to an LIP would be acceptable – to fulfill an important patient care need and when an applicant with a complete, "clean" application is awaiting review and approval of the medical staff executive committee and board.

						The following examples of a "patient care need" are given: • A physician becomes ill or takes a leave of absence and an LIP would need to cover his/her practice until he/she returns • A specific LIP has the necessary skills to provide care to a patient that an LIP currently privileged does not possess In order for an application to be considered "complete and clean" there must be verification of current licensure, relevant training or experience, current competence, ability to perform the privileges requested, and any other criteria required by the organization's medical staff bylaws. The National Practitioner Data Bank query results must have been obtained and evaluated. It is also required that the new applicant has a complete application with no current or previously successful challenge to licensure or registration, has not been subject to involuntary termination of medical staff appointment at another organization, and has not been subject to involuntary limitation, reduction, denial, or loss of clinical privileges. Medical staff bylaws, rules and regulations, or policies must describe the mechanism used for granting temporary privileges and must stipulate that, in an emergency, any medical staff member who has clinical privileges is permitted to provide any type of patient care necessary as a life-saving measure or to prevent serious harm—regardless of his or her medical staff status or clinical privileges—provided that the care provided is within the scope of the individual's license. The temporary status may also be granted to locum tenens physicians. These physicians are employed for a short-term, specific purpose, usually through an employment agency. These physicians typically complete an abbreviated application process or all or part of the primary-source verification may be delegated to the locum tenens company. All requirements for granting temporary privileges must be met prior to granting temporary privileges
Emergency Privileges	MS. 5.14.4.1	√			√	The JCAHO allows emergency privileges to be granted on a case-by-case basis when the hospital's emergency management plan has been activated, and the organization is

| | | | | | unable to handle the immediate patient needs.

The medical staff must

- identify in writing the individual(s) responsible for granting emergency privileges.

- describe in writing the responsibilities of the individual(s) responsible for granting emergency privileges.

- describe in writing a mechanism to manage the activities of individuals who receive emergency privileges. There is a mechanism to allow staff to readily identify these individuals.

- addresses the verification process as a high priority.

The verification process for the credentials and privileges of those granted emergency privileges must begin as soon as the immediate situation is under control. This privileging process must be identical to the process for granting temporary privileges to fulfill an important patient care need.

The CEO or president of the medical staff or his or her designee(s) *may* grant emergency privileges upon presentation of any of the following:

- A current picture hospital ID card

- A current license to practice and a valid picture ID issued by a state, federal or regulatory agency

- Identification indicating that the individual is a member of a Disaster Medical Assistance Team

- Identification indicating that the individual has been granted authority by a federal, state or municipal entity to render patient care in emergency circumstances

- Presentation by current hospital or medical staff member(s) with personal knowledge regarding practitioner's identity |

CHAPTER 3
Roles and Responsibilities in Credentialing

Chapter 3
Roles and Responsibilities in Credentialing

The chart included in this chapter highlights the responsibilities of each person involved in the credentialing process. Although accreditation standards and state and federal law assign some responsibilities to specific persons or the medical staff or governing body, the actual work may be completed by the medical staff services professional. In addition, current JCAHO standards are referenced. The chart is not meant to be all-inclusive. State and federal regulations may contain additional requirements. We suggest that you use this chart as a basis for understanding and strongly encourage you to review the appropriate standards in the appropriate accreditor manuals for more details.

Chapter 3

Credentialing and privileging roles	Associated *CAMH* Standard No.	Explanation
Role of medical staff	MS.5 through 5.16.1	The medical staff is self-governing and has responsibility for the quality of the professional services provided by individuals with clinical privileges. Typical medical staff credentialing responsibilities include • development of a general criteria for medical staff appointment to be contained in the bylaws and presenting it to the governing body for approval • developing specific, detailed policies, procedures, and rules and regulations regarding credentialing and privileging • reviewing applications for medical staff appointment and privileges and submitting its recommendations to the governing body
Role of medical staff services professional		Most of the credentialing responsibilities of the medical staff are facilitated by the medical staff services professional (MSSP). The MSSP is responsible for processing and maintaining the applicant's credentials files. For example, the typical MSSP may • prescreen to ensure the applicant meets minimum criteria necessary to apply • distribute and receive the application • ensure completenesss of the application within the specified time period • obtain all relevant documents (with the applicant's assistance, if necessary) • conduct primary source verification • prepare the file for review • update the credentials file at the time of reappointment • monitor access to the credentials file • obtain and process all information necessary for reappointment; • coordination of peer review • orientation of new medical staff leaders and credentials committee members
Role of medical executive committee	MS.2.3.1, MS. 2.5, and MS.3 – 3.1.7	The JCAHO requires the MEC to submit to the board recommendations regarding appointment, clinical privileges, reappointment, and corrective action, and to develop specific policies for the MEC's role in supervision of residents, termination of medical staff appointees, the fair hearing, investigation, appointment and clinical privileges delineation process.
Role of credentials committee	Not a JCAHO required committee, but standards MS.5 through MS.5.16.1 apply to credentialing.	The JCAHO standards do not require a credentials committee, but many hospitals utilize this committee to review and make recommendations to the MEC regarding staff appointment, reappointment, and clinical privileges. During the application process, a credentials committee member might be responsible for soliciting information from past practice settings and for conducting an interview. The credentials committee chair oversees the hospital's credentialing program, including the activities of the credentials committee. One responsibility is to ensure that the credentials committee works as effectively and efficiently as possible. Further, this chair ensures that all credentialing activities are in compliance with JCAHO standards, as well as with laws, and regulations. Usually this position reports directly to the MEC. In larger hospitals, each department may have its own credentials committee.
Role of human resources or personnel department	HR	Some experts suggest that hospitals utilize the skills in the human resources department to help process requests from non-

Roles and Responsibilities in Credentialing

Credentialing and privileging roles	Associated *CAMH* Standard No.	Explanation
		physician practitioners who are not eligible for medical staff appointment but who are permitted to provide clinical services, particularly for hospital-contracted employees. In many hospitals, the MSSP handles credentialing from nonphysician practitioners who are employed by MS appointees.
Role of department chair	MS.4.2.1.3 through 4.2.1.5, and MS.5.14.4	This role occurs only in a departmentalized hospital. In a nondepartmentalized hospital, the MEC typically performs the tasks listed here. The department chair is usually the first person outside of the medical staff office to see and review the complete credentials file. The department chair: • reviews the application and makes a recommendation to the credentials committee or in the absence of this committee, directly to the MEC • recommends privileging criteria and evaluates requests for privileges • determines the qualifications and competence of department or service personnel who are not LIPs, and who provide patient care services • may make phone calls to solicit information from past practice settings • may conduct an interview if the individual is applying for a position in his or her department (alternatively, the credentials committee may do this) • continuously reviews the performance of all practitioners with clinical privileges and specified services in his or her department and reports to the MEC
Role of the board	GO.2.2 through GO2.2.3, and GO 2.5	The governing body (board) of a hospital, as the JCAHO defines it, is the group, or agency that has ultimate authority and responsibility for establishing policy, maintaining care quality, and providing for organization management and planning. The board has two key functions in credentialing and privileging: • It formally approves the medical staff bylaws, which establish the framework for credentialing and privileging. The JCAHO requires that, at minimum, the bylaws contain mechanisms and criteria through which practitioners are appointed, reappointed, granted privileges, and permitted to renew privileges. Board policies must require the medical staff to review and revise policies and procedures as warranted and at least every three years. • It acts on the recommendations of the medical staff executive committee and issues a final and official decision regarding each request for appointment, reappointment, initial privileges, and renewal of privileges. The board assumes legal responsibility for the hospital and is ultimately responsible for approving all bylaws, policies, and procedures. To expedite the appointment and privileging requests, the Board may delegate a committee of at least two members to act on its behalf in reviewing credentialing decisions. The standards require this committee to "be consistent with the governing body bylaws as they relate to forming a governing body committee", which means that this committee should be allowed by and defined in the policies or

Chapter 3

Credentialing and privileging roles	Associated *CAMH* Standard No.	Explanation
		bylaws of the board. The governing body's bylaws must specify the criteria for delegation. Review the intent statements for standard MS5.1.1. for specific criteria that must be met before this expedited credentialing can occur.
Role of the chief executive officer (CEO)	GO.2.2 through GO2.2.3, GO 2.5, and MS.5.14.4	The CEO functions as a liaison between the medical staff and the board and is typically responsible for assuring the JCAHO standards for the governing body are met. The CEO (or the CEO's agent—often the medical staff office) assists in the credentialing process by ensuring that the application and its supporting documentation reach the appropriate individuals or groups at the appropriate steps of the process. The CEO or agent forwards the application to the MEC for submission to the board and notifies each applicant for appointment and privileges, the applicable department chair, and the MEC of the board's final decision. The CEO, or his designee, grants temporary privileges on the recommendation of either the applicable clinical department chairperson or the president of the medical staff The CEO also acts as the official representative of the hospital in contacting the applicant at certain stages of the application process.
Role of administration		Hospital administration is responsible for ensuring that qualified, trained personnel are providing medical staff services in the hospital. It provides the medical staff office with necessary resources, including salaries for personnel, office space, telephone systems, and postage service. It also often acts as a link between the medical staff and the governing body.
Role of the applicant		The applicant's primary responsibility is to ensure that the hospital receives, in a timely manner, all of the information needed to evaluate his or her application for medical staff appointment. The applicant must answer all application questions truthfully and completely and must appear for an interview, if required. An applicant should supply any supporting documents necessary to process his or her application. For example, an applicant should help there is difficulty obtaining reference letters and information about his or her work at other facilities. The applicant is responsible for ensuring that the hospital receives all requested information. Medical staff bylaws (or a similar document) should include a timeframe for providing a complete application, and statements that an application is not complete until all supporting documents and information have been received and that it is the applicant's responsibility to complete the application. By doing so, a hospital need only inform an applicant that no further progress on his or her application is possible until he or she contacts the references that have failed to respond to requests for information and obtains the necessary information.

CHAPTER 4
Managed Care Credentialing

Chapter 4
Managed Care Credentialing

The fundamental purpose of credentialing—establishing that applicants meet the minimum criteria for appointment and determining whether applicants are clinically competent to perform requested services—are relevant not only to hospitals, but also to other types of health care organizations, such as managed care organizations (MCOs). MCOs must select and retain qualified individuals to provide care to their members. Although primary-source verification processes are essentially the same across organizations, managed care raises a number of issues for credentialing and privileging specialists. Credentialing professionals working in hospitals or other freestanding health care organizations must be familiar with managed care basics because they will receive a variety of requests and communications from MCOs.

MCOs must be prepared to credential hundreds or even thousands of practitioners in a reasonable amount of time. Many of the practitioners an MCO credentials might not have a direct relationship with the MCO, but instead come onto the panel through a relationship with another organization; therefore, those responsible for credentialing in the MCO must collect and evaluate thousands of bits of information. Those carrying out credentialing also deal with the files of individuals whom they will never meet and who have little, if any, loyalty to the MCO.

A practitioner on an MCO's provider panel may be credentialed by a number of organizations. For example, an MCO credentials all members of its provider panel. Independent practice associations (IPAs), preferred provider organizations (PPOs), and hospitals that contract with the MCO may also credential these practitioners. Because each organization essentially repeats the credentialing process done by the organizations, MCOs commonly delegate the responsibility and authority for credentialing to avoid this duplication.

About managed care
Managed care involves coordinating and arranging the provision of health services and benefits. In managed care, a third party other than the traditional two involved parties—the doctor and the patient—exerts partial or total control over the provision of care. Typically, the third party involved is an organization, such as an employer, that is paying for the health care. Often, a third-party payer will use another organization, such as an MCO, to manage health care on its behalf.

There are many different types of MCOs, such as health maintenance organizations (HMOs), PPOs, and provider-sponsored organizations (PSOs), to name a few. Even an insurance company can carry out managed care when an employer or individual purchases a traditional health insurance policy. (Traditional health insurance is often referred to as indemnity insurance.)

Managed care accreditation and certification
The National Committee for Quality Assurance (NCQA) is the most widely used managed care accrediting organization. The NCQA, which was established in 1991, surveys and accredits 60% of all MCOs. It also accredits credentials verification organizations (CVOs), PPOs, and behavioral managed health care organizations. In addition, the NCQA has certification programs for CVOs and physician organizations.

Many employers and other purchasers of health care through MCOs are concerned with Health Employer Data and Information Set (HEDIS) scores. HEDIS is a standardized set of performance measures used to compare the performance of managed health care plans. The NCQA collects this information and uses it to calculate national performance statistics and benchmarks.

The Joint Commission on Accreditation of Healthcare Organizations (JCAHO) also accredits MCOs through its health care network accreditation program. It also offers accreditation programs for PPOs and behavioral health care organizations.

In addition, the American Accreditation Healthcare Commission (AAHCC)—also known as the Utilization Review Accreditation Commission, or URAC—was founded in 1990 to establish standards for the health care industry. URAC accredits hospitals, HMOs, PPOs, third-party administrators, and provider groups. Some states require HMOs to be accredited and waive state licensure inspection for accredited HMOs. But for most MCOs, the value of accreditation is mainly as an indication to the public of the MCO's devotion to quality care.

Credentialing requirements in managed care

The majority of Americans receive health care under the control of MCOs, and many health care practitioners earn a major part of their incomes from MCO payments. Federal and state laws and regulations increasingly require MCOs to conduct thorough primary-source credentialing. Health care purchasers, legislative leaders, and consumers pressure MCOs to thoroughly evaluate the qualifications of potential panel members, and all major accreditors require MCOs to have active, documented credentialing processes.

As a result of these regulations, providers must apply for membership on practitioner panels. Once a practitioner files an application, the MCO reviews his or her qualifications against the MCO's set requirements and need for providers. Although this sounds similar to the process hospitals use to credential appointees of their medical staffs, MCOs' process for establishing requirements for panel membership and for reviewing applications for panel appointment is quite different than that for hospitals because MCOs do not have a formal medical staff.

MCOs typically handle many more applications than most hospitals. However, MCO accreditation standards often require the timeframe for completing the credentialing process to be much shorter than it is for hospitals. For example, the NCQA requires all primary-source verification to be no older than 180 days. The MCO must reverify any information that is older than 180 days.

Unlike hospitals, MCOs seldom have direct face-to-face contact with applicants or other professionals who know applicants well enough to provide detailed information. Even when part of an MCO's application process involves having an MCO representative visit an applicant's office (referred to as a "site visit"), this contact focuses on the office environment rather than on the applicant's qualifications. Although an MCO may have physicians on its panel, these physicians are usually scattered over a wide geographic area and do not routinely review provider applications.

All accrediting agencies require MCOs to credential providers—either directly or through delegation. This requirement means a lot of paperwork for LIPs who are members of 10–20 managed care plans and therefore must complete a separate application and reapplication for each plan. Some physician offices have an employee who completes this paperwork. The Council for Affordable Quality Healthcare (CAQH), a not-for-profit alliance of health plans and networks, is working to reduce administrative burdens for physicians, patients, and payers. This organization has developed single-application credentialing that allows physicians and other providers to submit one credentialing application to satisfy the requirements of all participating health plans and networks. CAQH then gathers and stores the data from all providers and makes these electronic records available to authorized health plans and networks.

As MCOs continue to make decisions affecting patient care, they are being held liable by the courts for failure to manage the care they provide and for negligent selection of providers. In fact, managed care plans are increasingly facing the same negligent credentialing liability as hospitals.

Licensed independent practitioner status in managed care

There are some important differences between hospitals' definition of and managed care's definition of a licensed independent practitioner (LIP). Every state presently includes in this group physicians, dentists, and podiatrists, and some states include other professions as well, such as nurse anesthetists.

The JCAHO defines an LIP as "Any individual permitted by law and by the organization to provide care and services, without direction or supervision, within the scope of the individual's license, and consistent with individually granted clinical privileges."

Hospitals are free, however, to use a narrower definition than the JCAHO permits (unless state law prohibits it). Some hospitals limit the LIP group to physicians only. In these hospitals, the definition of an LIP is therefore relatively clear and covers a small group of professions. The determination of who is an LIP in a hospital is important because the JCAHO's credentialing and privileging standards apply to all LIPs, whether they are in private practice, hospital employees, or working under contract.

Outside hospitals (in private offices and facilities other than hospitals), there is great variability among states and even among organizations within the same state as to which professions can practice without medical supervision or direction (that is, which professions fall within the category of LIP). For example, PhD psychologists, counselors, therapists, nurse-midwives, nurse practitioners, and clinical dietitians are able to open offices and practice with varying degrees of independence in many states. Many MCOs pay for such professionals' services and include them on their practitioner panels. As a result, any JCAHO standards that deal with LIPs cover whichever of these professions that state law and MCOs accept as LIPs. For this reason, MCO credentialing and privileging must often deal with a far larger and more variable group than hospital credentialing and privileging in the same state.

Credentialing physicians versus credentialing nonphysician LIPs in managed care

Credentialing physicians is relatively standardized and simple. There is a limited group of medical schools, licensing agencies, training institutions, and certifying boards. Most of these organizations are well-established, easy to reach, and quick to respond to credentialing-related queries. In contrast, the process for credentialing members of many other health care professions has not been standardized. The universities, colleges, and training programs educating these professionals are numerous; licensing agencies vary widely among states; and clinical training and specialty board certification are extremely diverse. As a general rule, the same type of primary-source verification of credentials done for physicians should be done for other professions, as should the same type of review of clinical competence and clinical activity at reappointment time. It is often difficult to obtain data to review when recredentialing these providers as the services they provide are not typically included in the routine quality review performed for physicians. For that reason, recredentialing activities focus mainly on evaluations by peers, feedback received from patients, and sanctions and licensure restriction checks.

Because credentials and the access to credentialing information vary considerably among nonphysician professions, MCOs (and hospitals) may not be as confident in their credentialing of this group. Even achieving some modest level of confidence is going to be more time-consuming than physician credentialing because of the absence of data banks for these professions.

Chapter 4

MCOs' credentialing policies, procedures, and rules

MCOs should thoroughly review applicable laws, publications, guidelines, and accreditation standards to gain a sound knowledge of what a comprehensive credentialing system requires. They should design this system with the following objectives in mind:

- Member safety
- Consistency
- Objectivity
- Clinical competence

With these goals, knowledge of laws and standards, and a thorough assessment of the MCO's staffing needs, the MCO leaders can develop the credentialing requirements for membership in the practitioner panel, including the following:

- What information the MCO will require for application for panel membership
- The required level of education, training, and experience
- Each individual's roles and responsibilities
- Credentials processing time limits

The credentialing process as an administrative responsibility

The majority of MCOs involve LIPs (usually physicians) in the credentialing process. In an MCO, credentialing is an administrative responsibility-since administration determines the minimum requirements for membership on the practitioner panel. Often one or more LIPs are in the upper levels of administration, and overseeing credentialing is among their primary duties.

An MCO's administration typically uses a number of criteria for membership in addition to clinical competence, including criteria relating to the characteristics of the practitioner's practice, office staff, and office; the geographic location of the practice; and the MCO's need for the type of specialist or primary care practitioner at the time of application. Some MCOs identify the number of providers needed to service their patient population. After this number is reached, the panel may be closed and no more applications will be accepted.

An MCO's administration also reviews applications, verifies credentials, and monitors practitioners' performance. Decisions about applications typically go through the office of the medical director (or other senior physician), and this individual may use a committee of practitioners to assist in decision-making. Some states mandate the extent of physician involvement in decision-making and limit the factors MCOs can use to make determinations.

Some large MCOs are decentralized, meaning that many major functions, including credentialing, are done within each regional administration, rather than in MCO headquarters. In many decentralized MCOs, however, headquarters sets criteria and policies that are the responsibility of regional medical directors or similar officials.

MCOs may delegate credentialing to organizations with which they contract for the provision of services. For example, an MCO contracting with a medical group or an IPA to provide care might assign responsibility for credentialing to that group. In such a case, the MCO will establish credentialing, reporting, and oversight requirements that the group must follow. The MCO will then monitor how well the group does its job.

Delegated credentialing and outsourcing

The major organizations that accredit MCOs—the JCAHO, NCQA, and AAHCC/URAC—recognize and accept delegated credentialing. However, they do not allow MCOs to merely rely on subsidiary organizations to do the credentialing; they instead require MCOs to maintain oversight of the credentialing process (with the partial exception of the NCQA, as discussed below).

Although an MCO delegates the authority to act on its behalf, the MCO remains accountable for ensuring that the function is carried out properly. This MCO oversight is intended to ensure that the MCOs' credentialing requirements and policies are followed, even though the credentialing is done by other organizations. MCOs commonly delegate credentialing functions to physician medical groups, IPAs, hospitals/health care systems, and CVOs.

The JCAHO's requirements regarding the use of CVOs are spelled out in the intent statement for MS.5.4.3.1 through MS.5.4.3.2. The intent statement requires organizations to be confident in the completeness, accuracy, and timeliness of information provided by a CVO. To achieve this confidence, the organization should evaluate the agency providing the information initially and then periodically. Below is a summary of the "principles" that should guide such an evaluation:

- The CVO makes known what data and information it can provide.

- The CVO provides documentation describing how it collects data, develops information, and performs verifications.

- The CVO provides the user with sufficient information about database functions, including any limitations of information available from the agency (for example, practitioners not included in the database); the timeframe for responses to requests for information; and a summary overview of quality control processes relating to data integrity, security, transmission accuracy, and technical specifications.

- The user and CVO agree on the format for transmitting a practitioner's credentials information.

- The user can easily tell which information provided by the CVO is from a primary source and which is not.

- When the agency transmits information that can expire (such as licensure and board certification), it provides the date when the information was last updated from the primary source.

- The agency certifies that the information transmitted to the user accurately presents the information it obtained.

- The user can discern whether the information transmitted by the agency includes all primary-source information gathered by the agency and, if not, where additional information can be obtained.

- The user can engage the agency's quality control processes to resolve concerns about transmission errors, inconsistencies, or other data issues.

The NCQA offers an exception to the requirement for regular review as part of oversight of delegated credentialing. The NCQA waives its oversight requirement for MCOs that delegate their credentialing to NCQA-certified CVOs. However, CVO certification is done separately for each credentialing verification function (e.g., medical school graduation, licensure, etc.), so an MCO must make sure that the functions for which its CVO is NCQA-certified mesh with the functions it is delegating to the CVO. NCQA requires an MCO that delegates credentialing activities to demonstrate that it has not compromised its ability to evaluate structures and processes and to achieve improved performance.

URAC standards require the MCO to review the contractor's policies and procedures and establish criteria for the contractor to follow. These standards also require all contracts with a delegated entity to specify which elements will be delegated. Organizations must implement a mechanism for oversight of the delegated activity.

Subdelegation

The NCQA allows an MCO's delegate to give a third entity the authority to carry out part of the credentialing function that has been delegated by the MCO. For example, an MCO may delegate credentialing activities to a provider hospital organization that then delegates part of the credentialing function to the hospital. The hospital would be the subdelegate.

The delegate or the MCO must oversee the work performed by the subdelegate to make sure that the subdelegate meets both the MCO's and the NCQA's standards. In cases of subdelegation, the MCO is accountable for the performance of both the delegate and the subdelegate.

How an MCO oversees delegated credentialing

Because an MCO that delegates its credentialing remains responsible for its credentialing decisions, the MCO must ensure that the organization to which it delegates performs the credentialing well—a process called oversight. To oversee its delegated credentialing, an MCO typically has one of its experts visit each delegated organization at least annually to examine a sample of credentials files to ensure that they meet the applicable accreditors' standards.

Oversight typically consists of the following actions:

- An examination of the contracting organization's credentialing policy and procedure statements to be sure they are acceptable

- An examination of a sample of the completed credential files to be sure they comply both with the contractor's policies and with the MCO's requirements

- A test of the accuracy of the material in a sampling of credentials, often done by redoing the verification of the files in that sample

Confidentiality of information in delegated credentialing

Accreditation standards include requirements protecting patient information, including patient consent for release of information and the confidentiality of medical records. The NCQA's standards are very explicit about the protection of patient health information. Standard CR13 details the language that must appear in delegated contracts regarding the use, creation, and disclosure of protected patient information.

In addition, the Health Insurance Portability and Accountability Act of 1996 contains strict requirements concerning the security and privacy of health data.

Delegation raises the issue of authority to share confidential information among organizations. An MCO should ensure that appropriate language is included in contractual agreements with third parties to permit exchange of information. These statements will protect both the MCO and the organization to which it delegates. Serious penalties may be imposed for unauthorized release of information even if the release appears logical. The safest approach to release of information is to get consent from any practitioner whose information is to be shared. If an organization routinely uses a CVO, it may be advisable to include the name of the CVO in the release. Typically, an organization will secure practitioner consent by including a release of information statement in its application form. Note that as a result of federal law, data from the National Practitioner Data Bank or Healthcare Practitioner Data Bank cannot be shared with a third party even with the applicant's consent.

Liability in delegated credentialing

Accreditation issues aside, an MCO is ethically and legally responsible for ensuring the competence of its practitioners. Many MCOs consider credentialing a risk management issue. Although it might seem that the duplicate credentialing that organizations carry out is a terrible waste of resources, performing its own credentialing is still the best safeguard an organization has to protect the integrity of its practitioner panel.

In some network accreditation surveys, the JCAHO has allowed MCOs to accept a practitioner's appointment to the medical staff of a JCAHO-accredited hospital as sufficient evidence of satisfactory credentialing. However, even this is not as helpful as it may seem for several reasons:

1. The hospital will almost certainly not evaluate, as part of its credentialing process, some issues and items the MCO needs. For example, an MCO needs to consider a practitioner's office site review and the time it takes for a new patient to get an appointment, but medical staff appointment provides no information about these factors.

2. The hospital might have verified a practitioner's credentials as much as two years ago, so the verified information might not be current.

3. Simply verifying credentials does not provide all essential information concerning a practitioner. For example, a hospital might have uncovered challenges or adverse actions against a practitioner's license, but granted appointment anyway, unbeknownst to the MCO. Or, a practitioner may be currently under investigation, but no final review action has been taken.

4. Most important, JCAHO accreditation does not imply that a hospital's credentialing process is anything more than minimally acceptable. A hospital might be performing credentialing at a quality level far below what is acceptable to the MCO, yet achieve overall accreditation. In fact, the JCAHO might have found a hospital's credentialing to be out of compliance but the hospital has done well enough in other areas to achieve accreditation. The MCO would not learn about the credentialing noncompliance unless it reviewed the JCAHO accreditation report of the hospital.

This is not to say that a hospital cannot carry out the credentialing function under a delegated contract that spells out the exact needs of the MCO. However, hospitals and MCOs have different needs and different accreditation standards. As noted earlier, although an MCO may delegate the authority to act on its behalf, the MCO remains accountable for making sure the function is carried out properly.

Credentialing in hospital-owned MCOs or an MCO-owned hospital

If two parts of a single organization credential separately, they may well be duplicating efforts. This issue raises a difficult question. Generally, credentialing information should not be shared across the boundaries of an organization without consent from the applicant being credentialed, but it is not always easy to determine the exact boundaries in some modern health care organizations. Boundaries depend on such issues as ownership, bylaws, licensure, and state law, and will likely require legal consultation. Answering this question should involve individual research and legal consultation by organizations that are grappling with the issue.

Fair hearing and appeal requirements for MCOs

MCOs are not required to have anything like a set of bylaws to provide for semi-autonomous governance of the practitioner group—one of the purposes of hospital medical staff bylaws. Instead practitioners usually relate to an MCO through one of several available models. For example:

- Practitioners might be employees, in which case the relationship is based upon employment rules within the organization and federal and state employment law

- Practitioners might contract directly with the MCO, in which case the conditions stated in the contract and contract law prevail

- Practitioners might be members of a group that contracts with the MCO, in which case the contract deals with the MCO-practitioner group relationship, and the individual practitioner relates to the group in a manner determined by the group's organization

The JCAHO requires hospitals' bylaws to provide a fair hearing and appeal process for hospital medical staff appointees that allows the member to explain or defend him- or herself before the medical staff can take any significant adverse action. MCOs do not have this requirement. Therefore, the extent to which an MCO offers a fair hearing and appeal process depends on the type of relationship the MCO has with its practitioners; the provisions set out in the governing documents; and state law, if applicable. Many MCOs do not offer a fair hearing and appeal process to practitioners who are adversely affected by the MCO.

However, many MCO contracts offer practitioners the right to examine the information submitted in support of their credentialing applications and the right to correct any erroneous information.

Practitioner office audits and managed care credentialing

Many MCOs require an office visit or evaluation for some or all practitioners on their panels (often called office audits or site inspections) as part of the credentialing process. These visits are often conducted by a member of the MCO's quality improvement department, provider relations department, or similar unit who uses a checklist of items that must be examined for compliance with the MCO's standards. (Medical staff services professionals who credential on behalf of MCOs typically do not conduct site visits, but instead may use site visit documentation as part of practitioner applications.) Each office is rated on individual items (such as quality of clinical records, cleanliness, training, and attitudes of employees, etc.) and as a whole. Information from a practitioner's site visit is considered when determining whether the practitioner will be appointed to the MCO's practitioner panel. Site visits are usually repeated every two years, at reappointment, or as necessary in response to reports of difficulties or problems.

Differences among managed care accreditors regarding credentialing requirements

Although accreditation standards change all the time, at present there are no significant differences among the accreditation organizations' requirements. The NCQA does differ in its requirement regarding the timeliness of credentials verification, however, and this does sometimes produce a difference in credentialing procedures. Specifically, the NCQA requires that the verification of a credential must be no older than 180 days at the time of review. Thus, if the processing of a practitioner's application is delayed, some of the verifications might expire during the delay. The wisest course for an MCO to take when preparing for accreditation is to consult the latest set of the appropriate accreditor's credentialing standards (see Chapter 10: Credentialing and Privileging Resources for these accreditors' contact information).

Economic credentialing (or privileging)

Economic credentialing is the consideration of economic issues and information unrelated to quality of care or competency in the credentialing process. It can occur at two levels: 1) determining how many and what types of practitioners the practitioner panel should include, and 2) deciding whether a particular practitioner should be added to or continue on the panel.

The first level of economic credentialing deals with the question of how many practitioners are needed, given the number and type of members the MCO expects to serve. This question is important because on the one hand, credentialing and orienting a practitioner into the system are an expense to an MCO, so it is in the MCO's interest not to credential any more practitioners than will be needed; while on the other hand, an MCO with too few practitioners will have unhappy members because of difficulty in getting prompt service. Therefore, determining the number and distribution of practitioners is a critically important decision for the welfare of an MCO and its members.

Most MCOs develop plans that specify the numbers and types of practitioners they need, then follow their plans. Many times, this practice leads MCOs to turn away panel applicants because more practitioners are available than they need. As a result, when much of the medical care in a region is controlled by MCOs, some competent practitioners might find themselves without enough patients to make a living for reasons that are beyond their control, which strikes the practitioners as unfair.

The antithesis to this approach of limiting panel membership is called the "any willing provider" approach, which calls for MCOs to admit to their panels any practitioners who meet their established minimal requirements, and agree to provide services for the fees offered, regardless of specialty or practice characteristics. This approach forbids MCOs to discriminate against applicants for economic reasons. Many physicians and their organizations support the "any willing provider" approach, whereas many MCOs and their organizations oppose it. In some states, this difference has been or is being fought over in the state legislature.

The second level of economic credentialing involves looking at practice expenses per case or as a whole that individual practitioners generate for the MCO. This level of economic credentialing depends upon statistical analysis of the practice of each practitioner-often called a profile-and a comparison of the practitioner with the panel as a whole or with an appropriate subgroup (such as specialists in the same field). When a practitioner appears to be unduly expensive (compared to similar specialists), the practitioner might be denied continued membership on the provider panel. On the other hand, some practitioners may receive monetary rewards for being "low cost" providers. Some MCOs will withhold a certain percentage of money due the provider and payback this money as an incentive to keep costs low.

Opponents of this approach point out that the more expensive practitioners might be the ones providing the highest quality of care and by eliminating these individuals, the organization will be lowering its quality. Much of the opposition to economic credentialing among physician groups and others seems to stem from the fear that MCOs will use it to sacrifice quality of care to increase income. Proponents respond that economic credentialing is a negative and therefore unfair way to describe one aspect of utilization management, a time-honored part of managed care and an essential part of the cost saving that has made managed care so popular.

Profiling in economic credentialing

Profiling is the process of putting a practitioner's (or a hospital's or other clinical facility's) individual statistics together in one chart or table to facilitate the examination of the practitioner's record. A practitioner's profile often includes a statistical or graphic comparison of the practitioner with the averages for similar practitioners or averages for the whole panel. Because profiling is frequently a part of economic credentialing, many view it as a negative activity.

Undoubtedly, profiling can be used to eliminate practitioners who are willing to take the most difficult—and therefore expensive—cases, while protecting those practitioners who provide low-quality, inexpensive care. However, the profiling process can be applied to any kind of data-especially quality of care. For example, a non-economic profile for a practitioner might deal with the number of patient complaints per number of patients treated, average waiting time for a patient to get an appointment, average patient time spent in the practitioner's waiting room before being seen, etc. Overall, profiling is a neutral statistical process and can be used for good or bad purposes.

Three unique challenges of MCO credentialing

How to handle MCOs' requirement for admitting privileges if your hospital does not offer a privilege called "admitting privileges"

When MCOs (or other organizations) require admitting privileges, the concern is about the privilege practitioners have to admit patients to hospitals. MCOs once relied completely on the hospital to credentialing providers. When an MCO asked if the physician had admitting privileges, it was really questioning whether the hospital had credentialed the provider, found that he/she was competent, and allowed admitting privileges and staff appointment. This is no longer the case. When an MCO asks whether the physician has admitting privileges, this is exactly what it wants to know. There is a growing trend for physicians to limit their practice to office-based medicine and rely on another physician or hospitalist to care for patients admitted to the hospital. Some MCOs allow practice. However, some MCO continue to require that providers have admitting privileges at a contracted facility. Although some physicians limit their practice to outpatient services, they may need to admit a patient on occasion. (For example, a physician who performs surgery in a freestanding ambulatory center may need to admit a patient when faced with a postoperative problem). The easiest way for MCOs to get this information is to ask the hospital whether the physician can admit, rather than asking about admitting privileges or staff status. Although not usually the case, some nonphysician practitioners are privileged to admit patients.

Handling a high volume of requests from MCOs if you have staffing or legal issues

Depending on the number of providers on the medical staff, a hospital may receive hundreds of requests from MCOs for information about medical staff appointees. However, the hospital may not be staffed to handle the requests or may be advised by its attorney not to respond to requests for certain information.

Hospital medical staff offices that are asked to handle hundreds or even thousands of information requests per year have a workload crisis, especially if they are not staffed to do so. The initial response to these requests at some hospitals has been to refuse to respond or to respond with only minimal information. This practice penalizes medical staff appointees whose applications for membership on the panels of MCOs or similar organizations cannot be processed for lack of information. It also penalizes the public, because a hospital might possess negative information that an MCO should have to make an informed decision and possibly save the public from exposure to a practitioner whose skills are not acceptable. Hospitals are increasingly charging fees for releasing requested information to MCOs and others. This seems to be a fair way to deal with the problem, because fees can be used to pay for the staffing necessary to respond to such requests. Another option is for the hospital to give the MCO a list of medical staff appointees on a routine basis that is accompanied by a letter stating that all providers on the list are "in good standing." Many MCOs include this requirement in their contracts with hospitals. Although some hospitals do not agree with the use of such lists, they are widely accepted in most of the country.

The medical staff office seldom sees the contracts signed by the hospital and MCO even though the contract may include requirements for credentials verification or for delegation of credentialing functions. A contract between a hospital and MCO should specify what and how information is shared. The medical staff office should review these contracts to learn the exact requirements for sharing information.

Another issue is the hospital's potential liability if it releases negative information to the MCO about a medical staff appointee. Clearly, a hospital that possesses such information has an ethical responsibility to provide it to those who request it. It is important that this information be carefully worded to minimize liability and reflect facts, rather than opinions. This is a matter a hospital must discuss with its attorney. A safe rule would be to report the exact wording that was reported to the National Practitioner Data Bank.

Privileging in practitioners' private office settings
It would be difficult to adapt hospital privileging procedures to suit office privileging. In hospital settings, because hospital owners (i.e., the board) have legal control over privileging and everything else going on in the hospital, practitioners can be required to perform only approved procedures. In addition, nursing staff can easily monitor the use of privileges because they are involved in-or in a position to observe-most clinical activities. In private office settings, however, any procedure that a patient and practitioner agree on that is within the scope of the practitioner's license is legally permissible (unless there is a state law to the contrary). And even if an MCO limits what can be done in its panel practitioner offices (i.e., establish privileges), there usually is no observer analogous to the hospital nursing staff with an obligation to report noncompliance. An MCO that pays a practitioner on a fee-for-service basis can monitor the procedures for which the practitioner bills and can place limits on which procedures it will pay. However, if a patient decides to pay for a procedure outside of MCO coverage, the MCO has no way of knowing about it and no way of discouraging it. When an MCO pays a practitioner a monthly fee to care for a patient (i.e., capitation), the practitioner does not report individual office procedures to the MCO.

CHAPTER 5

Schools, Colleges, and Educational Programs

Chapter 5
Schools, Colleges, and Educational Programs

Education details a hospital should verify

Because education is usually the first step in professional preparation, a critical step in processing a practitioner's application is verifying that the applicant has completed an educational program at an accredited school. A hospital should be most concerned with an applicant's attendance and graduation; the details of an applicant's educational program or quality of work performed are generally not relevant to processing an application. A hospital will request information about an applicant's quality of work and clinical competence from an internship, residency program, or other later stages of training.

When a practitioner successfully completes an educational program, he or she usually receives a degree. Sometimes graduates earn certificates or other types of credentials instead. Equivalent programs at different schools—even within the same profession—might award different credentials to their graduates. It is important for credentials reviewers to realize that such differences in terminology do not necessarily indicate different levels of education. For instance, American allopathic medical schools give the MD (Doctor of Medicine) degree upon completion, osteopathic medical schools give the DO (Doctor of Osteopathy) degree, and some foreign medical schools award the MBBS (Bachelor of Medicine and Bachelor of Surgery) degree.

JCAHO requirements for verifying education

Because the Joint Commission on Accreditation of Healthcare Organizations (JCAHO) requires organizations to verify particular credentials through the primary source, a hospital must contact a school directly to confirm an applicant's education. The hospital may use a credentials verification organization (CVO) as long as the agency verifies, in writing, that it uses primary-source information. Once information regarding an applicant's education is obtained, it need not be verified again at reappointment. This information is considered static—meaning it does not change over time. Only major professional education needs to be verified. For example, one must verify medical school graduation for a physician but verification of college graduation is optional. Also, the JCAHO's requirement for primary-source verification is limited to those professionals going through the medical staff credentialing process, not those persons whose qualifications are evaluated through the human resources or personnel system. (However, it is certainly a good idea to do primary-source verification of applicants for all positions, even if it is not required.)

Good practice also requires organizations to make sure that the school or program from which each applicant graduated is accredited by the profession's recognized umbrella organization. For example, a hospital should make sure that all of its allopathic physician applicants graduated from medical colleges that the American Medical Association (AMA) recognizes.

Potential problems with verifying degrees and certificates

The JCAHO does not require organizations to verify degrees or certificates in writing—it allows the hospital to use a documented telephone conversation to verify an applicant's licensure, education, training and experience, competence,

Chapter 5

and peer references. According to the JCAHO, when verifying via the telephone, be sure to document the

- date of the conversation
- name and title of the person providing the information
- name of the organization when appropriate (e.g., the school, certifying board, employing organization, etc.)
- specific information provided
- date and signature of the person receiving the information

Many organizations seek written verification that practitioners did complete appropriate educational programs. In fact, some require that verifications include the official seals of the schools and colleges. There is some difference of opinion as to the importance of documenting medical school completion when a physician has completed a residency program. The National Committee for Quality Assurance allows the verification of a practitioner's highest education level to constitute verification of education previously achieved.

Obtaining official written verifications from schools is often a difficult and time-consuming task. Schools vary in how they handle requests for verifications. For some schools, hospitals must contact the office of the dean or the registrar, while in others, they must contact the particular educational program directly. Even when a hospital knows which office verifies degrees or certificates, it cannot be sure of the office's policy regarding verifications. For example, does the office provide telephone verifications? Does it accept faxed requests for verifications? Does it require a signed release of information form from each graduate in question? Does the office charge a fee per verification? In addition, verifying the medical school graduation of foreign or military graduates presents its own challenges.

All this uncertainty can add up to a great deal of frustration and confusion for those processing practitioner applications—not to mention considerably large phone bills from trying to find answers to questions regarding educational verifications. This chapter details the correct contact, explains each school's verification policy, and provides additional information (such as Web site links). Knowing this information will help ease the process of obtaining educational verifications and provide some answers to certain questions.

Chapter overview

This chapter is organized into nine sections that cover each of the following groups of practitioners:

- Allopathic physicians (this group has two sections—one for medical schools, and one for residency and internship programs)
- Osteopathic physicians
- Dentists
- Podiatrists
- Physician assistants
- Nurse anesthetists
- Nurse-midwives
- Chiropractors

Each section in this chapter includes separate entries for all of the accredited schools, colleges, and programs in the particular profession. Each school's entry includes information about how to contact the appropriate office and how that office verifies degrees or certificates—including details such as whether it provides telephone, fax, or electronic verifications to hospitals; allows hospitals to fax verification requests; charges a fee for verifications; and whether it requires a signed release of information form from each graduate in question.

In addition, one section includes information about how listed medical schools verify and maintain records of graduates who completed affiliated residency or internship programs. Some schools may also verify related residencies and internships. But in many cases, the hospitals at which residencies or internships are served are responsible for maintaining those records—typically the hospital's house staff office handles this task.

Guidelines for querying schools, colleges, and educational programs

The entries in this chapter include the specific policies of each office for verifying degrees or certificates. However, there are some general procedures that might help expedite verifications and ensure that they are sent to the appropriate person. Readers should consider the following points when requesting telephone or written verifications:

- Identify yourself clearly and state the purpose for your query when requesting telephone verifications
- Include self-addressed, stamped envelopes when requesting written verifications
- Provide any useful identification information—such as each graduate's name (including the name under which the graduate was registered, if applicable), graduation date, birth date, and Social Security number—to help an office retrieve records and information more quickly and easily
- Include some sort of direction on the envelope or fax cover sheet of requests for written verifications, such as the words "Attention: Degree verification request enclosed"
- Include clear and specific instructions that indicate where and to whom an office should mail or fax written verifications (a department, name, and title can help to ensure that the verification reaches the correct person)
- Include a photograph of each graduate in question to reduce the possibility of someone successfully adopting the identity of a graduate

A note

These guidelines and the specific information in the following sections will help hospitals expedite and ensure the accuracy of degree and certificate verifications. Although each office listed was contacted individually, policies and procedures sometimes change. We appreciate any updates, suggestions, and information readers might have in regard to any of the schools, colleges, and programs described in this chapter.

Hospitals might find that using a CVO is a good alternative for primary-source verification of education or school attendance. Information about an applicant's attendance and graduation is often most easily and inexpensively obtained by using a CVO. It is important, however, that those who use a CVO monitor the quality of the CVO's work. The hospital should ask the CVO to provide documentation, in writing, that they use only primary sources of information.

The JCAHO standards in the *Comprehensive Accreditation Manual for Hospitals* contain specific items that should be evaluated when choosing a CVO. Refer to the intent statement for M.S.5.4.3.1 and M.S.5.4.3.2 for details.

International medical schools

When we started to compile a list of international medical schools, we realized that there were quite a few obstacles:

- There are many international medical schools, but there is no organization that accredits medical schools worldwide.
- No organizations have a list of the international medical schools that graduate the greatest number of physicians who study or practice in the United States or Canada. The AMA, the Federation of State Medical Boards, and the Educational Commission for Foreign Medical Graduates—the agencies most likely to compile a listing of international schools that graduate the greatest number of physicians who go on to practice in the United States and Canada—do not record such information.
- Overseas communication and language barriers would result in incomplete information.
- The World Health Organization publishes the *World Directory of Medical Schools*—an economical, comprehensive listing of international schools.

Chapter 5

For these reasons, we simply listed directories of other sources of information regarding international medical schools. Please see the following resources for more details:

Organizations

American Medical Association
515 N. State Street
Chicago, ILLINOIS 60610
Telephone: 312/464-5000
Web site: www.ama-assn.org

Educational Commission for Foreign Medical Graduates
3624 Market Street
Philadelphia, PENNSYLVANIA 19104-2685
Telephone: 215/386-5900   Fax: 215/387-9963
Web site: www.ecfmg.org

Federation of State Medical Boards
Federation Place
400 Fuller Wiser Road, Suite 300
Euless, TEXAS 76039-3855
Telephone: 817/868-4000   Fax: 817/868-4099
Web site: www.fsmb.org

Published resources

Directory of Medical and Dental Schools Worldwide (1995)
(Note: Directory includes school telephone numbers)
U.S. Directory Service
Douglas Publications, Inc.
2807 N. Parham Road, Suite 200
Richmond, VIRGINIA 23294
Telephone: 804/762-9600 or 800/223-1797   Fax: 804/217-8999
E-mail: infor@douglaspublications.com
Web site: www.douglaspublications.com

World Directory of Medical Schools
World Health Organization
Avenue Appia 20
1211 Geneva 27
Switzerland
Telephone: (+00 41 22) 791 21 11   Fax: (+00 41 22) 791 31 11
Telex: 415 416
Telegraph: UNISANTE GENEVA
Web site: www.who.org

WHO Regional Office for the Americas/Pan American Health Organization
525 23rd Street, NW
Washington, DISTRICT OF COLUMBIA 20037

Telephone: 202/974-3000   Fax: 202/974-3663
E-mail: postmaster@paho.org
Web site: www.who.org
http://intranet.wpro.who.int/APPLICS/medschool/default.cfm (Use to search for schools)

Web resources

These Web sites list medical schools, but be advised that these sites are for reference only and are not for primary-source verification.

Yahoo! provides a list of international medical schools:

www.yahoo.com/Health/Medicine/Education/Medical_Schools/

The Union de Universidades de America Latina maintains a listing of links to Latin American schools:

www.unam.mx/udual/afiliacion/lista.htm

The Foundation for Advancement of International Medical Education and Research maintains the International Medical Education Directory:

http://imed.ecfmg.org/

Medical School Degrees, Residencies, Internships, and Fellowships

Alabama

University of Alabama School of Medicine
Verification of degrees MD only

Telephone:	Free of charge.
Written:	Written transcripts are $5 each. Mail requests, including signed release forms and physician's Social Security number and maiden name (if applicable). $5 for transcripts; $5 for certified diploma copies.
Electronic:	Not provided.

Medical Student Services Records Office
University of Alabama School of Medicine
Volker Hall P-100
1530 Third Avenue S (mailing address)
1670 University Boulevard (physical address)
Birmingham, ALABAMA 35294-0019
Telephone: 205/934-4964
Fax: 205/934-8724
Web site: www.uab.edu/uasom

University of Alabama School of Medicine
Verification of residencies and internships

Telephone:	Not provided.
Written:	Free of charge. Faxed upon request. Mail or fax requests, including signed release forms.
Electronic:	Not provided.

Graduate Medical Education Department
RWUH Room 190
University of Alabama School of Medicine
619 S. 19th Street
Birmingham, ALABAMA 35249
Telephone: 205/934-4793
Fax: 205/975-9279
E-mail: dbrown@uabmc.edu
Web site: www.main.uab.edu

University of South Alabama College of Medicine
Notes: Verifications of PA, nursing, or allied health degrees are not handled by this office.
Verification of degrees MD only

Telephone:	Not provided.
Written:	Free of charge. Mail or fax requests, including signed release forms.
Electronic:	Not provided.

Office of Student Records
University of South Alabama College of Medicine
1005 Medical Science Building
Mobile, ALABAMA 36688-0002
Telephone: 334/460-7180
Fax: 334/460-6761
E-mail: rsmith@jaguar1.usouthal.edu
Web site: www.usouthal.edu

University of South Alabama Hospitals
Notes: Fellowships must be verified through individual departments.
Verification of residencies and internships

Telephone:	Free of charge.
Written:	Free of charge. Faxed upon request in emergency situations only. Mail or fax requests, including signed release forms and physician's Social Security number.
Electronic:	Not provided.

> House Staff Office
> University of South Alabama Hospitals
> 2451 Fillingim Street
> Mobile, ALABAMA 36617
> Telephone: 251/471-7117
> Fax: 251/470-5884
> E-mail: bpendergrass@usamail.usouthal.edu

Arizona

University of Arizona College of Medicine
Verification of degrees MD only

Telephone:	Free of charge.
Written:	Free of charge. Faxed upon request. Mail or fax requests, including signed release forms.
Electronic:	Not provided.

> Office of Student Records
> Arizona Health Sciences Center
> University of Arizona College of Medicine
> PO Box 245026
> Tucson, ARIZONA 85724-5026
> Telephone: 520/626-6518
> Fax: 520/626-6300
> E-mail: cflint@u.arizona.edu
> Web site: www.medicine.arizona.edu/curricularaffairs/electives

University of Arizona College of Medicine
Verification of residencies and fellowships

Telephone:	Free of charge.
Written:	Free of charge. Faxed upon request. Mail or fax requests, including signed release forms and physician's specific program. Will forward written requests to appropriate residency program office.
Electronic:	Not provided.

> Office of Graduate Medical Education
> Arizona Health Sciences Center
> University of Arizona College of Medicine
> PO Box 245085
> Tucson, ARIZONA 85724-5085
> Telephone: 520/626-7878
> Fax: 520/626-0090
> Web site: www.medicine.arizona.edu/gme

Medical School Degrees, Residencies, Internships, and Fellowships

Arkansas

University of Arkansas for Medical Sciences
Verification of degrees, residencies, internships, and fellowships

Telephone: Free of charge.
Written: Free of charge. Faxed upon request. Mail or fax requests, including signed release forms.
Electronic: Not provided.

> House Staff Student Records Office
> University of Arkansas for Medical Sciences
> Mail Slot 552
> 4301 W. Markham Street
> Little Rock, ARKANSAS 72205
> Telephone: 501/686-5356
> Fax: 501/686-8160
> Web site: www.uams.edu

British Columbia

University of British Columbia Faculty of Medicine
Verification of residencies

Telephone: Not provided.
Written: $10 per verification; $15 for official letter of verification. Mail requests, including physician's name and year of graduation, and check made payable to University of British Columbia.
Electronic: Not provided.

> Dean's Office
> University of British Columbia Faculty of Medicine
> Room 317 2194 Health Sciences Mall
> Vancouver, BRITISH COLUMBIA V6T 1Z3
> CANADA
> Telephone: 604/875-4500 (undergraduate office)   604/822-2421 (Dean's office)
> Fax: 604/822-6061
> Web site: www.med.ubc.ca

University of British Columbia Faculty of Medicine
Verification of residencies

Telephone: Not provided.
Written: $10 per verification; $15 for official letter of verification. Mail requests, including physician's name and year of graduation, and check made payable to University of British Columbia.
Electronic: Not provided.

> University of British Columbia Faculty of Medicine
> 3100 910 W. Tenth Avenue
> Department of Surgery
> Vancouver, BRITISH COLUMBIA V5Z4E3
> CANADA
> Telephone: 604/875-4545   Fax: 604/875-4036
> Web site: www.surgery.ubc.ca

California

Charles R. Drew University of Medicine and Science College of Medicine
Verification of degrees

Telephone: Not provided.
Written: Free of charge. Faxed upon request. Mail or fax requests, including signed release forms and physician's year of graduation.
Electronic: Not provided.

> Office of Medical Student Affairs
> Charles R. Drew University of Medicine and Science College of Medicine
> 1731 E. 120th Street
> Los Angeles, CALIFORNIA 90059
> Telephone: 323/563-5956   Fax: 323/563-4957
> E-mail: phmiller@cdrewu.edu
> Web site: www.cdrewu.edu

Charles R. Drew University of Medicine and Science College of Medicine
Verification of residencies and internships

Telephone: Free of charge.
Written: Free of charge. Faxed upon request. Mail or fax requests, including signed release forms.
Electronic: Not provided.

> Charles R. Drew University of Medicine and Science College of Medicine
> Office of Postgraduate Medical Education
> Martin Luther King Hospital
> 1731 E. 120th Street
> Los Angeles, CALIFORNIA 90059
> Telephone: 323/563-4800   Fax: 323/569-0597
> Web site: www.cdrewu.edu

Keck School of Medicine of the University of Southern California
Verification of degrees

Telephone: Free of charge.
Written: Free of charge. Mail or fax requests, including signed release forms and physician's Social Security number. Please include exact name under which the student was registered.
Electronic: Not provided.

> 1975 Zonal Avenue KAM 100B
> Los Angeles, CALIFORNIA 90033
> Telephone: 323/442-2553   Fax: 323/442-2663
> Web site: www.usc.edu/schools/medicine

Loma Linda University Medical Center
Verification of residencies and internships

Telephone: Not provided.
Written: Free of charge. Faxed upon request, but will not have school's official seal. Mail or fax requests, including signed release forms.
Electronic: Not provided.

Medical School Degrees, Residencies, Internships, and Fellowships

House Staff Office
Loma Linda University Medical Center, Room A602
PO Box 2000
Loma Linda, CALIFORNIA 92354
Telephone: 909/558-8131   Fax: 909/558-0430
Web site: www.llu.edu/llumc/residency/train.htm

Loma Linda University School of Medicine
Verification of degrees

Telephone: Contact school for more information.
Written: Mail request. Include signed release form, and physician's Social Security number and exact name when enrolled in program and date of birth.
Electronic: Not provided.

Loma Linda University
School of Medicine
Attention: MD degree verification
Loma Linda, CALIFORNIA 92350
Telephone: 909/558-4729   800/422-4558 (front desk)
Fax: 909/558-0255
Web site: www.llu.edu/llu/medicine/index

Stanford University School of Medicine
Verification of degrees

Telephone: Free of charge.
Written: Free of charge. Faxed upon request. Mail or fax requests, including signed release forms.
Electronic: Not provided.

Stanford University School of Medicine
Department of Medicine, Room S101
Stanford, CALIFORNIA 94305-5109
Telephone: 650/723-5410   Fax: 650/498-6741
Web site: www.med.stanford.edu

UCLA Medical Center
Verification of internal medicine residencies, internships, and fellowships

Telephone: Not provided.
Written: $10 per verification. Faxed upon request. Mail or fax requests, including signed release forms.
Electronic: Not provided.
Department of Medicine
UCLA Medical Center, 32-115 CHS
Los Angeles, CALIFORNIA 90095-1736
Telephone: 310/825-7375   Fax: 310/825-5791
Web site: www.med.mcu.ech

University of California at Davis School of Medicine
Verification of degrees

Telephone: Not provided.
Written: Free of charge. Faxed upon request. Mail or fax requests, including signed release forms.

Electronic:	Not provided.

Office of Student Records
MS1-C Room 124
University of California at Davis School of Medicine
1 Shields Avenue
Davis, CALIFORNIA 95616
Telephone: 530/752-3105   Fax: 530/754-7295
Web site: www.medome.ucdavis.edu/ome

University of California at Davis School of Medicine
Verification of residencies and internships
Telephone:	Not provided.
Written:	Free of charge. Faxed upon request. Mail or fax requests, including signed release forms, and physician's dates of attendance and area of specialization.
Electronic:	Not provided.

University of California at Davis Medical Center
2730 Stockton Boulevard, Suite 2200
Sacramento, CALIFORNIA 95817
Telephone: 916/734-2756   916/734-5355 (main)
Fax: 916/734-8829
Web site: www.hr.ucdmc.ucdavis.edu

University of California at Los Angeles School of Medicine
Verification of degrees
Telephone:	Provide physician's name, year of graduation, and Social Security number.
Written:	Faxed upon request. Mail, phone, or fax requests, including signed release forms, Social Security number and physician's year of graduation.
Electronic:	Not provided.

Office of Student Affairs
University of California at Los Angeles School of Medicine
12-159 CHS
Box 951720
Los Angeles, CALIFORNIA 90095-1720
Telephone: 310/206-0973   Fax: 310/794-9574

University of California at Los Angeles School of Medicine
Notes: Also provides verification for internships.
Verification of surgical residencies
Telephone:	Not provided.
Written:	Free of charge. Faxed upon request. Mail or fax requests, including signed release forms.
Electronic:	Not provided.

Surgical Education Office
Department of Surgery
Box 951749
University of California at Los Angeles School of Medicine
10833 LeConte Avenue, Room 72-229 CHS

Los Angeles, CALIFORNIA 90095-1749
Telephone: 310/825-6557 (coordinator)   310/206-9291 (director of surgery education)
Fax: 310/267-0369
Web site: www.surgery.medsch.ucla.edu

University of California at San Diego School of Medicine
Notes: Transcripts: $6 per copy. Make check payable to U.C. Regents.
Verification of degrees MD only
Telephone: Free of charge.
Written: Free of charge. Faxed upon request. Mail or fax requests, including signed release forms.
Electronic: Not provided.

Office of Student Affairs
University of California at San Diego School of Medicine
9500 Gilman Drive
Mail Code 0606
La Jolla, CALIFORNIA 92093-0606
Telephone: 858/534-3700   Fax: 858/534-8556
E-mail: jkmorgan@ucsd.edu
Web site: www.ucsd.edu

University of California at San Diego School of Medicine
Verification of residencies and internships
Telephone: Free of charge.
Written: Free of charge. Faxed upon request. Mail or fax requests, including signed release forms. Will forward evaluation requests to appropriate departments.
Electronic: Not provided.

Graduate Medical Education
University of California at San Diego Medical Center
200 W. Arbor Drive
San Diego, CALIFORNIA 92103-8972
Telephone: 619/543-2699 (assistant director)   619/543-3684 (executive director)
Fax: 619/543-3676

University of California at San Francisco School of Medicine
Verification of residencies, internships, and fellowships
Telephone: Not provided.
Written: Free of charge. Faxed upon request. Mail or fax requests, including signed release forms and physicians specific program. Will forward requests to appropriate departments.
Electronic: Not provided.

Office of Graduate Medical Education
University of California at San Francisco School of Medicine
PO Box 0474
San Francisco, CALIFORNIA 94143-0474
Telephone: 415/476-4561
Fax: 415/502-4166
Web site: www.som.ucsf.edu/som

University of California Davis, Medical Center
Notes: Verification of residencies and internships completed after 1975.
Verification of residencies and internships
Telephone: Free of charge.
Written: Free of charge. Mail or fax requests, including signed release forms and physician's dates of residency.
Electronic: Free of charge.

> University of California Davis Medical Center
> Surgery Residency Office
> 2315 Stockton Boulevard, Room 6309
> Sacramento, CALIFORNIA 95817
> Telephone: 916/734-2724   Fax: 916/734-5633
> E-mail: gensurg.residency@ucdavis.edu
> Web site: www.surgery.ucdmc.ucdavis.edu

University of California Irvine, College of Medicine
Notes: Internships and residencies, fellowships and fifth pathways verified through Graduate Medical Education Office only (714/456-3526).
Verification of degrees, internships, and residencies
Telephone: Free of charge.
Written: Free of charge. Faxed upon request. Mail or fax requests, including signed release forms.
Electronic: Not provided.

> Office of Educational Affairs
> University of California, Irvine College of Medicine
> Building 802, Room 252
> Irvine, CALIFORNIA 92697-4089
> Telephone: 949/824-6138   Fax: 949/824-2083
> Web site: www.uci.edu

University of California San Francisco, School of Medicine
Verification of degrees
Telephone: Free of charge; prefer written request.
Written: Free of charge. Faxed upon request. Mail or fax requests, including signed release forms and physician's Social Security number and former name (if applicable).
Electronic: Not provided.

> Office of Admission and Registrar
> University of California San Francisco School of Medicine
> 500 Parnassus Avenue MU200-W
> San Francisco, CALIFORNIA 94143-0244
> Telephone: 415/476-4356 (transcripts)   415/476-8280 (registration)
> Fax: 415/476-9690
> Web site: saawww.ucsf.edu

University of Southern California School of Medicine
Verification of residencies, internships, and fellowships
Telephone: Not provided.
Written: Free of charge. Mail requests, including signed release forms.
Electronic: Not provided.

Medical School Degrees, Residencies, Internships, and Fellowships

Office of Graduate Medical Education
Los Angeles County USC Medical Center
Health Science Campus
1200 North State Street
Room 1102
Los Angeles, CALIFORNIA 90033
Telephone: 323/226-6931   Fax: 323/226-6651

Colorado

University of Colorado Health Sciences Center
Verification of degrees

Telephone:	Free of charge.
Written:	Free of charge. Faxed upon request. Mail or fax requests, including signed release forms.
Electronic:	Not provided.

Office of Student Admissions & Records
Campus Box A054
University of Colorado Health Sciences Center
4200 E. Ninth Avenue
Denver, COLORADO 80262
Telephone: 303/315-7676
Fax: 303/315-3358
E-mail: student.services@uchsc.edu
Web site: www.uchsc.edu

Connecticut

University of Connecticut School of Medicine
Verification of degrees

Telephone:	Free of charge. Limit one verification per call.
Written:	Free of charge. Faxed upon request. Mail or fax requests, including signed release forms.
Electronic:	Not provided.

Attention: Registrar
Office of the Registrar
University of Connecticut School of Medicine
263 Farmington Avenue
Farmington, CONNECTICUT 06030-1827
Telephone: 860/679-3125
Fax: 860/679-1902
E-mail: erdavis@uchu.edu
Web site: www.uchc.edu

University of Connecticut School of Medicine
Verification of residencies and internships

Telephone:	Free of charge.
Written:	Free of charge. Faxed upon request. Mail or fax requests, including signed release forms.
Electronic:	Not provided.

Attention: Residency verification
Office of Residency Administration MC 1925
University of Connecticut School of Medicine
263 Farmington Avenue
Farmington, CONNECTICUT 06030-1925
Telephone: 860/679-2147
Fax: 860/679-1282
Web site: medicine.uchc.edu

Yale-New Haven Hospital
Verification of residencies and internships

Telephone: Free of charge.
Written: Free of charge. Faxed upon request. Mail or fax requests, including signed release forms.
Electronic: Not provided.

Yale-New Haven Hospital
House Staff Office
Tompkins 209
20 York Street
New Haven, CONNECTICUT 06510
Telephone: 203/688-2259
Fax: 203/688-5599
E-mail: depaul@ynhh.org
Web site: www.yalenewhavenhospital.org

District of Columbia

George Washington University School of Medicine and Health Sciences
Verification of degrees

Telephone: Free of charge.
Written: Free of charge. Faxed upon request. Mail or fax requests.
Electronic: Free of charge. E-mail requests to msdalw@gwumc.edu.

Attention: Director of Student Services
George Washington University School of Medicine and Health Sciences
2300 Eye Street NW, Ross 716
Washington, DISTRICT OF COLUMBIA 20037
Telephone: 202-994-3502
Fax: 202-994-0926
E-mail: msdalw@gwumc.edu

George Washington University School of Medicine and Health Sciences
Verification of residencies and internships

Telephone: Not provided.
Written: Free of charge. Faxed upon request. Mail or fax requests, including signed release forms.
Electronic: Not provided.

Office of Graduate Medical Education
George Washington University Medical Center
2300 I Street NW, Suite 707

Washington, DISTRICT OF COLUMBIA 20037
Telephone: 202/994-1000
Fax: 202/994-1604
E-mail: gwgme@gwu.edu
Web site: www.gwumc.edu

Georgetown University School of Medicine
Verification of degrees

Telephone: Not provided.
Written: Mail, fax, or e-mail request. Letter of certification and transcript are $5 each. Include signed release form, and physician's Social Security number and exact name when enrolled in program.
Electronic: Not provided.

Office of Academic Records
School of Medicine
Georgetown University
Box 571418
Washington, DISTRICT OF COLUMBIA 20057-1421
Telephone: 202/687-1127   202/687-1856 (Records Clerk)
Fax: 202/687-7660
E-mail: medreg@georgetown.edu
Web site: www.dml.georgetown.edu/schmed/registrar

Howard University College of Medicine
Verification of degrees

Telephone: Free of charge. Provide physician's name and year of graduation.
Written: Free of charge. Faxed upon request. Mail or fax requests, including signed release forms and physician's year of graduation.
Electronic: Not provided.

Office of Academic Affairs
Howard University College of Medicine
520 West Street NW, Room 527
Washington, DISTRICT OF COLUMBIA 20059
Telephone: 202/806-6280
Fax: 202/806-7934
Web site: www.howard.edu

Howard University College of Medicine
Verification of residencies and internships

Telephone: Not provided.
Written: Free of charge. Mail requests, including signed release forms.
Electronic: Not provided.

Associate Dean for Academic Affairs
Howard University College of Medicine
520 W. Street NW
Washington, DISTRICT OF COLUMBIA 20059
Telephone: 202/806-6270   202/806-9494 (academic affairs)

Fax: 202/806-7934
Web site: www.howard.edu

Florida

Jackson Memorial Hospital
Verification of residencies and internships

Telephone: Free of charge.
Written: Free of charge. Faxed upon request. Mail or fax requests, including signed release forms.
Electronic: Response may be sent via e-mail.

Jackson Memorial Hospital
1611 NW 12th Avenue
Department of Physician's Services
E.T.O. 1004
Miami, FLORIDA 33136
Telephone: 305/585-6448
Fax: 305/585-2495
Web site: www.um-jmh.org

University of Florida College of Medicine
Verification of degrees MD only

Telephone: Free of charge.
Written: Free of charge. Mail or fax requests, including signed release forms.
Electronic: Not provided.

Office of Student Affairs
University of Florida Health Sciences Center
PO Box 100216
Gainesville, FLORIDA 32610
Telephone: 352/392-3071
Fax: 352/846-0622
E-mail: rleacock@dean.med.ufl.edu
Web site: www.ufl.edu

University of Florida College of Medicine
Verification of residencies and internships

Telephone: Free of charge.
Written: Free of charge. Faxed upon request. Mail or fax requests, including signed release forms.
Electronic: Not provided.

Attention: Residency verification request
Office of the Dean of Personnel
University of Florida College of Medicine
PO Box 103450
Gainesville, FLORIDA 32610
Telephone: 352/265-8014
Fax: 352/265-8018
E-mail: marj@dean.med.ufl.edu

University of Miami Medical School
Verification of degrees

Telephone: Free of charge.
Written: Free of charge. Mail requests, including signed release forms, and physician's Social Security number and date of birth.
Electronic: Not provided.

> Office of Student Affairs
> University of Miami Medical School
> PO Box 016960 (R-128)
> Miami, FLORIDA 33101
> Telephone: 305/547-6811
> Fax: 305/243-6757

University of South Florida College of Medicine
Verification of degrees MD only

Telephone: Free of charge.
Written: Free of charge. Faxed upon request. Mail or fax requests, including signed release forms. Phone requests in emergency situations only.
Electronic: Not provided.

> University of South Florida College of Medicine
> Office of the Registrar MDC32
> 12901 Bruce B. Downs Boulevard
> Tampa, FLORIDA 33612-4799
> Telephone: 813/974-0828
> Fax: 813/974-8181 or 813/974-4990
> E-mail: atsinney@hsc.usf.edu

University of South Florida College of Medicine
Verification of internal medicine residencies, internships, and fellowships

Telephone: Not provided.
Written: Free of charge. Faxed upon request. Mail or fax requests, including signed release forms. Phone requests in emergency situations only.
Electronic: Not provided.

> University of South Florida College of Medicine
> Graduate Medical Education
> 12901 Bruce B. Downs Boulevard, MDC41
> Tampa, FLORIDA 33612-4799
> Telephone: 813/974-9744
> Fax: 813/974-8359
> Web site: www.hsc.usf.edu

Georgia

Emory University School of Medicine
Verification of degrees

Telephone: Not provided.

Written: Free of charge. Mail or fax requests, including signed release forms.
Electronic: Not provided.

> Office of Medical Education
> Emory University School of Medicine
> 1440 Clifton Road, Room 309
> Atlanta, GEORGIA 30322
> Telephone: 404/727-5655
> Fax: 404/727-0045
> Web site: www.emory.edu

Medical College of Georgia
Verification of degrees
Telephone: Free of charge.
Written: Free of charge. Faxed upon request. Mail or fax requests, including signed release forms.
Electronic: Not provided.

> Office of the Registrar
> Medical College of Georgia
> Room AA171
> Augusta, GEORGIA 30912-7315
> Telephone: 706/721-2201
> Fax: 706/721-0186
> E-mail: registrar@mail.mcg.edu
> Web site: www.mcg.edu

Medical College of Georgia
Notes: Verification requests must go to individual departments. Call before submitting request.
Verification of residencies and internships
Telephone: Not provided.
Written: Not provided.
Electronic: Not provided.

> Medical College of Georgia
> Office of Graduate Medical Education AE-3042
> Augusta, GEORGIA 30912
> Telephone: 706/721-3052
> Fax: 706/721-7501
> E-mail: hwalp@mail.mcg.edu
> Web site: www.mcg.edu

Medical College of Georgia, Nursing Anesthesia Program
Verification of degrees
Telephone: Free of charge.
Written: Free of charge. Faxed upon request. Mail or fax requests, including signed release forms.
Electronic: Not provided.

> Office of the Registrar
> Medical College of Georgia

Medical School Degrees, Residencies, Internships, and Fellowships

AA171
1120 15th Street
Augusta, GEORGIA 30912-7315
Telephone: 706/721-2201
Fax: 706/721-0186
Web site: www.mcg.edu

Mercer University School of Medicine
Verification of degrees

Telephone: Free of charge. Provide physician's name and year of graduation.
Written: Free of charge. Faxed upon request, followed by mailed hard copy. Mail requests, including signed release forms and physician's year of graduation.
Electronic: Not provided.

Admissions Office
Mercer University School of Medicine
1550 College Street
Macon, GEORGIA 31207-0001
Telephone: 478/301-2542
Fax: 478/301-2547
Web site: www.merceruniversity.edu

Mercer University School of Medicine
Verification of residencies and internships

Telephone: Not provided.
Written: Free of charge. Faxed upon request. Mail or fax requests, including signed release forms.
Electronic: Not provided.

Mercer University School of Medicine
Office of Medical Education
Medical Center of Central Georgia
PO Box 6000
Macon, GEORGIA 31208
Telephone: 478/633-1061
Fax: 478/633-1578
Web site: www.mccg.org

Morehouse School of Medicine
Verification of degrees

Telephone: Free of charge.
Written: Free of charge. Faxed upon request. Mail or fax requests, including signed release forms.
Electronic: Not provided.

Office of the Registrar
Morehouse School of Medicine
720 Westview Drive
Atlanta, GEORGIA 30310-1495
Telephone: 404/752-1652
Fax: 404/752-1512
Web site: www.msm.edu

Morehouse School of Medicine
Verification of residencies and internships
Telephone: Not provided.
Written: Free of charge. Faxed upon request. Mail or fax requests, including signed release forms.
Electronic: Not provided.

> Attention: Residency verification request
> Graduate Medical Education Office
> Morehouse School of Medicine
> 720 Westview Drive SW
> Atlanta, GEORGIA 30310-1495
> Telephone: 404/752-1857
> Fax: 404/752-1088
> E-mail: boothb@msm.edu
> Web site: www.msm.edu

Hawaii

University of Hawaii School of Medicine
Notes: Also provides certification of licensure for out-of-state requests free of charge.
Verification of degrees, internships, and residencies
Telephone: Free of charge.
Written: Free of charge. Mail requests, including signed release forms.
Electronic: Not provided.

> Office of the Registrar
> University of Hawaii School of Medicine
> Biomedical Science Building B104
> 1960 E. West Road
> Honolulu, HAWAII 96822
> Telephone: 808/956-8300
> Fax: 808/956-9547
> Web site: hawaiimed.hawaii.edu

Illinois

Finch University of the Health Sciences/Chicago Medical School
Verification of degrees
Telephone: Free of charge.
Written: Free of charge. Faxed upon request in emergency situations only. Mail requests, including signed release forms.
Electronic: Not provided.

> Attention: Office of the Registrar
> Chicago Medical School
> Finch University of the Health Sciences
> 3333 Green Bay Road
> North Chicago, ILLINOIS 60064
> Telephone: 847/578-3229
> Fax: 847/578-3284

Medical School Degrees, Residencies, Internships, and Fellowships

E-mail: pratth@finchcms.edu
Web site: www.finchcms.edu

Finch University of the Health Sciences/Chicago Medical School
Verification of residencies and internships

Telephone: Free of charge. Mail or fax signed release form.
Written: Free of charge. Faxed upon request. Mail or fax requests, including signed release forms.
Electronic: Free of charge.

Office of Clinical Affairs
Finch University of the Health Sciences/Chicago Medical School
3333 Green Bay Road
North Chicago, ILLINOIS 60064
Telephone: 847/578-3241
Fax: 847/578-3320
Web site: www.finchcms.edu

Loyola University of Chicago, Stritch School of Medicine
Verification of degrees

Telephone: Free of charge.
Written: Free of charge. Faxed upon request. Mail or fax requests, including signed release forms.
Electronic: Not provided.

Office of the Registrar, Room 220
Loyola University of Chicago, Stritch School of Medicine
2160 S. First Avenue
Maywood, ILLINOIS 60153
Telephone: 708/216-3222
Fax: 708/216-8151
Web site: www.meddean.luc.edu

Loyola University of Chicago, Stritch School of Medicine
Verification of residencies and internships

Telephone: Not provided.
Written: Free of charge. Faxed upon request. Mail or fax requests, including signed release forms.
Electronic: Not provided.

Office of Graduate Medical Education
Loyola University of Chicago, Stritch School of Medicine
2160 S. First Avenue
Building 101, Room 1740
Maywood, ILLINOIS 60153
Telephone: 708/216-3769
Fax: 708/216-9033

Northwestern University, The Feinberg School of Medicine
Verification of degrees

Telephone: Not provided.
Written: Mail, fax, or e-mail request. Include signed release form, and physician's Social Security number and

Chapter 5

	exact name when enrolled in program.
Electronic:	Not provided.

Department of Medicine
Northwestern University, The Feinberg School of Medicine
251 E. Huron Street
Galter Pavilion, Suite 3-150
Chicago, ILLINOIS 60611
Telephone: 312/926-6895
Fax: 312/926-0239
Web site: www.nums.nwu.edu

OSF Saint Francis Medical Center
Notes: Verification of residencies and internships from 1940–1985. Phone verification is provided with faxed authorization.
Verification of residencies and internships

Telephone:	Not provided.
Written:	Free of charge. Faxed upon request. Mail or fax requests, including signed release forms and self-addressed, stamped envelope.
Electronic:	Provided upon faxed authorization.

OSF Saint Francis Medical Center
Attention: Credentialing
Professional Staff Office
530 N.E. Glen Oak Avenue
Peoria, ILLINOIS 61637
Telephone: 309/655-6899
Fax: 309/624-8933
E-mail: cathy.rupert@osfhealthcare.org
Web site: www.osfhealthcare.org

Pritzker School of Medicine at the University of Chicago
Verification of degrees

Telephone:	Not provided.
Written:	Free of charge. Faxed upon request. Mail or fax requests, including signed release forms.
Electronic:	Not provided.

Attention: Medical school verifications
Office of Medical Education
Pritzker School of Medicine at the University of Chicago
924 E. 57th Street, Suite 104
Chicago, ILLINOIS 60637
Telephone: 773/702-1939
Fax: 773/702-2598
E-mail: lponce@bsd.uchicago.edu
Web site: www.pritzker.bsd.uchicago.edu

Rush Presbyterian St. Luke's Medical Center
Verification of residencies and internships

Telephone:	Not provided.

Medical School Degrees, Residencies, Internships, and Fellowships

Written: Free of charge. Mail (preferred) or fax requests, including signed release forms.
Electronic: Not provided.

Office of Graduate Medical Education
Rush Presbyterian St. Luke's Medical Center
600 S. Paulina Street, Suite 524
Chicago, ILLINOIS 60612-3842
Telephone: 312/942-5495
Fax: 312/942-2333

Rush University, Rush Medical College
Verification of degrees
Telephone: Free of charge. Provide physician's name and Social Security number.
Written: Free of charge. Faxed upon request. Mail or fax requests, including signed release forms and physician's Social Security number.
Electronic: Not provided.

Office of the Registrar
Rush University
600 S. Paulina Street, Suite 440
Chicago, ILLINOIS 60612
Telephone: 312/942-5681
Fax: 312/942-2219
E-mail: registrar@rush.edu
Web site: www.rushu.rush.edu

Southern Illinois University School of Medicine
Verification of degrees
Telephone: Not provided.
Written: Free of charge. Faxed upon request in emergency situations only. Mail or fax requests, including signed release forms.
Electronic: Not provided.

Office of Student Affairs
Southern Illinois University School of Medicine
801 N Rutledge, Room 3080
Springfield, ILLINOIS 62794-9624
Telephone: 217/782-0890
Fax: 217/785-5538
E-mail: jlangley@siumed.edu
Web site: www.siumed.edu

Southern Illinois University School of Medicine, Office of Residency Affairs
Notes: Residency Affairs Office verifies dates of attendance and completion; forwards requests for more information to appropriate program director.
Verification of residencies and internships
Telephone: Free of charge.
Written: Free of charge. Faxed upon request. Mail or fax requests, including signed release forms.
Electronic: Not provided.

Office of Residency Affairs
Southern Illinois University School of Medicine
PO Box 19656
Springfield, ILLINOIS 62794-9656
Telephone: 217/782-8853
Fax: 217/785-0828
E-mail: ljones@siumed.edu

University of Illinois at Chicago
Verification of degrees
Telephone: Free of charge. Provide physician's Social Security number and date of birth.
Written: $4 fee per verification (payable to Univ. of Illinois at Chicago). Mail requests, including signed release forms, and physician's Social Security number and date of birth.
Electronic: Not provided.

Attention: Records
Office of Admissions and Records (MC 018)
University of Illinois at Chicago
PO Box 5220
1200 W. Harrison
Chicago, ILLINOIS 60680-5220
Telephone: 312/996-4350   312/355-0379 (hearing impaired)
Fax: 312/413-9719
E-mail: uicadmit@uic.edu
Web site: www.uic.edu.

University of Ilinois at Chicago, Graduate Medical Education
Notes: GME office verifies the dates of a residency or internship only. For information on privileges delineation or to complete a form, contact specific residency or internship programs directly.
Verification of residencies and internships
Telephone: Free of charge.
Written: Free of charge. Faxed upon request. Mail or fax requests, including signed release forms.
Electronic: Not provided.

Office of Graduate Medical Education (MC 675)
University of Illinois at Chicago College of Medicine
820 S. Wood Street
Chicago, ILLINOIS 60612
Telephone: 312/996-2933
Fax: 312/996-3050
E-mail: gme@uic.edu
Web site: www.uic.edu.gme.com

University of Illinois College of Medicine at Peoria
Verification of degrees
Telephone: Free of charge.
Written: Free of charge. Faxed upon request. Mail or fax requests, including signed release forms.
Electronic: Free of charge.

Medical School Degrees, Residencies, Internships, and Fellowships

> Office of Student Affairs
> University of Illinois College of Medicine at Peoria
> PO Box 1649
> One Illini Drive
> Peoria, ILLINOIS 61656
> Telephone: 309/671-8411
> Fax: 309/671-8480
> E-mail: asm@uic.edu

University of Illinois College of Medicine at Peoria
Notes: Verification of residencies and internships from 1985–present.
Verification of residencies and internships

Telephone:	Not provided.
Written:	Free of charge. Faxed upon request. Mail or fax requests, including signed release forms.
Electronic:	Not provided.

> Office of Graduate Medical Education
> University of Illinois College of Medicine at Peoria
> PO Box 1649
> Peoria, ILLINOIS 61656
> Telephone: 309/671-8450
> Fax: 309/671-8452
> Web site: www.uicomp.oic.edu

University of Illinois College of Medicine at Rockford
Verification of degrees

Telephone:	Not provided.
Written:	$5 per verification ($10 per verification if additional information is requested). Faxed upon request. Mail or fax requests, including signed release forms.
Electronic:	Not provided.

> Attention: Verification request, Allena Fortson
> Student and Alumni Affairs
> University of Illinois College of Medicine at Rockford
> 1601 Parkview Avenue
> Rockford, ILLINOIS 61107-1897
> Telephone: 815/395-5581
> Fax: 815/395-5867
> E-mail: allenam@uic.edu

University of Illinois College of Medicine at Rockford
Verification of residencies and internships

Telephone:	Free of charge.
Written:	Free of charge. Faxed upon request. Mail or fax requests, including signed release forms.
Electronic:	Free of charge.

> Residency Office
> University of Illinois College of Medicine at Rockford
> 1221 E. State Street

Rockford, ILLINOIS 61104
Telephone: 815/972-1037
Fax: 815/972-1092
E-mail: farionw@uic.edu/fprp.htm or brettr@uic.edu
Web site: www.uic.edu/fprp.htm

University of Illinois College of Medicine at Urbana
Verification of degrees

Telephone: Not provided.
Written: Free of charge. Faxed upon request. Mail or fax requests, including signed release forms.
Electronic: Not provided.

Office of Student Affairs
Medical Science Building Room 190
University of Illinois College of Medicine at Urbana
506 S. Mathews Avenue
Urbana, ILLINOIS 61801
Telephone: 217/333-5469
Fax: 217/244-4444
Web site: www.uiuc.edu

University of Illinois College of Medicine at Urbana
Verification of residencies and internships

Telephone: Need permission of resident.
Written: Free of charge. Faxed upon request. Mail or fax requests, including signed release forms.
Electronic: Not provided.

Internal Medicine Residency Program
University of Illinois at Urbana College of Medicine
611 W. Park Street
Urbana, ILLINOIS 61801
Telephone: 217/383-3110
Fax: 217/244-0621
Web site: www.med.uiuc.edu/residency

Indiana

Indiana University School of Medicine
Verification of degrees

Telephone: Free of charge. Web site verification is not encouraged.
Written: Free of charge. Faxed upon request. Mail or fax requests. Web site verification is not encouraged.
Electronic: Not provided.

Graduate Credentialing
Office of Medical Student Academic Affairs
Indiana University School of Medicine
635 Barnhill Drive, Room 160
Indianapolis, INDIANA 46202-5127
Telephone: 317/274-7895

Medical School Degrees, Residencies, Internships, and Fellowships

Fax: 317/278-4755
Web site: msaa.iusm.iu.edu

Indiana University School of Medicine
Verification of residencies and internships

Telephone:	Not provided.
Written:	Call Office of House Staff Affairs at 317/274-8282 for instructions on submitting request.
Electronic:	Not provided.

Office of House Staff Affairs
Fesler Hall Room 224
Indiana University School of Medicine
1120 South Drive
Indianapolis, INDIANA 46202-5114
Telephone: 317/274-8282
Web site: www.medicine.iu.edu

Iowa

University of Iowa Hospitals and Clinics
Verification of residencies and internships

Telephone:	Free of charge.
Written:	Free of charge. Faxed upon request. Mail or fax requests, including signed release forms.
Electronic:	Not provided.

Office of House Staff Affairs, Room 1303 JCP
University of Iowa Hospitals and Clinics
200 Hawkins Drive
Iowa City, IOWA 52242-1009
Telephone: 319/356-2256 (office of house staff affairs)   319/356-1616 (general information)
Fax: 319/384-6004
Web site: www.uihealthcare.com

University of Iowa, Roy J. & Lucille A. Carver College of Medicine
Verification of degrees MD only

Telephone:	Free of charge.
Written:	Free of charge. Faxed upon request. Mail or fax requests, including signed release forms.
Electronic:	Not provided.

Attention: Degree verification request
Office of Medical Student Affairs
University of Iowa, Roy J. & Lucille A. Carver College of Medicine
100 CMAB
Iowa City, IOWA 52242-1101
Telephone: 319/335-6823
Fax: 319/335-8049
Web site: www.medicine.uiowa.edu

Kansas

University of Kansas Medical Center
Notes: University of Kansas at Wichita School of Medicine does not verify medical degrees. Direct requests to the main Kansas University campus in Kansas City.

Verification of residencies and internships

Telephone: Free of charge.
Written: Free of charge. Mail or fax requests, including signed release forms.
Electronic: Not provided.

> University of Kansas Medical Center
> Office of the Registrar
> 3001 Student Center
> 3013 Rainbow Boulevard
> Kansas City, KANSAS 66160-7191
> Telephone: 913/588-6588   913/588-6594 (credentialing)   913/588-6595 (credentialing)
> Fax: 913/588-4697
> E-mail: kumcregistrar@kumc.edu
> Web site: www.kumc.edu

University of Kansas School of Medicine–Wichita
Notes: GME office verifies residencies that took place after 1989. To verify residencies that took place prior to or during 1989, contact the specific residency or internship program.

Verification of residencies and internships

Telephone: Free of charge.
Written: Free of charge. Faxed upon request. Mail or fax requests, including signed release forms.
Electronic: Not provided.

> Office of Graduate Medical Education
> University of Kansas School of Medicine–Wichita
> 1010 N. Kansas
> Wichita, KANSAS 67214-3199
> Telephone: 316/293-2665
> Fax: 316/293-1893
> E-mail: pvogelsa@kumc.edu
> Web site: www.kumc.edu

Kentucky

University of Kentucky College of Medicine

Verification of degrees

Telephone: Free of charge. Provide physician's Social Security number and year of graduation.
Written: Free of charge. Faxed upon request. Mail or fax requests, including signed release forms, and physician's Social Security number and year of graduation.
Electronic: Not provided.

> Office of Student Affairs
> Chandler Medical Center
> University of Kentucky College of Medicine
> 800 Rose Street MN-104

Medical School Degrees, Residencies, Internships, and Fellowships

Lexington, KENTUCKY 40536-0298
Telephone: 859/323-5261
Fax: 859/323-2076
Web site: www.mc.uky.edu.medicine

University of Kentucky College of Medicine
Verification of residencies and internships
Telephone: Free of charge with faxed signed release form.
Written: Free of charge. Faxed upon request. Mail or fax requests, including signed release forms.
Electronic: Not provided.

University of Kentucky College of Medicine
Chandler Medical Center
Office of Graduate Medical Education
800 Rose Street, Room HQ-101
Lexington, KENTUCKY 40536-0293
Telephone: 859/323-5871
Fax: 859/323-2054

University of Louisville School of Medicine
Verification of degrees
Telephone: Free of charge.
Written: Free of charge. Faxed upon request (depending on workload). Mail or fax requests, including signed release forms.
Electronic: Not provided.

Registrar's Office
University of Louisville
Louisville, KENTUCKY 40292
Telephone: 502/852-6522 (Registrar's Office)   502/852-5184 (School of Medicine)
Fax: 502/852-7088
E-mail: regoff@gwise.louisville.edu
Web site: www.louisville.edu

University of Louisville School of Medicine
Verification of residencies and internships
Telephone: Free of charge.
Written: Free of charge. Faxed upon request (depending on workload). Mail or fax requests, including signed release forms.
Electronic: Not provided.

Attention: Residency verification request
House Staff Office
Abell Administration Center Room 518
University of Louisville School of Medicine
323 E. Chestnut Street
Louisville, KENTUCKY 40202-3866
Telephone: 502/852-7105
Fax: 502/852-8866

Louisiana

Louisiana State University at New Orleans School of Medicine
Verification of degrees

Telephone: Free of charge.
Written: Free of charge. Faxed upon request. Mail or fax requests, including signed release forms.
Electronic: Not provided.

>Office of Student Affairs
>Louisiana State University at New Orleans School of Medicine
>1542 Tulane Avenue
>New Orleans, LOUISIANA 70112
>Telephone: 504/568-4874
>Fax: 504/568-8534
>E-mail: lmills1@lsuhsc.edu
>Web site: www.lsuhsc.edu

Louisiana State University at New Orleans School of Medicine
Verification of residencies and internships

Telephone: Not provided.
Written: Free of charge. Mail or fax requests. Include full name, date of birth, Social Security number, program specialty, and year of program.
Electronic: Not provided.

>Office of Graduate Medical Education
>Louisiana State University at New Orleans School of Medicine
>2020 Gravier Street, 1st Floor, Suite 102
>New Orleans, LOUISIANA 70112
>Telephone: 504/568-8686
>Fax: 504/599-1453
>E-mail: gme@lsumc.edu
>Web site: www.lsumc.edu

Louisiana State University at Shreveport School of Medicine
Verification of degrees

Telephone: Not provided.
Written: Free of charge. Faxed upon request. Mail or fax requests, including signed release forms.
Electronic: Not provided.

>Office of the Registrar
>Louisiana State University at Shreveport School of Medicine
>PO Box 33932
>Shreveport, LOUISIANA 71130-3932
>Telephone: 318/675-5205
>Fax: 318/675-4758
>E-mail: shvreg@lsuhsc.edu
>Web site: www.sh.lsuhsc.edu/registrar/ELECT_BK.PDF

Medical School Degrees, Residencies, Internships, and Fellowships

LSU Health Sciences Center School of Medicine at Shreveport
Verification of degrees MD only

Telephone: Free of charge.
Written: Free of charge. Faxed upon request. Mail or fax requests, including signed release forms.
Electronic: Not provided.

>Office of Medical Education
>Louisiana State University Medical Center
>1501 Kings Highway
>Shreveport, LOUISIANA 71130-3932
>Telephone: 318/675-5000 (main)   318/675-5068 (office of medical education)
>Fax: 318/675-5666
>E-mail: shvreg@lsuhsc.edu
>Web site: www.sh.sluhsc.edu/registrar

Tulane University School of Medicine
Notes: Transcript fees: $5 for first address, $2 each additional address (same fees for Dean's Letters); $5 fee to certify licensure forms; $8 fee if state requires a transcript; additional $10 handling fee in CA. All fees must be paid by the graduate.

Verification of degrees

Telephone: Free of charge.
Written: Free of charge. Faxed upon request in emergency situations only. Mail requests, including signed release forms and physician's year of graduation.
Electronic: Not provided.

>Attention: Degree verification request
>Graduate Medical Education SL 97
>Tulane University School of Medicine
>1430 Tulane Avenue
>New Orleans, LOUISIANA 70112
>Telephone: 504/584-1922
>Fax: 504/988-4599
>E-mail: jheine@tulane.edu

Tulane University School of Medicine
Verification of residencies, internships, and fellowships

Telephone: Not provided.
Written: $10 per verification if training was completed more than a year ago. Faxed upon request. Mail or fax requests, including signed release forms.
Electronic: Not provided.

>Attention: Helen Weisler
>SL 97
>Tulane University School of Medicine
>1430 Tulane Avenue
>New Orleans, LOUISIANA 70112
>Telephone: 504/584-1746
>Fax: 504/988-4599

The 2003 Credentialing and Privileging Desk Reference

Maryland

Johns Hopkins University School of Medicine
Verification of degrees, internships, and residencies

Telephone: Free of charge.
Written: Free of charge. Faxed upon request, followed by hard copy. Mail or fax requests, including signed release forms.
Electronic: Not provided.

Office of the Registrar
Johns Hopkins University School of Medicine
119 Medical Administration Building
720 Rutland Avenue
Baltimore, MARYLAND 21205
Telephone: 410/955-3080
Fax: 410/955-0826
Web site: infonet.welch.jhu.edu/son/teaching

Naval School of Health Sciences
Notes: Naval Hospital Oakland California closed in June 1995. Direct all verification requests to Registrar Naval School of Health Sciences.

Verification of degrees

Telephone: Free of charge.
Written: Free of charge. Mail request, including signed release forms.
Electronic: Not provided.

Commanding Officer
Attention: Registrar
Naval School of Health Sciences
8901 Wisconsin Avenue
Betheseda, MARYLAND 20889-5611
Telephone: 301/295-4818
Fax: 301/295-4823
E-mail: jfbehnke@nsh10.med.navy.mil
Web site: nshs.med.navy.mil

Uniformed Services University of the Health Sciences, S. Edward Hebert School of Medicine
Verification of degrees

Telephone: Free of charge. Provide your name, hospital name, physician's name, Social Security number, and date of graduation.
Written: Free of charge. Faxed upon request (followed by hard copy). Mail or fax requests, including signed release forms.
Electronic: Information available on our Web site.

Attention: Office of the Registrar
USUHS School of Medicine
4301 Jones Bridge Road
Bethesda, MARYLAND 20814-4799
Telephone: 301/295-3198

Medical School Degrees, Residencies, Internships, and Fellowships

Fax: 301/295-3545
Web site: www.usuhs.mil

Uniformed Services University of the Health Sciences School of Medicine
Notes: This office can only verify information about obstetrics and gynecology.
Verification of residencies and internships
Telephone: Not provided.
Written: Free of charge.
Electronic: Not provided.

USUHS School of Medicine
4301 Jones Bridge Road
Department of Obstetrics and Gynocology
Bethesda, MARYLAND 20814-4299
Telephone: 301/295-4390
Fax: 301/295-6240
E-mail: webmaster@usuhs.mil
Web site: www.usuhs.mil/obg

University of Maryland Baltimore
Verification of degrees
Telephone: Free of charge. Provide physician's Social Security number.
Written: Free of charge. Faxed upon request (depending on workload). Mail or fax requests including signed release forms and physician's Social Security number.
Electronic: Not provided.

Attention: Verification Office
Office of the Registrar
University of Maryland Baltimore
621 W. Lombard Street, Room 326
Baltimore, MARYLAND 21201
Telephone: 410/706-7480
Fax: 410/706-4053
Web site: www.admincomp.umaryland.edu/orr

University of Maryland Medical Systems
Verification of residencies, internships, fellowships, and affiliation
Telephone: Free of charge.
Written: Free of charge. Faxed upon request. Mail or fax requests, including signed release forms.
Electronic: Not provided.

University of Maryland Medical Systems
Medical Staff Services
29 S. Green Street, Suite 420
Baltimore, MARYLAND 21201-1544
Telephone: 410/328-2902
Fax: 410/328-6433

Massachusetts

Boston University School of Medicine
Verification of degrees

Telephone: Not provided.
Written: Free of charge. Mail requests, including signed release forms.
Electronic: Not provided.

> Office of the Registrar
> Boston University School of Medicine
> 715 Albany Street, Room A-414
> Boston, MASSACHUSETTS 02118
> Telephone: 617/638-4160
> Fax: 617/638-4155
> Web site: www.bumc.bu.edu/busm/reg

Harvard Medical School
Verification of degrees

Telephone: Free of charge.
Written: Free of charge. Mail requests, including signed release forms.
Electronic: Not provided.

> Harvard Medical School
> Registrar's Office
> 25 Shattuck Street, Room 213
> Gordon Hall
> Boston, MASSACHUSETTS 02115
> Telephone: 617/432-1515
> Web site: www.hms.harvard.edu/registrar

Harvard Medical School
Verification of residencies and internships

Telephone: Free of charge.
Written: Free of charge. Mail request, including signed release form.
Electronic: Not provided.

> Harvard Medical School
> Registrar's Office
> 25 Shattuck Street, Room 213
> Boston, MASSACHUSETTS 02115
> Telephone: 617/432-1515
> Web site: www.hms.harvard.edu/registrar

Tufts University School of Medicine
Verification of degrees

Telephone: Free of charge.
Written: Free of charge for verifications; $5 for transcripts. Mail requests, including signed release forms.
Electronic: Not provided.

Office of the Registrar
Tufts University School of Medicine
145 Harrison Avenue
Boston, MASSACHUSETTS 02111
Telephone: 617/636-6568
Fax: 617/636-0432
Web site: www.tufts.edu

Tufts University School of Medicine
Verification of degrees MD only
Telephone: Free of charge.
Written: Free of charge. Mail or fax requests, including signed release forms. $5 for transcripts.
Electronic: Not provided.

Tufts University School of Medicine
145 Harrison Avenue
Boston, MASSACHUSETTS 02111
Telephone: 617/636-6568
Fax: 617/636-0432
Web site: www.medicine.tufts.edu

University of Massachusetts Medical School
Verification of residencies and internships
Telephone: Free of charge.
Written: Free of charge. Mail or fax requests, including signed release forms.
Electronic: Not provided.

University of Massachusetts Medical School
55 Lake Avenue N
Worcester, MASSACHUSETTS 01655
Telephone: 508/856-2903
Fax: 508/856-6420
Web site: www.umassmed.edu

University of Massachusetts Medical School
Verification of degrees
Telephone: Free of charge.
Written: Free of charge. Mail or fax requests, including signed release forms.
Electronic: Not provided.

University of Massachusetts Medical School
55 Lake Avenue N
Worcester, MASSACHUSETTS 01655
Telephone: 508/856-2267   508/856-3927
Fax: 508/856-1899
Web site: www.umassmed.edu

Chapter 5

Michigan

Michigan State University College of Human Medicine

Note: This university has multiple listings over the next several pages. Each listing is for a specific department. You must apply to the correct department for verification requests.

Hematology/Oncology
Verification of surgical residencies and internships

Telephone:	Free of charge. Only for existing residencies; completed residencies must be verified by fax or mail.
Written:	Free of charge. Faxed upon request. Mail or fax requests, including signed release forms.
Electronic:	Not provided.

>Attention: Residency verification request
>Hematology/Oncology Department
>Michigan State University College of Human Medicine
>B424 Clinical Center
>138 Service Road
>East Lansing, MICHIGAN 48824
>Telephone: 517/353-8730
>Fax: 517/353-6392
>E-mail: mcmahon@msu.edu
>Web site: www.msu.edu

Internal Medicine
Verification of internal medicine residencies and internships

Telephone:	Not provided.
Written:	Free of charge. Mail requests, including signed release forms.
Electronic:	Not provided.

>Internal Medicine Residency Program
>B301 Clinical Center
>138 Service Road
>East Lansing, MICHIGAN 48824-1313
>Telephone: 517/353-5100
>Fax: 517/432-2759
>Web site: www.im.msu.edu

Medical Degree
Verification of degrees

Telephone:	Free of charge.
Written:	Free of charge. Faxed upon request (followed by hard copy). Mail or fax requests including signed release forms.
Electronic:	Not provided.

>Attention: Medical degree verification
>Office of Academic Programs
>A-254 Life Sciences Building
>Michigan State University College of Human Medicine
>East Lansing, MICHIGAN 48824

Medical School Degrees, Residencies, Internships, and Fellowships

>Telephone: 517/353-5440, Ext. 244
>Fax: 517/432-1051
>E-mail: nyquistm@msu.edu

Residency
Verification of surgical residencies and internships
Telephone: Free of charge. Only for existing residencies; completed residencies must be verified by fax or mail.
Written: Free of charge. Faxed upon request. Mail or fax requests, including signed release forms.
Electronic: Not provided.

>Attention: Residency verification request
>Michigan State University College of Human Medicine
>B424 Clinical Center
>138 Service Road
>East Lansing, MICHIGAN 48824
>Telephone: 517/353-8730
>Fax: 517/353-6392
>E-mail: linda.east@ht.msu.edu

Pediatric Residency
Verification of surgical residencies and internships
Telephone: Free of charge. Only for existing residencies; completed residencies must be verified by fax or mail.
Written: Free of charge. Faxed upon request. Mail or fax requests, including signed release forms.
Electronic: Not provided.

>Attention: Residency verification request
>Pediatric Residency Program
>Michigan State University College of Human Medicine
>PO Box 30480
>Lansing, MICHIGAN 48909
>Telephone: 517/346-2856   517/483-2856
>Fax: 517/374-4017
>E-mail: pedsres@msu.edu

Pediatrics
Verification of surgical residencies and internships
Telephone: Free of charge. Only for existing residencies; completed residencies must be verified by fax or mail.
Written: Free of charge. Faxed upon request. Mail or fax requests, including signed release forms.
Electronic: Not provided.

>Attention: Residency verification request
>Pediatrics Department
>Michigan State University College of Human Medicine
>B424 Clinical Center
>138 Service Road
>East Lansing, MICHIGAN 48824
>Telephone: 517/353-8730
>Fax: 517/353-6392
>E-mail: pedsres@msu.edu

Surgery
Verification of surgical residencies and internships
Telephone: Free of charge. Only for existing residencies; completed residencies must be verified by fax or mail.
Written: Free of charge. Faxed upon request. Mail or fax requests, including signed release forms.
Electronic: Not provided.

>Attention: Residency verification request
>Surgical Department
>Michigan State University College of Human Medicine
>B424 Clinical Center
>138 Service Road
>East Lansing, MICHIGAN 48824
>Telephone: 517/353-8730
>Fax: 517/353-6392

University of Michigan Hospitals and Health Centers
Notes: Offers Graduate Medical Education.
Verification of residencies and internships
Telephone: Free of charge.
Written: Free of charge. Faxed upon request. Mail or fax requests, including signed release forms.
Electronic: Not provided.

>University of Michigan Hospitals and Health Centers
>Graduate Medical Education
>1500 E. Medical Center Drive
>3107 Medical Science 1 Box 0610
>Ann Arbor, MICHIGAN 48109-0610
>Telephone: 734/764-3186
>Fax: 734/763-5889
>E-mail: chunter@med.umisch.edu

University of Michigan Medical School
Verification of degrees
Telephone: Not provided.
Written: Free of charge. Faxed upon request. Mail or fax requests, including signed release forms.
Electronic: Not provided.

>University of Michigan Medical School
>C5124 Medical Science One
>1301 Catherine Street
>Ann Arbor, MICHIGAN 48109-0611
>Telephone: 734/764-0219   Fax: 734/936-3510
>Web site: www.med.umich.edu/medschool

Wayne State University School of Medicine
Verification of degrees
Telephone: Free of charge.
Written: Free of charge. Faxed upon request. Mail or fax requests, including signed release forms and physician's year of graduation.
Electronic: Not provided.

Medical School Degrees, Residencies, Internships, and Fellowships

Office of Records and Registration
Wayne State University School of Medicine
1272 Scott Hall
540 E. Canfield Street
Detroit, MICHIGAN 48201
Telephone: 313/577-1470
Fax: 313/577-3434
E-mail: sdriscol@med.wayne.edu
Web site: www.med.wayne.edu

Wayne State University School of Medicine
Verification of MD and DO licenses

Telephone:	Free of charge.
Written:	Free of charge. Faxed upon request. Mail or fax requests, including signed release forms and physician's years.
Electronic:	Not provided.

Records and Registration
Wayne State University School of Medicine
540 E. Canfield Street
Room 1272
Detroit, MICHIGAN 48201
Telephone: 313/577-1470
Fax: 313/577-3434
E-mail: sdriscol@med.wayne.med.edu
Web site: www.med.wayne.edu

Minnesota

Mayo Graduate School of Medicine
Verification of residencies and fellowships

Telephone:	Free of charge.
Written:	Free of charge. Faxed upon request. Mail or fax requests, including signed release forms.
Electronic:	Not provided.

Attention: Residency verification
Office of Graduate Medical Education
Mayo Graduate School of Medicine
200 First Street SW
Rochester, MINNESOTA 55905
Telephone: 507/284-4339
Fax: 507/284-0999

Mayo Medical School
Verification of degrees

Telephone:	Free of charge.
Written:	Free of charge for verifications; $5 for transcripts. Faxed upon request. Mail or fax requests, including signed release forms.
Electronic:	Not provided.

Attention: Medical degree verification
Office of the Registrar
Mayo Medical School
200 First Street SW
Rochester, MINNESOTA 55905
Telephone: 507/284-3627
Fax: 507/284-2634
E-mail: bartz.delores@mayo.edu

University of Minnesota at Duluth School of Medicine
Notes: *University of Minnesota medical students attend the University of Minnesota at Duluth for the first two years, then complete their medical education at the University of Minnesota at Minneapolis.*
Annual report of licensed physicians
Telephone: Not provided.
Written: Free of charge.
Electronic: Free of charge.

University of Minnesota at Duluth School of Medicine
1035 University Drive
Duluth, MINNESOTA 55812
Telephone: 218/726-7571
Fax: 218/726-7383
E-mail: med@d.umn.edu
Web site: www.d.umn.edu/medweb

University of Minnesota at Minneapolis Medical School
Notes: *MD degrees only. Verification of residencies, internships and fellowships are done by departments.*
Verification of degrees
Telephone: Free of charge.
Written: Free of charge. Faxed upon request. Mail or fax requests, including signed release forms.
Electronic: Not provided.

Office of Student Affairs
University of Minnesota at Minneapolis Medical School
Mayo Mail Code 293
420 Delaware Street SE
Minneapolis, MINNESOTA 55455-0374
Telephone: 612/624-8101
Fax: 612/626-4200
Web site: www.med.umn.edu

University of Minnesota Medical School Twin Cities
Notes: *Call verification information phone number before submitting request.*
Verification of residencies and internships
Telephone: Free of charge. Provide physician's Social Security number.
Written: Free of charge. Mail requests, including signed release forms.
Electronic: Not provided.

Attention: Residency verification request

Human Resources Department
University of Minnesota
200 Donhowe Building
319 15th Avenue SE
Minneapolis, MINNESOTA 55455
Telephone: 612/625-2000   612/625-8328 (human resources)   612/624-8486 (residency information)
Web site: www.med.umn.edu

Mississippi

University of Mississippi Medical Center School of Medicine
Telephone: Not provided.
Written: Not provided.
Electronic: Not provided.

School of Medicine
Registrar's Office
2500 N. State Street
Jackson, MISSISSIPPI 39216-4505
Telephone: 601/984-1100
Fax: 601/984-1973
Web site: www.ums.edu

University of Mississippi Medical Center School of Medicine
Verification of degrees, internships, and residencies
Telephone: Free of charge.
Written: Free of charge. Mail or fax requests, including signed release forms.
Electronic: Not provided.

Student Services and Records
University of Mississippi Medical Center School of Medicine
2500 N. State Street
Jackson, MISSISSIPPI 39216-4505
Telephone: 601/984-1080
Fax: 601/984-1079
Web site: www.umsmed.edu

University of Mississippi Medical Center School of Health Related Professions
Telephone: Free of charge.
Written: Free of charge.
Electronic: Not provided.

School of Health Related Professions
2500 N. State Street
Jackson, MISSISSIPPI 39216
Telephone: 601/984-1080
Fax: 601/984-1079
Web site: www.umsmed.edu

Missouri

Barnes Jewish Hospital
Verification of residencies and internships

Telephone: Free of charge.
Written: Free of charge. All requests for verification must be submitted in writing. Must have name, date of birth, training specialty, dates of training, and hopsital trained at.
Electronic: Not provided.

> Attention: Residency verification request
> Office of Graduate Medical Education
> Barnes Jewish Hospital
> One Barnes Jewish Hospital Plaza MS Number 90-09355
> St. Louis, MISSOURI 63110
> Telephone: 314/362-1935
> Fax: 314/362-7491 (not to be used for verification)
> Web site: www.bjc.org/bjh.html

Saint Louis University School of Medicine
Verification of degrees MD only

Telephone: Not provided.
Written: Free of charge. Mail requests, including signed release forms. For residencies, include physician's start/end dates and specific department.
Electronic: Not provided.

> Office of the Registrar
> Saint Louis University School of Medicine
> 1402 S. Grand Boulevard
> Saint Louis, MISSOURI 63104
> Telephone: 314/577-8216
> Fax: 314/268-5093

University of Missouri at Columbia School of Medicine
Verification of degrees

Telephone: Not provided.
Written: $10 processing fee (to be placed in a medical student scholarship fund). Faxed upon request. Mail or fax requests, including signed release form.
Electronic: Not provided.

> Attention: Degree verification request
> Office of Medical Education
> Medical Science Building, Room MA-213
> University of Missouri at Columbia School of Medicine
> Columbia, MISSOURI 65212
> Telephone: 573/882-2923 (primary)   573/882-9219 (secondary)
> Fax: 573/884-2988
> Web site: www.missouri.edu

University of Missouri at Kansas City School of Medicine
Verification of degrees

Medical School Degrees, Residencies, Internships, and Fellowships

Telephone: Free of charge.
Written: Free of charge. Faxed upon request. Mail or fax requests, including signed release forms.
Electronic: Not provided.

>Office of Student Affairs
>UMKC School of Medicine
>2411 Holmes
>Kansas City, MISSOURI 64108
>Telephone: 816/235-1900
>Fax: 816/235-6579

University of Missouri at Kansas City School of Medicine
Verification of internal medicine residencies and internships
Telephone: Not provided.
Written: Free of charge. Faxed upon request. Mail or fax requests, including signed release forms and years of residency.
Electronic: Free of charge. E-mail requests to intmed@umkc.edu; include scanned release forms (as attachment).

>Internal Medicine Residency Program
>UMKC School of Medicine
>2411 Holmes
>Kansas City, MISSOURI 64108
>Telephone: 816/881-6212
>Fax: 816/881-6209
>E-mail: intmed@umkc.edu
>Web site: www.med.umkc.edu/residency/intmed

University of Missouri at Kansas City School of Medicine
Verification of surgical residencies and internships
Telephone: Not provided.
Written: Free of charge. Faxed upon request. Mail or fax requests, including signed release forms.
Electronic: Not provided.

>Department of Surgery
>Truman Medical Center
>UMKC School of Medicine
>2301 Holmes
>Kansas City, MISSOURI 64108
>Telephone: 816/556-3505 (Educational Coordinator)   816/556-3679 (main)
>Fax: 816/556-3347
>Web site: www.umkcsurgery.org

University of Missouri-Columbia School of Medicine
Verification of residencies and internships
Telephone: Not provided.
Written: Free of charge. Faxed upon request. Mail or fax requests, including signed release forms, and physician's years of residency and specific department.
Electronic: Not provided.

>Education Office

Department of Internal Medicine
University of Missouri-Columbia
MA-406 Health Sciences Center
One Hospital Drive
Columbia, MISSOURI 65212
Telephone: 573/882-6198
Fax: 573/884-5690
E-mail: im_house@health.missouri.edu
Web site: imed.missouri.edu

Washington University School of Medicine
Verification of degrees
Telephone: Free of charge.
Written: Free of charge. Faxed upon request. Mail or fax requests, including signed release forms.
Electronic: Not provided.

Attention: Degree verification request
Registrar Admissions Office
Washington University School of Medicine
660 S. Euclid
Campus Box 8107
St. Louis, MISSOURI 63110
Telephone: 314/362-6858
Fax: 314/362-4658
Web site: www.medicine.wustl.edu

Nebraska

Creighton University School of Medicine
Verification of degrees
Telephone: Free of charge. Must send signed release form previous to verification.
Written: Free of charge. Faxed upon request. Mail or fax requests, including signed release forms.
Electronic: Not provided.

Office of Student Affairs
Creighton University School of Medicine
2500 California Plaza
Omaha, NEBRASKA 68178
Telephone: 402/280-2905
Fax: 402/280-2599
Web site: www.creighton.edu

Creighton University School of Medicine
Verification of residencies and internships
Telephone: Free of charge.
Written: Free of charge. Faxed upon request. Mail or fax requests, including signed release forms.
Electronic: Not provided.

Office of Graduate Medical Education

Medical School Degrees, Residencies, Internships, and Fellowships

Creighton University School of Medicine
601 N. 30th Street, Suite 1609
Omaha, NEBRASKA 68131
Telephone: 402/280-4677   402/280-5250
Fax: 402/449-5641

University of Nebraska College of Medicine
Verification of residencies and internships

Telephone: Free of charge.
Written: Free of charge. Faxed upon request. Mail or fax requests, including signed release forms.
Electronic: Not provided.

Office of Graduate Medical Education
University of Nebraska Medical Center
984285 Nebraska Medical Center
Omaha, NEBRASKA 68198-4285
Telephone: 402/559-7426
Fax: 402/559-9232
Web site: www.unmc.edu

University of Nebraska Medical Center
Verification of degrees

Telephone: Free of charge.
Written: Free of charge. Mail or fax requests, including signed release forms.
Electronic: Not provided.

Academic Records
University of Nebraska Medical Center
984230 Nebraska Medical Center
Omaha, NEBRASKA 68198-4230
Telephone: 402/559-7391 (academic records)   402/559-7262 (Registrar)
Fax: 402/559-6796
Web site: www.unmc.edu

Nevada

University of Nevada School of Medicine
Verification of degrees

Telephone: Free of charge.
Written: Free of charge. Faxed upon request. Mail or fax requests, including signed release forms.
Electronic: Not provided.

Attention: MD degree verification request
Office of Student Affairs
Mail Stop 357
University of Nevada School of Medicine
Reno, NEVADA 89557
Telephone: 775/784-6063
Fax: 775/784-6194

E-mail: diane@scs.unr.edu
Web site: www.unr.edu/med

University of Nevada School of Medicine
Verification of residencies and internships

Telephone:	Free of charge.
Written:	Free of charge. Faxed upon request. Mail or fax requests, including signed release forms. Will forward requests to appropriate departments for verification.
Electronic:	Free of charge.

Attention: Residency verification
Office of Graduate Medical Education
University of Nevada School of Medicine
Administration, Room 332
Reno, NEVADA 89557
Telephone: 775/784-6844 (personnel office)
Fax: 775/784-6096
E-mail: olxon@med.unr.edu

New Hampshire

Dartmouth Medical School
Verification of degrees

Telephone:	Free of charge.
Written:	Free of charge. Faxed upon request. Mail or fax requests.
Electronic:	Not provided.

Office of the Registrar
Dartmouth Medical School
One Medical Center Drive
Lebanon, NEW HAMPSHIRE 03756
Telephone: 603/650-2248
Fax: 603/650-2244
E-mail: DMS.registrar@dartmouth.edu
Web site: www.dartmouth.edu/dms/registrar.htm

Office of Graduate Medical Education
Verification of residencies and internships
Telephone: Free of charge. Limited questions answered.
Written: Free of charge. Faxed upon request. Mail or fax requests, including signed release forms.
Electronic: Not provided.

> Dartmouth-Hitchcock Medical Center
> Office of Graduate Medical Education
> Building Three Level Five
> One Medical Center Drive
> Lebanon, NEW HAMPSHIRE 03756
> Telephone: 603/650-5748
> Fax: 603/650-5754
> E-mail: lisa.d.roderick@hitchcock.org
> Web site: www.hitchcock.org

New Jersey

New Jersey Medical School at the University of Medicine and Dentistry of New Jersey
Verification of degrees
Telephone: Free of charge.
Written: Free of charge. Faxed upon request. Mail or fax requests, including signed release forms.
Electronic: Not provided.

> Office of the Registrar
> New Jersey Medical School at UMDNJ
> 185 S. Orange Avenue
> Medical Sciences Building, Room B-640
> Newark, NEW JERSEY 07103-2714
> Telephone: 973/972-4640
> Fax: 973/972-6930
> Web site: www.umdnj.edu

New Jersey Medical School at the University of Medicine and Dentistry of New Jersey at Newark
Notes: GME office verifies residencies that took place prior to and during 1989. To verify residencies completed after 1989, contact the specific residency or internship program director.
Verification of residencies and internships
Telephone: Not provided.
Written: $30 fee for information prior to 1992. No charge for 1992 to present. Mail request, signed release form, and payment (made payable to UMDNJ). Request processing time: minimum 10 days.
Electronic: Not provided.

> Office of Graduate Medical Education
> New Jersey Medical School at UMDNJ
> 30 Bergen Street ADMC-1107
> Newark, NEW JERSEY 07107-3000
> Telephone: 973/972-6048
> Fax: 973/972-2229

Robert Wood Johnson Medical School at the University of Medicine and Dentistry of New Jersey at Piscataway
Verification of degrees

Telephone:	Free of charge.
Written:	Free of charge from crenentialing, $3 per verification from other sources. Mail or fax requests, including signed release forms.
Electronic:	Not provided.

> Office of the Registrar
> Robert Wood Johnson Medical School at UMDNJ at Piscataway
> 675 Hoes Lane
> Piscataway, NEW JERSEY 08854-5635
> Telephone: 732/235-4565
> Fax: 732/235-5078

Robert Wood Johnson Medical Schoolm at the University of Medicine and Dentistry of New Jersey at Piscataway
Verification of residencies and internships

Telephone:	Free of charge.
Written:	Free of charge. Mail or fax requests, including signed release forms.
Electronic:	Not provided.

> Robert Wood Johnson Medical School at UMDNJ at Piscataway
> 675 Hoes Lane
> Piscataway, NEW JERSEY 08854-5635
> Telephone: 732/235-4565
> Fax: 732/235-5078

New Mexico

University of New Mexico Health Sciences Center, School of Medicine
Verification of degrees

Telephone:	Free of charge. Provide physician's Social Security number.
Written:	Free of charge. Mail or fax requests, including signed release forms.
Electronic:	Free of charge.

> University of New Mexico Health Sciences Center
> School of Medicine
> Office of Student Affairs
> BMSB Room 107
> Albuquerque, NEW MEXICO 87131-5166
> Telephone: 505/272-3414 (general information)
> Fax: 505/272-8239
> E-mail: bkaputa@salud.unm.edu
> Web site: www.hsc.unm.edu/studaffairs

University of New Mexico Medical School
Verification of residencies and internships

Telephone:	Free of charge.
Written:	Free of charge. Faxed upon request. Mail or fax requests, including signed release forms.

Medical School Degrees, Residencies, Internships, and Fellowships

Electronic: Not provided

Graduate Medical Education
Health Sciences Center
University of New Mexico
Albuquerque, NEW MEXICO 87131-5156
Telephone: 505/272-6225
Fax: 505/272-5184
E-mail: jsparkma@salud.unm.edu
Web site: www.hsc.unm.edu/gme

New York

Albany Medical College
Verification of degrees

Telephone: Free of charge.
Written: Free of charge. Faxed upon request. Mail or fax requests, including signed release forms. $5 charge if student requires transcript.
Electronic: Not provided.

Office of Student Records
Albany Medical College
Mail Code 3
47 New Scotland Avenue
Albany, NEW YORK 12208
Telephone: 518/262-5523
Fax: 518/262-5887
Web site: www.amc.edu

Albany Medical College
Verification of residencies and internships

Telephone: Free of charge. Dates of residencies and internships only; no evaluation information without release forms.
Written: Free of charge. Faxed upon request. Mail or fax requests, including signed release forms.
Electronic: Not provided.

Office of Graduate Medical Education
Albany Medical Center Hospital Mail Code 50
43 New Scotland Avenue
Albany, NEW YORK 12208
Telephone: 518/262-3593
Fax: 518/262-6014
Web site: www.amc.edu

Albert Einstein College of Medicine of Yeshiva University
Verification of degrees

Telephone: Free of charge for issue date of degree only.
Written: Free of charge. Mail requests, including signed release forms, physician's Social Security number, date of birth, and maiden name (if applicable). Only physicians themselves can request verification by fax (must include signed release form).

Electronic: Not provided.

> Office of the Registrar
> Albert Einstein College of Medicine of Yeshiva University
> 1300 Morris Park Avenue
> Bronx, NEW YORK 10461
> Telephone: 718/430-2102
> Fax: 718/430-8840
> Web site: www.aecom.yu.edu

Columbia University College of Physicians and Surgeons
Verification of degrees
Telephone: Free of charge.
Written: Free of charge. Mail requests, including signed release forms, and physician's Social Security number, year of graduation, and maiden name (if applicable).
Electronic: Not provided.

> Attention: Registrar Services
> Columbia University, Student Administrative Services
> 630 W. 168th Street, Unit 45
> New York, NEW YORK 10032
> Telephone: 212/305-3992
> Fax: 212/305-1590
> Web site: www.columbia.edu

Kings County Hospital State University of New York at Brooklyn College of Medicine
Notes: Office verifies pre–1970 residencies and internships. Requests to verify those post–1970 will be forwarded to the appropriate department. Those that occurred after 1992 will be verified by the GME's Office at Downstate SUNY Brooklyn.
Verification of residencies and internships
Telephone: Not provided.
Written: Free of charge. Faxed upon request. Mail or fax requests, including signed release forms.
Electronic: Not provided.

> State University of New York at Brooklyn College of Medicine
> Office of House Staff Affairs
> Kings County Hospital
> 451 Clarkson Avenue
> Brooklyn, NEW YORK 11203
> Telephone: 718/245-2026
> Fax: 718/245-4062

Mount Sinai Hospital
Verification of residencies, internships, fellowships, and affiliation
Telephone: Not provided.
Written: Free of charge. Faxed upon request. Mail or fax requests, including signed release forms.
Electronic: Automated verification system available at Web site for residencies and internships completed on or after July 1, 1992. For verifications of prior training, send written requests.

> Medical Staff Services

Mount Sinai Hospital
One Gustave L. Levy Place
Box 1116
New York, NEW YORK 10029-6575
Telephone: 212/241-6114
Fax: 212/996-2230
E-mail: jpreolo@smtplink.mssm.edu
Web site: www.mssm.edu

Mount Sinai Medical Center
Verification of degrees
Telephone: Free of charge.
Written: Free of charge. Mail requests including signed release forms.
Electronic: Not provided.

Office of Registrar
Mount Sinai School of Medicine
One Gustave L. Levy Place
Box 1257
New York, NEW YORK 10029
Telephone: 212/241-6500 (main)   212/241-6691 (Registrar's office)
Fax: 212/369-6013
Web site: www.mountsinai.org

New York Medical College
Verification of degrees
Telephone: Free of charge.
Written: Free of charge. Mail requests, including signed release forms.
Electronic: Not provided.

Office of the Registrar
New York Medical College
Sunshine Cottage
Valhalla, NEW YORK 10595
Telephone: 914/594-4495
Web site: www.nymc.edu

New York Presbyterian Hospital
Notes: Medical Board Office does not verify residencies or internships if malpractice or competency is involved, but will refer hospitals to the appropriate program administrator.
Verification of residencies and fellowships
Telephone: Free of charge.
Written: Free of charge. Must include a signed release form.
Electronic: Not provided.

New York Weill Cornell Center
New York Presbyterian Hospital
Medical Board Office
525 E. 68th Street
New York, NEW YORK 10021

Telephone: 212/746-1802
Fax: 212/746-8673
Web site: www.nyp.org

New York Presbyterian Hospital, Columbia Presbyterian Campus
Verification of residencies and internships
Telephone: Not provided.
Written: Free of charge. Mail requests, including signed release forms.
Electronic: Not provided.

> New York Presbyterian Hospital
> Columbia Presbyterian Campus
> Medical House Staff Office
> 622 W. 168th Street, PH2-203
> New York, NEW YORK 10032
> Telephone: 212/305-1787
> Fax: 212/305-2057

New York University School of Medicine
Verification of degrees
Telephone: Free of charge.
Written: Free of charge. Mail requests, including physician's name, date of birth, and Social Security number.
Electronic: Not provided.

> Office of Registration
> New York University School of Medicine
> 550 First Avenue
> New York, NEW YORK 10016
> Telephone: 212/263-5291
> Fax: 212/263-5264
> Web site: www.med.nyu.edu

New York University School of Medicine
Verification of residencies and internships
Telephone: Free of charge.
Written: Free of charge. Faxed upon request. Mail or fax requests, including signed release forms.
Electronic: Not provided.

> Attention: House Staff Office
> New York University Medical Center
> 650 First Avenue, 3rd Floor
> New York, NEW YORK 10016
> Telephone: 212/263-5506
> Fax: 212/263-7002
> E-mail: catherine.griffin@med.nyu.edu
> Web site: www.nyu.med.edu

State University of New York at Buffalo School of Medicine
Verification of degrees
Telephone: Free of charge.

Medical School Degrees, Residencies, Internships, and Fellowships

Written: Free of charge. Faxed upon request. Mail or fax requests, including signed release forms.
Electronic: Not provided.

> Office of Medical Education
> State University of New York at Buffalo School of Medicine
> 40 Biomedical Education Building
> 3435 Main Street
> Buffalo, NEW YORK 14214
> Telephone: 716/829-2802
> Fax: 716/829-2798
> Web site: www.smbs.buffalo.edu/ome

State University of New York at Buffalo School of Medicine
Verification of residencies and internships

Telephone: Free of charge.
Written: Free of charge. Faxed upon request. Mail or fax requests, including signed release forms and physician's Social Security number.
Electronic: Not provided.

> Office of Graduate Medical Education and Resident Services
> State University of New York at Buffalo School of Medicine
> 3435 Main Street
> 117 Cary Hall
> Buffalo, NEW YORK 14214
> Telephone: 716/829-2012
> Fax: 716/829-3999
> E-mail: gme@buffalo.edu
> Web site: www.smbs.buffalo.edu/gme

State University of New York at Syracuse College of Medicine
Verification of residencies and internships

Telephone: Not provided.
Written: Free of charge. Faxed upon request. Mail or fax requests, including signed release forms.
Electronic: Not provided.

> State University of New York at Syracuse College of Medicine
> Office of Graduate Medical Education
> SUNY Upstate Medical University
> 750 E. Adams Street
> Syracuse, NEW YORK 13210
> Telephone: 315/464-7617
> Fax: 315/464-7619
> E-mail: henderss@upstate.edu
> Web site: www.upstate.edu/gme

State University of New York Downstate Medical Center
Verification of degrees

Telephone: Free of charge.
Written: Free of charge. Faxed upon request. Mail or fax requests, including signed release forms.

Electronic: Not provided.

> SUNY Downstate Medical Center
> Office of the Registrar
> Box 98
> 450 Clarkson Avenue
> Brooklyn, NEW YORK 11203-2098
> Telephone: 718/270-4551
> Fax: 718/270-7592
> E-mail: registrar@downstate.edu
> Web site: www.downstate.edu

State University of New York Stony Brook University
Verification of degrees

Telephone: Free of charge. Provide name and year of graduation.
Written: Free of charge. Faxed upon request. Mail or fax requests, including signed release forms, and physician's Social Security number and year of graduation.
Electronic: Not provided.

> Attention: Degree verification request
> Office of Medical Education
> SUNY Stony Brook School of Medicine
> Stony Brook, NEW YORK 11794-8432
> Telephone: 631/444-1030
> Fax: 631/444--9521
> Web site: www.uhmc.sunysb.edu

State University of New York Stony Brook University Hospital
Verification of residencies, internships, fellowships, and affiliation

Telephone: Free of charge.
Written: Free of charge. Faxed upon request. Mail or fax requests, including signed release forms.
Electronic: Not provided.

> Medical House Staff Services Department
> University Hospital 14-036
> SUNY Stony Brook
> Stony Brook, NEW YORK 11794-7718
> Telephone: 631/444-2754
> Fax: 631/444-6031
> E-mail: joyce.manolakes@sunysb.edu
> Web site: www.uhmc.sunysb.edu

State University of New York Upstate Medical University
Verification of degrees

Telephone: Free of charge. Can only verbally verify degrees of physicians who graduated from 1989 to present.
Written: Free of charge. Faxed upon request. Mail or fax requests, including signed release forms.
Electronic: Not provided.

Medical School Degrees, Residencies, Internships, and Fellowships

Attention: Office of the Registrar
SUNY Upstate Medical University
155 Elizabeth Blackwell Street
Syracuse, NEW YORK 13210
Telephone: 315/464-4604
Fax: 315/464-8822
E-mail: registrar@upstate.edu
Web site: www.upstate.edu/staffaffairs/registrar

University of Rochester School of Medicine and Dentistry
Verification of degrees

Telephone:	Free of charge.
Written:	Free of charge. Written requests should include self-addressed, stamped envelope.
Electronic:	Not provided.

Medical School Registrars Office
601 Elmwood Avenue
Box 601
Rochester, NEW YORK 14642
Telephone: 585/275-4541
Fax: 585/273-1016
Web site: www.urmc.rochester.edu

University of Rochester Strong Memorial Hospital
Verification of residencies and internships

Telephone:	Not provided.
Written:	Free of charge. Faxed upon request. Mail or fax requests, including signed release forms.
Electronic:	Not provided.

University of Rochester Strong Memorial Hospital
Office for Graduate Medical Education
601 Elmwood Avenue
Box 601
Rochester, NEW YORK 14642
Telephone: 585/275-4607
Fax: 585/473-5694

Weill Medical College of Cornell University
Verification of degrees

Telephone:	Not provided.
Written:	Free of charge. Faxed upon request. Mail or fax requests, including signed release forms.
Electronic:	Not provided.

Office of the Registrar
Weill Medical College of Cornell University
1300 York Avenue, Room C118
New York, NEW YORK 10021-4805
Telephone: 212/746-1055
Fax: 212/746-5981

Westchester Medical Center
Verification of residencies and internships

Telephone: Not provided.
Written: Free of charge. Mail requests, including signed release forms.
Electronic: Not provided.

>House Staff Office
>Westchester Medical Center
>Room 420, Elmwood Hall
>Valhalla, NEW YORK 10595
>Telephone: 914/493-7292   914/493-8076 (Medical Staff Office)
>Fax: 914/493-8575
>Web site: www.wcmc.com

North Carolina

Duke University Medical Center
Verification of residencies and internships

Telephone: Not provided.
Written: Free of charge. Faxed upon request. Mail or fax requests, including signed release forms.
Electronic: Not provided.

>Graduate Medical Education
>Duke University Medical Center
>Box 3951
>Durham, NORTH CAROLINA 27710
>Telephone: 919/684-3491
>Fax: 919/684-8565
>Web site: www.gme.duke.edu

Duke University School of Medicine
Verification of degrees

Telephone: Free of charge.
Written: Free of charge. Faxed upon request. Mail, phone, or fax requests.
Electronic: Not provided.

>Office of the Registrar
>Duke University School of Medicine
>PO Box 3878
>Duke S. Room 0119, Purple Zone
>Durham, NORTH CAROLINA 27710
>Telephone: 919/684-2304
>Fax: 919/684-2593
>E-mail: medreg@mc.duke.edu
>Web site: medschool.duke.edu

East Carolina University School of Medicine
Verification of residencies and internships

Telephone: Free of charge.

Medical School Degrees, Residencies, Internships, and Fellowships

Written: Free of charge. Faxed upon request. Mail or fax requests, including signed release forms.
Electronic: Free of charge.

> East Carolina University School of Medicine
> Pitt County Memorial Hospital
> Office of Graduate Medical Education
> 2100 Stantonburg Road
> PO Box 602A
> Greenville, NORTH CAROLINA 27835
> Telephone: 252/816-4268
> Fax: 252/816-8304
> E-mail: ariddick@pcmh.com
> Web site: www.uhseast.com

The Brody School of Medicine at East Carolina University
Verification of degrees
Telephone: Not provided.
Written: Free of charge. Faxed upon request. Mail or fax requests, including signed release forms.
Electronic: Not provided.

> Office of Student Admissions
> The Brody School of Medicine at East Carolina University
> Brody Building AD 52
> Greenville, NORTH CAROLINA 27858-4354
> Telephone: 252/816-2202
> Fax: 252/816-1926
> Web site: www.ecu.edu/med

University of North Carolina at Chapel Hill School of Medicine
Verification of degrees MD only
Telephone: Free of charge. Can only verify what is public record.
Written: Free of charge. Faxed upon request. Mail (preferred) or fax requests, including signed release forms and physician's Social Security number and year of graduation. $5 fee for transcripts.
Electronic: Not provided.

> Office of the Registrar
> UNC at Chapel Hill School of Medicine
> Campus Box 7000
> 121 MacNider Building
> Chapel Hill, NORTH CAROLINA 27599-7000
> Telephone: 919/962-8332 (Registrar's Office)
> Fax: 919/966-9930
> Web site: www.med.unc.edu

University of North Carolina at Chapel Hill School of Medicine
Notes: Web site for Medical School is www.med.unc.edu.
Verification of clinical privileges and hospital affiliation.
Telephone: Not provided.
Written: Free of charge. Faxed upon request. Mail or fax requests, including signed release forms.

Electronic: Not provided.

> Office of Medical Staff Services
> University of North Carolina Hospitals
> 101 Manning Drive
> Campus Box 7600
> Chapel Hill, NORTH CAROLINA 27514
> Telephone: 919/966-1520
> Fax: 919/843-0055
> Web site: www.unchealthcare.org

University of North Carolina at Chapel Hill School of Medicine
Verification of residencies and fellowships
Telephone: Not provided.
Written: Free of charge. Faxed upon request. Mail or fax requests, including signed release forms.
Electronic: Not provided.

> Office of Graduate Medical Education
> University of North Carolina Hospitals
> 1107A First Floor, West Wing
> Campus Box 7600
> Chapel Hill, NORTH CAROLINA 27514
> Telephone: 919/966-1072
> Fax: 919/966-0290

Wake Forest University School of Medicine
Verification of degrees
Telephone: Free of charge.
Written: Free of charge. Faxed upon request. Mail or fax requests, including signed release forms.
Electronic: Not provided.

> Office of Student Services
> Wake Forest University School of Medicine
> Medical Center Boulevard
> Winston-Salem, NORTH CAROLINA 27157-1085
> Telephone: 336/716-4271
> Fax: 336/716-5807
> E-mail: lsnyder@wfubmc.edu
> Web site: www.wfubmc.edu

North Dakota

University of North Dakota School of Medicine and Health Sciences
Verification of degrees MD only
Telephone: Free of charge.
Written: Free of charge. Faxed upon request. Mail or fax requests, including signed release forms.
Electronic: Not provided.

> University of North Dakota School of Medicine and Health Sciences

Office of Student Affairs
501 N. Columbia Road
Box 9037
Grand Forks, NORTH DAKOTA 58203
Telephone: 701/777-4221   701/777-2840 (Marilyn Martin)
Fax: 701/777-4942
E-mail: mmartin@medicine.nodak.edu
Web site: www.med.und.nodak.edu/

Ohio

Case Western Reserve University School of Medicine
Verification of degrees

Telephone: Not provided.
Written: Free of charge. $5 fee for transcripts.
Electronic: Automated verification system available at Web site. To obtain a user name and password for your hospital/organization, contact CWRU Registar's Office (registrar@po.cwru.edu).

Office of the Registrar
Case Western Reserve University School of Medicine
10900 Euclid Avenue
Room T408
Cleveland, OHIO 44106-4920
Telephone: 216/368-5497 (Medical School Registrar's Office)   216/368-4311 (University Registrar's Office)
Fax: 216/368-8711 (university)   216/368-4621 (medical school)
E-mail: registrar@po.cwru.edu
Web site: www.cwru.edu/default.html

Medical College of Ohio
Verification of degrees

Telephone: Free of charge.
Written: Mail or fax request. Include signed release form, and physician's Social Security number and exact name when enrolled in program.
Electronic: Not provided.

Medical College of Ohio
3045 Arlington Avenue, Room 114
Toledo, OHIO 43614-5805
Telephone: 419/383-4198
Fax: 419/383-4003
E-mail: registrar@mco.edu
Web site: www.mco.edu

Medical College of Ohio at Toledo
Notes: Office will verify residencies and internships that took place before 1970. Requests to verify later residencies and internships will be forwarded to the appropriate department.
Verification of residencies and internships

Telephone: Not provided.
Written: Free of charge. Mail or fax requests, including signed release forms.
Electronic: Not provided.

    Office of Graduate Medical Education
    Medical College of Ohio at Toledo
    3045 Arlington Avenue
    Third Floor, Mulford Library Building
    Toledo, OHIO 43614-5805
    Telephone: 419/383-4244
    Fax: 419/383-6100
    Web site: www.mco.edu

Northeastern Ohio Universities College of Medicine
Verification of degrees
Telephone: Free of charge.
Written: Free of charge. Faxed upon request. Mail or fax requests, including signed release forms.
Electronic: Not provided.

    Office of the Registrar and Student Services
    Northeastern Ohio Universities College of Medicine
    4209 State Route 44
    PO Box 95
    Rootstown, OHIO 44272
    Telephone: 330/325-2511
    Fax: 330/325-5905
    Web site: www.neoucom.edu

Northeastern Ohio Universities College of Medicine
Verification of licenses
Telephone: Not provided.
Written: Free of charge. Mail or fax requests, including signed release forms.
Electronic: Not provided.

    Northeastern Ohio Universities College of Medicine
    Attention: Student Services
    PO Box 95
    Rootstown, OHIO 44272-0095
    Telephone: 330/325-6478
    Fax: 330/325-5905
    Web site: www.neoucom.edu

Ohio State University College of Medicine and Public Health
Verification of degrees
Telephone: Free of charge.
Written: Free of charge. Faxed upon request. Mail or fax requests, including signed release forms.
Electronic: Not provided.

    Office of Student Affairs

Medical School Degrees, Residencies, Internships, and Fellowships

Ohio State University College of Medicine and Public Health
370 West Ninth Avenue
Room 209, Meiling Hall
Columbus, OHIO 43210
Telephone: 614/-292-5674
Fax: 614/292-1544
Web site: www.osu.edu

Ohio State University Medical Center
Verification of residencies, internships, fellowships, and affiliation

Telephone: Not provided.
Written: Free of charge. Mail requests, including signed release forms and self-addressed, stamped envelope. Mail to: Room 588, Building 13, 1375 Perry Street, Columbus, OH 43201.
Electronic: Not provided.

Office of the Medical Staff Affairs
410 W. Tenth Avenue
Ohio State University Medical Center
Columbus, OHIO 43210
Telephone: 614/293-8000
Web site: www.osumedcenter.edu

University Hospital/University of Cincinnati College of Medicine
Verification of residencies, internships, and fellowships

Telephone: Not provided.
Written: Free of charge. Mail requests, including signed release forms, name and dates of resident's program, and self-addressed, stamped envelope. Minimum four-week response.
Electronic: Not provided.

Office of Graduate Medical Education
The University Hospital
234 Goodman Street
ML# 0796
Cincinnati, OHIO 45219-2316
Telephone: 513/584-4118
Fax: 513/584-3778
E-mail: trauthd@healthall.com
Web site: www.intranethealth.healthall.com

University Hospitals of Cleveland
Verification of residencies and internships

Telephone: Free of charge.
Written: Free of charge. Faxed upon request. Mail or fax requests, including signed release forms. Please send performance evaluation requests directly to departments.
Electronic: Not provided.

University Hospitals of Cleveland
Residency Office
11100 Euclid Avenue
Cleveland, OHIO 44106

Chapter 5

>Telephone: 216/844-3887
>Fax: 216/844-1949
>E-mail: jean.siebert@uhhs.com

University of Cincinnati College of Medicine
Verification of degrees

Telephone: Free of charge.
Written: Free of charge. Mail or fax requests, including signed release forms.
Electronic: Not provided.

>Office of Student Affairs
>University of Cincinnati College of Medicine
>231 Albert Sabin Way
>Cincinnati, OHIO 45267-0552
>Telephone: 513/558-5575
>Fax: 513/558-1100
>Web site: www.uc.edu

Wright State University School of Medicine
Verification of degrees

Telephone: Free of charge.
Written: Free of charge. Faxed upon request. Mail or fax requests, including signed release forms.
Electronic: Free of charge.

>Office of Student Affairs/Admissions
>Wright State University School of Medicine
>PO Box 1751
>Dayton, OHIO 45401
>Telephone: 937/775-2934
>Fax: 937/775-3322
>Web site: www.med.wright.edu

Wright State University School of Medicine
Verification of residencies and internships

Telephone: Not provided.
Written: Free of charge. Mail or fax requests, including signed release forms.
Electronic: Not provided.

>Faculty and Clinical Affairs
>Wright State University School of Medicine
>PO Box 927
>Dayton, OHIO 45401-0927
>Telephone: 937/775-2033
>Fax: 937/775-3256
>E-mail: som_fca@wright.edu
>Web site: www.med.wright.edu/fca

Oklahoma

University of Oklahoma at Tulsa College of Medicine
Verification of degrees, internships, and residencies

Telephone:	Free of charge.
Written:	Free of charge. Faxed upon request. Mail or fax requests, including signed release forms.
Electronic:	Free of charge. E-mail requests for verification of degrees to Darla-Puckett@ouhsc.edu. E-mail requests for verification of internships and residencies to Karen-Gregorovic@ouhsc.edu.

> Office of Residency and Student Affairs
> Unicersity of Oklahoma College of Medicine Tulsa
> 4502 E. 41st Street
> Tulsa, OKLAHOMA 74135
> Telephone: 918/660-3000
> Fax: 918/660-3084
> Web site: www.tulsa.ouhsc.edu

University of Oklahoma Health Sciences Center at Oklahoma City
Verification of residencies and internships

Telephone:	Free of charge.
Written:	Free of charge. Mail requests, including department name and signed release forms. Will fax in emergency situations only.
Electronic:	Not provided.

> University of Oklahoma Health Sciences Center at Oklahoma City
> Admissions and Records
> BSEB Room 200
> PO Box 26901
> Oklahoma City, OKLAHOMA 73190
> Telephone: 405/271-1537 (records)   405/271-2359 (switchboard)   405/271-8001 (verification of residencies, internships, and fellowships)
> Fax: 405/271-2480
> E-mail: ouhsc.admissions@ouhsc.edu
> Web site: www.admissions.ouhsc.edu

University of Oklahoma Health Sciences Center at Oklahoma City
Verification of degrees

Telephone:	Free of charge.
Written:	Free of charge. Faxed upon request in emergency situations only. Mail, phone, or fax requests.
Electronic:	Not provided.

> OUHSC Office of Admission and Records
> BSEB200
> PO Box 26901
> Oklahoma City, OKLAHOMA 73190-0001
> Telephone: 405/271-2359
> Fax: 405/271-2480
> Web site: www.ouhsc/admission.edu

Oregon

Oregon Health & Science University
Verification of residencies and internships

Telephone: Free of charge.
Written: Free of charge. Mail or fax requests, including signed release forms.
Electronic: Not provided.

> Office of Graduate Medical Education
> Oregon Health & Science University
> 3181 S.W. Sam Jackson Park Road, Mail Code L579
> Portland, OREGON 97201
> Telephone: 503/494-8652
> Fax: 503/494-8513
> Web site: www.ohsu.edu

Oregon Health & Sciences University School of Medicine
Verification of degrees

Telephone: Free of charge.
Written: Free of charge. Faxed upon request. Mail or fax requests, including signed release forms. Fee charged for state licensures and certifications.
Electronic: Not provided.

> Office of the Registrar
> Oregon Health & Sciences University School of Medicine
> 3181 S.W. Sam Jackson Park Road
> Mail Code L109
> Portland, OREGON 97201
> Telephone: 503/494-7800
> Fax: 503/494-4629
> Web site: www.ohsu.edu

Pennsylvania

Jefferson Medical College
Verification of degrees

Telephone: Free of charge.
Written: Free of charge. Faxed upon request. Mail or fax requests, including signed release forms.
Electronic: Not provided.

> University Office of the Registrar
> Jefferson Medical College
> 1015 Walnut Street
> Curtis Building, Room G22
> Philadelphia, PENNSYLVANIA 19107-5099
> Telephone: 215/503-8734
> Fax: 215/923-6974
> Web site: www.tju.edu

MCP Hahnemann University Hospital
Notes: Contact specific residency or internship programs directly. Graduate Medical Education Office (215/842-6806) will provide correct phone number and address.
Verification of residencies and internships

Telephone: Not provided.
Written: Free of charge.
Electronic: Not provided.

    MCP Hahnemann University Hospital
    3300 Henry Avenue
    Graduate Medical Education
    Philadelphia, PENNSYLVANIA 19129
    Telephone: 215/842-6806   215/842-6343 (verifications)
    Fax: 215/843-7345

MCP Hahnemann University School of Medicine
Notes: Hospitals seeking verifications of degrees awarded by the combined program of Allegheny University Hahnemann School of Medicine and the Medical College of Pennsylvania (1995 or after) should contact MCP Hahnemann's Office of the Registrar.
Verification of degrees

Telephone: Free of charge.
Written: Free of charge; $6 for transcript copy. Mail or fax requests, including signed release forms.
Electronic: Not provided.

    Office of the Registrar
    MCP Hahnemann University School of Medicine
    2900 Queen Lane
    Philadelphia, PENNSYLVANIA 19129-1096
    Telephone: 215/991-8207
    Fax: 215/843-5243
    E-mail: jerri.simmons@drexel.edu
    Web site: www.mcphu.edu

Pennsylvania State University College of Medicine
Notes: Also verifications of Physician Assistant
Verification of degrees
Telephone: Not provided.
Written: Free of charge. Faxed upon request. Mail or fax requests, including Social Security number, year of graduation, and signed release forms.
Electronic: Not provided.

    Office of Student Affairs H-060
    Pennsylvania State University College of Medicine
    Milton S. Hershey Medical Center
    500 University Drive
    Hershey, PENNSYLVANIA 17033
    Telephone: 717/531-4103
    Fax: 717/531-6225
    E-mail: studentaffairs@hmc.psu.edu
    Web site: www.hmc.psu.edu

Pennsylvania State University College of Medicine
Verification of residencies and internships
Telephone: Free of charge.
Written: Free of charge. Faxed upon request. Mail or fax requests, including signed release forms.
Electronic: Not provided.

    Graduate Medical Education MC H088
    Milton S. Hershey Medical Center
    PO Box 850
    Hershey, PENNSYLVANIA 17033
    Telephone: 717/531-1692
    Fax: 717/531-2077
    Web site: www.hmc.psu.edu

Temple University Hospital
Verification of residencies and internships
Telephone: Not provided.
Written: Free of charge. Faxed upon request. Mail or fax requests, including signed release forms.
Electronic: Not provided.

    Graduate Medical Education
    Temple University Hospital
    Broad and Ontario Streets
    Philadelphia, PENNSYLVANIA 19140
    Telephone: 215/707-3804
    Fax: 215/707-5886

Temple University School of Medicine
Verification of degrees
Telephone: Free of charge.
Written: Free of charge. Mail or fax requests, including signed release forms.

Medical School Degrees, Residencies, Internships, and Fellowships

Electronic: Not provided.

> Office of Faculty and Student Records
> Medical Research Building, Room 106
> Temple University School of Medicine
> 3420 N. Broad Street
> Philadelphia, PENNSYLVANIA 19140
> Telephone: 215/707-3949
> Fax: 215/707-2940
> E-mail: ofsr@temple.edu
> Web site: www.temple.edu

Thomas Jefferson University Hospital
Verification of residencies and internships

Telephone: Free of charge.
Written: Free of charge. Faxed upon request. Mail or fax requests, including signed release forms.
Electronic: Not provided.

> House Staff Office
> Thomas Jefferson University Hospital
> 111 S. 11th Street, Suite 2160
> Gibbon Building
> Philadelphia, PENNSYLVANIA 19107
> Telephone: 215/955-6610
> Fax: 215/955-3995
> Web site: www.jeffersonhealth.org

University Health Center of Pittsburgh
Notes: Provides verification of fellowships as well as residencies and internships.
Verification of residencies and internships

Telephone: Free of charge.
Written: Free of charge. Faxed upon request. Mail or fax requests, including signed release forms.
Electronic: Not provided.

> Attention: Director GME
> Office of Graduate Medical Education
> University Health Center of Pittsburgh
> 121 Meyran Avenue, Second Floor
> Pittsburgh, PENNSYLVANIA 15213
> Telephone: 412/647-5815
> Fax: 412/647-5809
> E-mail: coopermr@msx.upmc.edu

University of Pennsylvania Health System
Notes: Also does verification of hospital affiliates.
Verification of residencies and internships

Telephone: Not provided.
Written: Free of charge. Mail or fax requests, including signed release forms and self-addressed, stamped envelopes.
Electronic: Not provided.

Department of Medical Affairs and Graduate Medical Education
Hospital of the University of Pennsylvania
3624 Market Street, Suite 560W
Philadelphia, PENNSYLVANIA 19104
Telephone: 215/662-2286
Fax: 215/349-5800
Web site: www.uphsnet.med.upenn.edu

University of Pennsylvania School of Medicine
Verification of degrees

Telephone:	Free of charge.
Written:	Free of charge. Faxed upon request. Mail or fax requests, including signed release forms.
Electronic:	Not provided.

Office of the Registrar
University of Pennsylvania School of Medicine
100 Stemmler Hall
3450 Hamilton Walk
Philadelphia, PENNSYLVANIA 19104-6087
Telephone: 215/898-4646
Fax: 215/898-0833

University of Pittsburgh School of Medicine
Verification of degrees MD only

Telephone:	Free of charge. Social Security number required.
Written:	Free of charge. Mail or fax requests, including signed release forms.
Electronic:	Not provided.

Office of Student Affairs
University of Pittsburgh School of Medicine
3550 Terrace Street
M-218 Scaife Hall
Pittsburgh, PENNSYLVANIA 15261
Telephone: 412/648-9040
Fax: 412/624-0290
E-mail: joann@medschool.pit.edu
Web site: www.dean-med.pit.edu

Puerto Rico

Ponce School of Medicine
Notes: Registrar's Office only verifies medical degrees.
Verification of degrees

Telephone:	Free of charge.
Written:	Free of charge. Mail or fax requests, including signed release forms.
Electronic:	Not provided.

Attention: Registrar's Office
Ponce School of Medicine
PO Box 7004

Medical School Degrees, Residencies, Internships, and Fellowships

Ponce, PUERTO RICO 00732-7004
Telephone: 787/840-2575, Ext. 2126 (registrar's office)
Fax: 787/259-1931
Web site: www.psm.edu

Universidad Central del Caribe, School of Medicine
Notes: Registrar's Office will forward residency or internship verification requests to the appropriate departments.
Verification of degrees, internships, and residencies
Telephone: Not provided.
Written: Free of charge. Mail or fax requests, including signed release forms.
Electronic: Not provided.

> Office of the Registrar
> School of Medicine
> Universidad Central del Caribe
> Ramon Ruiz Arnau University Hospital
> Call Box 60327
> Bayamon, PUERTO RICO 00960-6032
> Telephone: 787/798-3001, Ext. 237
> Fax: 787/778-0794
> E-mail: icordero@uccaribe.edu
> Web site: www.uccaribe.edu

University of Puerto Rico
Notes: Registrar's Office will forward residency or internship verification requests to the appropriate departments.
Verification of degrees, internships, and residencies
Telephone: Not provided.
Written: Free of charge. Faxed upon request. Mail or fax requests, including signed release forms.
Electronic: Not provided.

> Office of the Registrar
> Medical Sciences Campus
> University of Puerto Rico
> PO Box 365067
> San Juan, PUERTO RICO 00936-5067
> Puerto Rico
> Telephone: 787/758-2525
> Fax: 787/756-7044
> Web site: www.rcm.upr.edu

Quebec

Universite de Montreal Faculte de Medecine
Verification of degrees, internships, and residencies
Telephone: Not provided.
Written: Mail or fax requests, including signed release forms.
Electronic: Available on Web site for a fee.

> Attention: Verification request

Office of Postgraduate Medical Education
Universite de Montreal Faculte de Medecine
2900 Boulevard Edouard Montpetit
PO Box 6128 Sucursale Centre-Ville
Montreal, QUEBEC H3C 3J7
CANADA
Telephone: 514/343-6859
Fax: 514/343-2068
Web site: www.umontreal.ca

Rhode Island

Brown Medical School
Verification of degrees
Telephone: Not provided.
Written: Free of charge. Faxed upon request. Mail or fax requests including signed release forms.
Electronic: Not provided.

Office of Medical Student Affairs
Brown Medical School
Box G-A2
97 Waterman Street
Providence, RHODE ISLAND 02912
Telephone: 401/863-2441
Fax: 401/863-3801
E-mail: donna_arruda@brown.edu
Web site: www.brown.edu

Brown Medical School
Notes: Contact specific residency or internship programs directly.
Verification of degrees MD only
Telephone: Not provided.
Written: Free of charge. Mail or fax requests, including signed release forms.
Electronic: Not provided.

Brown Medical School
97 Waterman Street
Box G
Providence, RHODE ISLAND 02912
Telephone: 401/863-2441
Fax: 401/863-3801

South Carolina

Medical University of South Carolina College of Medicine
Verification of degrees
Telephone: Information provided through Student National Clearing House.
Written: Information provided through Student National Clearing House.
Electronic: Not provided.

Medical School Degrees, Residencies, Internships, and Fellowships

>Office of Enrollment Services
>MUSC College of Medicine
>41 Bee Street
>PO Box 250203
>Charleston, SOUTH CAROLINA 29425
>Telephone: 843/792-3281
>Fax: 843/792-3764
>Web site: www.musc.edu/es

Medical University of South Carolina College of Medicine
Verification of residencies, internships, and fellowships

Telephone:	Free of charge. Written request is preferred.
Written:	Free of charge. Faxed upon request. Mail or fax requests, including signed release forms.
Electronic:	Not provided.

>Attention: Credentials Coordinator
>Office of Graduate Medical Education
>MUSC College of Medicine
>169 Ashley Avenue, Room 202, Main Hospital
>PO Box 250333
>Charleston, SOUTH CAROLINA 29425
>Telephone: 843/792-2575
>Fax: 843/792-9295
>Web site: www.musc.edu/gme

University of South Carolina School of Medicine
Verification of degrees MD only

Telephone:	Free of charge.
Written:	Free of charge. Faxed upon request. Mail or fax requests, including signed release forms.
Electronic:	Not provided.

>University of South Carolina School of Medicine
>Office of the Registrar
>Admissions and Enrollment Services
>Columbia, SOUTH CAROLINA 29208
>Telephone: 803/733-3325
>Fax: 803/733-3328
>E-mail: mills@med.sc.edu
>Web site: www.med.sc.edu

South Dakota

University of South Dakota School of Medicine
Verification of degrees MD only

Telephone:	Not provided.
Written:	Free of charge. Faxed upon request. Mail or fax requests, including signed release forms.
Electronic:	Not provided.

>Attention: Degree verification request, Kay Austin

The 2003 Credentialing and Privileging Desk Reference

Office of Medical Student Affairs
University of South Dakota School of Medicine
414 E. Clark Street
Lee Medical Building, Room 105
Vermillion, SOUTH DAKOTA 57069-2390
Telephone: 605/677-4256
Fax: 605/677-5109
E-mail: kaustin@usd.edu
Web site: med.usc.edu

University of South Dakota School of Medicine
Verification of residencies and internships
Telephone: Not provided.
Written: Free of charge. Mail or fax requests. All written verifications must be accompanied by a written form.
Electronic: Not provided.

University of South Dakota School of Medicine
1400 W. 22nd Street
Sioux Falls, SOUTH DAKOTA 57105-1570
Telephone: 605/357-1300
Fax: 605/357-1311
Web site: www.med.usd.edu

Tennessee

East Tennessee State University College of Medicine
Verification of degrees MD only
Telephone: Free of charge.
Written: Free of charge. Faxed upon request. Mail or fax requests, including signed release forms.
Electronic: Not provided.

Attention: Degree verification request
Office of Student Affairs Records
Quillen College of Medicine
East Tennessee State University
PO Box 70580
Johnson City, TENNESSEE 37614
Telephone: 423/439-2032 (Assistant Registrar)   423/439-2104 (Technical Clerk)
Fax: 423/439-2110
E-mail: plummerc@etsu.edu
Web site: www.qcom.etsu.edu/sacom

East Tennessee State University College of Medicine
Notes: Office of Finance and Administration will forward requests to appropriate department, but prefers hospitals contact departments directly.
Verification of residencies and internships
Telephone: Free of charge.
Written: Free of charge. Mail requests, including signed release forms.
Electronic: Not provided.

Medical School Degrees, Residencies, Internships, and Fellowships

Quillen College of Medicine
East Tennessee State University
PO Box 70420
Johnson City, TENNESSEE 37614
Telephone: 423/439-6373
Fax: 423/439-8854
E-mail: shipley@etsu.edu
Web site: www.etsu.edu

Meharry Medical College
Verification of degrees
Telephone: Not provided.
Written: Free of charge; $2 if official seal is required. Faxed upon request. Mail or fax requests, including signed release forms, and physician's Social Security number and year of graduation.
Electronic: Not provided.

Office of Admissions and Records
Meharry Medical College
1005 D. B. Todd Jr. Boulevard
Nashville, TENNESSEE 37208
Telephone: 615/327-6223
Fax: 615/327-6228
E-mail: admissions@mmc.edu
Web site: www.mmc.edu

Meharry Medical College School of Medicine
Verification of residencies and internships
Telephone: Free of charge.
Written: Free of charge. Faxed upon request. Mail or fax requests, including signed release forms.
Electronic: Not provided.

Office of Graduate Medical Education
Meharry Medical College
1005 D. B. Todd Jr. Boulevard
Nashville, TENNESSEE 37208
Telephone: 615/327-5973
Fax: 615/321-2939
Web site: www.patton.mmt.edu

University of Tennessee Health Science Center
Verification of degrees
Telephone: Not provided.
Written: Free of charge. Mail or fax requests.
Electronic: Not provided.

Attention: Degree verification request
Office of the Registrar
University of Tennessee Health Science Center
790 Madison Avenue, Suite 119

Memphis, TENNESSEE 38163
Telephone: 901/448-5560
Fax: 901/448-7772
Web site: www.utmem.edu

University of Tennessee Health Science Center
Verification of residencies and internships

Telephone: Free of charge.
Written: Free of charge. Faxed upon request. Mail or fax requests, including signed release forms.
Electronic: Not provided.

Office of Graduate Medical Education
University of Tennessee Health Science Center
956 Court Avenue, Box 19A
Memphis, TENNESSEE 38163
Telephone: 901/448-5364 (main)   901/448-5560 (Registrar's Office)
Fax: 901/448-7543
Web site: www.utmem.edu/gme

Vanderbilt University Medical Center
Verification of residencies and internships

Telephone: Not provided.
Written: Free of charge. Faxed upon request. Mail or fax requests, including signed release forms.
Electronic: Not provided.

Office of Graduate Medical Education
Vanderbilt University Medical Center
2601 The Vanderbilt Clinic
Nashville, TENNESSEE 37232-5283
Telephone: 615/322-4916
Fax: 615/343-1496
Web site: www.mc.vanderbilt.edu/gme

Vanderbilt University, Office of the University Registrar
Verification of degrees

Telephone: Free of charge.
Written: Free of charge. Faxed upon request. Mail or fax requests, including signed release forms.
Electronic: Not provided.

Attention: Degree verification request
Office of the University Registrar
Vanderbilt University
PD 505
Nashville, TENNESSEE 37203
Telephone: 615/322-7701
Fax: 615/343-7709
Web site: www.vanderbilt.edu

Medical School Degrees, Residencies, Internships, and Fellowships

Texas

Baylor College of Medicine
Verification of degrees

Telephone:	Free of charge.
Written:	Free of charge. Faxed upon request. Mail or fax requests, including signed release forms, name of program, maiden name (if applicable), and self-addressed, stamped envelopes.
Electronic:	Not provided.

Office of the Registrar
Baylor College of Medicine
One Baylor Plaza, Suite 108M
Houston, TEXAS 77030
Telephone: 713/798-4600 (student affairs)   713/798-7766 (registrar's office)
Fax: 713/798-6368
E-mail: registrar@bcm.tmc.edu
Web site: www.bcm.tmc.edu

Baylor College of Medicine
Verification of residencies and internships

Telephone:	Free of charge.
Written:	Free of charge. Mail no faxes.
Electronic:	Not provided.

Attention: Residency/fellowship verification
Office of Graduate Medical Education S103
Baylor College of Medicine
One Baylor Plaza
Houston, TEXAS 77030
Telephone: 713/798-4608
Fax: 713/798-4334
Web site: www.bcm.tmc.edu

Texas A&M University System Health Science Center College of Medicine
Verification of degrees

Telephone:	Not provided.
Written:	Free of charge. Faxed upon request in emergency situations only. Mail or fax requests, including signed release forms.
Electronic:	Not provided.

Texas A&M University System Health Science Center College of Medicine
Office of Student Affairs and Admissions
159 Reynolds Medical Building
College Station, TEXAS 77843-1114
Telephone: 979/845-7743
Fax: 979/845-5533
Web site: www.tamushsc.tamu.edu

The 2003 Credentialing and Privileging Desk Reference

Texas A&M University System Health Science Center College of Medicine
Notes: Verifies MD licenses only
Verification of MD and DO licenses
Telephone: Not provided.
Written: Free of charge. Faxed upon request. Mail or fax requests, including signed release forms. (Please include name of MD.)
Electronic: Not provided.

>Texas A&M University System Health Science Center College of Medicine
>159 Joe H. Reynolds Medical Building
>College Station, TEXAS 77843-1114
>Telephone: 979/845-7743
>Fax: 979/845-5533
>E-mail: med-stu-aff@tamu.edu
>Web site: www.tamushsc.tamu.edu

Texas Tech University Health Sciences Center
Verification of degrees
Telephone: Free of charge. Provide physician's name and Social Security number.
Written: Free of charge. Faxed upon request. Mail or fax requests, including physician's Social Security number. Must include signed release form.
Electronic: Not provided.

>Office of the Registrar, 3B310
>Texas Tech University Health Sciences Center
>3601 Fourth Street (Mail stop) 8310
>Lubbock, TEXAS 79430
>Telephone: 806/743-2300
>Fax: 806/743-3027
>E-mail: leanne.ball@ttmc.ttuhsc.edu

Texas Tech University School of Medicine
Verification of residencies and internships
Telephone: Not provided
Written: Written verification with faxed or mail signed release form.
Electronic: Not provided.

>Office of Graduate Medical Education
>Texas Tech University Health Sciences Center
>3601 Fourth Street
>Lubbock, TEXAS 79430
>Telephone: 806/743-2978
>Fax: 806/743-1599
>E-mail: kathy.wright@ttmc.ttuhsc.edu
>Web site: www.remedy.ttuhsc.edu/gme

University of Texas Health Science Center at Houston
Notes: Certificate program in Dental Hygiene will be changing to a degree program in the near future.
Verification of degrees, internships, and residencies

Medical School Degrees, Residencies, Internships, and Fellowships

Telephone: Free of charge. Some files indicate physician in question must submit signed release forms before hospitals can request verifications.
Written: Free of charge. Faxed upon request. Mail or fax requests, including signed release forms and physician's Social Security number.
Electronic: Not provided.

> University of Texas Health Science Center at Houston
> Office of the Registrar
> PO Box 20036
> Houston, TEXAS 77225
> Telephone: 713/500-3361
> Fax: 713/500-3356
> Web site: www.registrar.uth.tmc.edu

University of Texas Health Science Center at San Antonio
Verification of degrees
Telephone: Free of charge. Provide physician's Social Security number.
Written: Free of charge. Faxed upon request. Mail or fax requests, including physician names, degrees, Social Security numbers, and signed release forms.
Electronic: Not provided.

> Office of the Medical Registrar
> University of Texas Health Science Center at San Antonio
> 7703 Floyd Curl Drive
> San Antonio, TEXAS 78229-3900
> Telephone: 210/567-2665
> Fax: 210/567-2645
> E-mail: wrightlc@uthscsa.edu
> Web site: www.uthscsa.edu

University of Texas Health Science Center at San Antonio
Notes: Hospitals must directly contact specific residency or internship programs; Registrar's Office will forward hospitals to the appropriate department.
Verification of degrees MD only
Telephone: Free of charge.
Written: Free of charge. Mail or fax requests, including signed release forms. No verifications after 1990.
Electronic: Information available on verification Web site.

> University of Texas Health Science Center at San Antonio
> 7703 Floyd Curl Drive
> San Antonio, TEXAS 78229-3900
> Telephone: 210/567-2665   703/742-7791 (verification)
> Fax: 210/567-2645
> Web site: www.uthscsa.edu (general information)   www.studentclearinghouse.org (verification)

University of Texas Medical Branch at Galveston
Verification of degrees
Telephone: Free of charge.
Written: Free of charge. Mail or fax requests, including signed release forms, and physician's Social Security number and maiden name (if applicable).

Electronic: Not provided.

> Office of Enrollment Services
> University of Texas Medical Branch at Galveston
> Ashbell Smith Building, Room 1206
> 301 University Boulevard
> Galveston, TEXAS 77555-1312
> Telephone: 409/772-1215
> Fax: 409/772-4466
> Web site: www.utmb.edu

University of Texas Medical Branch at Galveston
Notes: House Staff Office will fax or e-mail hospitals a list of departments and contacts; hospitals must contact specific residency or internship programs directly.
Verification of residencies and fellowships
Telephone: Not provided.
Written: Free of charge.
Electronic: Not provided.

> House Staff Office
> University of Texas Medical Branch at Galveston
> 301 University Boulevard
> Galveston, TEXAS 77555-0462
> Telephone: 409/772-5285
> Fax: 409/772-9785
> Web site: www.utmb.edu

University of Texas Southwestern Medical Center at Dallas School of Medicine
Verification of degrees
Telephone: Free of charge.
Written: Free of charge. Mail requests, including signed release forms.
Electronic: Not provided.

> Attention: Medical degree verification
> Office of the Registrar
> University of Texas Southwestern Medical Center at Dallas School of Medicine
> 5323 Harry Hines Boulevard
> Dallas, TEXAS 75390-9096
> Telephone: 214/648-2670
> Fax: 214/648-3289
> E-mail: admissions@utsouthwestern.edu
> Web site: www.utsouthwestern.edu

University of Texas Southwestern Medical Center at Dallas School of Medicine
Verification of residencies and internships
Telephone: Not provided.
Written: Free of charge. Faxed upon request. Mail or fax requests, including signed release forms.
Electronic: Not provided.

Medical School Degrees, Residencies, Internships, and Fellowships

University of Texas Southwestern Medical Center at Dallas School of Medicine
House Staff Office
Parkland Memorial Hospital
5201 Harry Hines Boulevard
Dallas, TEXAS 75235
Telephone: 214/590-1398
Fax: 214/590-1403
E-mail: njjohn@parknet.pmh.org

Utah

University of Utah School of Medicine
Verification of degrees

Telephone: Free of charge. Must be accompanied by signed release form.
Written: Free of charge. Faxed upon request. Mail or fax requests, including signed release forms.
Electronic: Not provided.

Attention: Degree verification request
Room 1C101
University of Utah School of Medicine
30 N. 1900 E
Salt Lake City, UTAH 84132-2101
Telephone: 801/581-7201
Fax: 801/585-3300
Web site: www.med.utah.edu

University of Utah School of Medicine
Notes: GME office cannot verify information regarding medical skills or professional competence. Forward these requests to the department under which the training was completed.

Verification of residencies, internships, and fellowships

Telephone: Free of charge.
Written: Free of charge. Faxed upon request. Mail or fax requests, including signed release forms.
Electronic: Not provided.

Office of Graduate Medical Education
University of Utah Hospital
30 N. 1900 E
1C412 University Medical Center
Salt Lake City, UTAH 84132-2115
Telephone: 801/581-2401
Fax: 801/585-2507
E-mail: grad.mededuc@hsc.utah.edu
Web site: www.med.utah.edu/som/education/gme

Vermont

University of Vermont College of Medicine
Verification of degrees

Telephone: Free of charge.

Chapter 5

Written: Free of charge. Faxed upon request. Mail or fax requests, including signed release forms.
Electronic: Not provided.

    Attention: Medical degree verification
    University of Vermont College of Medicine
    Office of Student Affairs, E215 Given
    89 Beaumont Avenue
    Burlington, VERMONT 05405
    Telephone: 802/656-2150
    Fax: 802/656-9377
    E-mail: eve.greene@uvm.edu
    Web site: www.med.uvm.edu

University of Vermont College of Medicine

Notes: Hospitals should contact specific departments for the most accurate information. For those residents who served years ago, the GME Office can only verify dates of attendance, not dates of completion.

Verification of residencies and internships

Telephone: Not provided.
Written: Fees apply. Mail requests, including signed release forms.
Electronic: Not provided.

    University of Vermont College of Medicine
    Office of Graduate Medical Education
    MCHV Campus, Smith 132
    Fletcher Allen Health Care/Medical Center Hospital of Vermont
    111 Colchester Avenue
    Burlington, VERMONT 05401
    Telephone: 802/656-3131(Undergraduate Office)   802/656-9736 (Registrar)
    Fax: 802/847-4503
    Web site: www.vermontmednet.org

Virginia

Eastern Virginia Medical School

Verification of degrees

Telephone: Free of charge.
Written: Free of charge. Mail or fax requests, including signed release forms and year of graduation. Use official Eastern Virginia Medical School transcript request forms (available via Office of the Registrar) for transcipt requests.
Electronic: Not provided.

    Attention: Student Records Coordinator
    Office of the Registrar
    Eastern Virginia Medical School
    PO Box 1980
    700 Olney Road
    Norfolk, VIRGINIA 23507
    Telephone: 757/446-5244   Fax: 757/446-5817
    E-mail: grayjh@evms.edu
    Web site: www.evms.edu

Medical School Degrees, Residencies, Internships, and Fellowships

Eastern Virginia Medical School
Notes: Office verifies only dates of attendance and completion, but will forward requests for further information to the specific department.

Verification of residencies and internships

Telephone:	Not provided.
Written:	Free of charge. Faxed upon request. Mail or fax requests, including signed release forms.
Electronic:	Not provided.

>Attention: Residency verification request
>Office of Graduate Medical Education
>Eastern Virginia Medical School
>358 Mowbray Arch
>Norfolk, VIRGINIA 23507
>Telephone: 757/446-6190
>Fax: 757/446-6195
>Web site: www.mevms.edu

Medical College of Virginia Hospitals
Verification of residencies and internships

Telephone:	Not provided.
Written:	Free of charge. Faxed upon request. Mail or fax requests, including signed release forms.
Electronic:	Not provided.

>Office of Graduate Medical Education
>Medical College of Virginia Hospitals
>MCV Box 980-257
>Richmond, VIRGINIA 23298
>Telephone: 804/828-9783
>Fax: 804/828-5613
>E-mail: mpierce@ncun-vcu.edu

University of Virginia School of Medicine
Verification of degrees

Telephone:	Not provided.
Written:	Provided free of charge but would prefer use of Degree Check option; available on Web site.
Electronic:	Prefer use of Degree Check option; accessible at website.

>University of Virginia School of Medicine
>Certification Officer
>Office of the University Registrar
>Carruthers Hall
>PO Box 400203
>1001 N. Emmet Street
>Charlottesville, VIRGINIA 22904-4203
>Telephone: 434/924-4122
>Fax: 434/924-4156
>E-mail: certify@virginia.edu
>Web site: www.med.virginia.edu/medicine/student.affairs/verify.html

University of Virginia School of Medicine
Verification of degrees, internships, and residencies

Telephone:	Free of charge.
Written:	Free of charge. Faxed upon request. Mail or fax requests, including signed release forms.
Electronic:	Not provided.

> Attention: Residency verification request
> Medical Staff Residency Office
> University of Virginia Health System
> Box 800291
> Charlottesville, VIRGINIA 22908-0001
> Telephone: 804/924-8145
> Fax: 804/924-0401
> E-mail: ma6n@virginia.edu
> Web site: hscvirginia.edu/med.cnr/depts/msro/health/housestaff

Virginia Commonwealth University School of Medicine, Medical College of Virginia Campus
Verification of degrees

Telephone:	Free of charge.
Written:	Free of charge. Faxed upon request. Mail or fax requests, including signed release forms. $5 fee for transcripts.
Electronic:	Not provided.

> Attention: Medical degree verification–Louise C. Mitchell
> Registrar, School of Medicine
> Virginia Commonwealth University School of Medicine, Medical College of Virginia Campus
> PO Box 980565
> Richmond, VIRGINIA 23298-0565
> Telephone: 804/828-9793
> Fax: 804/828-5115
> E-mail: lcmitche@vcu.edu

Washington

University of Washington School of Medicine
Verification of degrees MD only

Telephone:	Free of charge.
Written:	Free of charge. Mail requests, including signed release forms and self-addressed, stamped envelope.
Electronic:	Available for 1983–present at www.sdb.admin.washington.edu/graduatedir/public/graduatedir.asp.

> Attention: MD Degree Certification
> Office of Academic Affairs
> University of Washington School of Medicine
> Box 356340
> Seattle, WASHINGTON 98195-6340
> Telephone: 206/543-5560
> Fax: 206/616-3341
> E-mail: askuwsom@u.washington.edu
> Web site: www.washington.edu

University of Washington School of Medicine
Verification of residencies and internships

Telephone: Free of charge.
Written: Free of charge; recommended to check Web site for proper mail routing information, as well as proper department fax number.
Electronic: Not provided. Encouraged to use Web site to locate proper residency or fellowship program for increased response.

> University of Washington School of Medicine
> Department of GME
> PO Box 356340
> Seattle, WASHINGTON 98195
> Telephone: 206/543-0065
> Fax: 206/685-3314
> Web site: www.washington.edu

West Virginia

Marshall University Joan C. Edwards School of Medicine
Verification of degrees, internships, and residencies

Telephone: Free of charge.
Written: Free of charge. Faxed upon request. Mail or fax requests.
Electronic: Not provided.

> Ms. Karen Bledsoe
> Attention: Dean's Office
> Marshall University Joan C. Edwards School of Medicine
> 1600 Medical Center Drive
> Huntington, WEST VIRGINIA 25701-3655
> Telephone: 304/691-1704
> Fax: 304/691-1726
> E-mail: bledsoe@marshall.edu
> Web site: www.musom.marshall.edu

West Virginia University Hospitals, Inc.
Notes: Coordinator has records dating back to 1970. If the office cannot locate the physician's record, it will contact the appropriate department.

Verification of residencies, internships, and fellowships

Telephone: Free of charge with a signed faxed release of information form.
Written: Free of charge. Faxed upon request. Mail or fax requests, including signed release forms.
Electronic: Not provided.

> Attention: House Staff Coordinator
> Office of Graduate Medical Education
> West Virginia University School of Medicine
> House Staff Office
> PO Box 9001
> Morgantown, WEST VIRGINIA 26506-9001
> Telephone: 304/293-0672

Chapter 5

Fax: 304/293-4973
E-mail: lhardy@hsc.wvu.edu
Web site: www.hsc.wvu.edu/som/gme

West Virginia University School of Medicine
Verification of degrees MD only
Telephone: Not provided.
Written: Free of charge. Faxed upon request (followed by hard copy, if requested). Mail or fax requests, including signed release forms.
Electronic: Not provided.

Office of Student Services
West Virginia University School of Medicine
1146 Health Science Center
PO Box 9111
Morgantown, WEST VIRGINIA 26506-9111
Telephone: 304/293-2408
Fax: 304/293-7814
Web site: www.hsc.wvu.edu/som/students

Wisconsin

Medical College of Wisconsin
Verification of degrees
Telephone: Not provided.
Written: Free of charge. Mail requests, including signed release forms and physician's year of graduation.
Electronic: Not provided.

Office of the Registrar
Medical College of Wisconsin
8701 Watertown Plank Road
Milwaukee, WISCONSIN 53226
Telephone: 414/456-8733
Fax: 414/456-6506
Web site: www.mcw.edu/acad/registrar

Medical College of Wisconsin
Verification of residencies, internships, and fellowships
Telephone: Free of charge.
Written: Free of charge. Faxed upon request. Mail or fax requests, including signed release forms.
Electronic: Not provided.

Office of Graduate Medical Education
Medical College of Wisconsin, Affiliated Hospitals
8701 Watertown Plank Road
Milwaukee, WISCONSIN 53226
Telephone: 414/456-4575
Fax: 414/456-6528
E-mail: gme@mcw.edu
Web site: www.mcw.edu/gme

University of Wisconsin Medical School
Verification of MD degrees

Telephone:	Free of charge.
Written:	Free of charge. Faxed upon request in emergency situations only. Mail requests, including signed release forms.
Electronic:	Not provided.

Attention: Medical degree verification
University of Wisconsin Medical School
Office of Student Services Room 1143
1300 University Avenue
Madison, WISCONSIN 53706-1532
Telephone: 608/263-4912 (medical school verification only)
Fax: 608/262-2327

Osteopathic Medical Schools

Arizona

Arizona College of Osteopathic Medicine, Midwestern University
Annual report of licensed physicians

Telephone:	Free of charge.
Written:	Free of charge.
Electronic:	Free of charge.

Office of the Registrar
Arizona College of Osteopathic Medicine, Midwestern University
19555 N. 59th Avenue
Glendale, ARIZONA 85308
Telephone: 623/572-3200 (main)   623/572-3325
Fax: 623/572-3337
E-mail: cschen@arizona.midwestern.edu
Web site: www.midwestern.edu

California

Touro University, College of Osteopathic Medicine
Notes: First graduating class: 2001.
Annual report of licensed physicians

Telephone:	Not provided.
Written:	Not provided.
Electronic:	Not provided.

Touro University, College of Osteopathic Medicine
1210 Scott Street
San Francisco, CALIFORNIA 94115
Telephone: 415/292-0584
Fax: 415/292-0439
Web site: www.ccpm.edu

Florida

Nova Southeastern University, College of Osteopathic Medicine
Verification of degrees

Telephone:	Not provided.
Written:	Free of charge. Faxed upon request. Mail or fax requests, including signed release forms.
Electronic:	Not provided.

Nova Southeastern University, College of Osteopathic Medicine
Attention: Registrar's Office
3301 College Avenue
Fort Lauderdale, FLORIDA 33314
Telephone: 954/262-7249
Fax: 954/262-7265
E-mail: nsuregistrar@nova.edu
Web site: www.nova.edu

Illinois

Midwestern University, Chicago College of Osteopathic Medicine
Verification of degrees
Telephone: Free of charge.
Written: Free of charge. Faxed upon request. Mail or fax requests, including signed release forms.
Electronic: Not provided.

> Office of the Registrar
> Chicago College of Osteopathic Medicine
> Midwestern University
> 555 31st Street
> Downers Grove, ILLINOIS 60515
> Telephone: 630/515-6074
> Fax: 630/515-7140
> Web site: www.midwestern.edu

Iowa

Des Moines University Osteopathic Medical Center
Verification of degrees
Telephone: Free of charge.
Written: Free of charge. Faxed upon request for $10 per verification. Mail or fax requests, including signed release forms.
Electronic: Not provided.

> Office of the Registrar
> Des Moines University Osteopathic Medical Center
> 3200 Grand Avenue
> Des Moines, IOWA 50312
> Telephone: 515/271-1460
> Fax: 515/271-1578
> E-mail: registrar@dmu.edu
> Web site: www.dmu.edu

Kentucky

Pikeville College, School of Osteopathic Medicine
Annual report of licensed physicians
Telephone: Not provided.
Written: Not provided.
Electronic: Not provided.

> School of Osteopathic Medicine
> Pikeville College
> 147 Sycamore Street
> Pikeville, KENTUCKY 41501
> Telephone: 606/218-5250 (general information)   606/218-5400 (School of Medicine switchboard)
> Fax: 606/218-5442
> Web site: www.pc.edu

Osteopathic Medical Schools

Maine

University of New England, College of Osteopathic Medicine
Verification of degrees

Telephone: Free of charge.
Written: Free of charge. Faxed upon request. Mail or fax requests, including signed release forms.
Electronic: Not provided.

> Office of the Registrar
> College of Osteopathic Medicine
> University of New England
> 11 Hills Beach Road
> Biddeford, MAINE 04005
> Telephone: 207/283-0171, Ext. 2473 (Registrar's office)
> Fax: 207/294-5927
> E-mail: uneregistrar@une.edu
> Web site: www.une.edu

Michigan

Michigan State University, College of Osteopathic Medicine
Verification of degrees

Telephone: Free of charge.
Written: Free of charge. Faxed upon request (followed by hard copy if requested). Mail or fax requests, including signed release forms.
Electronic: Not provided.

> Michigan State University, College of Osteopathic Medicine
> Student Services Office
> C-103 E. Fee Hall
> East Lansing, MICHIGAN 48824-1316
> Telephone: 517/353-7741
> Fax: 517/432-1976
> E-mail: ander178@msu.edu
> Web site: www.com.msu.edu

Missouri

The University of Health Sciences, College of Osteopathic Medicine
Verification of degrees

Telephone: Not provided.
Written: Free of charge. Faxed upon request. Mail or fax requests, including signed release forms.
Electronic: Not provided.

> The University of Health Sciences
> College of Osteopathic Medicine
> Attention: GME S. Newby
> 1750 Independence Boulevard
> Kansas City, MISSOURI 64106

Telephone: 816/283-2364
Fax: 816/460-0556
E-mail: snewby@uhs.edu

New Jersey

University of Medicine and Dentistry of New Jersey, School of Osteopathic Medicine
Verification of degrees

Telephone:	Free of charge.
Written:	Free of charge. Faxed upon request. Mail or fax requests, including signed release forms.
Electronic:	Not provided.

Office of the Registrar
School of Osteopathic Medicine
University of Medicine and Dentistry of New Jersey
Academic Center
One Medical Center Drive, Suite 210
Stratford, NEW JERSEY 08084-1501
Telephone: 856/566-7055
Fax: 856/566-6895
Web site: www.som.umdnj.edu/index

New York

New York College of Osteopathic Medicine, of New York Institute of Technology
Notes: Transcripts are $4 per copy.
Verification of degrees

Telephone:	Free of charge.
Written:	Free of charge. Faxed upon request. Mail or fax requests, including signed release forms.
Electronic:	Not provided.

New York College of Osteopathic Medicine
New York Institute of Technology
PO Box 8000
Old Westbury, NEW YORK 11568
Telephone: 516/686-3777
Fax: 516/686-3835
Web site: www.nyit.edu

Ohio

Ohio University, College of Osteopathic Medicine
Verification of degrees

Telephone:	Free of charge. Limit five verifications per call.
Written:	Free of charge. Faxed upon request. Mail or fax requests, including signed release forms.
Electronic:	Not provided.

Ohio University, College of Osteopathic Medicine
Chubb Hall
Registrar's Office
Athens, OHIO 45701
Telephone: 740/593-4201
Fax: 740/593-4184
Web site: www.ohiou.edu

Oklahoma

Oklahoma State University, Center for Health Sciences Verification of degrees

Telephone: Free of charge.
Written: Free of charge for verifications; $3 for transcripts. Faxed upon request. Mail or fax requests, including signed release forms.
Electronic: Free of charge.

Student Affairs Office
College of Osteopathic Medicine
Oklahoma State University
1111 W. 17th Street
Tulsa, OKLAHOMA 74107-1898
Telephone: 918/561-8459
Fax: 918/561-8243
E-mail: bartlem@chs.okstate.edu
Web site: www.healthsciences.okstate.edu

Pennsylvania

Lake Erie College of Osteopathic Medicine

Notes: First graduating class: 1997.

Annual report of licensed physicians

Telephone: Not provided.
Written: Free of charge. Mail requests, including physician names and signed release forms.
Electronic: Not provided.

Student Affairs Office
Lake Erie College of Osteopathic Medicine
1858 West Grandview Boulevard
Erie, PENNSYLVANIA 16509
Telephone: 814/866-8123
Fax: 814/866-8123
Web site: www.lecom.edu

Philadelphia College of Osteopathic Medicine

Verification of degrees

Telephone: Free of charge.
Written: Free of charge. Faxed upon request. Mail or fax requests, including signed release forms.
Electronic: Not provided.

Office of the Registrar
Philadelphia College of Osteopathic Medicine
4170 City Avenue
Philadelphia, PENNSYLVANIA 19131-1694
Telephone: 215/871-6700
Fax: 215/871-6719
E-mail: registrar@pcom.edu
Web site: www.pcom.edu

Texas

University of North Texas Health Science Center at Fort Worth, Texas College of Osteopathic Medicine
Verification of degrees

Telephone:	Free of charge.
Written:	Free of charge. Faxed upon request. Mail or fax requests, including signed release forms.
Electronic:	Free of charge.

Office of the Registrar
Texas College of Osteopathic Medicine
University of North Texas Health Science Center, Fort Worth
3500 Camp Bowie Boulevard
Fort Worth, TEXAS 76107-2699
Telephone: 817/735-2201 (Registrar)   817/735-2000 (main)
Fax: 817/735-2568
E-mail: bbelton@hsc.unt.edu
Web site: www.hsc.unt.edu

Canadian Medical Schools

Alberta

University of Alberta, Faculty of Medicine and Dentistry
Verification of degrees, internships, and residencies

Telephone:	Not provided.
Written:	Free of charge. Mail requests, including signed release forms and self-addressed, stamped envelopes.
Electronic:	Free of charge via e-mail.

Faculty of Medicine and Dentistry
Room 245, Medical Sciences Building
University of Alberta
Edmonton, ALBERTA T6G 2H7
CANADA
Telephone: 780/492-5913
Fax: 780/492-9531
E-mail: silvia.franklin@ualberta.ca
Web site: www.ualberta.com

Calgary

University of Calgary, Faculty of Medicine
Verification of degrees

Telephone:	Not provided.
Written:	Free of charge for institutions. Graduates must pay a fee for verification; call for specific amount.
Electronic:	Not provided.

Office of the Associate Dean for Undergraduate Medical Education
University of Calgary
3330 Hospital Drive NW
Calgary, ALBERTA T2N 4N1
CANADA
Telephone: 403/220-3843 (Office of the Associate Dean)
Fax: 403/270-2681
Web site: www.med.ucalgary.ca/cren/welcome.htm

University of Calgary, Faculty of Medicine
Notes: Contact specific residency or internship programs directly.
Verification of residencies and internships

Telephone:	Not provided.
Written:	Free of charge.
Electronic:	Not provided.

Faculty of Medicine
University of Calgary
3330 Hospital Drive NW
Calgary, ALBERTA T2N 1N4
CANADA
Telephone: 403/220-5110 (main line)   403/220-6848 (administrative and faculty services)

Fax: 403/283-4740
Web site: www.ucalgary.ca

British Columbia

University of British Columbia, Faculty of Medicine
Verification of degrees

Telephone: Not provided.
Written: $15 for first verification; $10 each additional verification. Faxed upon request for additional $10 per verification. Mail requests, including receipt deadline date, signed release form, and check (made payable to the University of British Columbia).
Electronic: Not provided.

> Office of Undergraduate Education in the Faculty of Medicine
> Jim Pattison Pavilion, Room 3250
> University of British Columbia
> 910 W. Tenth Avenue
> Vancouver, BRITISH COLUMBIA V5Z 4E3
> CANADA
> Telephone: 604/875-4500
> Fax: 604/875-5611
> Web site: www.med.ubc.ca

University of British Columbia, Faculty of Medicine
Verification of degrees

Telephone: Not provided.
Written: $10 per verification; $15 for official letter of verification. Mail requests, including physician's name and year of graduation, and check made payable to University of British Columbia.
Electronic: Not provided.

> University of British Columbia, Faculty of Medicine
> 3250-910 W. Tenth Avenue
> Vancouver, BRITISH COLUMBIA V5Z 4E3
> CANADA
> Telephone: 604/875-4500
> Fax: 604/875-5611
> E-mail: drota@interchange.ubc.ca
> Web site: www.med.ubc.ca

Manitoba

University of Manitoba, Faculty of Medicine
Verification of degrees

Telephone: Not provided.
Written: Fee subject to change; call for more information. Mail requests, including signed release forms and payment.
Electronic: Not provided.

> Attention: Degree verification request
> Office of Medical Education, S204

Canadian Medical Schools

University of Manitoba
753 McDermot Avenue
Winnipeg, MANITOBA R3E 0W3
CANADA
Telephone: 204/789-3568
Fax: 204/789-3929
Web site: www.umanitoba.ca/faculties/medicine/education

University of Manitoba Faculty of Medicine
Verification of residencies and internships

Telephone: Not provided.
Written: Fee subject to change; call for more information. Mail requests, including signed release forms and payment.
Electronic: Not provided.

Attention: Residency verification request
Office of Postgraduate Medical Education, S204
University of Manitoba
753 McDermot Avenue
Winnipeg, MANITOBA R3E 0W3
Canada
Telephone: 204/789-3290
Fax: 204/789-3929
Web site: www.umanitoba.ca

Newfoundland

Memorial University of Newfoundland, Faculty of Medicine
Verification of degrees

Telephone: Free of charge.
Written: $25 per verification. Faxed upon request. Mail or fax requests, including signed release forms.
Electronic: Not provided.

Office of Student Affairs
Faculty of Medicine
Memorial University of Newfoundland
300 Prince Philip Drive
Saint Johns, NEWFOUNDLAND A1B 3V6
CANADA
Telephone: 709/777-6690
Fax: 709/777-8296
E-mail: mdray@mun.ca
Web site: www.med.mun.ca

Memorial University of Newfoundland, Faculty of Medicine
Verification of residencies and internships

Telephone: Not provided.
Written: $25 per verification. Faxed upon request for $5 fee. Mail or fax requests, including signed release forms.

Chapter 5

Electronic: Not provided.

> Office of Postgraduate Medical Studies
> Faculty of Medicine
> Memorial University of Newfoundland
> 300 Prince Philip Drive
> Saint Johns, NEWFOUNDLAND A1B 3V6
> CANADA
> Telephone: 709/777-6680
> Fax: 709/777-8377
> E-mail: pgms@mun.ca
> Web site: www.med.mun.ca/pgme

Nova Scotia

Dalhousie University Faculty of Medicine
Notes: For MD verifications, please contact Sharon Graham at 902/494-1848 or sharon.graham@dal.ca.
Verification of degrees, internships, and residencies
Telephone: Not provided.
Written: $50 per verification. Faxed upon request. Mail requests, including signed release forms and payment.
Electronic: Not provided.

> Office of Postgraduate Medical Education
> Dalhousie University
> 5849 University Avenue, Room C126
> Halifax, NOVA SCOTIA B3H 4H7
> CANADA
> Telephone: 902/494-2362 (When leaving a message, please don't leave toll-free numbers)
> E-mail: denise.mitchell@dal.ca
> Web site: www.medicine.dal.ca

Ontario

McMaster University School of Medicine
Verification of degrees
Telephone: Not provided.
Written: $8 per verification. Faxed back upon request for additional $5 within Canada or $10 to the U.S. Mail or fax requests, including signed release forms and payment (MC, Visa, check, or money order payable to McMaster Univ. Registrar's Office).
Electronic: Not provided.

> Office of the Registrar
> Gilmour Hall, Room 108
> McMaster University School of Medicine
> 1280 Main Street, W.
> Hamilton, ONTARIO L8S 4L8
> CANADA
> Telephone: 905/525-9140, Ext 24796
> Fax: 905/527-1105

McMaster University School of Medicine
Verification of residencies and internships

Telephone:	Not provided.
Written:	$8 per verification. Fax requests an additional $5 within Canada or $10 to the U.S. Mail or fax requests, including signed release forms and payment (MC, Visa, or check or money order payable to McMaster Univ. Registrar's Office).
Electronic:	Not provided.

Office of the Registrar
1200 Main Street, W.
Hamilton, ONTARIO L8N 3Z5
CANADA
Telephone: 905/525-9140, Ext. 22235 (admissions office)
Fax: 905/528-4727
Web site: www.fhs.mcmaster.ca

Queens University Faculty of Health Sciences
Verification of degrees

Telephone:	Not provided.
Written:	Free of charge. Mail requests, including signed release forms.
Electronic:	Not provided.

Office of Undergraduate Medical Education
Queens University Faculty of Health Sciences
69 Barrie Street
Kingston, ONTARIO K7L 3N6
CANADA
Telephone: 613/533-2542
Fax: 613/533-3190
E-mail: dj6@post.queensu.ca
Web site: www.queensu.ca

Ottawa

University of Ottawa Faculty of Medicine
Verification of degrees

Telephone:	Not provided.
Written:	$15–$70 per verification, depending on details requested (call for specific fees). Mail requests, including signed release forms and payment.
Electronic:	Not provided.

Office of Undergraduate Medical Education
University of Ottawa Faculty of Medicine
451 Smyth Road
Ottawa, ONTARIO K1H 8M5
CANADA
Telephone: 613/562-5800 ext. 8427 613/562-5400
Fax: 613/562-5457

E-mail: pgme@uottawa.ca
Web site: www.uottawa.ca

University of Ottawa Faculty of Medicine
Notes: Verifications provided only upon receipt of request form, along with certified check or money order. Processing time is 4–6 weeks. Urgent requests processed in 48 hours- additional $25 fee required.

Verification of residencies and internships

Telephone: Not provided.
Written: $35 to $70 per verification. $35 fee if only dates and program completed are required; $70 fee if a detailed assessment is required (rotations, evaluations, etc.). Mail requests, including signed authorization to release information, and payment.
Electronic: Not provided.

Office of Postgraduate Medical Education
University of Ottawa Faculty of Medicine
451 Smyth Road
Ottawa, ONTARIO K1H 8M5
CANADA
Telephone: 613/562-5413
Fax: 613/562-5420
E-mail: pgme@uottawa.ca
Web site: www.uottawa.ca

Toronto

University of Toronto Faculty of Medicine
Verification of degrees MD only

Telephone: Free of charge; prefer written request.
Written: Call for more information. Mail requests, including signed release forms, payment, and each physician's student identification number, year of graduation, and maiden name (if applicable). $6.90 fee; checks payable to University of Toronto.
Electronic: Not provided.

Registrar's Office
Medical Sciences Building, Room 2124
1 Kings College Circle
Toronto, ONTARIO M5S 1A8
CANADA
Telephone: 416/946-8236 (credentialing, undergraduate only)
Fax: 416/978-4194
E-mail: stella.miller@utoronto.ca
Web site: www.library.utoronto.ca/medicine

University of Toronto Faculty of Medicine
Verification of degrees, internships, and residencies

Telephone: Not provided.
Written: Fee varies; call for more information. Mail requests, including signed release forms, payment, and each physician's student ID number, year of graduation, and maiden name (if applicable).

Canadian Medical Schools

Electronic: Not provided.

> Office of Postgraduate Medical Education
> 500 University Avenue, 2nd Floor
> University of Toronto Faculty of Medicine
> Toronto, ONTARIO M5G2C1
> CANADA
> Telephone: 416/978-6976
> Fax: 416/978-7144
> E-mail: postgrad.med@utoronto.ca
> Web site: www.library.utoronto.ca/medicine

University of Western Ontario, Faculty of Medicine and Dentistry
Verification of degrees

Telephone: Free of charge.
Written: $4 for written. $6 for fax.
Electronic: Provided through e-mail free of charge.

> Attention: Degree verification request
> Undergraduate Medical Education
> Programs Department
> Stevenson Lawson Building Room 155
> University of Western Ontario
> London, ONTARIO N6A 5B8
> CANADA
> Telephone: 519/661-2111 ext. 84859 (Registrar)
> Fax: 519/661-3388
> E-mail: contact@uwo.ca
> Web site: www.registrar.uwo.ca

University of Western Ontario, Faculty of Medicine and Dentistry
Verification of residencies and internships

Telephone: Not provided.
Written: $50 for verification of residency training dates only; $75 for verification of training dates express processing. $75 verification of performance and training date, $100 for express processing. Mail or fax requests, including signed released forms.
Electronic: Not provided.

> Postgraduate Medical Education
> Faculty of Medicine and Dentistry
> Medical Sciences Building, Room M106
> University of Western Ontario
> London, ONTARIO N6A 5C1
> CANADA
> Telephone: 519/661-2019
> Fax: 519/661-3797
> E-mail: gerry.niles@fmd.uwo.ca
> Web site: www.med.uwo.ca/postgrad/pge.htm

Quebec

McGill University, Faculty of Medicine
Verification of degrees, internships, and residencies

Telephone: Not provided.
Written: $50 fee for written. Mail or fax requests, including signed release forms. Allow 4–6 weeks response time.
Electronic: Not provided.

> Postgraduate Medical Education Office
> McGill University Faculty of Medicine
> 3655 Promenade Sir William Osler
> Montreal, QUEBEC H3G 1Y6
> CANADA
> Telephone: 514/398-1458
> Fax: 514/398-3595
> E-mail: postgrad@med.mcgill.ca
> Web site: www.med.mcgill.ca/postgrad

Universite de Montreal, Faculte de Medecine
Verification of degrees, internships, and residencies

Telephone: Not provided.
Written: Mail or fax requests, including signed release forms. Must have date when residency was completed.
Electronic: Information available on Web site.

> Attention: Verification Request
> Office of Postgraduate Medical Education
> Universite de Montreal Faculte de Medecine
> 2900 Boulevard Edouard Montpetit
> PO Box 6128 Sucursale Centre Ville
> Montreal, QUEBEC H3C3J7
> CANADA
> Telephone: 514/343-6267
> Fax: 514/343-2068 Attention: Verification request
> Web site: www.umontreal.ca

Universite de Sherbrooke, Faculte de Medecine
Verification of degrees

Telephone: Not provided.
Written: Free of charge. Mail requests including signed release forms.
Electronic: Not provided.

> Attention: Verification request
> Office of Postgraduate Medical Education
> Faculte de Medecine
> Universite de Sherbrooke
> 3001 12th Avenue N.
> Sherbrooke, QUEBEC J1H 5N4
> CANADA
> Telephone: 819/564-5206

Fax: 819/564-5293
E-mail: llemieux@couriieri.usherb.ca
Web site: www.usherb.ca

Universite Laval, Faculte de Medecine
Verification of degrees, internships, and residencies

Telephone: Free of charge.
Written: Duties will be charged. Mail or fax requests, including signed release forms.
Electronic: Not provided.

Studies Management Coordinator
Faculte de Medecine, Local 1239
Pavillon Ferdinand-Vandry
Universite Laval
Sainte-Foy, QUEBEC G1K 7P4
CANADA
Telephone: 418/656-7459
Fax: 418/656-2915
Web site: www.fmed.ulaval.ca/postmd

Saskatchewan

University of Saskatchewan, College of Medicine
Verification of degrees

Telephone: Not provided.
Written: $40 per verification. Provide written release form.
Electronic: Information available on our Web site.

Office of Undergraduate Medical Education
College of Medicine
University of Saskatchewan
A204, Health Sciences Building
Saskatoon, SASKATCHEWAN S7N 5E5
CANADA
Telephone: 306/966-8556
Fax: 306/966-2601
E-mail: shepard@admin.usask.ca

University of Saskatchewan, College of Medicine
Verification of residencies and internships

Telephone: Not provided.
Written: $40 to verify program dates; $50 to obtain performance appraisals. Additional fees apply for courier or fax services. Call for more information. Mail requests, including signed release forms.
Electronic: Not provided.

Office of Postgraduate Medical Education
College of Medicine
University of Saskatchewan

A204, Health Sciences Building
107 Wiggins Road
Saskatoon, SASKATCHEWAN S7N 5E5
CANADA
Telephone: 306/966-8555
Fax: 306/966-2601
E-mail: rlo450@duke.usask.ca
Web site: www.usask.ca/medicine

Dental Schools

Alabama

University of Alabama School of Dentistry
Verification of degrees

Telephone: Free of charge.
Written: Free of charge. Faxed upon request. Mail or fax requests, including signed release forms.
Electronic: Information available on our Web site.

> Office of the Registrar
> University of Alabama School of Dentistry
> 1530 Third Avenue S., SDB-125
> Birmingham, ALABAMA 35294-0007
> Telephone: 205/934-3387
> Fax: 205/934-0209
> E-mail: cindye@uab.edu
> Web site: www.dental.uab.edu

California

Loma Linda University School of Dentistry
Verification of degrees

Telephone: Provided. Call University Records 909/558-4508 for information.
Written: Provided. Call University Records 909/558-4508 for information.
Electronic: Provided. Call University Records 909/558-4508 for information.

> Academic Affairs Office
> Loma Linda University School of Dentistry
> 11092 Anderson Street
> Loma Linda, CALIFORNIA 92350
> Telephone: 909/558-4601   909/558-4508 (university records)
> Fax: 909/558-4211
> Web site: www.llu.edu

University of California at Los Angeles (UCLA) School of Dentistry
Verification of degrees

Telephone: Not provided.
Written: Free of charge. Faxed upon request. Mail or fax requests, including signed release forms and dentist's year of graduation.
Electronic: Not provided.

> Office of Student and Alumni Affairs
> University of California at Los Angeles School of Dentistry
> CHS, Room A0-111
> 10833 Leconte Avenue
> Los Angeles, CALIFORNIA 90095-1762
> Telephone: 310/825-9789
> Fax: 310/825-9808
> E-mail: chess@dent.ucla.edu
> Web site: www.dent.ucla.edu

University of California San Francisco School of Dentistry
Verification of degrees

Telephone:	Free of charge. Limit 10 verifications per call.
Written:	Free of charge. Faxed upon request. Mail or fax requests, including signed release forms. Give two weeks notice.
Electronic:	Free of charge. E-mail requests to tuttler@dentistry.ucsf.edu.

Office of the Dean
University of California San Francisco School of Dentistry
707 Parnassus Avenue, Suite D4010
San Francisco, CALIFORNIA 94143-0636
Telephone: 415/476-1101
Fax: 415/476-3448
E-mail: tuttler@dentistry.ucsf.edu
Web site: www.ucsf.edu/dent

University of Southern California School of Dentistry
Verification of degrees

Telephone:	Free of charge.
Written:	$3 fee for verifications. $7 for official copy of transcripts, $5 for unofficial transcripts.
Electronic:	Not provided.

Office of Academic Affairs
University of Southern California School of Dentistry
925 W. 34th Street, Room 218
Los Angeles, CALIFORNIA 90089-0641
Telephone: 213/740-1001
Fax: 213/740-2376
Web site: www.usc/edu/hsc/dental

University of the Pacific School of Dentistry
Verification of degrees

Telephone:	Free of charge.
Written:	Free of charge. Faxed upon request. Mail or fax requests, including signed release forms.
Electronic:	Not provided.

Office of Academic Affairs
University of the Pacific School of Dentistry
2155 Webster Street
San Francisco, CALIFORNIA 94115
Telephone: 415/929-6437
Fax: 415/929-6654

Colorado

University of Colorado School of Dentistry
Verification of degrees

Telephone: Not provided.
Written: Free of charge. Faxed upon request. Mail or fax requests, including signed release forms.
Electronic: Not provided.

> Office of Academic Affairs
> University of Colorado School of Dentistry
> 4200 E. Ninth Avenue, Box C-284
> Denver, COLORADO 80262
> Telephone: 303/315-8891
> Fax: 303/315-0472
> E-mail: jill.blanchard@uchsc.edu
> Web site: www.uchsc.edu/sd/sd

Connecticut

University of Connecticut School of Dental Medicine
Verification of degrees

Telephone: Free of charge.
Written: Free of charge. Mail or fax requests, including signed release forms, dentist's Social Security number, year of graduation, and maiden name (if applicable).
Electronic: Not provided.

> Office of Records & Registration
> University of Connecticut School of Dental Medicine
> 263 Farmington Avenue
> Farmington, CONNECTICUT 06030-1827
> Telephone: 860/679-3125
> Fax: 860/679-1902
> E-mail: erdavis@uchc.edu
> Web site: www.uconn.edu

District of Columbia

Howard University College of Dentistry
Verification of degrees

Telephone: Not provided.
Written: Free of charge. Faxed upon request. Mail or fax requests, including signed release forms.
Electronic: Not provided.

> Office of the Dean
> Howard University College of Dentistry
> 600 W. Street NW
> Washington, DISTRICT OF COLUMBIA 20059
> Telephone: 202/806-0400   202/806-0445 (dean's office)
> Fax: 202/806-0354

Florida

University of Florida College of Dentistry
Verification of degrees

Telephone: Free of charge.
Written: Free of charge. Faxed upon request. Mail or fax requests, including signed release forms.
Electronic: Not provided.

>Office of Education
>University of Florida College of Dentistry
>Box 100407
>Gainesville, FLORIDA 32610-0407
>Telephone: 352/392-2949
>Fax: 352/846-3818
>E-mail: tdolan@dental.ufl.edu
>Web site: www.dental.ufl.edu

Georgia

Medical College of Georgia School of Dentistry
Verification of degrees

Telephone: Free of charge.
Written: Free of charge. Faxed upon request. Mail or fax requests, including signed release forms.
Electronic: Not provided.

>Office of Students, Admissions, and Alumni
>Medical College of Georgia School of Dentistry
>1459 Laney Walker Boulevard
>Augusta, GEORGIA 30912-1000
>Telephone: 706/721-2813
>Fax: 706/721-6276
>E-mail: chanes@mail.mcg.edu

Illinois

Southern Illinois University, School of Dental Medicine
Verification of degrees

Telephone: Free of charge.
Written: Free of charge. Faxed upon request. Mail or fax requests, including signed release forms.
Electronic: Not provided.

>Admissions Office
>Southern Illinois University, School of Dental Medicine
>2800 College Avenue
>Alton, ILLINOIS 62002
>Telephone: 618/474-7170
>Fax: 618/474-7249

Dental Schools

University of Illinois at Chicago College of Dentistry
Verification of degrees

Telephone: Free of charge. Limited verifications.
Written: Free of charge. Faxed upon request. Mail or fax requests.
Electronic: Not provided.

> Office of Academic Affairs
> University of Illinois at Chicago College of Dentistry
> 801 S. Paulina Street
> Chicago, ILLINOIS 60612
> Telephone: 312/996-2896
> Fax: 312/413-9050
> Web site: www.uic.edu

Indiana

Indiana University School of Dentistry
Verification of degrees

Telephone: Free of charge.
Written: Free of charge. Faxed upon request. Mail or fax requests, including signed release forms.
Electronic: E-mail requests to rkasberg@iupui.edu

> Student Affairs Office
> Indiana University School of Dentistry
> 1121 W. Michigan Street
> Indianapolis, INDIANA 46202
> Telephone: 317/274-8173
> Fax: 317/274-2419
> Web site: www.iusd.iupui.edu

Iowa

The University of Iowa College of Dentistry
Verification of degrees

Telephone: Free of charge.
Written: Free of charge. Faxed upon request in emergency situations only. Mail requests, including signed release forms. Fax requests in emergency situations only.
Electronic: Not provided.

> Office of the Dean
> The University of Iowa College of Dentistry
> Dental Science Building
> Iowa City, IOWA 52242
> Telephone: 319/335-9650
> Fax: 319/335-7155
> Web site: www.dentistry.uiowa.edu

Kentucky

University of Kentucky College of Dentistry
Verification of degrees

Telephone:	Free of charge.
Written:	Free of charge. Faxed upon request. Mail or fax requests, including signed release forms and dentist's year of graduation.
Electronic:	Free of charge. E-mail requests to dehaney@pop.uky.edu.

Office of Admissions and Student Affairs
University of Kentucky College of Dentistry
D-155 Chandler Medical Center
Lexington, KENTUCKY 40536-0297
Telephone: 859/323-6071
Fax: 859/257-5550
E-mail: dange2@e-mail.uky.edu
Web site: www.mc.uky.edu/dentistry

University of Louisville School of Dentistry
Verification of degrees

Telephone:	Free of charge.
Written:	Free of charge. Faxed upon request. Mail or fax requests, including signed release forms.
Electronic:	E-mail requests to sherry.kennedy@louisville.edu.

Sherry Kennedy Academic Coordinator
University of Louisville School of Dentistry
Health Sciences Center, Room 227
Louisville, KENTUCKY 40292
Telephone: 502/852-1207
Fax: 502/852-7163
E-mail: sherry.kennedy@louisville.edu
Web site: www.louisville.edu

Louisiana

Louisiana State University Health Sciences Center
Verification of degrees

Telephone:	Free of charge. Limit five verifications per call.
Written:	Free of charge. Faxed upon request in emergency situations only. Mail or fax requests, including signed release forms.
Electronic:	Not provided.

Office of the Registrar
LSU Health Sciences Center
433 Bolivar Street
Room 117
New Orleans, LOUISIANA 70112
Telephone: 504/568-4829

Fax: 504/568-5545
Web site: www.lsuhsc.edu

Maryland

University of Maryland, Baltimore College of Dental Surgery
Verification of degrees

Telephone:	Free of charge. Provide dentist's name, Social Security number, and year of graduation.
Written:	Free of charge. Faxed upon request. Mail or fax requests, including signed release forms.
Electronic:	Not provided.

Attention: Verification Request
Office of Academic Affairs
University of Maryland
666 W. Baltimore Street
Room 4-A-11
Baltimore, MARYLAND 21201
Telephone: 410/706-7483   (Academic affairs) 410/706-7461   (Deans office)
Fax: 410/706-0406
E-mail: alhoo1@dental.umaryland.edu
Web site: www.dental.umaryland.edu/homepage/default.asp

Massachusetts

Boston University Goldman School of Dental Medicine
Verification of degrees

Telephone:	Free of charge.
Written:	Free of charge. Faxed upon request. Mail or fax requests, including signed release forms.
Electronic:	Not provided.

Office of Admissions and Student Services
Boston University Goldman School of Dental Medicine
100 E. Newton Street, Room G305
Boston, MASSACHUSETTS 02118
Telephone: 617/638-4708
Fax: 617/638-4798
Web site: www.bu.edu

Harvard School of Dental Medicine
Verification of degrees

Telephone:	Not provided.
Written:	Free of charge. Faxed upon request. Mail or fax (preferred) requests, including signed release forms.
Electronic:	Not provided.

Office of Dental Education
Harvard School of Dental Medicine
188 Longwood Avenue
Boston, MASSACHUSETTS 02115

Telephone: 617/432-1447
Fax: 617/432-3881
Web site: www.hsdm.med.harvard.edu

Tufts University School of Dental Medicine
Verification of degrees

Telephone:	Free of charge.
Written:	Free of charge. Faxed upon request. Mail or fax requests, including signed release forms and dentist's year of graduation.
Electronic:	Verification available through e-mail.

Office of Registrar
Tufts University School of Dental Medicine
One Kneeland Street DHS-7, Room 742
Boston, MASSACHUSETTS 02111
Telephone: 617/636-6543 (Main Registrar)
Fax: 617/636-0309
Web site: www.tufts.edu

Michigan

University of Detroit Mercy School of Dentistry
Verification of degrees

Telephone:	Free of charge.
Written:	Free of charge. Faxed upon request. Mail or fax requests, including signed release forms.
Electronic:	Not provided.

Office of the Registrar
University of Detroit Mercy School of Dentistry
8200 W. Outer Drive
PO Box 19900
Detroit, MICHIGAN 48219-0900
Telephone: 313/494-6616
Fax: 313/494-6627

University of Michigan School of Dentistry
Verification of degrees

Telephone:	Free of charge.
Written:	Free of charge. Faxed upon request. Mail or fax requests.
Electronic:	Free of charge. E-mail requests to barant@umich.edu.

Office of Academic Affairs
University of Michigan School of Dentistry
1011 N. University, Room G226
Ann Arbor, MICHIGAN 48109-1078
Telephone: 734/764-1512
Fax: 734/647-6805
E-mail: barant@umich.edu
Web site: www.dent.umich.edu

Dental Schools

Minnesota

University of Minnesota
Verification of degrees

Telephone: Free of charge.
Written: Free of charge. Mail requests, including signed release forms.
Electronic: Not provided.

> University of Minnesota
> Office of the Dean
> 15-209 MOOS Tower
> 515 Delaware Street SE
> Minneapolis, MINNESOTA 55455
> Telephone: 612/625-9982 (Dean's office)   612/625-5333 (Registrar's office)
> Fax: 612/626-2654
> Web site: www.dentistry.umn.edu

Mississippi

The University of Mississippi Medical Center School of Dentistry

Telephone: Not provided.
Written: Free of charge.
Electronic: Not provided.

> School of Dentistry
> 2500 N. State Street
> Jackson, MISSISSIPPI 39216
> Telephone: 601/984-6000
> Fax: 601/984-1973
> Web site: www.umc.edu

University of Mississippi School of Dentistry
Verification of degrees

Telephone: Free of charge.
Written: Free of charge. Mail or fax requests, including signed release forms and dentist's Social Security number.
Electronic: Not provided.

> Office of Registrar and Student Records
> University of Mississippi Medical Center
> 2500 N. State Street
> Jackson, MISSISSIPPI 39216-4505
> Telephone: 601/984-1080
> Fax: 601/984-1079

Missouri

University of Missouri-Kansas City School of Dentistry
Verification of degrees

Telephone: Free of charge.

Written: Free of charge. Faxed upon request. Mail or fax requests, including signed release forms and dentists Social Security number.
Electronic: Not provided.

> Office of Student Programs
> University of Missouri, Kansas City School of Dentistry
> 650 E. 25th Street
> Kansas City, MISSOURI 64108
> Telephone: 816/235-2080
> Fax: 816/235-2157
> E-mail: beardd@umkc.edu
> Web site: www.umkc.edu/dentistry

Nebraska

Creighton University School of Dentistry
Verification of degrees
Telephone: Free of charge.
Written: Free of charge. Faxed upon request. Mail or fax requests, including signed release forms.
Electronic: Not provided.

> Office of the Registrar
> Creighton University School of Dentistry
> 2500 California Plaza
> Omaha, NEBRASKA 68178
> Telephone: 402/280-5060   402/280-2702 (Registrar's office)
> Fax: 402/280-5094
> Web site: www.cudental.edu

New Jersey

University of Medicine and Dentistry of New Jersey
Verification of degrees
Telephone: Free of charge.
Written: Free of charge. Faxed upon request. Mail or fax requests, including signed release forms.
Electronic: Free of charge. E-mail requests to lamettjw@umdnj.edu.

> Office of the Registrar
> University of Medicine and Dentistry of New Jersey
> 110 Bergen Street
> Newark, NEW JERSEY 07103
> Telephone: 973/972-4728 (Registrar's office)   973/972-4536 (Dean's office)
> Fax: 973/972-0309
> E-mail: lamettjw@umdnj.edu
> Web site: www.umdnj.edu/njdsweb

Dental Schools

New York

Columbia University School of Dental and Oral Surgery
Verification of degrees

Telephone: Not provided.
Written: Free of charge. Mail requests, including signed release forms, and each dentist's Social Security number, year of graduation and maiden name (if applicable).
Electronic: Not provided.

> Attention: Registrar Services
> Columbia University Student Administrative Services
> 630 W. 168th Street, Room 141, Box 45
> PNS 3-458
> New York, NEW YORK 10032
> Telephone: 212/305-8334
> Fax: 212/305-7134
> Web site: www.columbiasdoc.com

New York University College of Dentistry
Verification of degrees

Telephone: Not provided.
Written: Free of charge. Faxed upon request. Mail or fax requests, including dentist's name, Social Security number, years of graduation, and signed release forms.
Electronic: Not provided.

> Attention: Registrar
> New York University College of Dentistry
> 345 E. 24th Street
> New York, NEW YORK 10010
> Telephone: 212/998-9819
> Fax: 212/995-4240
> Web site: www.nyu.edu

State University of New York at Buffalo School of Dental Medicine
Verification of degrees

Telephone: Not provided.
Written: Free of charge. Faxed upon request. Mail or fax requests, including signed release forms.
Electronic: Not provided.

> Office of Student Affairs
> State University of New York at Buffalo School of Dental Medicine
> 327 Squire Hall
> 3435 Main Street
> Buffalo, NEW YORK 14214
> Telephone: 716/829-2839
> Fax: 716/833-3517
> E-mail: falter@buffalo.edu

North Carolina

University of North Carolina School of Dentistry
Verification of degrees

Telephone: Free of charge in emergency situations only.

Written: Free of charge. Faxed upon request in emergency situations only. Mail or fax requests, including signed release forms.

Electronic: Free of charge. E-mail requests to terry_barker@dentistry.unc.edu.

Office of Academic Affairs
University of North Carolina School of Dentistry
Old Dental Building Room 170E
Campus Box 7450
Chapel Hill, NORTH CAROLINA 27599-7450
Telephone: 919/966-4451
Fax: 919/966-5795
Web site: www.dent.unc.edu

Ohio

Case Western Reserve University School of Dentistry
Verification of degrees

Telephone: Not provided.

Written: $5 per verification. Mail requests, including signed release forms.

Electronic: Automated verification system available at Web site for students who graduated during 1993 or later.

Office of the Registrar
Case Western Reserve University School of Dentistry
2123 Abington Road
Cleveland, OHIO 44106-4905
Telephone: 216/368-3256
Fax: 216/368-6771
E-mail: bas3@po.cwru.edu
Web site: www.cwru.edu/dental/dent.html

Ohio State University College of Dentistry
Verification of degrees

Telephone: Free of charge. Limit two verifications per call. Degree confirmation only.

Written: Free of charge if mailed. Mail or fax requests, including signed release forms.

Electronic: Not provided.

Office of the Registrar
Ohio State University College of Dentistry
PO Box 182357
Columbus, OHIO 43218-2357
Telephone: 614/292-7768
Fax: 614/292-7619
Web site: www.dent.ohio-state.edu

Oklahoma

University of Oklahoma Health Sciences Center College of Dentistry
Verification of degrees

Telephone: Free of charge.
Written: Free of charge. Faxed upon request. Mail or fax requests, including signed release forms.
Electronic: Free of charge. E-mail requests to carla-lawson@ouhsc.edu.

Office of the Dean
University of Oklahoma Health Sciences Center College of Dentistry
PO Box 26901
Oklahoma City, OKLAHOMA 73190-3042
Telephone: 405/271-5444
Fax: 405/271-3423
E-mail: carla-lawson@ouhsc.edu
Web site: www.ouhsc.edu

Oregon

Oregon Health & Science University
Verification of degrees

Telephone: Free of charge.
Written: Free of charge. Faxed upon request. Mail or fax requests, including signed release forms.
Electronic: Free of charge. E-mail requests to badzinsk@ohsu.edu.

Office of Admissions and Student Affairs
OHSU School of Dentistry
611 Southwest Campus Drive
Portland, OREGON 97201-3097
Telephone: 503/494-5274
Fax: 503/494-6244
E-mail: badzinsk@ohsu.edu
Web site: www.ohsu.edu/sod

Pennsylvania

Temple University School of Dentistry
Verification of degrees

Telephone: Free of charge.
Written: Free of charge. Faxed upon request. Mail or fax requests, including signed release forms.
Electronic: Not provided.

Office of Academic Affairs
Temple University School of Dentistry
3223 N. Broad Street
Philadelphia, PENNSYLVANIA 19140
Telephone: 215/707-2800
Fax: 215/707-8174

University of Pennsylvania School of Dental Medicine
Verification of degrees
Telephone: Provided for credentialing agencies.
Written: Free of charge. Faxed upon request. Mail or fax requests, including signed release forms.
Electronic: Not provided.

> Office of Student Services
> University of Pennsylvania School of Dental Medicine
> 4001 Spruce Street
> Philadelphia, PENNSYLVANIA 19104-6003
> Telephone: 215/898-8940
> Fax: 215/898-5243

University of Pittsburgh, School of Dental Medicine
Verification of degrees
Telephone: Free of charge.
Written: $2 per verification. Mail requests.
Electronic: Not provided.

> Registrar's office
> University of Pittsburgh
> G-3 Thackeray Hall
> Pittsburgh, PENNSYLVANIA 15260
> Telephone: 412/624-7660   412/624-7635
> Fax: 412/624-9782
> E-mail: registrar@registrar.pitt.edu

Puerto Rico

University of Puerto Rico School of Dentistry
Verification of degrees
Telephone: Not provided.
Written: Free of charge. Mail or fax requests.
Electronic: Not provided.

> Office of the Registrar
> School of Dentistry
> Medical Sciences Campus
> University of Puerto Rico
> G.PO Box 365067
> San Juan, PUERTO RICO 00936-5067
> Telephone: 787/758-2525, Ext. 1105

South Carolina

Medical University of South Carolina College of Dental Medicine
Verification of degrees
Telephone: Free of charge.
Written: Free of charge. Faxed upon request. Mail or fax requests, including signed release forms.

Dental Schools

Electronic: Not provided.

> Office of the Dean
> Medical University of South Carolina College of Dental Medicine
> 173 Ashley Avenue
> Charleston, SOUTH CAROLINA 29425
> Telephone: 843/792-3811
> Fax: 843/792-1376
> E-mail: dechampr@musc.edu
> Web site: www.musc.edu

Tennessee

Meharry Medical College School of Dentistry
Verification of degrees

Telephone: Not provided.
Written: Free of charge. Faxed upon request. Mail or fax requests, including signed release forms.
Electronic: Not provided.

> Office of Admissions and Records
> Meharry Medical College School of Dentistry
> 1005 D. B. Todd Boulevard
> Nashville, TENNESSEE 37208
> Telephone: 615/327-6223
> Fax: 615/327-6228
> Web site: www.mmc.edu

University of Tennessee College of Dentistry
Verification of degrees

Telephone: Free of charge. Provide dentist's Social Security number and date of birth.
Written: Free of charge. Faxed upon request. Mail or fax requests, including signed release forms, and dentist's Social Security number and date of birth.
Electronic: Not provided.

> Office of Student Affairs
> University of Tennessee College of Dentistry
> 875 Union Avenue
> Memphis, TENNESSEE 38163
> Telephone: 901/448-6200
> Fax: 901/448-1625
> Web site: www.utmem.edu

Texas

Baylor College of Dentistry, Texas A&M University Health Science Center
Verification of degrees

Telephone: Not provided.
Written: Free of charge. Mail requests, including signed release forms.

Electronic: Not provided.

> Office of Admissions and Student Records
> Baylor College of Dentistry
> Texas A & M University Health Science Center
> PO Box 660677
> Dallas, TEXAS 75266-0677
> Telephone: 214/828-8230
> Fax: 214/874-4567
> E-mail: admissions@tambcd.edu
> Web site: www.tambcd.edu

University of Texas Health Science Center at San Antonio
Verification of degrees

Telephone: Free of charge. Limit five verifications per call.
Written: Free of charge. Faxed upon request. Mail or fax requests, including signed release forms.
Electronic: Not provided.

> Office of the Registrar
> University of Texas Health Science Center at San Antonio
> 7703 Floyd Curl Drive
> San Antonio, TEXAS 78229
> Telephone: 210/567-2674
> Fax: 210/567-2685
> E-mail: eblen@uthsca.edu
> Web site: www.uthscsa.edu

University of Texas, Health Science Center at Houston
Verification of degrees

Telephone: Free of charge.
Written: Free of charge. Mail or fax requests, including signed release forms.
Electronic: Not provided.

> Office of the Registrar
> University of Texas, Health Science Center at Houston-
> PO Box 20036
> Houston, TEXAS 77225
> Telephone: 713/500-3361 (Registrar's office)   713/500-4151
> Fax: 713/500-3356
> E-mail: studentaffairs@db.uth.tmc.edu
> Web site: www.uth.tmc.edu

Virginia

Virginia Commonwealth University School of Dentistry
Verification of degrees

Telephone: Not provided.
Written: $5 per verification. Faxed upon request. Mail or fax requests, including signed release forms.
Electronic: Not provided.

Office of the Dean
Virginia Commonwealth University School of Dentistry
PO Box 980566
Richmond, VIRGINIA 23298-0566
Telephone: 804/828-9184
Fax: 804/828-6072
E-mail: cssnyder@vcu.edu
Web site: www.dentistry.vcu.edu

Washington

University of Washington School of Dentistry
Verification of degrees
Telephone: Free of charge.
Written: Free of charge. Faxed upon request. Mail or fax requests, including signed release forms. Three days processing time for inquiries regarding pre-graduation dates prior to 1982.
Electronic: Verification available thru www.washington.edu/graduatedir/public/graduatedir.asp.

Office of the Dean
University of Washington School of Dentistry
Box 356365
D-322 Health Sciences Center
Seattle, WASHINGTON 98195-6365
Telephone: 206/543-5982 (Dean's office)   206/685-9484 (Student verification services)
Fax: 206/616-2612
Web site: www.dental.washington.edu

West Virginia

West Virginia University School of Dentistry
Verification of degrees
Telephone: Free of charge.
Written: Free of charge. Faxed upon request. Mail or fax requests, including signed release forms.
Electronic: Not provided.

Office of the Dean
West Virginia University School of Dentistry
Robert C. Byrd Health Science Center
PO Box 9400
Morgantown, WEST VIRGINIA 26506
Telephone: 304/293-2521
Fax: 304/293-2859

Wisconsin

Marquette University School of Dentistry
Verification of degrees
Telephone: Free of charge.
Written: Free of charge. Faxed upon request. Mail or fax requests, including signed release forms.

Electronic: Not provided.

> Marquette University School of Dentistry
> PO Box 1881
> Milwaukee, WISCONSIN 53201-1881
> Telephone: 414/288-7034
> Fax: 414/288-1773
> Web site: www.marquette.edu

Podiatry Schools

Podiatry Schools

California

California College of Podiatric Medicine
Verification of degrees

Telephone: Free of charge.
Written: $5 per verification. Mail requests, including signed release forms and payment.
Electronic: Not provided.

>Office of the Registrar
>California College of Podiatric Medicine
>1210 Scott Street
>San Francisco, CALIFORNIA 94115
>Telephone: 415/292-0414
>Fax: 415/292-0439
>E-mail: smarshal@ccpm.edu

Florida

Barry University, School of Graduate Medical Sciences
Verification of degrees

Telephone: Free of charge.
Written: Free of charge. Faxed upon request in emergency situations only. Mail requests, including signed release forms.
Electronic: Not provided.

>Office of the Registrar
>Adrian Hall, Room 108
>Barry University
>11300 NE Second Avenue
>Miami Shores, FLORIDA 33161
>Telephone: 305/899-3860
>Fax: 305/899-3946
>E-mail: registrar@mail.barry.edu
>Web site: www.barry.edu

Illinois

Dr. William M. Scholl College of Podiatric Medicine
Verification of degrees

Telephone: Free of charge. Only verifies year of graduation.
Written: Free of charge. Mail requests, including signed release forms.
Electronic: Not provided.

>Office of the Registrar
>Dr. William M. Scholl College of Podiatric Medicine
>1001 N. Dearborn Street
>Chicago, ILLINOIS 60610
>Telephone: 800/843-3059
>Web site: scholl.edu

Chapter 5

Ohio

Ohio College of Podiatric Medicine
Verification of degrees

Telephone: Free of charge.

Written: Free of charge. Faxed upon request in emergency situations only. Mail or fax requests, including signed release forms. Give plenty of notice.

Electronic: Free of charge. E-mail requests to address listed.

> Student Records Office
> Ohio College of Podiatric Medicine
> 10515 Carnegie Avenue
> Cleveland, OHIO 44106-3081
> Telephone: 216/707-8054
> Fax: 216/707-8097
> E-mail: shastings@ocpm.edu
> Web site: www.ocpm.edu

Pennsylvania

Temple University School of Podiatric Medicine
Verification of degrees

Telephone: Not provided.

Written: Free of charge. Faxed upon request in emergency situations only. Mail or fax requests, including signed release forms.

Electronic: Not provided.

> Office of the Registrar
> Temple University School of Podiatric Medicine
> Eighth and Race Streets
> Philadelphia, PENNSYLVANIA 19107
> Telephone: 215/625-5444
> Fax: 215/627-2815
> Web site: www.temple.edu

Chiropractic Schools

Australia

Macquarie University, Department of Chiropractic
Annual report of licensed physicians

Telephone: Not provided.
Written: Not provided.
Electronic: Not provided.

> Department of Chiropractic
> Building E7A, Suite 222
> Macquarie University, New South Wales 02109
> AUSTRALIA
> Telephone: +61-2-9850-9380
> Fax: +61-2-9850-9389
> E-mail: chiro@mq.edu.au
> Web site: www.chiro.mq.edu.au

Royal Melbourne Institute of Technology Chiropractic Unit
Annual report of licensed physicians

Telephone: Not provided.
Written: Not provided.
Electronic: Not provided.

> Dept. of Chiropractic Osteopathy and Complementary Medicine
> Royal Melbourne Institute of Technology
> GPO Box 71
> Bundoora 03083
> AUSTRALIA
> Telephone: 011-61-3-9925-7596
> Fax: 011-61-3-9467-2794

California

Life Chiropractic College West
Verification of degrees

Telephone: Not provided.
Written: Free of charge. Faxed upon request. Mail or fax requests, including signed release forms.
Electronic: Information available at our Web site.

> Office of the Registrar
> Life Chiropractice College West
> 25001 Industrial Boulevard
> Haywood, CALIFORNIA 94545
> Telephone: 510/780-4500
> Fax: 510/780-4525
> E-mail: info@lifewest.edu
> Web site: www.lifewest.edu

Palmer College of Chiropractic West
Verification of degrees
Telephone: Not provided.
Written: $25 per verification. Mail requests, including signed release forms and payment.
Electronic: Not provided.

> Office of the Registrar
> Palmer College of Chiropractic West
> 90 E. Tasman Drive
> San Jose, CALIFORNIA 95134
> Telephone: 408/944-6024
> Fax: 408/944-6032
> Web site: www.palmer.edu

Southern California University of Health Sciences, Los Angeles College of Chiropractic
Notes: Also home to College of Acupuncture and Oriental Medicine.
Verification of degrees
Telephone: Not provided.
Written: $20 per verification. Mail requests, including signed release forms and payment.
Electronic: Not provided.

> Southern California University of Health Sciences
> Office of the Registrar   Attention: Credentialing request
> Los Angeles College of Chiropractic
> PO Box 1166
> 16200 E. Amber Valley Drive
> Whittier, CALIFORNIA 90609-1166
> Telephone: 562/947-8755 ext. 7212
> Fax: 562/902-3306
> E-mail: registrar@scuhs.edu
> Web site: www.scuhs.edu

Canada

Canadian Memorial Chiropractic College
Verification of degrees
Telephone: Free of charge.
Written: Free of charge. Faxed upon request. Mail or fax requests, including signed release forms.
Electronic: Not provided.

> Office of the Registrar
> Canadian Memorial Chiropractic College
> 1900 Bayview Avenue
> Toronto, ONTARIO M4G 3E6
> Canada
> Telephone: 416/482-2340
> Fax: 416/488-0470
> Web site: www.cmcc.ca

Chiropractic Schools

Connecticut

University of Bridgeport College of Chiropractic
Verification of degrees

Telephone:	Not provided.
Written:	Free of charge. Faxed upon request. Mail or fax requests, including signed release forms.
Electronic:	Not provided.

Associate of Academic Affairs
College of Chiropractic
University of Bridgeport
75 Linden Avenue
Bridgeport, CONNECTICUT 06601
Telephone: 203/576-4336
Fax: 203/576-4351
E-mail: aonorato@bridgeport.edu
Web site: www.bridgeport.edu

England (UK)

Anglo-European College of Chiropractic
Annual report of licensed physicians

Telephone:	Not provided.
Written:	Not provided.
Electronic:	Not provided.

Attention: Academic Registrar
Academic Registry
Anglo-European College of Chiropractic
13-15 Parkwood Road
Bournemouth, Dorset BH5 2DF
ENGLAND
Telephone: +44(0) 1202 436200
Fax: +44(0) 1202 436312
E-mail: aecc@aecc-chiropractic.ac.uk

Georgia

Life University
Notes: Please check with Life University regarding accreditation for those who graduated in or after 2002.
Verification of degrees

Telephone:	Not provided.
Written:	$20 per verification. Mail requests, including signed release forms and payment. Fax available with credit card payment only.
Electronic:	Not provided.

Life University
Attention: Registrars Office
1269 Barclay Circle
Marietta, GEORGIA 30060

Telephone: 770/426-2780
Fax: 770/426-2872
Web site: www.life.edu

Indiana

Northwestern Health Sciences University
Verification of degrees

Telephone: Free of charge. Provide chiropractor's name, Social Security number, and student identification number.
Written: Free of charge. Faxed upon request. Mail or fax requests, including signed release forms.
Electronic: Not provided.

> Office of the Registrar
> Northwestern Health Sciences University
> 2501 W. 84th Street
> Bloomington, INDIANA 55431-1599
> Telephone: 612/888-4777, Ext. 440
> Fax: 612/888-6713

Iowa

Palmer College of Chiropractic
Notes: Requires a 30-day turnaround time after receipt of written verification request.
Verification of degrees

Telephone: Not provided.
Written: $30 per verification. Mail or fax requests, including signed release forms and payment.
Electronic: Not provided.

> Attention: Bridgett M. Lance, Academic Records Coordinator
> Office of the Registrar
> Palmer College of Chiropractic
> 1000 Brady Street
> Davenport, IOWA 52803-5287
> Telephone: 563/884-5685
> Fax: 563/884-5864
> E-mail: lance_b@palmer.edu
> Web site: www.palmer.edu

Missouri

Cleveland Chiropractic College
Verification of degrees

Telephone: Not provided.
Written: Free of charge. Faxed upon request. Mail or fax requests, including signed release forms.
Electronic: Not provided.

> Office of Student Services
> Cleveland Chiropractic College
> 6401 Rockhill Road
> Kansas City, MISSOURI 64131

Chiropractic Schools

Telephone: 816/501-0100
Fax: 861/361-0272
Web site: www.cleveland.edu

Logan College of Chiropractic
Verification of degrees

Telephone: Not provided.
Written: Free of charge. Faxed upon request. Mail or fax requests, including signed release forms.
Electronic: Not provided.

Office of the Registrar
Logan College of Chiropractic
1851 Schoettler Road
PO Box 1065
Chesterfield, MISSOURI 63006-1065
Telephone: 636/227-2100, Ext. 139
Fax: 636/207-2431
Web site: www.logan.edu

New York

New York Chiropractic College
Verification of degrees

Telephone: Not provided.
Written: Free of charge. Faxed upon request. Mail or fax requests, including signed release forms, and chiropractor's Social Security number and date of graduation.
Electronic: Not provided.

New York Chiropractic College
PO Box 800
2360 State Route 89
Seneca Falls, NEW YORK 13148-0800
Telephone: 315/568-3000
Fax: 315/568-3015
E-mail: enrollnow@nycc.edu
Web site: www.nycc.edu

Oregon

Western States Chiropractic College
Verification of degrees

Telephone: Not provided.
Written: Free of charge. Faxed upon request. Mail or fax requests.
Electronic: Not provided.

Office of the Registrar
Western States Chiropractic College
2900 NE 132nd Avenue
Portland, OREGON 97230

Telephone: 503/251-5706
Fax: 503/251-5723
E-mail: registrar@wschiro.edu
Web site: www.wschiro.edu

South Carolina

Sherman College of Straight Chiropractic
Verification of degrees

Telephone:	Free of charge.
Written:	Free of charge. Faxed upon request. Mail or fax requests, including signed release forms.
Electronic:	Free of charge. E-mail requests to cnendel@sherman.edu.

Office of the Registrar
Sherman College of Straight Chiropractic
PO Box 1452
Spartanburg, SOUTH CAROLINA 29304
Telephone: 864/578-8770
Fax: 864/599-4860
E-mail: cnendel@sherman.edu
Web site: www.sherman.edu

Texas

Parker College of Chiropractic
Verification of degrees

Telephone:	Not provided.
Written:	$20 per verification. Mail requests, including signed release forms and payment.
Electronic:	Not provided.

Office of the Registrar
Parker College of Chiropractic
2500 Walnut Hill Lane
Dallas, TEXAS 75229
Telephone: 972/438-6732
Fax: 214/902-2412
E-mail: lknight@parkercc.edu

Texas Chiropractic College
Verification of degrees

Telephone:	Not provided.
Written:	$25 per verification. Faxed upon request. Mail or fax requests, including signed release forms.
Electronic:	Not provided.

Office of the Registrar
Texas Chiropractic College
5912 Spencer Highway

Pasadena, TEXAS 77505-1699
Telephone: 281/998-6015
Fax: 281/991-4871
E-mail: mbowman@txchiro.edu
Web site: www.txchiro.edu

Physician Assistant Programs

Physician Assistant Programs

Alabama

University of Alabama at Birmingham, Surgical Physician Assistant Program
Verification of degrees

Telephone: Free of charge; prefer written request.
Written: Free of charge. Faxed upon request. Mail or fax requests, including signed release forms.
Electronic: Free of charge. E-mail requests to wilsonc@shrp.uab.edu.

> Surgical Assistant Program
> School of Health Related Professions
> University of Alabama at Birmingham
> Richard M. Scrushy Building
> 1705 University Boulevard
> Birmingham, ALABAMA 35294-1212
> Telephone: 205/934-4605
> Fax: 205/934-3780
> Web site: www.uab.edu/surgicalpa

California

Charles R. Drew University of Medicine and Science, Physician Assistant Program
Verification of degrees

Telephone: Not provided.
Written: Free of charge. Faxed upon request. Mail or fax requests, including signed release forms, and physician assistant's Social Security number and year of graduation.
Electronic: Not provided.

> College of Allied Health
> Charles R. Drew University of Medicine and Science
> 1731 E. 120th Street
> Los Angeles, CALIFORNIA 90059
> Telephone: 323/563-5879
> Fax: 323/-563-4833
> Web site: www.cdrewu.edu

Stanford University/Foothill College School of Medicine, Primary Care Associate Program
Verification of degrees

Telephone: Not provided.
Written: Free of charge. Faxed upon request. Mail or fax requests, including signed release forms.
Electronic: Visit Web site for more information.

> Primary Care Associate Program
> Stanford University School of Medicine
> 703 Welch Road, Suite F-1
> Palo Alto, CALIFORNIA 94304-1760
> Telephone: 650/723-7043
> Fax: 650/723-9692
> Web site: www.stanford.edu/dept/medsm/pca/tosc.html

University of California-Davis Medical Center, Family Nurse Practitioner/Physician Assistant Program
Verification of degrees

Telephone: Provided for graduation date only.
Written: Free of charge. Faxed upon request. Mail or fax requests, including signed release forms.
Electronic: Provided for graduation date only.

> Family Nurse Practitioner/Physician Assistant Program
> Department of Family and Community Medicine
> University of California-Davis Medical Center
> 2516 Stockton Boulevard, Room 254
> Sacramento, CALIFORNIA 95817
> Telephone: 916/734-3551
> Fax: 916/452-2112
> E-mail: isabel.schmitz@ucdmc.ucdavis.edu
> Web site: www.fnppa.ucdavis.edu

University of Southern California Keck School of Medicine, Primary Care Physician Assistant Program
Verification of degrees

Telephone: Not provided.
Written: Free of charge. Faxed upon request. Mail or fax requests, including signed release forms.
Electronic: Not provided.

> Primary Care Physician Assistant Program
> University of Southern California Keck School of Medicine
> 1000 S. Freemont Avenue
> Building A6, Room 6429
> Alhambra, CALIFORNIA 91803
> Telephone: 626/457-4255
> Fax: 626/457-4260
> Web site: www.usc.edu/medicine/pa

Western University of Health Sciences
Verification of degrees

Telephone: Free of charge.
Written: Free of charge and faxed upon request. Mail or fax requests, including signed release forms.
Electronic: Not provided.

> Western University of Health Sciences
> Student Affairs Office
> 309 E. Second Street
> Pomona, CALIFORNIA 91766-1854
> Telephone: 909/623-6116 (main campus)   909/469-5340 (Student Affairs)
> Fax: 909/469-5425
> Web site: www.westernu.edu

Physician Assistant Programs

Colorado

University of Colorado Health Science Center, Child Health Associate/Physician Assistant Program
Verification of certificates

Telephone:	Not provided.
Written:	Free of charge. Faxed upon request. Mail or fax requests, including signed release forms, and physician assistant's Social Security number and year of graduation.
Electronic:	Not provided.

Child Health Associate/Physician Assistant Program
University of Colorado Health Science Center
Box F-543
PO Box 6508
Aurora, COLORADO 80045-0508
Telephone: 303/315-7963
Fax: 303/724-1350
E-mail: chapa-info@uchsc.edu
Web site: www.uchsc.edu/chapa

Connecticut

Yale University School of Medicine, Physician Associate Program
Verification of degrees

Telephone:	Free of charge.
Written:	Free of charge. Faxed upon request. Mail or fax requests, including signed release forms and physician assistant's year of graduation.
Electronic:	Not provided.

Physician Associate Program
Yale University School of Medicine
47 College Street, Suite 220
New Haven, CONNECTICUT 06510
Telephone: 203/785-2860
Fax: 203/785-3601
E-mail: janet.liscio@yale.edu
Web site: www.info.med.yale.edu/phyassoc

District of Columbia

George Washington University, Physician Assistant Program
Verification of degrees

Telephone:	Not provided.
Written:	Free of charge. Faxed upon request. Mail or fax requests, including signed release forms.
Electronic:	Not provided.

> George Washington University
> 2175 K Street NW, Suite 820
> Washington, DISTRICT OF COLUMBIA 20037
> Telephone: 202/530-2390   202/530-2389 (Director)
> Fax: 202/530-2360
> Web site: www.gwu.edu/gwu_pa

Howard University, Physician Assistant Program
Verification of degrees

Telephone:	Not provided.
Written:	Free of charge. Mail or fax requests, including signed release forms.
Electronic:	Not provided.

> Physician Assistant Department
> Division of Allied Health Sciences
> Howard University
> Annex II Room 119
> 6th and Bryant Streets NW
> Washington, DISTRICT OF COLUMBIA 20059
> Telephone: 202/806-7536
> Fax: 202/806-4476
> E-mail: mbarnard@howard.edu
> Web site: www.howard.edu

Florida

Nova Southeastern University, Physician Assistant Program
Verification of degrees

Telephone:	Free of charge in emergency situations only; prefer written request.
Written:	Free of charge. Faxed upon request. Mail or fax requests, including signed release forms.
Electronic:	Not provided.

> Office of the Registrar
> College of Allied Health
> Nova Southeastern University
> 3301 College Avenue
> Fort Lauderdale, FLORIDA 33314
> Telephone: 954/262-7271

Fax: 954/262-7265
E-mail: djeanne@nova.edu
Web site: www.nova.edu

University of Florida, Physician Assistant Program
Notes: All information except degree awarded and date awarded requires signed release form.
Verification of degrees
Telephone: Free of charge.
Written: Free of charge.
Electronic: Not provided.

Physician Assistant Program
University of Florida
PO Box 100176
Gainesville, FLORIDA 32610-0176
Telephone: 352/265-7955
Fax: 352/265-7996
E-mail: heikkpj@medicine.ufl.edu
Web site: www.med.ufl.edu/pap/apply

Georgia

Emory University School of Medicine, Physician Assistant Program
Verification of degrees
Telephone: Free of charge.
Written: Free of charge. Faxed upon request. Mail or fax requests, including signed release forms.
Electronic: Not provided.

Physician Assistant Program
Emory University School of Medicine
1462 Clifton Road NE, Suite 280
Atlanta, GEORGIA 30322
Telephone: 404/727-7825
Fax: 404/727-7836
Web site: www.pa.emory.edu

Medical College of Georgia, Physician Assistant Program
Verification of degrees
Telephone: Free of charge.
Written: Free of charge. Faxed upon request. Mail or fax requests, including signed release forms and physician assistant's Social Security number.
Electronic: Not provided.

Office of the Registrar AA 171
Medical College of Georgia
Augusta, GEORGIA 30912-7315
Telephone: 706/721-2201
Fax: 706/721-0186
E-mail: registrar@mail.mcg.edu
Web site: www.mcg.edu

Idaho

Idaho State University, Physician Assistant Program
Annual report of licensed physicians

Telephone: Not provided.
Written: Free of charge.
Electronic: Not provided.

> Physician Assistant Program
> Idaho State University
> 1021 Red Hill Road, Room 207
> Campus Box 8253
> Pocatello, IDAHO 83209
> Telephone: 208/282-4726
> Fax: 208/282-4969
> E-mail: kingnore@isu.edu
> Web site: www.isu.edu/paprog

Illinois

American Association of Medical Assistants
Annual report of licensed physicians

Telephone: Not provided.
Written: Not provided.
Electronic: Information available on our Web site.

> American Association of Medical Assistants
> 20 N. Wacker Drive, Suite 1575
> Chicago, ILLINOIS 60606-2903
> Telephone: 312/899-1500
> Fax: 312/899-1259
> Web site: www.aama-ntl.org

Finch University of Health Sciences, Chicago Medical School
Verification of degrees

Telephone: Free of charge.
Written: Free of charge. Faxed upon request in emergency situations only. Mail requests, including signed release forms. Fax requests in emergency situations only.
Electronic: Not provided.

> Office of the Registrar
> Chicago Medical School
> Finch University of Health Sciences
> 3333 Green Bay Road
> North Chicago, ILLINOIS 60064
> Telephone: 847/578-3229
> Fax: 847/578-3284
> E-mail: pratth@finchcms.edu
> Web site: www.suhscms.edu

Physician Assistant Programs

Malcolm X College, Physician Assistant Program
Verification of degrees

Telephone: Free of charge.
Written: Free of charge. Faxed upon request. Mail or fax requests, including signed release forms. Fee charged for transcripts. Call for prices.
Electronic: Not provided.

Physician Assistant Program
Malcolm X College
1900 W. Van Buren Street, Room 3241
Chicago, ILLINOIS 60612
Telephone: 312/850-7268
Fax: 312/850-3538
Web site: www.ccc.edu

Midwestern University
Verification of degrees

Telephone: Free of charge.
Written: Free of charge. Faxed upon request. Mail or fax requests, including signed release forms. Give plenty of notice.
Electronic: Not provided.

Office of the Registrar
Midwestern University
555 31st Street
Downers Grove, ILLINOIS 60515
Telephone: 630/515-6074
Fax: 630/515-7140
E-mail: rstell@midwestern.edu
Web site: www.midwestern.edu

Southern Illinois University, Physician Assistant Program
Notes: Pending accreditation as of May 2002.
Annual report of licensed physicians

Telephone: Not provided.
Written: Free of charge.
Electronic: Not provided.

Physician Assistant Program
Southern Illinois University
Lindegren Hall 129, Mail Code 6516
Carbondale, ILLINOIS 62901-6516
Telephone: 618/453-1151
Fax: 618/453-7216
E-mail: pawebmaster@som.siu.edu
Web site: www.mccoy.lib.siu.edu.~paprogram

Indiana

University of Saint Francis (formerly Lutheran College of Health Professions)
Verification of degrees

Telephone: Free of charge.
Written: Free of charge. Mail requests, including physician assistant names and Social Security numbers.
Electronic: Free of charge.

> Physician Assistant Program
> University of Saint Francis
> 2701 Spring Street
> Fort Wayne, INDIANA 46808
> Telephone: 260/434-7657
> Fax: 260/434-7585
> E-mail: kgraham@sf.edu
> Web site: www.sf.edu

Iowa

Des Moines University, Osteopathic Medical Center
Verification of degrees

Telephone: Free of charge.
Written: Free of charge if mailed. Faxed upon request for $10 per verification. Mail or fax requests, including signed release forms.
Electronic: Not provided.

> Registrar's Office
> Des Moines University, Osteopathic Medical Center
> 3200 Grand Avenue
> Des Moines, IOWA 50312
> Telephone: 515/271-1460
> Fax: 515/271-1578
> E-mail: registrar@dmu.edu
> Web site: www.dmu.edu

University of Iowa College of Medicine, Physician Assistant Program
Verification of degrees

Telephone: Free of charge.
Written: Free of charge. Faxed upon request. Phone, mail, or fax requests.
Electronic: Free of charge. E-mail requests to janet-steenlage@uiowa.edu.

> Physician Assistant Program
> University of Iowa College of Medicine
> 5167 Westlawn
> Iowa City, IOWA 52242-1008
> Telephone: 319/335-8922
> Fax: 319/335-8923
> E-mail: diane-rosene@uiowa.edu
> Web site: www.medicine.uiowa.edu/pa/pa.htm

Kansas

Wichita State University, Physician Assistant Program
Verification of degrees

Telephone: Free of charge.
Written: Free of charge. Faxed upon request. Mail requests, including signed release forms. Fax requests in emergency situations only.
Electronic: Not provided.

Physician Assistant Program
College of Health Professions
Campus Box 43
Wichita State University
Wichita, KANSAS 67260-0043
Telephone: 316/978-3011
Fax: 316/978-3025
E-mail: Accessed through Web site.
Web site: www.witchita.edu

Kentucky

University of Kentucky, Physician Assistant Program
Verification of degrees

Telephone: Free of charge.
Written: Free of charge. Faxed upon request, followed by a mailed hard copy. Mail or fax requests, including signed release forms.
Electronic: Not provided.

Physician Assistant Studies
University of Kentucky Medical Center
121 Washington Avenue, Suite 118
Lexington, KENTUCKY 40536-0003
Telephone: 859/323-1100, Ext. 226
Fax: 859/323-5986
Web site: www.uky.edu

Maryland

Naval School of Health Sciences, Physician Assistant Program
Verification of degrees

Telephone: Free of charge.
Written: Free of charge. Mail requests, including signed release forms.
Electronic: Not provided.

Commanding Officer
Attention: Registrar
Naval School of Health Sciences
8901 Wisconsin Avenue

Betheseda, MARYLAND 20889-5611
Telephone: 301/295-4818
Fax: 301/295-4823
E-mail: jfbehnke@nsh10.med.navy.mil
Web site: www.nshs.med.navy.mil

The Community College of Baltimore County, Physician Assistant Program
Verification of degrees
Telephone: Free of charge.
Written: Free of charge. Faxed upon request. Mail or fax requests, including signed release forms.
Electronic: Free of charge.

Physician Assistant Program
CCBC Essex
7201 Rossville Boulevard
Baltimore, MARYLAND 21237
Telephone: 410/780-6159
Fax: 410/780-6405
Web site: ccbc.cc.md.us

Massachusetts

Northeastern University Physician Assistant Program
Notes: Offers a two-year graduate program for Master's Degree in Physician Assistant studies.
Verification of degrees
Telephone: Free of charge.
Written: Free of charge. Mail requests, including signed release forms.
Electronic: Not provided.

Physician Assistant Program
Northeastern University
202 Robinson Hall
Boston, MASSACHUSETTS 02115
Telephone: 617/373-3195
Web site: www.neu.edu/bouve/department/pa/pap.html

Michigan

University of Detroit Mercy Physician Assistant Program
Verification of degrees
Telephone: Free of charge.
Written: Free of charge. Mail or fax requests including signed release forms.
Electronic: Not provided.

Office of the Registrar
University of Detroit Mercy
4001 W. McNichols
PO Box 19900
Detroit, MICHIGAN 48219-0900

Physician Assistant Programs

Telephone: 313/993-3313
Fax: 313/993-3317
E-mail: registrar@udmercy.edu
Web site: www.udmercy.edu

Western Michigan University, Physician Assistant Program
Verification of degrees MD only

Telephone:	Free of charge. Limit three verifications per call.
Written:	Free of charge. Mail requests, including signed release forms and as much information as possible.
Electronic:	Not provided.

Western Michigan University
Office of the Registrar
1903 W. Michigan Avenue
Kalamazoo, MICHIGAN 49008
Telephone: 616/387-4300
Web site: www.wmich.edu/registrar

Missouri

Saint Louis University, Physician Assistant Program
Verification of degrees

Telephone:	Free of charge.
Written:	Free of charge. Faxed upon request. Mail or fax requests, including signed release forms.
Electronic:	Not provided.

Physician Assistant Program
School of Allied Health Professions
Saint Louis University
3437 Caroline Street
Saint Louis, MISSOURI 63104
Telephone: 314/577-8521
Fax: 314/577-8503
Web site: www.slu.edu

Nebraska

Interservice Physician Assistant Program
Notes: Program at Fort Sam Houston in San Antonio. Active duty military students must complete one year at Army's Academy of Health Care Sciences; then one year at military or affiliated medical facilities. University of Nebraska awards B.S. degrees.

Verification of degrees

Telephone:	Free of charge.
Written:	Free of charge. Faxed upon request. Mail or fax requests.
Electronic:	Verification available via e-mail.

Physician Assistant Program
University of Nebraska Medical Center
984300 Nebraska Medical Center
Omaha, NEBRASKA 68198-4300

Telephone: 402/559-2742
Fax: 402/559-5356
E-mail: aflaski@unmc.edu

University of Nebraska Medical Center, Physician Assistant Program
Verification of degrees

Telephone:	Free of charge.
Written:	Free of charge. Faxed upon request. Mail or fax requests.
Electronic:	Free of charge.

Physician Assistant Program
University of Nebraska Medical Center
984300 Nebraska Medical Center
Omaha, NEBRASKA 68198-4300
Telephone: 402/559-9495
Fax: 402/559-5356
E-mail: nsimmons@unmc.edu
Web site: unmc.edu/alliedhealth/pa

New Jersey

American Association of Surgical Physician Assistants
Verification of membership

Telephone:	Not provided.
Written:	Not provided.
Electronic:	Not provided.

American Association of Surgical Physician Assistants
PO Box 867
Bernardsville, NEW JERSEY 07924
Telephone: 888/882-2772
Fax: 732/805-9582
E-mail: theaaspa@aol.com
Web site: www.aaspa.com

University of Medicine and Dentistry of New Jersey at Piscataway, Physician Assistant Program
Verification of degrees

Telephone:	Not provided.
Written:	Free of charge. Faxed upon request. Mail or fax requests including signed release forms.
Electronic:	Not provided.

Physician Assistant Program
University of Medicine and Dentistry of New Jersey
675 Hoes Lane
Piscataway, NEW JERSEY 08854-5635
Telephone: 732/235-4445
Fax: 732/235-4820
Web site: www2.umdnj.edu/paweb

Physician Assistant Programs

University of Medicine and Dentistry of New Jersey, Physician Assistant Program
Annual report of licensed physicians

Telephone: Free of charge.
Written: Free of charge. Mail or fax requests, including signed release forms.
Electronic: Not provided.

> University of Medicine and Dentristy of New Jersey
> 65 Bergen Street
> University Heights
> Newark, NEW JERSEY 07107-3001
> Telephone: 973/972-5954
> Fax: 973/972-7157
> Web site: www.umdnj.edu

New Mexico

The University of New Mexico School of Medicine, Physician Assistant Program
Notes: Provisional accreditation: April 1997. First graduating class: 1999.
Annual report of licensed physicians

Telephone: Not provided.
Written: Not provided.
Electronic: Free of charge.

> Physician Assistant Program
> Department of Family and Community Medicine
> The University of New Mexico School of Medicine
> 2400 Tucker NE
> Albuquerque, NEW MEXICO 87131-5241
> Telephone: 505/272-9678
> Fax: 505/272-9828
> E-mail: paprogram@salud.unm.edu
> Web site: hsc.unm.edu/pap/

New York

Albany Hudson Valley, Physician Assistant Program
Verification of degrees

Telephone: Not provided.
Written: Free of charge. Faxed upon request. Mail or fax requests, including signed release forms.
Electronic: Not provided.

> Physician Assistant Program
> Albany Medical College
> 47 New Scotland Avenue
> Albany, NEW YORK 12208-3479
> Telephone: 518/262-5251
> Fax: 518/262-6698
> E-mail: dalsr@mail.amc.edu
> Web site: www.hvcc.edu

CUNY Harlem Hospital Center, Physician Assistant Program
Verification of degrees

Telephone: Free of charge. Must speak with Director.
Written: Free of charge. Mail requests, including signed release forms.
Electronic: Not provided.

> Physician Assistant Program
> CUNY Harlem Hospital Center
> 506 Lenox Avenue
> WP Building, Room 609
> New York, NEW YORK 10037
> Telephone: 212/939-2525
> Fax: 212/939-2529
> E-mail: paprog@ccny.cuny.edu
> Web site: www.cuny.edu

D'Youville College, Physician Assistant Program
Verification of degrees

Telephone: Free of charge.
Written: Free of charge. Faxed upon request. Mail or fax requests, including signed release forms.
Electronic: Not provided.

> Office of the Registrar
> D'Youville College
> 320 Porter Avenue
> Buffalo, NEW YORK 14201
> Telephone: 716/881-7626
> Fax: 716/881-7622
> E-mail: smithwb@dyc.edu
> Web site: www.dyc.edu

Rochester Institute of Technology, Physician Assistant Program
Verification of degrees

Telephone: Free of charge.
Written: Free of charge. Faxed upon request. Mail or fax requests, including signed release forms and physician assistant's Social Security number.
Electronic: Not provided.

> Office of the Registrar
> George Eastman Building
> Rochester Institute of Technology
> 27 Lomb Memorial Drive
> Rochester, NEW YORK 14623-5603
> Telephone: 716/475-2821
> Fax: 716/475-7005
> E-mail: 605ask@rit.edu
> Web site: www.rit.edu

Sisters of Charity Medical Center, Physician Assistant Program
Verification of degrees
Telephone: Not provided.
Written: Free of charge. Faxed upon request. Mail or fax requests, including signed release forms.
Electronic: Not provided.

>Physician Assistant Program
>Sisters of Charity Medical Center
>Bayley Seton Campus
>75 Vanderbilt Avenue
>Staten Island, NEW YORK 10304-3850
>Telephone: 718/354-5570
>Fax: 718/354-6146

State University of New York at Stony Brook, School of Health Technology & Management, Physician Assistant Program
Verification of degrees
Telephone: Free of charge. Please include year of graduation.
Written: Free of charge. Faxed upon request. Mail or fax requests, including signed release forms.
Electronic: Free of charge. E-mail requests to bhoos@notes.cc.sunysb.edu or aperrino@notes.cc.sunysb.edu.

>Physician Assistant Program
>School of Health Technology & Management
>SUNY-Stony Brook
>HSC L2-052
>Stony Brook, NEW YORK 11794-8202
>Telephone: 631/444-3190
>Fax: 631/444-7621
>E-mail: paprogram@notes.cc.sunysb.edu
>Web site: www.uhmc.sunysb.edu/shtm

SUNY Downstate Medical Center
Verification of degrees
Telephone: Not provided.
Written: Free of charge. Faxed upon request. Mail or fax requests, including signed release forms.
Electronic: Not provided.

>Registrar's Office
>SUNY Downstate Medical Center
>450 Clarkson Avenue
>Box 98
>Brooklyn, NEW YORK 11203
>Telephone: 718/270-4551 (Registrar's Office)
>Fax: 718/270-7592
>E-mail: sls.downstate@edu/registrar
>Web site: www.downstate.edu

The Brooklyn Hospital Center Long Island University, Physician Assistant Program

Notes: Degree programs offered for Bachelor of Science, Physician Assistant.

Verification of degrees

Telephone:	Free of charge.
Written:	Free of charge. Faxed upon request. Mail or fax requests, including signed release forms.
Electronic:	Not provided.

Physician Assistant Program
Brooklyn Hospital Center Long Island University
121 DeKalb Avenue
Brooklyn, NEW YORK 11201
Telephone: 718/260-2780
Fax: 718/260-2790
E-mail: tbhcpap@aol.com
Web site: www.liu.edu

Touro College, Physician Assistant Program

Verification of degrees

Telephone:	Not provided.
Written:	Free of charge. Mail requests including signed release forms.
Electronic:	Not provided.

Physician Assistant Program
Division of Health Sciences
Touro College
1700 Union Boulevard, Room 212
Bayshore, NEW YORK 11706
Telephone: 631/665-1600
Fax: 632/665-6086
Web site: www.touro.edu

Weill Cornell Medical College, Physician Assistant Program

Verification of degrees

Telephone:	Not provided.
Written:	Free of charge. Faxed upon request. Mail or fax requests, including signed release forms, and physician assistant's Social Security number, date of birth, and year of graduation.
Electronic:	Not provided.

Physician Assistant Program
Weill Cornell Medical College
1300 York Avenue, Box 195, Room F1917
New York, NEW YORK 10021
Telephone: 212/746-5134
Fax: 212/746-0407
Web site: www.med.cornell.edu/pa

North Carolina

Duke University Medical Center, Physician Assistant Program
Verification of degrees

Telephone:	Free of charge.
Written:	Free of charge. Faxed upon request (followed by mailed hard copy). Mail, phone, or fax requests.
Electronic:	Information available on our Web site.

Department of Community & Family Medicine
Duke University Medical Center
DUMC 3848
Durham, NORTH CAROLINA 27710
Telephone: 919/681-3155
Fax: 919/681-3371
E-mail: paadmission@mc.duke.edu
Web site: www.pa.mc.duke.edu

Wake Forest University Health Sciences, Physician Assistant Program
Verification of degrees

Telephone:	Free of charge.
Written:	Free of charge. Faxed upon request. Mail or fax requests, including signed release forms.
Electronic:	Not provided.

Physician Assistant Program
Wake Forest University Health Sciences
111 Chestnut Street-Victoria Hall
Winston-Salem, NORTH CAROLINA 27101
Telephone: 336/716-2023
Fax: 336/716-4432
E-mail: kscales@wsubmc.edu
Web site: www.wfmbmc.edu

North Dakota

University of North Dakota School of Medicine, Physician Assistant Program
Verification of certificates

Telephone:	Free of charge.
Written:	Free of charge. Faxed upon request. Mail or fax requests, including signed release forms.
Electronic:	Provided if signed release waiver from student.

Physician Assistant Program
Department of Community Medicine and Rural Health
University of North Dakota School of Medicine
PO Box 9037
Grand Forks, NORTH DAKOTA 58202-9037
Telephone: 701/777-2344
Fax: 701/777-2389
E-mail: mcdaniel@medicine.nodak.edu
Web site: www.med.und.nodak.edu

Ohio

Cuyahoga Community College, Physician Assistant Program
Verification of degrees

Telephone:	Not provided.
Written:	Free of charge. Faxed upon request. Mail or fax requests, including signed release forms, and physician assistant's year of graduation and student number.
Electronic:	Not provided.

Physician Assistant Program
Cuyahoga Community College
11000 Pleasant Valley Road
Parma, OHIO 44130
Telephone: 216/987-5363
Fax: 216/987-5066
Web site: www.tri-c.cc.oh.us

Kettering College of Medical Arts, Physician Assistant Program
Verification of degrees

Telephone:	Free of charge.
Written:	Free of charge. Faxed upon request. Mail or fax requests, including signed release forms and physician assistant's Social Security number.
Electronic:	Not provided.

Registrar's Office
Kettering College of Medical Arts
3737 Southern Boulevard
Kettering, OHIO 45429
Telephone: 937/395-8628 (Admissions Office)   800/433-KCMA (toll-free)
Fax: 937/395-8338
Web site: www.kcma.edu

Oklahoma

University of Oklahoma at Oklahoma City, Physician Assistant Program
Verification of degrees

Telephone:	Free of charge.
Written:	Free of charge. Faxed upon request in emergency situations only. Mail or fax requests, including signed release forms, physician assistant's Social Security number and year of graduation.
Electronic:	Not provided.

Records Department, BSE 200
University of Oklahoma Health Sciences Center
PO Box 26901
Oklahoma City, OKLAHOMA 73190
Telephone: 405/271-1537 (student records, grades, transcripts.)   405/271-3282 (admissions)
405/271-2359 (general)
Fax: 405/271-2480
Web site: www.admissions.ouhsc.edu

Pennsylvania

Chatham College, Physician Assistant Program
Notes: Initial accreditation: April 1997.
Verification of degrees
Telephone: Free of charge. Prefer written requests.
Written: Free of charge. Mail requests, including signed release forms.
Electronic: Free of charge. E-mail requests to freeman@chatham.edu or becker@chatham.edu.

> Physician Assistant Program
> Chatham College
> Woodland Road
> Pittsburgh, PENNSYLVANIA 15232
> Telephone: 412/365-1412
> Fax: 412/365-1623
> E-mail: parks@chatham.edu
> Web site: www.chatham.edu

Duquesne University, Physician Assistant Program
Verification of degrees
Telephone: Free of charge.
Written: Free of charge. Faxed upon request. Mail or fax requests, including physician assistant names, Social Security numbers, and signed release forms.
Electronic: Not provided.

> Office of the Registrar
> Duquesne University
> 600 Forbes Avenue
> Pittsburgh, PENNSYLVANIA 15282-0299
> Telephone: 412/396-6212
> Fax: 412/396-5622
> Web site: www.duq.edu

Kings College, Physician Assistant Program
Verification of degrees
Telephone: Not provided.
Written: Free of charge. Mail or fax requests, including signed release forms.
Electronic: Not provided.

> Physician Assistant Program
> Kings College
> 133 N. River Street
> Wilkes-Barre, PENNSYLVANIA 18711
> Telephone: 570/208-5853
> Fax: 570/208-6018
> E-mail: sesedon@kings.edu
> Web site: web.kings.edu

MCP Hahnemann University, Physician Assistant Program
Verification of degrees
Telephone: Not provided.
Written: Free of charge. Faxed upon request. Mail or fax requests, including signed release forms and physician assistant's Social Security number, year of graduation, and maiden name (if applicable).
Electronic: Information available on our Web site.

Physician Assistant Program
College of Nursing and Health Professions
MCP Hahnemann University
245 N. 15th Street, MS 504
Bellet Building, 8th Floor
Philadelphia, PENNSYLVANIA 19102-1192
Telephone: 215/762-7135
Fax: 215/762-1164
Web site: www.mcphu.edu

Saint Francis de Sales. Physician Assistant Program
Annual report of licensed physicians
Telephone: Free of charge.
Written: Free of charge. Must include signed release form.
Electronic: Not provided.

Physician Assistant Program
De Sales University
2755 Station Avenue
Center Valley, PENNSYLVANIA 18034-9568
Telephone: 610/282-1100, Ext. 1474
Fax: 610/282-1893
Web site: www.desales.edu

Saint Francis University of Pennsylvania, Physician Assistant Program
Verification of degrees
Telephone: Not provided.
Written: Free of charge. Faxed upon request. Mail or fax requests, including signed release forms and physician assistant's year of graduation.
Electronic: Not provided.

Department of Physician Assistant Sciences
Saint Francis University of Pennsylvania
PO Box 600
Loretto, PENNSYLVANIA 15940-0600
Telephone: 814/472-3130
Fax: 814/472-3137
Web site: www.francis.edu

South Dakota

University of South Dakota School of Medicine, Physician Assistant Studies Program
Verification of degrees

Telephone: Free of charge.
Written: Free of charge. Faxed upon request. Mail or fax requests, including signed release forms.
Electronic: Not provided.

> Physician Assistant Program
> University of South Dakota School of Medicine
> 414 E. Clark Street
> Vermillion, SOUTH DAKOTA 57069-2390
> Telephone: 605/677-5128
> Fax: 605/677-6569
> E-mail: usdpa@usd.edu
> Web site: www.usd.edu/pa

Tennessee

Trevecca Nazarene University, Physician Assistant Program
Verification of degrees

Telephone: Free of charge with faxed release form signed by physician.
Written: Free of charge. Faxed upon request. Mail or fax requests, including signed release forms.
Electronic: Not provided.

> Attention: Director
> Physician Assistant Program
> Trevecca Nazarene College
> 333 Murfreesboro Road
> Nashville, TENNESSEE 37210-2877
> Telephone: 615/248-7739
> Fax: 615/248-1622
> Web site: www.trevecca.edu

Texas

Baylor College of Medicine, Physician Assistant Program
Verification of degrees

Telephone: Free of charge.
Written: Free of charge. Faxed upon request. Mail or fax requests, including signed release forms, self-addressed, stamped envelopes, and physician assistants program and maiden name (if applicable).
Electronic: Not provided.

> Office of the Registrar
> Baylor College of Medicine
> One Baylor Plaza, Suite M108
> Houston, TEXAS 77030
> Telephone: 713/798-7766 (main)   713/798-3374 (Physician Assistants recorder)

Fax: 713/798-1518
E-mail: registrar@bcm.tmc.edu
Web site: www.bcm.tmc.edu

Interservice Physician Assistant Program
Verification of degrees

Telephone:	Free of charge.
Written:	Free of charge. Faxed upon request. Mail or fax requests, including signed release forms.
Electronic:	Not provided.

Attention: Degree verification request
MCCS HMP PA Branch
CMD-AMEDD C&S
U.S. Army
3151 Scott Road, Suite 1202
Fort Sam Houston, TEXAS 78234-6138
Telephone: 210/221-7791   210/221-1004 (Secretary)
Fax: 210/221-8493
E-mail: fortsamhouston@army.mil
Web site: www.fortsamhouston.amedd.army.mil

University of North Texas Health Science Center at Fort Worth
Annual report of licensed physicians

Telephone:	Free of charge.
Written:	Free of charge.
Electronic:	Information available on Web site.

Physician Assistant Studies
University of North Texas Health Science Center at Fort Worth
3500 Camp Bowie Boulevard
Fort Worth, TEXAS 76107-2699
Telephone: 817/735-2301 (Physician Assistant Studies)
Fax: 817/735-2529
E-mail: martinj@hsc.unt.edu
Web site: www.hsc.unt.edu/departments/physicianassistantstudies

University of Texas Medical Branch at Galveston, Physician Assistant Program
Verification of degrees

Telephone:	Free of charge. Collect calls will not be accepted.
Written:	Free of charge. Faxed upon request. Mail or fax requests, including signed release forms. Postage must be provided.
Electronic:	Not provided.

Physician Assistant Program
School of Allied Health Sciences
University of Texas Medical Branch at Galveston
301 University Boulevard
Galveston, TEXAS 77555-1145
Telephone: 409/772-3046

Fax: 409/772-9710
Web site: www.sahs.utmb.edu/programs/pas

University of Texas Southwestern Medical Center at Dallas, Physician Assistant Program
Verification of degrees
Telephone: Free of charge.
Written: Free of charge. Mail requests, including signed release forms.
Electronic: Not provided.

Office of Registrar
University of Texas Southwestern Medical Center at Dallas
5323 Harry Hines Boulevard
Dallas, TEXAS 75390-9162
Telephone: 214/648-5617
Fax: 214/648-3289
E-mail: admisssions@utsouthwestern.edu
Web site: www.utsouthwestern.edu

Utah

University of Utah School of Medicine, Physician Assistant Program
Verification of residencies and degrees
Telephone: Not provided.
Written: Free of charge. Faxed upon request. Mail or fax requests, including signed release forms.
Electronic: Not provided.

Physician Assistant Program
University of Utah School of Medicine
375 Chiepta Way, Suite A
Salt Lake City, UTAH 84108
Telephone: 801/581-7766
Fax: 801/581-5807
Web site: www.utah.edu/upap

Virginia

American Academy of Physician Assistants
Notes: They also provide verification of physician assistant certificates.
Annual report of licensed physicians
Telephone: Free of charge.
Written: Free of charge.
Electronic: Not provided.

American Academy of Physician Assistants
950 N. Washington Street
Alexandria, VIRGINIA 22314-1552
Telephone: 703/836-2272
Fax: 703/684-1924
E-mail: aapa@aapa.org
Web site: www.aapa.org

Association of Physician Assistant Programs
Notes: *Only conducts verification regarding accreditation of specific physician assistant programs.*
Annual report of licensed physicians
Telephone: Not provided.
Written: Free of charge.
Electronic: Information available on our Web site.

> Association of Physician Assistant Programs
> 950 N. Washington Street
> Alexandria, VIRGINIA 22314-1552
> Telephone: 703/548-5538
> Fax: 703/684-1924
> E-mail: apap@aapa.org
> Web site: www.apap.org

College of Health Sciences, Physician Assistant Program
Notes: *Provisional accreditation: April 1997. First graduating class: 1999.*
Annual report of licensed physicians
Telephone: Not provided.
Written: Free of charge.
Electronic: Not provided.

> Physician Assistant Program
> College of Health Sciences
> 920 S. Jefferson Street
> Roanoke, VIRGINIA 24016
> Telephone: 540/985-4016
> Fax: 540/224-4551
> E-mail: pa@health.chs.edu
> Web site: www.chs.edu

Washington

University of Washington/MEDEX Northwest, Physician Assistant Program
Verification of degrees
Telephone: Free of charge with faxed release form signed by physician assistant.
Written: Free of charge. Faxed upon request. Mail, phone, or fax requests, including signed release forms.
Electronic: Not provided.

> Physician Assistant Program
> University of Washington/MEDEX Northwest
> 4245 Roosevelt Way NE
> Seattle, WASHINGTON 98105-6920
> Telephone: 206/598-2600
> Fax: 206/598-5195
> E-mail: medex@u.washington.edu
> Web site: www.washington.edu/medical/som/depts/medex

West Virginia

Alderson Broaddus College, Physician Assistant Program
Verification of degrees
Telephone: Free of charge.
Written: Free of charge. Faxed upon request. Mail or fax requests, including signed release forms.
Electronic: Not provided.

Physician Assistant Program
Alderson Broaddus College
PO Box 2036
500 College Hill Drive
Phillipi, WEST VIRGINIA 26416
Telephone: 304/457-6283
Fax: 304/457-6308
E-mail: holt_m@ab.edu
Web site: www.ab.edu

Wisconsin

Marquette University, Physician Assistant Program
Notes: *Provisional accreditation: April 1997. First graduating class: 1999. Presently fully accredited.*
Verification of degrees
Telephone: Free of charge.
Written: Free of charge. Mail or fax requests, including signed release forms.
Electronic: Not provided.

Physician Assistant Program
Marquette University
PO Box 1881
1700 Building
Milwaukee, WISCONSIN 53201-1881
Telephone: 414/288-5688
Fax: 414/288-7951
Web site: www.marquette.edu

University of Wisconsin Madison Medical Sciences Center, Physician Assistant Program
Verification of degrees
Telephone: Not provided.
Written: Free of charge. Faxed upon request. Mail or fax requests, including signed release forms.
Electronic: Not provided.

Medicine School Health Profession Programs
Student Services Admissions Office
University of Wisconsin Madison Medical Sciences Center
1300 University Avenue, Room 1070
Madison, WISCONSIN 53706
Telephone: 608/263-6800
Fax: 608/263-6434

UW La Crosse Gundersen Mayo Physician Assistant Program

Notes: Initial accreditation: April 1997. First graduating class: October 1997.

Annual report of licensed physicians

Telephone: Not provided.
Written: Not provided.
Electronic: Available on Web site free of charge.

Physician Assistant Program
University of Wisconsin LaCrosse
1725 State Street, 4th Floor HSC
LaCrosse, WISCONSIN 54601-3767
Telephone: 608/785-6620
Fax: 608/785-6647
E-mail: paprogram@uwlax.edu
Web site: www.uwlax.edu/pastudies

Nursing Schools

Alabama

University of Alabama at Birmingham School of Nursing, Graduate Program
Verification of degrees

Telephone:	Free of charge.
Written:	Free of charge. Mail or fax requests, including signed release forms.
Electronic:	Not provided.

Graduate Program
University of Alabama at Birmingham School of Nursing
MB-108
1530 Third Avenue S
Birmingham, ALABAMA 35294-1210
Telephone: 205/934-0610
Fax: 205/975-6142
E-mail: studaffr@son.uab.edu
Web site: www.uab.edu/son

Arizona

Arizona State University College of Nursing
Verification of Degrees

Telephone:	Not provided
Written:	Free of charge. Mail or fax requests.
Electronic:	Not provided.

Arizona State University College of Nursing
Tempe, ARIZONA 85287
Telephone: 480/965-2987   Fax: 480/965-8468
E-mail: nursing@asu.edu
Web site: www.nursing.asu.edu

California

University of Southern California Department of Nursing
Verification of degrees

Telephone:	Not provided.
Written:	Mail requests, including signed release forms.
Electronic:	Not provided.

University of Southern California Department of Nursing
Center for Health Professions
1540 Alcazar Street
CHP-Room 222
Los Angeles, CALIFORNIA 90089
Telephone: 212/740-7444
Web site: usc.edu/nursing

Georgia

Emory University, Nell Hodgson Woodruff School of Nursing
Verification of degrees

Telephone: Free of charge.
Written: Free of charge. Faxed upon request in emergency situations only. Mail or fax requests, including signed release forms.
Electronic: Not provided.

> Attention: Director
> Student Affairs Office
> Nell Hodgson Woodruff School of Nursing
> Emory University
> 1520 Clifton Road
> Atlanta, GEORGIA 30322
> Telephone: 404/727-3500 (main)   404/727-6915 (Student Services)
> Fax: 404/727-9668
> E-mail: nhallor@emory.edu
> Web site: www.nursing.emory.edu

Illinois

Southern Illinois University Edwardsville
Verification of degrees

Telephone: Not provided.
Written: Free of charge. Faxed upon request. Mail or fax requests, including signed release forms.
Electronic: Not provided.

> Southern Illinois University Edwardsville
> Registrar's Office
> Rensleman Hall
> Edwardsville, ILLINOIS 62026-1066
> Telephone: 618/650-2080 (Registrar)   618/650-3956 (Nursing)
> Fax: 618/650-5013
> E-mail: nursing@siue.edu
> Web site: www.register.siue.edu

Mississippi

University of Southern Mississippi
Verification of degrees

Telephone: Free of charge.
Written: Free of charge. Mail request.
Electronic: Not provided.

> Office of the University Registrar
> University of Southern Mississippi
> Box 5006
> Hattiesburg, MISSISSIPPI 39406-5006

Telephone: 601/266-5006
Fax: 601/266-5816
Web site: www.registrar.usm.edu

New York

University at Buffalo School of Nursing, Nurse Practitioner Advanced Certificate Program
Verification of degrees

Telephone: Free of charge.
Written: Free of charge. Faxed upon request. Mail or fax requests, including signed release forms and nurse practitioner's Social Security number.
Electronic: Free of charge.

> Student Affairs Office
> University at Buffalo School of Nursing, Nurse Practitioner Advanced Certificate Program
> 1040 Kimball Tower
> 3435 Main Street
> Buffalo, NEW YORK 14214
> Telephone: 716/829-2537
> Fax: 716/829-2021
> E-mail: nurse-studentaffairs@buffalo.edu
> Web site: www.nursing.buffalo.edu

Pennsylvania

Clarion University School of Nursing
Verification of degrees

Telephone: Not provided.
Written: Free of charge. Mail or fax signed request.
Electronic: Not provided.

> Office of the Registrar
> Clarion University of Pennsylvania
> 122 Carrier Administrattion
> 840 Wood Street
> Clarion, PENNSYLVANIA 16214-1232
> Telephone: 814/676-2229
> Fax: 814/393-2039
> E-mail: dbills@clarion.edu
> Web site: www.clarion.edu

Nurse Anesthesia (CRNA) Programs

Alabama

Anesthesia at Southeast Alabama Medical Center
Notes: No longer serving as a medical school. Previous attendance or degrees may still be verified. Location now used as clinical rotation site only.

Verification of degrees

Telephone: Free of charge.
Written: Free of charge. Faxed upon request (followed by hard copy). Mail or fax requests, including signed release forms and nurse anesthetist's date of graduation.
Electronic: Not provided.

> Department of Anesthesia
> Southeast Alabama Medical Center
> PO Drawer 6987
> Dothan, ALABAMA 36302
> Telephone: 334/793-8105
> Fax: 334/712-3705
> E-mail: jkelly@samc.org

University of Alabama Birmingham, Nurse Anesthetist Program

Verification of degrees

Telephone: Not provided.
Written: Free of charge. Faxed upon request. Mail or fax requests, including signed release forms.
Electronic: Not provided.

> Nurse Anesthetist Program
> University of Alabama Birmingham
> 1530 Third Avenue S, Suite 230 RMSB
> Birmingham, ALABAMA 35294-1212
> Telephone: 205/934-3209
> Fax: 205/934-3212
> Web site: www.uab.edu/mna

California

Kaiser Permanente School of Anesthesia

Verification of degrees

Telephone: Not provided.
Written: Free of charge. Faxed upon request. Mail or fax requests, including signed release forms.
Electronic: Not provided.

> Kaiser Permanente School of Anesthesia
> 100 S. Los Robles, Suite 550
> Pasadena, CALIFORNIA 91188
> Telephone: 626/564-3000
> Fax: 626/564-3099
> Web site: www.kpsan.org

Samuel Merritt College, Graduate Program of Nurse Anesthesia
Verification of degrees

Telephone: Free of charge with Social Security number.
Written: Free of charge. Faxed upon request. Mail or fax requests, including signed release forms and nurse anesthetist's Social Security number.
Electronic: Not provided.

> Registrar's Office
> Samuel Merritt College
> 370 Hawthorne Avenue
> Oakland, CALIFORNIA 94609
> Telephone: 510/869-6130
> Fax: 510/869-6204
> E-mail: registrar@samuelmerritt.edu
> Web site: www.samuelmerritt.edu

University of Southern California, Program of Nurse Anesthesia
Verification of degrees

Telephone: Free of charge. Only for nurse anesthetists who graduated 1997 to present.
Written: $5 per verification (payable to USC). Mail requests, including signed release forms, each nurse anesthetist's Social Security number or student identification number, date of birth, dates of attendance, name of program, and enrolled name.
Electronic: Not provided.

> University of Southern California Program of Nurse Anesthesia
> Attention: Verification Department
> University of Southern California
> 1540 E. Alcazar Street CHP222
> Los Angeles, CALIFORNIA 90033
> Telephone: 323/442-2001 (general information)
> Fax: 323/442-2090
> E-mail: uscnurse@usc.edu
> Web site: www.usc.edu

Connecticut

Hospital of Saint Raphael, School of Nurse Anesthesia
Verification of degrees

Telephone: Free of charge.
Written: Free of charge. Faxed upon request. Mail or fax requests, including signed release forms, and nurse anesthetist's Social Security number and maiden name (if applicable).
Electronic: Not provided.

> School of Nurse Anesthesia
> Hospital of Saint Raphael
> 1423 Chapel Street
> New Haven, CONNECTICUT 06511
> Telephone: 203/789-3351 (School of Nurse Anesthesia)
> Fax: 203/789-3352
> E-mail: hsrsna@snet.net

New Britain School of Nurse Anesthesia
Verification of degrees

Telephone: Free of charge.
Written: Free of charge. Faxed upon request. Mail, phone, or fax requests, including signed release forms.
Electronic: Free of charge via e-mail.

> New Britain School of Nurse Anesthesia
> 100 Grand Street
> New Britain, CONNECTICUT 06050
> Telephone: 860/224-5612
> Fax: 860/826-4992
> E-mail: dwood@nbgh.org
> Web site: www.nbgh.org

Southern Connecticut State University/Bridgeport Hospital, Nurse Anesthesia Program
Verification of degrees

Telephone: Not provided.
Written: Free of charge. Faxed upon request. Mail or fax requests, including signed release forms, and nurse anesthetist's year of graduation.
Electronic: Not provided.

> Attention: Director, Nurse Anesthesia Program
> Southern Connecticut State University/Bridgeport Hospital
> 267 Grant Street
> Bridgeport, CONNECTICUT 06610-0120
> Telephone: 203/384-4746
> Fax: 203/384-3855

District of Columbia

Georgetown University School of Nursing, Nurse Anesthesia Program
Verification of licenses

Telephone: Not provided.
Written: Provided. Call for fee information.
Electronic: Not provided.

> Nurse Anesthesia Program
> Georgetown University School of Nursing
> Box 571107
> 3700 Reservoir Road NW
> Washington, DISTRICT OF COLUMBIA 20057-1107
> Telephone: 202/687-4612
> Fax: 202/687-2128
> E-mail: jasinskd@georgetown.edu
> Web site: www.georgetown.edu

Florida

Barry University, Master of Science in Anesthesia Program
Verification of degrees

Telephone: Not provided.
Written: Free of charge. Faxed upon request. Mail or fax requests, including signed release forms.
Electronic: Not provided.

> Master of Science in Anesthesia Program
> Barry University School of Natural and Health Science
> 11300 N.E. Second Avenue
> Miami Shores, FLORIDA 33161-6695
> Telephone: 305/899-3230
> Fax: 305/899-3366
> Web site: www.barry.edu

Gooding Institute of Nurse Anesthesia at Bay Medical Center
Verification of degrees

Telephone: Free of charge.
Written: Free of charge. Mail requests, including signed release forms.
Electronic: Not provided.

> Gooding Institute of Nurse Anesthesia
> Bay Medical Center
> 615 N. Bonita Avenue
> Panama City, FLORIDA 32401
> Telephone: 850/747-6918
> Fax: 850/747-6115
> E-mail: gooding@baymedical.org
> Web site: www.baymedical.org

Illinois

Decatur Memorial Hospitals/Bradley University/Nurse Anesthesia Program
Verification of degrees

Telephone: Not provided.
Written: Free of charge. Faxed upon request. Mail or fax requests, including signed release forms.
Electronic: Not provided.

> Nurse Anesthesia Program
> Decatur Memorial Hospitals/Bradley University
> 2300 N. Edward Street
> Decatur, ILLINOIS 62526-4193
> Telephone: 217/876-2578
> Fax: 217/876-2587
> Web site: www.dmhcares.org

Ravenswood Hospital Medical Center School of Anesthesia, DePaul University, Graduate Program in Nurse Anesthesia

Verification of degrees

Telephone: Free of charge.

Written: Free of charge. Faxed upon request. Mail or fax requests, including signed release forms, and nurse anesthetist's Social Security number and year of graduation.

Electronic: Not provided.

> Graduate Program in Nurse Anesthesia
> Ravenswood Hospital Medical Center School of Anesthesia, DePaul University
> 4550 N. Winchester Avenue
> Chicago, ILLINOIS 60640-5205
> Telephone: 773/878-4300 ext 5286
> Fax: 773/279-3115
> E-mail: ravenswoodsa@rhmc.com
> Web site: www.rhmc.com

Rush University College of Nursing, Nurse Anesthesia Program

Verification of degrees

Telephone: Free of charge with Social Security number.

Written: Free of charge. Faxed upon request. Graduates themselves must mail or fax requests, including release forms, Social Security number, full name, and year graduated.

Electronic: Not provided.

> Office of the Registrar
> Rush University
> 600 S. Paulina Street, Suite 440
> Chicago, ILLINOIS 60612
> Telephone: 312/942-5681
> Fax: 312/942-2219
> E-mail: registrar_office.rushu@edu
> Web site: www.rushu.rush.edu

Southern Illinois University at Edwardsville School of Nursing, Nurse Anesthesia Specialization

Verification of degrees

Telephone: Not provided.

Written: Free of charge. Faxed upon request. Mail or fax requests, including signed release forms.

Electronic: Not provided.

> Office of the Dean
> School of Nursing
> Southern Illinois University at Edwardsville
> Alumni Hall, Room 2333
> Edwardsville, ILLINOIS 62026-1066
> Telephone: 618/650-3959
> Fax: 618/650-3854
> Web site: www.siue.edu

Chapter 5

Iowa

Department of Veterans Affairs, Drake University
Verification of degrees

Telephone: Free of charge.
Written: Free of charge. Faxed upon request. Mail, phone, or fax requests.
Electronic: Not provided.

> Office of the Registrar
> Department of Veterans Affairs, Drake University
> 2507 University Avenue
> Des Moines, IOWA 50311
> Telephone: 515/271-3901
> Fax: 515/271-3977
> Web site: www.drake.edu

University of Iowa College of Nursing, Anesthesia Nursing Program
Verification of degrees

Telephone: Not provided.
Written: Free of charge. Mail requests, including signed release forms.
Electronic: Not provided.

> Anesthesia Nursing Program
> Department of Anesthesia
> University of Iowa
> 200 Hawkins Drive
> Room 6441 JCP
> Iowa City, IOWA 52242-1079
> Telephone: 319/384-7354
> Fax: 319/384-7286
> E-mail: nursing-anesthesia@uiowa.edu
> Web site: www.anesth.uiowa.edu/srna/

Kansas

University of Kansas Medical Center Program of Nurse Anesthesia Education
Verification of degrees

Telephone: Not provided.
Written: Free of charge. Faxed upon request. Mail or fax requests on letterhead stationary, including signed release forms, and nurse anesthetist's Social Security number and year of graduation.
Electronic: Not provided.

> Program of Nurse Anesthesia Education
> University of Kansas Medical Center
> 3901 Rainbow Boulevard
> Kansas City, KANSAS 66160-7604
> Telephone: 913/588-6612
> Fax: 913/588-3334
> Web site: www.kumc.edu/sah/nurseanesthesia

Kentucky

Trover Foundation/Murray State University, Program of Anesthesia
Verification of degrees
Telephone: Free of charge.
Written: Free of charge. Faxed upon request. Mail, phone, or fax requests.
Electronic: Not provided.

> Program of Anesthesia
> Trover Foundation/Murray State University
> 435 N. Kentucky Avenue, Suite A
> Madisonville, KENTUCKY 42431-1768
> Telephone: 270/824-3460
> Fax: 270/824-3469
> E-mail: anesprog@trover.org
> Web site: www.crnaky.com

Louisiana

Medical Center of Louisiana at New Orleans
Notes: Contact Louisiana State University for information regarding nurse anesthesia program; 504/568-4123.
Verification of degrees
Telephone: Not provided.
Written: Free of charge. Faxed upon request. Mail or fax requests, including signed release forms, and nurse anesthetist's Social Security number, year of graduation, and maiden name (if applicable).
Electronic: Not provided.

> Department of Anesthesia
> Charity Hospital
> 1532 Tulane Avenue
> New Orleans, LOUISIANA 70112
> Telephone: 504/903-2816
> Fax: 504/903-0937
> E-mail: ch/xusna@mail.com
> Web site: www.lsuhsc.edu

Maine

University of New England, School of Nurse Anesthesia
Verification of degrees
Telephone: Free of charge.
Written: Free of charge. Faxed upon request. Mail or fax requests, including signed release forms.
Electronic: Not provided.

> Office of the Registrar
> University of New England
> 716 Stevens Avenue
> Portland, MAINE 04103

Chapter 5

Telephone: 207/797-7261
Fax: 207/797-7225
Web site: www.une.edu

Maryland

Durham Regional Hospital, School of Anesthesia for Nurses
Notes: Durham Regional Hospital School of Anesthesia for Nurses closed in September 1994. Direct verification requests to the Watts School of Nursing at Durham Regional Hospital.
Annual report of licensed physicians
Telephone: Not provided.
Written: Not provided.
Electronic: Not provided.

>4301 Jones Bridge Road
>Bethesda, MARYLAND 20814
>Fax: 301-295-1722

The Naval School of Health Sciences, Navy Nurse Corps Anesthesia Program
Verification of degrees
Telephone: Free of charge.
Written: Free of charge. Faxed upon request. Mail or fax requests, including signed release forms, and nurse anesthetist's passport date.
Electronic: Not provided.

>Commanding Officer
>Attention: Registrar
>The Naval School of Health Sciences
>8901 Wisconsin Avenue
>Bethesda, MARYLAND 20889-5611
>Telephone: 301/295-4818
>Fax: 301/295-4823
>E-mail: jfbehnke@nsh10.med.navy.mil
>Web site: www.nshs.med.navy.mil

Uniformed Services University of the Health Sciences, Graduate School of Nursing, Nurse Anesthesia Program
Verification of degrees
Telephone: Free of charge.
Written: Free of charge. Faxed upon request. Mail, phone, or fax requests.
Electronic: Not provided.

>Nurse Anesthesia Program
>Graduate School of Nursing
>Uniformed Services University of the Health Sciences
>4301 Jones Bridge Road
>Bethesda, MARYLAND 20814
>Telephone: 301/295-0979 (main)   301/295-1206 (Nurse Anesthesia Program)
>Fax: 301/295-1722

Nurse Anesthesia (CRNA) Programs

United States Air Force Graduate Program of Nurse Anesthesia
Verification of degrees
Telephone: Not provided.
Written: Free of charge. Mail or fax requests, including signed release forms.
Electronic: Not provided.

> United States Air Force, Graduate Program of Nurse Anesthesia
> Uniform Services University of Health Services
> 4301 Jones Bridge Road
> Bethesda, MARYLAND 20814
> Telephone: 301/295-0979
> Fax: 301/295-1722
> Web site: www.usuhs.mil

United States Air Force Graduate Program of Nurse Anesthesia
Notes: Program moved in December 1998. Contact the U.S. Air Force Graduate Program of Nurse Anesthesia at the Uniformed Services University of Health Services in Maryland for verification information.
Annual report of licensed physicians
Telephone: Not provided.
Written: Not provided.
Electronic: Not provided.

> Attention: United States Air Force Graduate Program of Nurse Anesthesia
> 4301 Jones Bridge Road
> Bethesda, MARYLAND 20814
> Telephone: 301/295-0979
> Fax: 301/295-1722

Massachusetts

Berkshire Medical Center School of Anesthesia
Notes: Verification provided through Human Resources.
Verification of degrees
Telephone: Not provided.
Written: Free of charge. Faxed upon request. Mail or fax requests, including signed release forms.
Electronic: Not provided.

> Berkshire Medical Center, Human Resources
> 725 North Street
> Pittsfield, MASSACHUSETTS 01201
> Telephone: 413/447-2786
> Fax: 413/447-2091

Northeastern University Graduate School of Nursing/Nurse Anesthesia Program
Verification of degrees
Telephone: Free of charge.
Written: Free of charge. Mail or fax requests, including nurse names and Social Security numbers, and signed release forms.
Electronic: Not provided.

Nurse Anesthesia Program
Northeastern University Graduate School of Nursing
205 Robinson Hall
360 Huntington Avenue
Boston, MASSACHUSETTS 02115
Telephone: 617/373-7962
Fax: 617/373-8675
Web site: www.neu.edu

Michigan

Henry Ford Hospital, University of Detroit, Mercy Graduate Program of Nurse Anesthesia
Verification of degrees
Telephone: Not provided.
Written: Free of charge. Faxed upon request. Mail or fax requests including signed release forms.
Electronic: Not provided.

Graduate Program of Nurse Anesthesia
University of Detroit Mercy
2799 W. Grand Boulevard, CFP Room 303
Detroit, MICHIGAN 48202
Telephone: 313/916-2934
Fax: 313/916-2606
E-mail: schanes@hfhs.org
Web site: www.hfhs.org

Oakland University/William Beaumont Hospital, Education Program in Nurse Anesthesia
Verification of degrees
Telephone: Not provided.
Written: Free of charge. Mail requests, including signed release forms.
Electronic: Not provided.

Nurse Advising Office
School of Nursing
Oakland University
447 O'Dowd Hall
Rochester, MICHIGAN 48309-4401
Telephone: 248/370-4068
Fax: 248/370-2996
E-mail: nursinginfo@oakland.edu
Web site: www2.oakland.edu/nursing

Saint Joseph Mercy Oakland, University of Detroit, Mercy Graduate Program of Nurse Anesthesiology
Verification of degrees
Telephone: Not provided.
Written: Free of charge. Faxed upon request. Mail or fax requests, including signed release forms, and nurse anesthetist's year of graduation and maiden name (if applicable).
Electronic: Not provided.

Saint Joseph Mercy Oakland
PO Box 436011
44405 Woodward Avenue
Pontiac, MICHIGAN 48341-6011
Telephone: 248/858-6593
Fax: 248/858-6599
E-mail: doschm@trinity-health.org
Web site: ids.udmercy.edu/naprogram

University of Michigan-Flint/Hurley Medical Center Anesthesia Program
Verification of degrees

Telephone:	Free of charge in emergency situations only.
Written:	Free of charge. Faxed upon request. Mail or fax requests including signed release forms.
Electronic:	Not provided.

Anesthesia Program
University of Michigan-Flint/Hurley Medical Center
One Hurley Plaza
Flint, MICHIGAN 48503
Telephone: 810/257-9264
Fax: 810/760-0839
Web site: www.hurleymc.com/education/anesthes/index.htm

Wayne State University Eugene Applebaum College of Pharmacy and Health Sciences Detroit Receiving Hospital, Department School of Nurse Anesthesia
Verification of degrees

Telephone:	Not provided.
Written:	Free of charge. Mail requests, including signed release forms, and nurse anesthetist's Social Security number and year of graduation.
Electronic:	Not provided.

School of Nurse Anesthesia
Wayne State University Eugene Applebaum College of Pharmacy and Health Sciences Detroit Receiving Hospital
4201 Saint Antoine, Room 2V
Detroit, MICHIGAN 48201
Telephone: 313/745-3610
Fax: 313/993-7729

Minnesota

Mayo School of Health Sciences Nurse Anesthesia Program
Verification of degrees

Telephone:	Not provided.
Written:	Free of charge for verifications; $5 for transcripts. Faxed upon request. Mail, phone, or fax requests, including signed release forms.
Electronic:	Not provided.

Nurse Anesthesia (CRNA) Masters Program
Mayo School of Health Sciences
Siebens Eleven
200 First Street SW
Rochester, MINNESOTA 55905
Telephone: 507/284-3678   800/626-9041 (toll-free)
Fax: 507/284-0656
E-mail: kray@mayo.edu
Web site: www.mayo.edu

Minneapolis School of Anesthesia
Verification of degrees
Telephone: Free of charge.
Written: Free of charge. Faxed upon request, followed by hard copy. Mail or fax requests, including signed release forms. Follow faxed requests with hard copy.
Electronic: Not provided.

Minneapolis School of Anesthesia
6715 Minnetonka Boulevard
St. Louis Park, MINNESOTA 55426-3499
Telephone: 952/925-5222
Fax: 952/925-6004

Minneapolis VA School of Anesthesia
Verification of degrees
Telephone: Free of charge.
Written: Free of charge. Faxed upon request. Mail or fax requests, including signed release forms and nurse anesthetist's Social Security number.
Electronic: Not provided.

Minneapolis VA School of Anesthesia
One Veterans Drive, 112A
Minneapolis, MINNESOTA 55417-2399
Telephone: 612/725-2000, Ext. 3392
Fax: 612/970-5887

Saint Mary's University, Graduate Program in Nurse Anesthesia
Notes: Formerly Abbott Northwestern Hospital; Saint Mary's keeps Abbotts student records as well as student records for Northwestern Hospital.
Verification of degrees
Telephone: Not provided.
Written: Free of charge for verifications; $3 for transcripts. Faxed upon request. Mail or fax requests, including signed release forms.
Electronic: Not provided.

Graduate Program in Nurse Anesthesia
Saint Mary's University
2500 Park Avenue
Minneapolis, MINNESOTA 55404
Telephone: 612/728-5133

Fax: 612/728-5167
E-mail: mmoody@smumn.edu
Web site: www.smumn.edu

Missouri

Southwest Missouri School of Anesthesia
Verification of degrees
Telephone: Free of charge with release form signed by nurse anesthetist.
Written: Free of charge. Faxed upon request. Mail, phone, or fax requests, including signed release forms and nurse anesthetist's Social Security number.
Electronic: Not provided.

Southwest Missouri School of Anesthesia
1235 East Cherokee
Springfield, MISSOURI 65804
Telephone: 417/885-6890
Fax: 417/885-6895
E-mail: as14293@sprg.smhs.com

Truman Medical Center, School of Nurse Anesthesia
Verification of degrees
Telephone: Not provided.
Written: Free of charge. Faxed upon request. Mail or fax requests, including signed release forms and nurse anesthetist's Social Security number.
Electronic: Not provided.

School of Nurse Anesthesia
Truman Medical Center
2301 Holmes Street
Kansas City, MISSOURI 64108
Telephone: 816/556-3216
Fax: 816/556-3963
E-mail: tmcanes@tmcned.org
Web site: www.med.umkc.edu/crna

Nebraska

Bryan LGH Medical Center, University of Kansas, School of Nurse Anesthesia
Verification of degrees
Telephone: Not provided.
Written: Free of charge. Faxed upon request, followed by hard copy. Mail or fax requests, including signed release forms, and nurse anethetist's Social Security number, year of graduation, and maiden name (if applicable). Follow faxed requests with hard copy.
Electronic: Not provided.

School of Nurse Anesthesia
Bryan LGH Medical Center
1600 S. 48th Street
Lincoln, NEBRASKA 68506-1299

Telephone: 402/481-3135
Fax: 402/481-8404
E-mail: mgibson@bryanlgh.org
Web site: www.bryanlgh.org

New Jersey

Our Lady of Lourdes Medical Center, Nurse Anesthesia Program
Verification of degrees

Telephone: Free of charge.
Written: Free of charge. Faxed upon request. Mail or fax requests, including signed release forms.
Electronic: Not provided.

Nurse Anesthesia Program
Our Lady of Lourdes Medical Center
Attention: Anesthesia Department
1600 Haddon Avenue
Camden, NEW JERSEY 08103
Telephone: 856/757-3897 (Nurse Anesthesia Department)
Fax: 856/968-2568
E-mail: roddend@lourdesnet.org

New York

Albany Medical College Center for Nurse Anesthesiology
Verification of degrees

Telephone: Not provided.
Written: Free of charge. Faxed upon request. Mail or fax requests, CRNA name, year of graduation, and signed release forms.
Electronic: Not provided.

Center for Nurse Anesthesiology
Albany Medical College
47 New Scotland Avenue, MC-131
Albany, NEW YORK 12208
Telephone: 518/262-4303
Fax: 518/262-5170
E-mail: amcnap@mail.amc.edu

Columbia University School of Nursing, Program in Nurse Anesthesia
Verification of degrees

Telephone: Not provided.
Written: Free of charge. Mail requests, including signed release forms, and CRNA name, anesthetist's Social Security number, year of graduation, and maiden name (if applicable).
Electronic: Not provided.

Attention: Registrar Services
Columbia University, Student Administrative Services
650 W. 168th Street, Room 141, Box 45
New York, NEW YORK 10032

Nurse Anesthesia (CRNA) Programs

Telephone: 212/305-3992
Fax: 212/305-1590
Web site: www.columbia.edu

Harlem Hospital, Anesthesia School for Nurses
Verification of degrees
Telephone: Not provided.
Written: Free of charge. Faxed upon request. Mail or fax requests, including signed release forms.
Electronic: Not provided.

Anesthesia School for Nurses
Harlem Hospital
506 Lenox Avenue
New York, NEW YORK 10037-1801
Telephone: 212/939-3575
Fax: 212/939-3574

Kings County Hospital Center, School of Anesthesia for Nurses
Verification of degrees
Telephone: Not provided.
Written: Free of charge. Mail requests, including signed release forms.
Electronic: Not provided.

School of Anesthesia for Nurses
Kings County Hospital Center
450 Clarkson Avenue
Brooklyn, NEW YORK 11203-2054
Telephone: 718/270-7656 (School of Anesthesia)   718/245-4409 (main)
Fax: 718/270-7636
E-mail: varirao@netmail.hscbklyn.edu
Web site: www.hscbklyn.edu

State University of New York Downstate Medical Center
Notes: School offers Masters degrees and certificate programs.
Verification of degrees
Telephone: Free of charge; prefer written request.
Written: Free of charge. Mail or fax requests, including signed release forms and nurse-midwife's maiden name (if applicable).
Electronic: Not provided.

Midwifery Education Program
SUNY Downstate Medical Center
450 Clarkson Avenue, Box 1227
Brooklyn, NEW YORK 11203
Telephone: 718/270-7740
Fax: 718/270-7634
Web site: www.downstate.edu/chrp/midwif

University at Buffalo School of Nursing, Nurse Anesthesia Program
Verification of degrees

Telephone: Free of charge.
Written: Free of charge. Faxed upon request. Mail or fax requests, including signed release forms and nurse anesthetist's Social Security number.
Electronic: Free of charge.

Student Affairs Office
University at Buffalo School of Nursing, Nurse Anesthesia Program
1040 Kimball Tower
3435 Main Street
Buffalo, NEW YORK 14214
Telephone: 716/829-2537
Fax: 716/829-2021
E-mail: nurse-studentaffairs@buffalo.edu
Web site: nursing.buffalo.edu

North Carolina

Carolinas Healthcare System, UNC–Charlotte
Verification of degrees

Telephone: Free of charge.
Written: $5 fee. Mail or fax requests, including signed release forms and each nurse anesthetist's Social Security number, year of graduation, and maiden name (if applicable).
Electronic: Not provided.

Nurse Anesthesia Program
Carolinas Healthcare System, UNC-Charlotte
PO Box 32861
1200 Blythe Boulevard
Charlotte, NORTH CAROLINA 28232-2861
Telephone: 704/355-2375
Fax: 704/355-7263
E-mail: jhall@carolinashealthcare.org
Web site: www.carolinas.org

Durham Regional Hospital, Watts School of Nursing
Verification of degrees

Telephone: Free of charge.
Written: Free of charge. Faxed upon request. Mail or fax requests including signed release forms. $5 for transcripts.
Electronic: Not provided.

Watts School of Nursing
Durham Regional Hospital
3643 N. Roxboro Street
Durham, NORTH CAROLINA 27704
Telephone: 919/470-7348 (School of Nursing)
Fax: 919/470-7346
Web site: drh.duhs.duke.edu/wattsson

Nurse Anesthesia (CRNA) Programs

North Dakota

University of North Dakota, Specialization in Anesthesia Masters Program
Verification of degrees

Telephone: Free of charge.

Written: Free of charge. Faxed upon request. Mail or fax requests, including signed release forms, and nurse anesthetist's Social Security number and year of graduation.

Electronic: Not provided.

> Office of the Registrar
> University of North Dakota
> PO Box 8382
> Grand Forks, NORTH DAKOTA 58202-8382
> Telephone: 701/777-2711   800/CAL-LUND (Central Operator)
> Fax: 701/777-2696
> Web site: www.und.edu

Ohio

Case Western Reserve University/Mt. Sinai Medical Center/Cleveland Clinic Foundation, Frances Payne Bolton School of Nursing, School of Nurse Anesthesia
Verification of degrees

Telephone: Not provided.

Written: $5 per verification that requires searching. Faxed upon request. Mail or fax requests, including signed release forms, and each nurse anesthetist's Social Security number and year of graduation.

Electronic: Automated verification system available at Web site to verify degrees awarded within past 12–15 years. Username: degree; password: 2verif. Access to Web site is currently limited to credentialing agencies.

> Attention: Degree verification request
> Office of the Registrar
> Pardee Hall, Room 223
> Case Western Reserve University
> 10900 Euclid Avenue
> Cleveland, OHIO 44106-4904
> Telephone: 800/825-2540, Ext. 2183
> Fax: 216/368-8711
> Web site: www.cwru.edu/provost/registrar/degweb.html

St. Elizabeth Health Center, School for Nurse Anesthetists, Inc.
Verification of degrees

Telephone: Not provided.

Written: Free of charge for verifications; $3 for transcripts. Faxed upon request. Mail or fax requests, including signed release forms.

Electronic: Not provided.

> School for Nurse Anesthetists
> St. Elizabeth Health Center
> 1044 Belmont Avenue
> PO Box 2165

Youngstown, OHIO 44501-1790
Telephone: 330/480-3444
Fax: 330/480-5202
Web site: www.belpark.net/crnaschool

The University of Akron College of Nursing Anesthesia Track
Verification of degrees

Telephone:	Free of charge.
Written:	Free of charge. Faxed upon request. Mail or fax requests, including signed release forms and nurse anethetist's Social Security number.
Electronic:	Not provided.

Attention: Enrollment verification request
Office of the University Registrar
The University of Akron
Akron, OHIO 44325-6208
Telephone: 330/972-8300
Fax: 330/972-6097
E-mail: registrar@uakron.edu
Web site: www.uakron.edu

University of Cincinnati Nurse Anesthesia Program
Verification of degrees

Telephone:	Free of charge.
Written:	Free of charge. Faxed upon request. Mail or fax requests, including signed release forms.
Electronic:	Not provided.

Office of the Registrar
Mail Location 150
PO Box 210150
University of Cincinnati
Cincinnati, OHIO 45221-0150
Telephone: 513/556-6517
Fax: 513/556-6579
Web site: www.uc.edu/registrar

Pennsylvania

Hamot Medical Center School of Anesthesia
Verification of degrees

Telephone:	Not provided.
Written:	Faxed upon request. Mail or fax requests, including signed release forms and payment. Call first for fee.
Electronic:	Not provided.

School of Anesthesia
Hamot Medical Center
201 State Street
Erie, PENNSYLVANIA 16550

Nurse Anesthesia (CRNA) Programs

Telephone: 817/877-2938
Fax: 817/877-6070
E-mail: steve.anderson@hamot.org
Web site: www.hamotschoolofanesthesia.com

Lankenau Hospital School of Nurse Anesthesia
Verification of degrees

Telephone:	Free of charge.
Written:	Free of charge. Faxed upon request. Mail or fax requests, including signed release forms.
Electronic:	Not provided.

School of Nurse Anesthesia
Lankenau Hospital
100 Lancaster Avenue
Wynnewood, PENNSYLVANIA 19096
Telephone: 610/645-2145
Fax: 610/645-3411
E-mail: wildgustb@mlhs.org
Web site: www.villanova.edu

MCP Hahnemann University, Graduate Program of Nurse Anesthesia
Verification of degrees

Telephone:	Free of charge. Provide nurse anesthetist's Social Security number. Only for nurse anesthetists who graduated 1983 to present.
Written:	Free of charge. Faxed upon request. Mail or fax requests, including signed release forms.
Electronic:	Not provided.

Office of the Registrar
MCP Hahnemann University
Broad and Vine Streets
Mail Stop 445
Philadelphia, PENNSYLVANIA 19102-1192
Telephone: 215/762-7602
Fax: 215/762-4313

Montgomery Hospital, School of Anesthesia
Verification of degrees

Telephone:	Free of charge.
Written:	$2 per verification. Mail or fax requests, including signed release forms and payment.
Electronic:	Not provided.

School of Anesthesia at Montgomery Hospital
1301 Powell Street
PO Box 992
Norristown, PENNSYLVANIA 19404-0992
Telephone: 610/270-2139
Fax: 610/270-2318
E-mail: philacrna@aol.com

Nazareth Hospital, School of Nurse Anesthesiology
Notes: School is affiliated with and issues certificates through St. Joseph's University.
Verification of certificates
Telephone: Free of charge.
Written: Free of charge. Faxed upon request. Mail or fax requests, including signed release forms, and nurse anesthetist's Social Security number and year of graduation.
Electronic: Not provided.

> School of Nurse Anesthesiology
> Nazareth Hospital
> 2601 Holme Avenue
> Philadelphia, PENNSYLVANIA 19152-2096
> Telephone: 215/335-6217
> Fax: 215/335-6668
> E-mail: jwoods@che-east.org

Pennsylvania Hospital, School of Nurse Anesthesia
Verification of degrees
Telephone: Not provided.
Written: Free of charge. Faxed upon request. Mail or fax requests, including signed release forms.
Electronic: Not provided.

> School of Nurse Anesthesia
> Pennsylvania Hospital
> 700 Spruce Street, Suite 402
> Philadelphia, PENNSYLVANIA 19107-6192
> Telephone: 215/829-3320
> Fax: 215/829-8757
> Web site: www.med.upenn.edu/pahosp/pahpe/nurse_anesth/index.html

Saint Francis Medical Center, LaRoche College, School of Anesthesia
Verification of degrees
Telephone: Free of charge. Unofficial.
Written: Faxed upon request. Mail or fax requests, including signed release forms, and nurse anesthetist's year of graduation and maiden name (if applicable). $15 fee.
Electronic: Not provided.

> Attention: Director
> School of Anesthesia
> Saint Francis Medical Center, LaRoche College
> 400 45th Street
> Pittsburgh, PENNSYLVANIA 15201-1198
> Telephone: 412/622-4369
> Fax: 412/688-3883
> E-mail: loefflera@sfhs.edu
> Web site: www.sfhs.edu/library/schools.anesth

University of Pittsburgh School of Nursing, Nurse Anesthesia Program
Verification of degrees

Telephone: Not provided.
Written: Free of charge. Faxed upon request. Mail or fax requests, including signed release forms.
Electronic: Not provided.

> Nurse Anesthesia Program
> University of Pittsburgh School of Nursing
> 3500 Victoria Street
> 336 Victoria Building
> Pittsburgh, PENNSYLVANIA 15261
> Telephone: 412/624-4860
> Fax: 412/383-7227
> E-mail: napcrna@pitt.edu
> Web site: www.pitt.edu/nap

Westmoreland Latrobe Hospitals, LaRoche College School of Anesthesia
Verification of degrees

Telephone: Free of charge.
Written: Free of charge. Faxed upon request. Mail or fax requests, including signed release forms.
Electronic: Not provided.

> School of Anesthesia
> Westmoreland Latrobe Hospitals, LaRoche College
> 532 W. Pittsburgh Street
> Greensburg, PENNSYLVANIA 15601
> Telephone: 724/832-4144
> Fax: 724/832-4164
> E-mail: bighoward@aol.com

Puerto Rico

InterAmerican University of Puerto Rico
Verification of degrees

Telephone: Not provided.
Written: Free of charge. Mail requests, including signed release forms.
Electronic: Not provided.

> Graduate Program in Nurse Anesthesiology
> Nursing Department
> InterAmerican University of Puerto Rico
> PO Box 4050
> Arecibo, PUERTO RICO 00614-4050
> Telephone: 787/878-5475
> Fax: 787/880-1624
> E-mail: jons@arecibo.inter.edu

University of Puerto Rico
Verification of degrees
Telephone: Not provided.
Written: Free of charge. Faxed upon request. Mail or fax requests, including release forms signed by nurse anesthetists.
Electronic: Not provided.

>Office of the Registrar, School of Nursing
>Medical Sciences Campus
>University of Puerto Rico
>GPO 365067
>San Juan, PUERTO RICO 00936-5067
>Telephone: 787/758-2525, Ext. 5224
>Fax: 787/756-7944

Quebec

Faculty of Medicine of University of Montreal
Notes: School of Nurse Anesthesia no longer exists. Direct verification requests to Director of Human Resources.
Verification of degrees
Telephone: Free of charge.
Written: Service charges. Mail or fax requests, including signed release forms.
Electronic: Not provided.

>Attention: Director
>Human Resources Department
>Eastern Maine Medical Center
>PO Box 6128, Station Centre-ville
>Montreal, QUEBEC H3C 3J7
>CANADA
>Telephone: 514/343-6111, Ext. 4131   514/343-6267 (Medicine of University of Montreal)
>Fax: 514/343-2068, Attention: Verification request

Rhode Island

Memorial Hospital of Rhode Island, School of Nurse Anesthesia
Verification of degrees
Telephone: Free of charge.
Written: Free of charge. Faxed upon request. Mail or fax requests, including signed release forms.
Electronic: Not provided.

>Attention: Program Director
>School of Nurse Anesthesia
>Memorial Hospital of Rhode Island
>111 Brewster Street
>Pawtucket, RHODE ISLAND 02860
>Telephone: 401/729-2485
>Fax: 401/729-3476
>E-mail: foster@ids.net
>Web site: www.mhri.org/anes

Saint Joseph Hospital, School of Anesthesia for Nurses
Verification of degrees

Telephone: Not provided.
Written: Free of charge. Faxed upon request. Mail or fax requests, including signed release forms.
Electronic: Not provided.

School of Anesthesia for Nurses
Saint Joseph Hospital
200 High Service Avenue
North Providence, RHODE ISLAND 02904-5113
Telephone: 401/456-3639
Fax: 401/752-8140
E-mail: saintjoes@aol.com

South Carolina

Medical University of South Carolina, Anesthesia for Nurses Program
Notes: All information is obtained through National Student Clearing House. Call for specific information.
Verification of degrees

Telephone: Free of charge.
Written: Provided through National Student Clearing House.
Electronic: Not provided.

Attention: Degree verification request
Enrollment Services
Medical University of South Carolina
41 Bee Street
PO Box 250203
Charleston, SOUTH CAROLINA 29425-2714
Telephone: 843/792-5396
Fax: 843/792-3764
Web site: www.musc.edu

Palmetto Richland Memorial Hospital/USC/PRMH Graduate Program in Nurse Anesthesia
Verification of degrees

Telephone: Free of charge.
Written: Free of charge. Faxed upon request. Mail or fax requests, including signed release forms, and nurse anesthetist's Social Security number, year of graduation, and maiden name (if applicable).
Electronic: Not provided.

Graduate Program in Nurse Anesthesia
Richland Memorial Hospital/USC
Five Richland Medical Park, Suite 221
Columbia, SOUTH CAROLINA 29203
Telephone: 803/434-6344
Fax: 803/434-4099
E-mail: kwilliam@richmed.medpark.sc.edu
Web site: www.med.sc.edu:88/mnuran.htm

South Dakota

Avera McKennan University and Health Systems
Verification of degrees

Telephone:	Not provided.
Written:	Free of charge. Graduates themselves must mail requests, including signed release forms.
Electronic:	Not provided.

Attention: Degree verification request
School of Anesthesia for Registered Nurses
McKennan Hospital University of South Dakota
800 E. 21st Street
Sioux Falls, SOUTH DAKOTA 57117-5045
Telephone: 605/322-8000
Fax: 605/322-8885
Web site: www.averamckennan.org

Mount Marty College, Graduate Program in Nurse Anesthesia
Verification of degrees

Telephone:	Free of charge.
Written:	Free of charge. Faxed upon request. Mail or fax requests.
Electronic:	Not provided.

Office of the Registraar
Mount Marty College
1105 W. Eight Street
Yankton, SOUTH DAKOTA 57078
Telephone: 605/668-1515 (Registrar's Office)   605/322-8090 (Program Director, Graduate Programs)
Fax: 605/322-8095
E-mail: msna@mtmc.edu
Web site: www.mtmc.edu

Tennessee

Erlanger Medical Center, School of Nurse Anesthesia
Verification of degrees

Telephone:	Not provided.
Written:	Free of charge. Faxed upon request. Mail or fax requests, including signed release forms.
Electronic:	Not provided.

School of Nurse Anesthesia
Erlanger Medical Center
975 E. Third Street
Chattanooga, TENNESSEE 37403-2112
Telephone: 423/778-7760
Fax: 423/778-6659
E-mail: wilsonst@erlanger.org
Web site: www.erlanger.org

Middle Tennessee School of Anesthesia
Verification of degrees
Telephone: Not provided.
Written: Free of charge. Mail requests, including signed release forms, and nurse anesthetist's Social Security number, year of graduation, and maiden name (if applicable).
Electronic: Not provided.

>Middle Tennessee School of Anesthesia
>315 Hospital Drive
>Madison, TENNESSEE 37116-6414
>Telephone: 615/868-6503
>Fax: 615/868-9885
>Web site: www.mtsa.edu

University of Tennessee Medical Center, Nurse Anesthesia Concentration
Notes: Transcript information requests require a signed and dated letter from the graduate. It must include your Social Security number, phone number, exact name by which you were known while in the program, and name and address of the person receiving the information.
Verification of degrees
Telephone: Not provided.
Written: Free of charge. Mail requests, including signed release forms.
Electronic: Not provided.

>University of Tennessee Medical Center, Nurse Anesthesia Concentration
>1924 Alcoa Highway
>Drawer U-109
>Knoxville, TENNESSEE 37920-6999
>Telephone: 865/544-9222
>Fax: 865/544-6852

Texas

Baylor College of Medicine, Graduate Program in Nurse Anesthesia
Verification of degrees
Telephone: Free of charge.
Written: Free of charge. Faxed upon request. Mail or fax requests, including signed release forms, self-addressed, stamped envelopes, and nurse anesthetist's program and maiden name (if applicable).
Electronic: Not provided.

>Office of the Registrar
>Baylor College of Medicine
>One Baylor Plaza, Suite M-108
>Houston, TEXAS 77030
>Telephone: 713/798-7766
>Fax: 713/798-7951
>E-mail: registrar@bcm.tmc.edu
>Web site: www.bcm.tmc.edu

U.S. Army Graduate Program in Anesthesia Nursing
Notes: For information about the program or its clinical sites, contact the U.S. Army Graduate Program in Anesthesia Nursing.
Annual report of licensed physicians
Telephone: Not provided.
Written: Not provided.
Electronic: Not provided.

>   Academy of Health Sciences
>   Department of Academic Support MCCS-HST
>   2250 Stanley Road, Suite 223
>   Fort Sam Houston, TEXAS 78234-6150
>   Telephone: 210/221-6219 (main office)   210/221-8426 (second line)   210/221-8066 (third line)
>   Fax: 210/221-8711
>   Web site: www.cs.amedd.army.mil/crna

University of Texas Health Science Center, Houston School of Nursing
Verification of degrees
Telephone: Free of charge.
Written: Free of charge. Faxed upon request. Mail or fax requests, including signed release forms.
Electronic: Not provided.

>   Office of the Registrar
>   University of Texas Health Science Center
>   PO Box 20036
>   Houston School of Nursing
>   Houston, TEXAS 77225
>   Telephone: 713/500-3361
>   Fax: 713/500-3356
>   Web site: www.uthouston.edu

Virginia

DePaul Medical Center Bonsecour
Notes: School no longer offers nurse anesthesia program. Last graduating class: 1997.
Verification of degrees
Telephone: Not provided.
Written: Free of charge. Mail or fax requests, including signed release forms.
Electronic: Not provided.

>   School of Nurse Anesthesia
>   DePaul Medical Center Bonsecour
>   150 Kingsley Lane
>   Attention: Human Resources
>   Norfolk, VIRGINIA 23505-4602
>   Telephone: 757/889-5241
>   Fax: 757/889-5222
>   Web site: www.bonsecourshamptonroads.org

Old Dominion University School of Nursing, Nurse Anesthesia Program
Verification of degrees
Telephone: Not provided.
Written: Free of charge. Faxed upon request. Mail or fax requests, including signed release forms.
Electronic: Information available on our Web site.

>Old Dominion University School of Nursing
>4608 Hampton Boulevard
>Technology Building
>Norfolk, VIRGINIA 23529-0500
>Telephone: 757/683-4297
>Fax: 757/683-5253
>E-mail: oduson@odu.edu
>Web site: web.odu.edu

Virginia Commonwealth University, Department of Nurse Anesthesia
Verification of degrees
Telephone: Free of charge.
Written: Free of charge. Faxed upon request. Mail or fax requests, including signed release forms.
Electronic: Information available on Web site.

>Department of Nurse Anesthesia
>Virginia Commonwealth University
>PO Box 980226
>Richmond, VIRGINIA 23298-0226
>Telephone: 804/828-9808
>Fax: 804/828-0581
>E-mail: mdfallac@hsc.vcu.edu
>Web site: views.vcu.edu/sahp/rngas

West Virginia

Charleston Area Medical Center, School of Nurse Anesthesia
Verification of degrees
Telephone: Not provided.
Written: $25 verification fee, upon request with written consent. $10 transcript fee for written verification.
Electronic: Not provided.

>School of Nurse Anesthesia
>Charleston Area Medical Center
>Robert C. Byrd Building, Room 2041
>3110 MacCorkle Avenue SE
>Charleston, WEST VIRGINIA 25304
>Telephone: 304/388-9950
>Fax: 304/388-9955
>E-mail: barbara.riffle@camc.org
>Web site: www.camcinstitute.org/anesthesia

United Hospital Center/LaRoche College, Nurse Anesthesia Program
Notes: School of Anesthesia closed in August 1997. Direct requests to United Hospital Center.
Verification of degrees
Telephone: Not provided.
Written: Free of charge. Mail requests, including signed release forms.
Electronic: Not provided.

> Attention: Degree verification request
> PO Box 1680
> United Hospital Center/LaRoche College
> Clarksburg, WEST VIRGINIA 26302-1680
> Telephone: 304/624-2315
> Fax: 304/624-2308

Wisconsin

Franciscan Skemp Healthcare, School of Anesthesia
Verification of degrees
Telephone: Free of charge.
Written: Free of charge. Faxed upon request. Mail, or fax requests.
Electronic: Not provided.

> Attention: Director
> Franciscan Skemp Healthcare, School of Anesthesia
> 700 West Avenue S
> La Crosse, WISCONSIN 54601
> Telephone: 608/785-0940
> Fax: 608/791-9799
> Web site: fshweb.mayo.edu

Nurse-Midwifery Programs

California

California Family Health Council, Inc.
Notes: This contact information is for the Training Division.
Verification of certificates

Telephone:	Free of charge.
Written:	$15 per verification. Faxed upon request. Mail or fax requests. Mail payment.
Electronic:	Not provided.

> Attention: Anita Aguirre, Director of Clinical EPA
> A Division of CFAC
> 492 Division Street
> Campbell, CALIFORNIA 95008
> Telephone: 408/374-3720
> Fax: 408/374-7385
> E-mail: epa@cfhc.org
> Web site: www.cfhc.org

Charles R. Drew University of Medicine and Science College of Allied Health
Verification of certificates

Telephone:	Not provided.
Written:	Free of charge. Mail requests, including signed release forms.
Electronic:	Not provided.

> Nurse-Midwifery Education Program
> College of Allied Health Sciences
> Charles R. Drew University of Medicine and Science
> 1731 E. 120th Street
> Los Angeles, CALIFORNIA 90059
> Telephone: 323/563-4951
> Fax: 323/357-3601 or 323/563-5871
> E-mail: frcushen@cdrewu.edu or almcghee@cdrewu.edu
> Web site: www.cdrewu.edu

UCSD Nurse-Midwifery Education Program
Verification of degrees

Telephone:	Free of charge.
Written:	Free of charge. Faxed upon request. Mail, phone, or fax requests, including signed release forms.
Electronic:	Free of charge

> University of California, San Diego
> 9500 Gilman Drive, Department 0809
> La Jolla, CALIFORNIA 92093-0809
> Telephone: 619/543-5480
> Fax: 619/543-7757

Chapter 5

UCSF Interdepartmental Nurse-Midwifery Education Program
Notes: Program's headquarters located at UCSF School of Nursing. Direct requests for verifications and/or information to the UCSF Nurse-Midwifery Education Program.

Verification of degrees

Telephone:	Not provided.
Written:	Free of charge. Include signed release form.
Electronic:	Free of charge.

> Office Of Student Affairs
> Two Koret Way
> Room N319X
> Box 0602
> San Francisco, CALIFORNIA 94143-0602
> Telephone: 415/476-1435
> Fax: 415/476-9707
> Web site: nurseweb.ucsf.edu

UCSF/SFGH Interdepartmental Nurse-Midwifery Education Program
Verification of certificates

Telephone:	Not provided.
Written:	Free of charge. Faxed upon request. Mail or fax requests, including signed release forms and date of graduation.
Electronic:	Not provided.

> UCSF/SFGH Interdepartmental Nurse-Midwifery Education Program
> SFGH Ward 6D
> 1001 Potrero Avenue
> San Francisco, CALIFORNIA 94110
> Telephone: 415/206-5106
> Fax: 415/206-3112
> E-mail: baorellin@oobgyn.ucss.edu
> Web site: www.ucss.edu

University of Southern California, Nurse-Midwifery Education Program
Verification of degrees

Telephone:	Free of charge via automated verification system; calls limited to three minutes. Input each student's ID number (same as Social Security number). Only for nurse midwives who graduated 1980 to present.
Written:	$5 per verification. Mail requests, including payment, signed release forms, and each nurse-midwife's Social Security number, date of birth, dates attended, and date of graduation.
Electronic:	Not provided.

> Verifications Department
> Office of the Registrar
> University of Southern California
> University Park
> Los Angeles, CALIFORNIA 90089-0912
> Telephone: 213/740-9230 (general information)   213/743-1516 (automated verification system)
> 213/743-1516 (verification degree or transcript)
> Fax: 888/777-3230

Colorado

University of Colorado Health Sciences Center
Verification of degrees

Telephone: Not provided.
Written: $30 charge. Faxed upon request. Mail or fax requests, including signed release forms.
Electronic: Not provided.

> University of Colorado Health Sciences Center
> School of Nursing, Office of Admissions and Student Support
> 4200 E. Ninth Avenue
> Campus Box C-288-6
> Denver, COLORADO 80262
> Telephone: 303/315-5592
> Fax: 303/315-8660
> E-mail: son.oasis@uchsc.edu
> Web site: www.uchsc.edu/nursing

Connecticut

Yale University, Nurse-Midwifery Program
Verification of degrees

Telephone: Free of charge.
Written: Free of charge. Faxed upon request. Mail or fax requests for verifications. Mail requests for transcripts, including signed release forms.
Electronic: Not provided.

> Nurse-Midwifery Program
> School of Nursing
> Yale University
> 100 Church Street S
> PO Box 9740
> New Haven, CONNECTICUT 06536-0740
> Telephone: 203/785-2389
> Fax: 203/737-5409
> Web site: www.nursing.yale.edu

District of Columbia

Georgetown University Graduate Program in Nurse-Midwifery
Verification of degrees

Telephone: Free of charge.
Written: Free of charge. Faxed upon request. Mail or fax requests, including signed release forms.
Electronic: Not provided.

> Georgetown University
> School of Nursing
> Graduate Program in Nurse-Midwifery
> 3700 Reservoir Road NW

Washington, DISTRICT OF COLUMBIA 20057
Telephone: 202/687-4772
Fax: 202/784-3128
Web site: www.georgetown.edu

Florida

University of Miami, School of Nursing
Notes:
Verification of degrees
Telephone: Free of charge.
Written: Free of charge. Faxed upon request. Mail or fax requests, including signed release forms.
Electronic: Not provided.

Office of Student Admissions and Records
University of Miami
PO Box 248025
Coral Gables, FLORIDA 33124-4616
Telephone: 305/284-4323
Fax: 305/284-2507
E-mail: admission@miami.edu
Web site: www.miami.edu-nur.

University of Miami/Jackson Memorial Medical Center, Nurse-Midwifery Precertification Program
Verification of certificates
Telephone: Not provided.
Written: Free of charge. Faxed upon request. Mail, phone, or fax requests, including signed release forms.
Electronic: Not provided.

University of Miami
School of Nursing
PO Box 248153
5801 Red Road
Coral Gables, FLORIDA 33124-3850
Telephone: 305/284-3666 (School of Nursing)   305/284-6256 (Nurse-Midwifery department)
Fax: 305/284-5686
Web site: www.miami.edu/nur

Georgia

Emory University, Nell Hodgson Woodruff School of Nursing
Verification of degrees
Telephone: Free of charge.
Written: Free of charge. Faxed upon request in emergency situations only. Mail or fax requests, including signed release forms.
Electronic: Not provided.

Attention: Director
Student Affairs Office
Nell Hodgson Woodruff School of Nursing

Emory University
1520 Clifton Road
Atlanta, GEORGIA 30322
Telephone: 404/727-3500
Fax: 404/727-8509
E-mail: kstark@nurse.emory.edu

Kentucky

Frontier School of Midwifery and Family Nursing
Verification of certificates

Telephone: Free of charge.
Written: Free of charge. Faxed upon request. Mail or fax requests, including signed release forms and nurse-midwife's Social Security number.
Electronic: Not provided.

Office of the Registrar
Frontier School of Midwifery and Family Nursing
PO Box 528
195 School Street
Hyden, KENTUCKY 41749
Telephone: 606/672-2312
Fax: 606/672-3776
E-mail: jlwoods@midwives.org
Web site: www.midwives.org

Massachusetts

Baystate Medical Center Nurse-Midwifery Education Program
Verification of certificates

Telephone: Free of charge.
Written: Free of charge. Faxed upon request. Mail or fax requests, including signed release forms.
Electronic: Not provided.

Nurse-Midwifery Education Program
Baystate Medical Center
759 Chestnut Street
Springfield, MASSACHUSETTS 01199
Telephone: 413/794-4448
Fax: 413/794-8770
E-mail: midwifery@bhs.org
Web site: www.bhs.org

Boston University School of Public Health, Nurse-Midwifery Education Program
Notes: Also offers graduate program for careers in Public Health.
Verification of degrees

Telephone: Free of charge.
Written: Free of charge. Faxed upon request. Mail or fax requests, including signed release forms.
Electronic: Not provided.

Attention: Director
Nurse-Midwifery Education Program
Boston University School of Public Health
715 Albany Street T5, W
Boston, MASSACHUSETTS 02118
Telephone: 617/638-5012
Fax: 617/638-5370
Web site: www.bu.edu

Michigan

University of Michigan School of Nursing, Nurse-Midwifery Education Program
Verification of degrees

Telephone: Not provided.
Written: Free of charge. Faxed upon request. Mail or fax requests, including signed release forms.
Electronic: Free of charge.

Nurse-Midwifery Education Program
University of Michigan School of Nursing
400 N. Ingalls Room 3320
Ann Arbor, MICHIGAN 48109-0482
Telephone: 734/763-3710
Fax: 734/615-8764
E-mail: crothers@umich.edu
Web site: www.personal.umich.edu~dswalker/umhome.htm

Minnesota

University of Minnesota School of Nursing Nurse-Midwifery Program
Verification of degrees

Telephone: Free of charge. Provide nurse-midwife's Social Security number.
Written: Free of charge. Mail or fax requests, including signed release forms and nurse-midwife's Social Security number.
Electronic: Not provided.

University of Minnesota School of Nursing
Nurse-Midwifery Program
6-101 Weaver-Densford Hall
308 Harvard Street SE
Minneapolis, MINNESOTA 55455
Telephone: 612/624-4454
Fax: 612/624-3174
E-mail: nurseoss@umn.edu
Web site: www.nursing.umn.edu

New Jersey

University of Medicine and Dentistry of New Jersey-Newark, School of Health-Related Professions
Verification of certificates

Telephone: Free of charge.
Written: Free of charge. Faxed upon request. Mail or fax requests, including signed release forms.
Electronic: Not provided.

> Attention: Program Director
> School of Health-Related Professions
> University of Medicine and Dentistry of New Jersey-Newark
> 65 Bergen Street
> Newark, NEW JERSEY 07107-3001
> Telephone: 201/972-4249
> Fax: 201/972-7403
> E-mail: diegmaek@umdnj.edu

New Mexico

University of New Mexico College of Nursing
Verification of degrees

Telephone: Not provided.
Written: Free of charge. Mail requests, including signed release forms.
Electronic: Not provided.

> Nurse-Midwifery Program
> University of New Mexico College of Nursing
> Nursing/Pharmacy Building
> Albuquerque, NEW MEXICO 87131-5688
> Telephone: 505/272-1184
> Fax: 505/272-8901
> E-mail: midwyfe@unm.edu
> Web site: www.hsc.unm.edu/consg

New York

Columbia University, Graduate Program in Nurse-Midwifery
Verification of degrees

Telephone: Free of charge.
Written: Free of charge. Mail requests, including signed release forms, and nurse-midwife's Social Security number, year of graduation, and maiden name (if applicable).
Electronic: Not provided.

> Attention: Registrar's Office
> Columbia University Student Administrative Services
> 630 W. 168th Street, Unit 45

Chapter 5

New York, NEW YORK 10032
Telephone: 212/305-3992
Fax: 212/305-1590
E-mail: sashs@columbia.edu
Web site: www.columbia.edu

New York University, Nurse-Midwifery Education Program
Verification of degrees
Telephone: Not provided.
Written: Free of charge. Mail requests, including signed release forms, and nurse-midwife's Social Security number and date of graduation. Requests will be forwarded to Records Office.
Electronic: Not provided.

Nurse-Midwifery Education Program
New York University
246 Green Street
New York, NEW YORK 10003-6677
Telephone: 212/998-5895
Fax: 212/995-4384
E-mail: pb8@nyu.edu
Web site: www.nyu.edu/education/nursing

North Central Bronx Hospital
Notes: For something other than a degree verification (e.g., transcript), please contact the Columbia University School of Nursing. (This program is no longer in operation.)
Verification of precertification
Telephone: Free of charge. Limit two verifications per call.
Written: Free of charge. Mail requests, including release form signed by nurse-midwife.
Electronic: Not provided.

Nurse-Midwifery Precertification Program
Department of OB/GYN
N. Central Bronx Hospital
3424 Kossuth Avenue, Room 14805
Bronx, NEW YORK 10467
Telephone: 718/519-3155   718/519-2141 (OB/GYN)
Fax: 718/519-3154

State University of New York at Stony Brook School of Nursing, Pathways to Midwifery Program
Verification of degrees
Telephone: Free of charge. Please include year of graduation.
Written: Free of charge. Mail or fax requests, including signed release forms.
Electronic: Not provided.

State University of New York at Stony Brook School of Nursing, Pathways to Midwifery Program
Student Affairs Office
SUNY-Stony Brook School of Nursing

Nurse-Midwifery Programs

Health Sciences Center, Level II
Stony Brook, NEW YORK 11794-8240
Telephone: 631/444-3200
Fax: 631/444-6628

State University of New York Downstate Medical Center, Midwifery Education Program
Verification of degrees

Telephone: Free of charge; prefer written request.
Written: Free of charge. Mail or fax requests, including signed release forms and nurse-midwife's maiden name (if applicable).
Electronic: Not provided.

Midwifery Education Program
SUNY Downstate Medical Center
450 Clarkson Avenue, Box 1227
Brooklyn, NEW YORK 11203
Telephone: 718/270-7740
Fax: 718/270-7634

University of Rochester School of Nursing
Notes: As of 2000, they no longer offer the Midwifery Program.
Verification of degrees

Telephone: Free of charge.
Written: Free of charge. Faxed upon request. Mail or fax requests, including signed release forms.
Electronic: Not provided.

University of Rochester School of Nursing
601 Elmwood Avenue, Box SON
Rochester, NEW YORK 14642
Telephone: 585/275-2375
Fax: 585/756-8299
Web site: www.urmc.rochester.edu

North Carolina

East Carolina University School of Nursing,
Verification of degrees

Telephone: Not provided.
Written: Free of charge. Graduates themselves must mail requests, including signed release forms.
Electronic: Not provided.

Office of the Registrar
East Carolina University School of Nursing
Greenville, NORTH CAROLINA 27858-4353
Telephone: 252/328-6747   252/328-6075 (School of Nursing)   252/328-4302 (Nurse-Midwifery Program)
Fax: 252/328-4300
E-mail: mossn@mail.ecu.edu
Web site: www.ecu.edu

Ohio

Case Western Reserve University, Frances Payne Bolton School of Nursing, Nurse-Midwifery Program
Verification of degrees

Telephone: Not provided.
Written: Free of charge. Faxed upon request. Mail or fax requests, including signed release forms, and nurse-midwife's Social Security number and year of graduation.
Electronic: Not provided.

> Registrar's Office
> Case Western Reserve University
> 2121 Abington Road
> Cleveland, OHIO 44106-4904
> Telephone: 216/368-4700 (main)   800/825-2540
> Fax: 216/368-3542
> E-mail: webmaster@fpb.cwru.edu
> Web site: www.fpb.cwru.edu

Ohio State University College of Nursing, Nurse-Midwifery Education Program
Verification of degrees

Telephone: Not provided.
Written: Free of charge. Faxed upon request. Mail or fax requests, including signed release forms.
Electronic: Not provided.

> Student Affairs
> Ohio State University College of Nursing
> 1585 Neil Avenue
> Columbus, OHIO 43210-1289
> Telephone: 614/292-4041
> Fax: 614/292-9399
> Web site: www.con-ohio.state.edu

University of Cincinnati, Nurse-Midwifery Education Program
Verification of degrees

Telephone: Free of charge.
Written: Free of charge. Mail requests, including signed release forms.
Electronic: Not provided.

> Nurse-Midwifery Education Program
> College of Nursing and Health
> University of Cincinnati
> 3110 Vine Street, ML 0038
> Cincinnati, OHIO 45221
> Telephone: 513/558-5282
> Fax: 513/558-2142
> Web site: www.uc.edu

Oregon

Oregon Health & Science University, School of Nursing
Verification of degrees

Telephone: Free of charge.
Written: Free of charge. Faxed upon request. Mail or fax requests, including signed release forms.
Electronic: Not provided.

> Attention: Program Director
> Oregon Health & Sciences University, School of Nursing
> 3181 S.W. Sam Jackson Park Road
> Portland, OREGON 97201-3098
> Telephone: 503/494-3822
> Fax: 503/494-3878
> E-mail: howec@ohfu.edu
> Web site: www.ohfu.edu

Pennsylvania

Institute of Midwifery, Women, and Health
Verification of certificates

Telephone: Free of charge.
Written: Free of charge.
Electronic: Information available on Web site.

> Institute of Midwifery, Women, and Health
> Philadelphia University
> 222 Hayward Hall
> School House Lane & Henry Avenue
> Philadelphia, PENNSYLVANIA 19144
> Telephone: 215/951-2525
> Fax: 215/951-2526
> Web site: www.instituteofmidwifery.org

University of Pennsylvania School of Nursing, Nurse-Midwifery Program
Verification of degrees

Telephone: Not provided.
Written: Free of charge. Faxed upon request. Mail or fax requests, including signed release forms on official stationary only.
Electronic: Not provided.

> Student Information Office
> University of Pennsylvania School of Nursing
> 420 Guardian Drive
> Philadelphia, PENNSYLVANIA 19104-6096
> Telephone: 215/898-4544
> Fax: 215/898-7399
> E-mail: nursinginfo@nursing.upenn.edu
> Web site: www.nursing.upenn.edu

Rhode Island

University of Rhode Island College of Nursing, Nurse-Midwife Program
Notes: Students are eligible for certification by the American College of Midwives.
Verification of degrees
Telephone: Free of charge.
Written: Free of charge. Faxed upon request. Mail, phone, or fax requests, including signed release forms.
Electronic: Not provided.

> University of Rhode Island College of Nursing
> White Hall
> Two Heathman Road
> Kingston, RHODE ISLAND 02881
> Telephone: 401/874-5328
> Fax: 401/874-2061
> E-mail: jmercer@uri.edu
> Web site: www.uri.edu/nursing

South Carolina

Medical University of South Carolina, Anesthesia for Nurses Program
Verification of degrees
Telephone: Not provided.
Written: Not provided.
Electronic: Not provided.

> Attention: Degree verification request
> Enrollment Services
> Medical University of South Carolina
> 41 Bee Street
> PO Box 250203
> Charleston, SOUTH CAROLINA 29425-2714
> Telephone: 843/792-3281
> Fax: 843/792-3764
> Web site: www.musc.edu/es

Texas

Baylor College of Medicine, Nurse-Midwifery Education Program
Verification of degrees
Telephone: Free of charge.
Written: Free of charge. Faxed upon request. Mail or fax requests, including signed release forms.
Electronic: Not provided.

> Office of the Registrar
> Baylor College of Medicine

Nurse-Midwifery Programs

One Baylor Plaza, Suite M-108
Houston, TEXAS 77030
Telephone: 713/798-7766
Fax: 713/798-1518
E-mail: registrar@bcm.tmc.edu
Web site: www.bcm.tmc.edu

Parkland School of Nurse-Midwifery
Verification of certificates

Telephone: Not provided.
Written: Free of charge. Mail requests, including nurse-midwife names, Social Security numbers, and signed release forms.
Electronic: Not provided.

Parkland School of Nurse-Midwifery
Parkland Health & Hospital System
MS 6017A
5201 Harry Hines Boulevard
Dallas, TEXAS 75235
Telephone: 214/590-2580
Fax: 214/590-0436
E-mail: mbruck@parknet.pmh.org
Web site: www.swmed.edu/home_pages/parkland/midwifery/midwifehome.html

University of Texas Medical Branch-Galveston
Verification of degrees

Telephone: Free of charge.
Written: Free of charge. Mail or fax requests, including signed release forms, and nurse-midwife's Social Security number and maiden name (if applicable).
Electronic: Not provided.

Attention: Degree verification request
Enrollment Services
University of Texas Medical Branch-Galveston
Ashbell Smith Building, Room 1206
Galveston, TEXAS 77555-1312
Telephone: 409/772-1215
Fax: 409/772-4466
Web site: www.utmb.edu

University of Texas-El Paso/Texas Tech University, Collaborative Nurse-Midwifery Program at Texas Tech University Health Science Center
Verification of degrees

Telephone: Free of charge.
Written: Free of charge. Faxed upon request. Mail or fax requests, including signed release forms.
Electronic: Not provided.

Attention: Director Collaborative Nurse-Midwifery Program

Chapter 5

Department of OB/GYN
Texas Tech University Health Science Center
University of Texas El Paso/Texas Tech University
4800 Alberta Avenue
El Paso, TEXAS 79905
Telephone: 915/545-6490
Fax: 915/545-6549
E-mail: midwifery@ttmcelp.ttuhse.edu

Utah

University of Utah College of Nursing, Graduate Program in Nurse-Midwifery
Verification of degrees

Telephone: Free of charge. Provide nurse-midwife's Social Security number.
Written: Free of charge. Faxed upon request. Mail, phone, or fax requests.
Electronic: Not provided.

Office of the Registrar
University of Utah
201 S. 1460 E, Room 250N
Salt Lake City, UTAH 84112-9056
Telephone: 801/581-8965
Fax: 801/585-9151
E-mail: registrar@saff.utah.edu
Web site: www.saff.utah.edu

Washington

University of Washington School of Nursing, Nurse-Midwifery Education Program
Verification of degrees

Telephone: Not provided.
Written: Free of charge. Faxed upon request. Mail or fax requests, including signed release forms.
Electronic: Not provided.

Attention: Degree verification request
Director
University of Washington School of Nursing
Box 357262
Seattle, WASHINGTON 98195-7262
Telephone: 206/543-8241
Fax: 206/543-6656
E-mail: midwife@u.washington.edu
Web site: www.son.washington.edu

Wisconsin

Marquette University College of Nursing
Verification of degrees
Telephone: Free of charge.
Written: Free of charge. Faxed upon request. Mail or fax requests, including signed release forms.
Electronic: Not provided.

> Associate Dean of Graduate Programs
> Marquette University College of Nursing
> PO Box 1881
> Milwaukee, WISCONSIN 53201-1881
> Telephone: 414/288-3810 (Associate Dean)   414/288-38420 (Midwifery department)
> Fax: 414/288-1597
> E-mail: karen.nest@marquette.edu
> Web site: www.marquette.edu/nursing

Ramsey Clinic, Nurse-Midwifery Precertification Program
Notes: Program closed in 1998. Please refer verification and other questions to the American College of Nurse-Midwives (ACNM) in Washington, DC (202/728-9860).
Verification of precertification
Telephone: Not provided.
Written: Not provided.
Electronic: Not provided.

CHAPTER 6
Licensing Agencies

Chapter 6
Licensing Agencies

How licensure is regulated

A license is the authority a government agency grants an individual to practice a profession. Almost all health care professionals are regulated through the licensure process. (In a few states, some health care professions are not licensed, but often are recognized through some sort of national testing and certification by a specialty organization.) Hospitals should verify the licenses (or, when appropriate, the national certification) of all health care practitioners. Current licensure is the minimum requirement for practicing a health care profession in a state where that profession is licensed. Practicing without a license—or even with an expired license—is usually considered a serious crime.

The federal government is not involved in professional licensure; each state establishes its own requirements and practices (with the exception of the federal Drug Enforcement Agency certificate). For this reason, a license is technically valid only within the state that issues it, although states commonly accept licenses issued by other states as evidence of completion of some (or all) of their own requirements (called partial reciprocity or complete reciprocity, respectively). For example, a licensing agency in one state might waive the written examination requirement for an applicant who passed a similar examination in another state. (There are a few governmental organizations that are not states but act like states for many purposes, including issuing licenses. Good examples of this are the District of Columbia and the Commonwealth of Puerto Rico.)

Each state has one or more agencies concerned with health care professional licensing. There are often subagencies devoted to each profession, usually led by a board of professionals and public representatives. These agencies establish regulations that define the scope of professions—what members of the profession are authorized to do—and ensure that all licensed members of the profession are competent to practice.

The details of licensure differ among states and even among professions in the same state. In fact, some professions are licensed in some states and not in others. Generally, licensure of physicians, dentists, and podiatrists is similar throughout the United States. But there are significant variations among states regarding the scope of nursing practice and the licensure of psychologists and social workers. Therefore, it is essential that credentialing personnel responsible for verifying licensure become familiar with the licensure details of their own states for each of the professions they credential.

It is important to note that an organization should verify licensure as a separate credential; it cannot assume a practitioner is licensed simply because the practitioner holds some other type of credential. For example, regarding medical licensure, although some state medical licensing agencies recognize diplomas awarded by the National Board of Medical Examiners (NBME) and/or certificates awarded by the Educational Commission for Foreign Medical Graduates (ECFMG) as evidence of having fulfilled some requirements for medical licensure—typically medical school graduation and the licensing examination—these credentials are not the equivalent of licensure (each state additionally requires a licensure application, fee, and sometimes other evidence of qualifications for full licensure). Thus, organizations might choose to verify NBME or ECFMG status, but are not required to do so by the Joint Commission on Accreditation of Healthcare Organizations (JCAHO). Proof of existence of NBME or ECFMG does not substitute for verification of licensure.

JCAHO requirements for license verification

Organizations are required by the Joint Commission on Accreditation of Healthcare Organizations (JCAHO)—and, typically, by state law—to be certain that all health care professionals practicing independently within their walls (who can be licensed) are currently licensed. (Other types of accredited organizations are required by state law to ensure that health care professionals are licensed, but state requirements might vary for different types of organizations.) In fact, licensure is one of the credentials the JCAHO requires to be verified with the primary source—the state licensing agency. The JCAHO makes no distinction among professions; credentialing professionals must use the same degree of detailed scrutiny when credentialing all licensed independent practitioners—both physicians and nonphysicians. JCAHO surveyors are instructed to notify JCAHO headquarters immediately if they find a hospital permitting an unlicensed practitioner to practice. This situation can then lead to severe penalties.

When a practitioner holds licenses in several states, the organization should verify the status of all licenses upon reappointment to ensure that the practitioner has not been disciplined in any other state. Typically, licensure action occurring in one state will trigger action in all states. Although such verification practices go beyond JCAHO requirements, they ensure that the organization is aware of any professional problems an applicant has encountered.

The significance of licensure

What, exactly, does a license mean in regard to an individual's competence? It says a practitioner possesses the minimum knowledge and experience to do the job. But unfortunately, current licensure does not always guarantee current competence.

An initial licensure requirement for most professions includes graduation from a recognized professional school or program—a logical criterion, since it can be assumed that graduates are adequately competent at the time of graduation. Licensing agencies also usually require applicants to pass an examination focusing on facts relevant to professional practice. Although neither schooling nor an examination truly indicates practical skills, few licensing agencies test the practical skills of applicants. Further, although graduation from a professional school is required, there is never any time limit on the acceptability of graduation. Obviously, an individual who graduated 30 years prior to licensure application might have knowledge and skills that are out of date.

Generally, renewal of licensure for most professions has only minimal requirements. These typically include paying a fee, attending continuing education courses, and avoiding disciplinary action. Unlike initial licensure, renewal does not presume to test a practitioner's competence in any way. Thus, even an individual who graduated many years ago and has not practiced certain professional skills for a long time may still qualify for a license renewal to use those skills. Many retired physicians maintain licensure through their lifetime, even though no longer actively practicing medicine.

Licenses generally allow individuals to practice in all aspects of a profession. For example, a psychiatrist who has not practiced in any other branch of medicine for many years is still licensed to perform surgery, just as a licensed surgeon may practice psychiatry and a nurse who has exclusively performed geriatric nursing for many years is still authorized by his or her state license to work in the newborn nursery.

State licensing agencies are not required to check credentials against any particular standards. As a result, some licensing agencies fail to adequately verify the credentials of applicants. The result is that individuals are sometimes able to obtain licenses fraudulently, without meeting all necessary requirements—most typically, the completion of professional training. A recent case described in newspaper headlines was that of an individual who had repeatedly received a state medical license but who had never graduated from medical school. The state had never verified the individual's claim.

Organizations cannot be sure that an individual who possesses a license is actually the person named on the license. Most state licensing agencies do not verify the identity of applicants by a fingerprint check, so it is possible that a person could successfully assume the identity of a licensed practitioner. Although such a situation is uncommon, organizations cannot afford the chance of employing a fraudulent practitioner. Some states are far more conscientious about checking credentials than others, but no comparative statistics are available. Do not assume that any state licensing agency thoroughly verifies credentials. A computer-savvy person with a quality printer can easily duplicate a license and other certificates.

Finally, current licensure does not always accurately indicate the presence or absence of disciplinary charges against a practitioner. Most licensing agencies treat any pending charges against a practitioner as completely confidential until final adjudication. Therefore, it is possible for an individual to be in the investigation or final stages of loss of license for incompetence or unethical behavior, but still maintain a license in good standing. Again, this underscores the need for hospitals to verify other credentials, obtain peer recommendations, and verify hospital appointment and privileges.

Licensure limitations

Licensed practitioners are accountable for practicing only within the authority granted by virtue of their licenses and are expected to comply with all state laws and regulations. Many state licensing agencies place limits on licenses. These limits might be specific to the individual in question—for example, a physician who has been disciplined for improper prescribing of controlled drugs may be forbidden to write prescriptions for such drugs—or they might apply to an entire profession—for example, in many states, advance practice nurses are able to practice only under the supervision of physicians.

When a health care profession as a whole has limited licenses, the members are often referred to as limited license professionals—those who, unlike physicians, may practice only under medical direction or supervision. Nurses and physician assistants, for example, are typical limited license professionals. The status of limited license professionals, however, is not always clear and varies among states and even by practice sites within the same state. For example, in some states, nurses cannot practice in hospitals without physician direction, but may practice independently outside hospitals. It is important that credentialing staff be familiar with state licensure limitations, which are outlined in the relevant state professional practice laws.

Verifying licensure

A critical part of processing an application is verifying that the applicant is currently licensed in the state in which you are located and that no restrictions have been placed on the license. Obtaining an applicant's history of disciplinary actions from the state licensing agency is equally important. It is also common to investigate an applicant's licensure history in every state in which he or she has practiced.

Obtaining a complete picture of an applicant's licensure history is sometimes difficult. Until recently, state licensing agencies commonly did not share applicants' licensure information with each other. It was possible for an individual disciplined in one state—even to the point of loss of license—to simply apply for a license in another state and start again with a fresh record. Although licensing agencies today usually investigate the out-of-state records of applicants, one cannot assume this is always the case. In fact, even a recent granting of a new state license does not necessarily mean an applicant had no problems in other states. For example, it is still possible for an individual to obtain a new state license when actions against his or her license in another state are not fully settled, or when an adverse decision occurred years ago. Some organizations require applicants to list all the states in which they have held licenses, and their licensure history in each. If a credentialer does not verify the licensure information that an applicant provides with other sources (such as the Federation of State Medical Boards [FSMB]), the credentialer may not learn of licensure history an applicant may have omitted. It is good practice to consider whether the physician was licensed in any state in which he or she worked or trained.

The best way of obtaining a complete picture of an applicant's licensure history is to consult multiple sources, rather than relying on any one source for all information. For this reason, a hospital should check the licensure histories of applicants by contacting any or all of the individual state licensing agencies, the National Practitioner Data Bank (NPDB), Health Integrity Protection Data Bank (HIPDB) and/or the FSMB. (Note: Hospitals are not allowed to query the HIPDB unless they have designated themselves as an entity providing a policy of health insurance. Some hospitals that provide insurance to their employees through a self-insurance program are eligible to query, but this information is kept separate from the physician's credentials file.)

In principle, the NPDB provides information about the licensure actions against a practitioner in all states in which the practitioner has practiced. In reality, however, information from the NPDB must be evaluated with several cautions in mind. First, the NPDB did not begin operations until 1989, so it does not have records for earlier events. Second, the NPDB's information is gathered through other agencies, so its records have the potential to be incomplete. In fact, on November 30, 2000, the General Accounting Office (GAO) criticized the reliability of the NPDB, pointing to underreporting by malpractice insurers, hospitals, and other health care providers. The GAO study found that a significant amount of the data in the NPDB was "incomplete, inappropriate, inconsistent, and even inaccurate." The report urged the Health Resources and Services Administration to beef up enforcement of the regulations that govern the data bank. In addition, the GAO recommended that the secretary of Health and Human Services seek legislative remedies to repair the flaws in the data bank. Similarly, the FSMB depends upon other agencies for its information, so it, too, may have incomplete files. The FSMB, however, does maintain data from the early 1900s on and also has a reputation for providing complete reports on practitioners.

How to use this chapter

Because so many physician licensing examinations have been developed, it is difficult to understand when each is used, and for what purpose. To help clarify the confusion surrounding physician licensing examinations, the first section of this chapter discusses the history, purpose, and current status of each.

The remainder of this chapter includes information on how to query state licensing agencies. Most state licensing agencies disclose the current licensure status of any professional to the public. Due to the public outcry for information, more states now release information concerning licensure disciplinary actions. Because hospitals must verify the licensure status of a large number of health care professionals during the course of a year, some licensing agencies offer special provisions for hospitals, such as online verification, a special telephone number, or an annual printed list of licensees. However, the means by which this information is provided varies from state to state and from agency to agency. For example, a licensing agency might or might not

- verify licensure over the telephone
- require written requests for licensure verifications
- charge a fee for written verifications
- publish a directory of licensed practitioners

Consider the following when requesting a telephone and/or written verification:

- Identify yourself clearly and state the purpose of your query when requesting telephone verifications

- Include self-addressed, stamped envelopes when requesting written verifications (unless your state uses a computer-generated envelope)

- Provide any useful information—such as the name (and maiden name, if applicable), license number, birth date, and Social Security number of the practitioners in question—to help an office retrieve the records and information more quickly and easily

- Include some sort of direction on the envelope or fax cover sheet of a verification request, such as the words "Attention: License verification request enclosed"

- Include clear and specific instruction as to where and to whom an agency should mail or fax written verifications (a department, name, and/or title can help to ensure that the verification reaches the correct person)

The listings provide information regarding how to contact all state licensing agencies for the following professionals:

- Physicians
- Dentists
- Podiatrists
- Physician assistants
- Psychologists
- Nurse anesthetists and nurse-midwives
- Chiropractors

Every agency listed was contacted directly, so each entry is current at the time of publication.

Physician licensing examinations

Background

Because licensure is a state function, there is no national license or standardized procedure for licensing in the United States. In recent years, however, progress has been made toward establishing uniform national standards and procedures for physician licensure, while still leaving ultimate licensing decisions to individual state licensing agencies. This progress has produced several important and complex changes in physician licensure examinations.

There are several physician licensing examinations, so the details of each can be confusing. It is essential that those responsible for evaluating physicians' credentials fully understand what these licensing examinations mean and how they can verify licensing examination credentials. The following pages discuss the main licensing examinations that credentialing personnel are likely to encounter and provide addresses and telephone numbers for readers to obtain more information. Note that several of the examinations described here are no longer available, but many physicians currently practicing have these credentials.

Licensure examinations offered by individual states

Years ago, each state had its own medical licensure examination. This system had several major drawbacks:

- Great variability among states in the extent of medical knowledge tested

- Unfairness in testing applicants who moved into new states—perhaps many years after graduating from medical school—whose clinical skills were good, but whose knowledge of basic medical sciences was out of date

- Great expense and burden to physicians who needed licenses in several states

Gradually, over the years, states stopped requiring or even offering state-sponsored licensure exams and instead have relied upon the national examinations described below. Nevertheless, there are still many currently active practitioners whose licenses are based upon state-specific examinations. These individuals may not have any of the national credentials. They may nevertheless have licenses in more than one state either through "reciprocity," where one state has recognized the license of another state; or through taking the individual examination of each state that has issued a license.

National Board of Medical Examiners

For many years, the NBME administered a three-part examination that was designed to be completed immediately after (or very shortly before) the end of the first year of postgraduate medical school education. Individuals who passed the exam became NBME diplomates. The NBME exam was advantageous for diplomates because the first two parts could be taken during medical school—while the material was fresh—and the final part could be taken shortly after graduation. Passing the three phases of the exam conferred lifetime status on successful candidates. In addition, at the time of examination, candidates did not need to designate any particular location for future licensure or practice, and could use NBME status to obtain licensure anywhere that the diplomate status was recognized—even many years after successfully completing the exam. NBME diplomates were thus given full or partial credit in many states for meeting some or all licensing examination requirements. Although NBME diplomate status was awarded for lifetime, some states that accepted NBME status for examination requirements did limit recognition to a specified period after examination.

The NBME examination was administered for the last time in May 1994. It has been replaced with the United States Medical Licensing Examination (USMLE).

Educational Commission for Foreign Medical Graduates

For many years, the ECFMG administered its own examination to graduates of medical schools located outside the United States, Puerto Rico, and Canada to assess their readiness to enter residency or fellowship programs within the United States. Those passing the exam became ECFMG-certified. The ECFMG also offered the Foreign Medical Graduate Examination in the Medical Sciences (FMGEMS) as part of its examination process.

Today, the ECFMG no longer administers its own examination or the FMGEMS. ECFMG processes USMLE and Clinical Skills Assessment Exam (CSA) applications for international medical students and graduates. It also proctors the CSA and reviews all documents associated with a student's final medical diploma. (see USMLE below). Although the USMLE is a three-part examination, the ECFMG only requires that candidates successfully complete the first two parts to be eligible for ECFMG certification. ECFMG certification is universally accepted in the United States and qualifies a graduate to apply for residencies and licensure in all 50 states and in U.S. territories.

To be eligible for certification by ECFMG, candidates must meet the following requirements:

- Graduate from a medical school outside of the United States, Canada, or Puerto Rico that is listed in the World Directory of Medical Schools (published by the World Health Organization) at the time of graduation. All documents provided to the ECFMG are verified directly with appropriate officials of the foreign medical schools.

- Pass Step 1 (basic medical) and Step 2 (clinical) of the USMLE within a seven-year period.

- Pass the English language proficiency test. ECFMG no longer administers the ECFMG English Test, although a passing performance is valid for two years from the date passed. To satisfy the English language proficiency requirement for ECFMG certification or to revalidate the Standard ECFMG Certificate, applicants must now take the Test of English as a Foreign Language. Information and application materials are available at www.toefl.org.

- Pass the CSA. The CSA is a one-day exam that requires examinees to demonstrate clinical proficiency, spoken English language proficiency, and appropriate interpersonal skills. This requirement only pertains to those certified by the ECFMG after June 30, 1998.

The JCAHO accepts verification from the ECFMG as a designated equivalent source for verification of a physician's graduation from a foreign medical school.

Fifth Pathway

The Fifth Pathway program was developed to help United States students who attend foreign medical schools circumvent the social service obligations of a foreign institution (some foreign medical schools require the student to remain in the country for a period of time serving the population as part of their training) and return to the United States to continue their professional education.

The Fifth Pathway program is attractive to students because it saves them one year in their application for graduate medical education in comparison with ECFMG. It also gives students a year of supervised training in an American hospital instead of a foreign one. However, it is not accepted in all states.

To receive Fifth Pathway certification, the student must pass Steps 1 and 2 of the USMLE, have favorable evaluations from Fifth Pathway program supervisors, and complete other administrative requirements.

Visa Qualifying Examination (VQE)

Federal law requires those applying for visas to enter the United States to pursue graduate medical education or work as physicians to pass a medical competence examination. The two-day VQE was one such examination, but is no longer administered. Applicants for visas now must pass Steps 1 and 2 of the USMLE, or demonstrate they have passed Parts I and II of the NBME examination or the FMGEMS (although the latter two exams are no longer offered, as described above).

Federation Licensing Examination (FLEX)

The FLEX was a three-day examination developed by the FSMB for individual state licensing agencies to administer. Its purpose was to facilitate national uniformity in licensure examinations, although ultimate licensing decisions remained with the individual state licensing agencies. The FLEX was last administered in December 1993. It also has been replaced by the USMLE. The FSMB still maintains records of FLEX scores.

Post-Licensure Assessment System (PLAS)

The Post-Licensure Assessment System (PLAS) is a joint program of the FSMB and NBME that was established in 1998 to provide services to medical licensing agencies for assessing the ongoing competency of licensed physicians. PLAS is comprised of the Special Purpose Examination (SPEX) program and the Assessment Center Program (see below). Its goal is to provide a standardized, national program for assisting state medical boards in ensuring that only qualified, competent physicians are licensed to practice medicine.

SPEX

The SPEX is a one-day exam that was developed on behalf of the FSMB to evaluate the medical competence of individuals who currently hold, or have previously held, a valid unrestricted license to practice medicine in the United States or Canada. This includes physicians seeking licensure reinstatement or reactivation after a period of professional inactivity, physicians seeking reciprocity, physicians applying for licensure by endorsement who are several years out of medical school, or physicians involved in disciplinary proceedings. Initially introduced in the spring of 1988, SPEX became part of the Post-Licensure Assessment System in 1998. Because relatively few physicians take the SPEX, a credentialer should always ask why a physician took it. The answer to this question might reveal an adverse action against a license that the applicant had not otherwise mentioned.

In order to take the SPEX exam, individuals must meet the following criteria:

- Physicians must hold or have held an unrestricted medical license in a U.S. or Canadian jurisdiction
- Self-nominated applicants must hold a current, unrestricted medical license to practice medicine in a U.S. or Canadian jurisdiction
- Eligibility requirements for board-sponsored applicants are established by the individual licensing boards pursuant to their statutory and regulatory provisions

The Institute for Physician Evaluation

The Institute for Physician Evaluation (IPE) is a joint service offered by the FSMB and the NBME for the evaluation of physicians' clinical competency. The IPE is designed to meet the needs of hospitals, state medical boards, medical organizations, and individual physicians in determining areas of strengths and weaknesses of the physician. Assessment protocols (including data regarding a physician's clinical competence, abilities, and medical knowledge) are combined with personalized and standardized testing modalities to produce an in-depth analysis of a physician's strengths and weaknesses in clinical practice. The outcome report of these assessments can be used to design an educational program for the physician.

The USMLE

As mentioned above, the USMLE recently replaced the NBME, ECFMG, and FSMB examinations. Thus, any physician required to take a licensing examination for practice in the United States now only needs to take the USMLE.

The USMLE is a three-part examination. Step 1 tests knowledge of basic medical science, and is typically taken in the second year of medical school. Step 2 assesses knowledge of clinical science, and is usually taken in the final year of medical school. Step 3 tests physicians' ability to apply clinical knowledge, is administered under the auspices of individual state licensing agencies only, and is typically taken during the first year of postgraduate education. In order to obtain their license, examinees must demonstrate a proficiency in each step. The level of proficiency required to meet the minimum passing level for each USMLE Step exam is reviewed periodically and adjusted.

Those eligible to take Steps 1 and 2 of the USMLE include enrollees or graduates of accredited United States or Canadian medical schools, accredited United States osteopathic schools, and overseas medical schools (enrollees or graduates of the latter must be deemed eligible for the exam by the ECFMG). To take Step 3 of the USMLE, candidates must have an MD or DO degree, have successfully passed Steps 1 and 2 of the exam, and meet any other requirements of the individual licensing authority sponsoring the Step 3 exam. In addition, Step 3 applicants who are graduates of foreign medical schools must be certified by the ECFMG or have successfully completed a "fifth pathway" program—one year of supervised clinical education in a United States medical school.

Successful completion of the USMLE does not confer any clinical authority, but is a major step toward the award of licensure in any United States jurisdiction. During the current transition from the previous examination options discussed above to the single USMLE, physicians may have partially completed one of the old examination options and be in the process of completing licensure requirements by finishing the USMLE.

Credentialers can contact the ECFMG, FSMB, and NBME at the addresses and telephone numbers below for more information on licensure examinations:

Educational Commission for Foreign Medical Graduates
3624 Market Street, 4th Floor
Philadelphia, PENNSYLVANIA 19104-2685
Telephone: 215/386-5900   Fax: 215/387-9963
Web site: www.ecfmg.org

Licensing Agencies

Federation of State Medical Boards of the United States, Inc.
Federation Place
400 Fuller Wiser Road, Suite 300
Euless, TEXAS 76039-3855
Telephone: 817/868-4000 Fax: 817/868-4099
Web site: www.fsmb.org

National Board of Medical Examiners
3750 Market Street
Philadelphia, PENNSYLVANIA 19104
Telephone: 215/590-9700 Fax: 215/590-9457
Web site: www.nbme.org

Medical Licensing Agencies

Alabama

Alabama State Board of Medical Examiners
Verification of licenses

Telephone:	Not provided.
Written:	Free of charge. Mail requests, including physician assistant names and license numbers (if known).
Electronic:	Automated verification system available at Web site, www.albme.org.

Board of Medical Examiners
PO Box 946
848 Washington Avenue
Montgomery, ALABAMA 36101-0946
Telephone: 334/242-4116
Fax: 334/242-4155
Web site: www.albme.org

Alabama State Board of Medical Examiners
Notes: Hard copy of Directory of Licensed Physicians is no longer in print. To obtain, must contact licensure commission: through special request. Fee for directory is $55.

Directory of licensed physicians

Telephone:	Not provided.
Written:	Provided free of charge. Exception would be if this is the original licensing agency. Need release of endorsement form. Fee is $10.
Electronic:	Information available on Web site.

Medical Licensure Commission
Board of Medical Examiners
PO Box 887
Montgomery, ALABAMA 36101
Telephone: 334/833-0710   334/242-4116 (switchboard)
Fax: 334/242-4155
Web site: www.albme.org

Alaska

Alaska State Medical Board
Directory of licensed physicians

Telephone: Free of charge.

Written: $20 per copy. Mail requests and check made payable to State of Alaska.

Electronic: Automated verification system available at Web site. No disciplinary information.

> Division of Occupational Licensing
> Alaska State Medical Board
> PO Box 110806
> Juneau, ALASKA 99811-0806
> Telephone: 907/465-2756 (applicants A-K)   907/465-2541 (applicants L-Z)
> Fax: 907/465-2974
> E-mail: license@dced.state.ak.us
> Web site: www.dced.state.ak.us/occ/

Alaska State Medical Board
Verification of MD and DO licenses

Telephone: Free of charge. Limit five verifications per call.

Written: $20 per verification made payable to the State of Alaska. Mail requests, including physician names and license numbers (if known), and payment.

Electronic: Automatic verification system available at Web site. No disciplinary information available.

> Division of Occupational Licensing
> Alaska State Medical Board
> PO Box 110806
> Juneau, ALASKA 99811-0806
> Telephone: 907/465-2534   907/465-2756
> Fax: 907/465-2974
> E-mail: license@dced.state.ak.us
> Web site: www.dced.state.akus/occ/home.htm

Arizona

Arizona Board of Osteopathic Examiners in Medicine and Surgery
Annual report of licensed physicians

Telephone: Free of charge.

Written: $5 per verification. Mail requests, including physician's name and license number (if known), and payment.

Electronic: Not provided.

> Arizona Board of Osteopathic Examiners in Medicine and Surgery
> 9535 E. Doubletree Ranch Road
> Scottsdale, ARIZONA 85258-5539
> Telephone: 480/657-7703
> Fax: 480/657-7715
> E-mail: information@azosteoboard.org
> Web site: www.azosteoboard.org

Medical Licensing Agencies

Arizona State Board of Medical Examiners
Directory of licensed physicians

Telephone: Free of charge. Limit two verifications per call.
Written: $5 per copy. Mail requests and payment.
Electronic: Automated verification system available at Web site. Also available on disk for $100 (dial Ext. 2778 for more information). Mail requests and payment.

Arizona Board of Medical Examiners
9545 E. Doubletree Ranch Road
Scottsdale, ARIZONA 85258
Telephone: 480/551-2700
Fax: 480/551-2704
E-mail: questions@bomex.org
Web site: www.azdocinfo.com

Arizona State Board of Medical Examiners
Verification of MD licenses

Telephone: Free of charge. Limit two verifications per call.
Written: $5 per verification. Mail requests, including physician names and license numbers (if known).
Electronic: Available through Web site at www.azdocinfo.com. Database of licensed physicians available via disk.

Arizona Board of Medical Examiners
9545 E. Doubletree Ranch Road
PO Box 6200
Scottsdale, ARIZONA 85261
Telephone: 480/551-2700
Fax: 480/551-2704
E-mail: questions@bomex.org
Web site: www.azdocinfo.com

Arkansas

Arkansas State Medical Board
Directory of licensed physicians

Telephone: Not provided.
Written: $20 per copy. Mail requests and payment.
Electronic: Fees vary by level.

Arkansas State Medical Board
2100 River Front Drive
Little Rock, ARKANSAS 72202-1793
Telephone: 501/296-1802
Fax: 501/296-1805
E-mail: office@armedicalboard.org
Web site: www.armedicalboard.org

Arkansas State Medical Board
Verification of MD and DO licenses

Telephone: Not provided.
Written: $15 per verification. Mail requests, including physician names and payment (check or money order).
Electronic: Modem verification service. Call for more information.

Chapter 6

Arkansas State Medical Board
2100 River Front Drive
Little Rock, ARKANSAS 72202-1793
Telephone: 501/296-1802
Fax: 501/296-1805
E-mail: office@armedicalboard.org
Web site: www.armedicalboard.org

California

Medical Board of California
Verification of licenses

Telephone: Free of charge. Limit three verifications per call.
Written: Call for fee information. Mail requests, including each physician's full name, office address, city/town of practice, and license number (if known).
Electronic: Automated verification system available at Web site.

License Verification
Medical Board of California
1426 Howe Avenue, Suite 54
Sacramento, CALIFORNIA 95825-3236
Telephone: 916/263-2382
Fax: 916/263-2944
Web site: www.medbd.ca.gov

Medical Board of California
Directory of licensed physicians

Telephone: Free of charge. Limit three verifications per call.
Written: Free of charge. Limit three per month.
Electronic: Free of charge. Unlimited on the Web site.

License Verification
Medical Board of California
1426 Howe Avenue, Suite 54
Sacramento, CALIFORNIA 95825-3236
Telephone: 916/263-2382
Fax: 916/263-2944
E-mail: webmaster@medbd.ca.gov
Web site: www.medbd.ca.gov

Medical Board of California
Verification of MD licenses

Telephone: Free of charge. Limit three verifications per call.
Written: Free of charge. Mail requests, including physician's full name, address of record, city/town of practice, and license number (if known).
Electronic: Automated verification system available at Web site.

License Verification
Medical Board of California
1426 Howe Avenue, Suite 54
Sacramento, CALIFORNIA 95825-3236

Telephone: 916/263-2382
Fax: 916/263-2944
Web site: www.medbd.ca.gov

Osteopathic Medical Board of California
Verification of DO licenses

Telephone: Free of charge.
Written: Free of charge. Mail requests, including physician names and self-addressed, stamped envelopes.
Electronic: Free of charge at Web site.

Osteopathic Medical Board of California
2720 Gateway Oaks Drive, Suite 350
Sacramento, CALIFORNIA 95833-3500
Telephone: 916/263-3100
Fax: 916/263-3117
E-mail: angie_burton@dca.ca.gov
Web site: www.docboard.org/cx

Colorado

Colorado State Board of Medical Examiners
Verification of MD and DO licenses

Telephone: Free of charge. Call automated verification system number; limit three verifications per call.
Written: Free of charge. Mail or fax requests, including physician names and license numbers (if known).
Electronic: Automated verification system available at Web site.

Board of Medical Examiners
1560 Broadway, Suite 1300
Denver, COLORADO 80202-5140
Telephone: 303/894-7690 (general information)   303/894-7434 (automated verification system)
Fax: 303/894-7692
Web site: www.dora.state.co.us/medical

Connecticut

Connecticut Department of Public Health
Verification of MD and DO licenses

Telephone: Free of charge. Limit five verifications per call.
Written: Free of charge. Limit 10 verifications per query. Faxed upon request. Mail or fax requests, including physician names and license numbers (if known), and Connecticut release forms (upon request). Separate MD and DO verification requests.
Electronic: Automated verification system available at Web site.

Division of Licensure and Registration
Department of Public Health
410 Capitol Avenue MS 12MQA
PO Box 340308
Hartford, CONNECTICUT 06134
Telephone: 860/509-7603
Fax: 860/509-7607 and 860/509-8457
Web site: www.ct-clic.com

Delaware

Delaware Board of Medical Practice
Directory of licensed physicians

Telephone: Not provided.
Written: $10 per copy. Mail requests and payment.
Electronic: Not provided.

> Delaware Board of Medical Practice
> 861 Silver Lake Boulevard
> Cannon Building, Suite 203
> Dover, DELAWARE 19904
> Telephone: 302/744-4511
> Fax: 302/739-2711
> E-mail: swolfe@state.de.us
> Web site: www.professionallicensing.state.de.us

Delaware Board of Medical Practice
Verification of MD and DO licenses

Telephone: Not provided.
Written: $10 per verification. Mail requests, including physician's name and license number (if known), and payment.
Electronic: Not provided.

> Delaware Board of Medical Practice
> 861 Silver Lake Boulevard, Suite 203
> Cannon Building
> Dover, DELAWARE 19904
> Telephone: 302/744-4500
> Fax: 302/739-2711
> Web site: www.professionallicensing.state.de.us

District of Columbia

Department of Health
Directory of licensed physicians

Telephone: Not provided.
Written: $50 per MD verification. $20 per verification of other professions.
Electronic: Not provided.

> Department of Health
> Office of Professional Licensing
> 825 N. Capital Street NE
> Room 2224
> Washington, DISTRICT OF COLUMBIA 20002
> Telephone: 202/442-9200
> Fax: 202/442-9431
> Web site: www.dchealth.gov

Medical Licensing Agencies

Department of Health
Verification of MD and DO licenses

Telephone: Free of charge. Limit of three verifications per day. Do not give license number over the phone.

Written: $50 per MD verification; all other requests are $20. Mail requests, including physician names and license numbers (if known), and payment.

Electronic: Not provided.

> Department of Health
> Health Care Licensing
> 825 N. Capital Street NE, Room 2224
> Washington, DISTRICT OF COLUMBIA 20002
> Telephone: 202/442-9200
> Fax: 202/442-9431
> Web site: www.dchealth.dc.gov

Florida

Division of Medical Quality Assurance
Verification of MD and DO licenses

Telephone: Free of charge. Limit three verifications per call. Call 850/488-0595, Ext. 0.

Written: $25 per verification. Mail requests, including physician names and license numbers (if known), and payment.

Electronic: Automated verification system available at Web site. Click on director, then health, then quick click on credentialing.

> Division of Medical Quality Assurance
> Bureau of Operations
> HMQAO/Bin C10
> 4052 Bald Cypress Way
> Credentialing Unit
> Tallahassee, FLORIDA 32399-3260
> Telephone: 850/245-4094
> Fax: 850/414-7754
> Web site: www.myflorida.com

Florida Board of Medicine

Notes: Licensee information/Exam Candidate information. Exam dates must be obtained directly from the licensing board office scheduling the exam. Exam candidate list or exam statistics: $21 per profession and exam date. Processing time: 4–6 weeks.

Listing of licensed physicians

Telephone: Free of charge.

Written: Medical Professionals paper printout: $101.54 (up to four professions for four counties or entire state). Checks payable to Dept. of Health; submit payment prior to processing of order.

Electronic: $52.64 for CD or disk (limit four professions per four counties or state of Florida). Extracted data have ASCII comma-delimited file. Consumer has 60 days to report media damages; after 60 days consumer must resubmit payment for replacements.

> HMQAMS Client Services
> Licensee Data Center
> Florida Board of Medicine
> 4052 Bald Cypress Way, Bin C99
> Tallahassee, FLORIDA 32399-0864
> Telephone: 850/245-4444, Ext. 3567

Chapter 6

Fax: 850/414-0864
Web site: www.doh.state.fl.us/MQA

Florida Board of Medicine
Notes: Certified Nurse Assistant data cannot be extracted by county. Please expect a 4–6 week processing time. Data are current as of the processing date.

Verification of licenses

Telephone: Free of charge. Call 850/488-0595 (Call Center).
Written: Registered Nurse paper printout: $334.04 (up to four counties or entire state). Certified Nurse Assistant paper printout: $409.04 (entire state). Call for more information.
Electronic: RN CDs or diskettes: $52.64 (limit four professions per four counties); Certified Nurse Assistant CDs or diskettes: $74.44 (for entire state). Extracted data have ASCII comma-delimited file. Call for more information.

Department of Health
Client Services Unit
PO Box 6320
Tallahassee, FLORIDA 32310-6320
Telephone: 850/245-4444, Ext. 3561 or 3562
Fax: 850/414-0864
E-mail: corey_benedict@doh.state.fl.us
Web site: www.doh.state.fl.us/MQA

Georgia

Georgia Composite State Board of Medical Examiners
Notes: Certification to another state board: $25 for Medical, $15 for Physicians Assistants, $10 for Acupuncture and Respiratory.

Directory of licensed physicians

Telephone: Free of charge.
Written: Not provided.
Electronic: Free of charge.

Composite State Board of Medical Examiners
2 Peach Tree Street NW, 36th Floor
Atlanta, GEORGIA 30303
Telephone: 404/656-3913
Fax: 404/656-9723
Web site: www.medicalboard.state.ga.us

Georgia Composite State Board of Medical Examiners
Verification of MD and DO licenses

Telephone: Free of charge. Limit three verifications per call.
Written: $25 per verification. Mail or fax requests, including physician names and license numbers (if known).
Electronic: Not provided.

Composite State Board of Medical Examiners
2 Peachtree Street NW, 36th Floor
Atlanta, GEORGIA 30303
Telephone: 404/656-3913   404/656-3914

Fax: 404/656-9723
E-mail: medicalboard@dch.state.ga.us
Web site: www.medicalboard.state.ga.us

Guam

Guam Board of Medical Examiners
Directory of licensed physicians

Telephone:	Not provided.
Written:	Not provided.
Electronic:	Not provided.

Guam Board of Medical Examiners
Department of Public Health and Social Services
PO Box 2816
Hagatna, GUAM 96932
Telephone: 671-475-0263
Fax: 671-477-2930
Web site: mail.admin-gov.gu/pubhealth

Hawaii

Hawaii Board of Medical Examiners

Notes: Verifications are done through Consumer Resource Center, 235 S. Beretania Street, 9th Floor, Honolulu, HAWAII 96813.

Verification of MD and DO licenses

Telephone:	Free of charge. Provide physician's license number.
Written:	Not provided.
Electronic:	Not provided.

Board of Medical Examiners
1010 Richards Street
Honolulu, HAWAII 96813
Telephone: 808/587-3295 (verifications) 808/586-3000 (licensing)
Web site: www.state.hi.us/dcca/pvl

Hawaii Board of Medical Examiners
Roster of licensed physicians

Telephone:	Call 808/587-3222 (Consumer Research Center).
Written:	$111 per roster; does not include names or addresses. Mail requests and payment.
Electronic:	Not provided.

Board of Medical Examiners
PO Box 3469
Honolulu, HAWAII 96801
Telephone: 808/586-2708
Fax: 808/586-2689
E-mail: medical@dcca.state.hi.us
Web site: www.state.hi.us/dcca/pvl

Idaho

Idaho State Board of Medicine
Notes: Primary verification is for physicians; physician assistants and other health professionals also verified.
Verification of licenses

Telephone:	Free of charge. Limit three verifications per day.
Written:	$20 per verification. Mail or fax requests, including physician names and license numbers (if known), self-addressed, stamped envelope, and payment.
Electronic:	Not provided.

Idaho State Board of Medicine
1755 Westgate Drive
Suite 140
Boise, IDAHO 83704
Telephone: 208/327-7000
Fax: 208/327-7005
E-mail: info@bom.state.id.us
Web site: www.bom.state.id.us

Idaho State Board of Medicine
Verification of MD and DO licenses

Telephone:	Free of charge. Limit three verifications per call.
Written:	$20 per verification. Mail requests, including physician names and license numbers (if known), and payment.
Electronic:	Not provided.

Idaho State Board of Medicine
1755 Westgate Drive, Suite 140
Boise, IDAHO 83704
Telephone: 208/327-7000
Fax: 208/327-7005
E-mail: tsolt@bom.state.id.us
Web site: www.bom.state.id.us

Idaho State Board of Medicine
Roster of licensed physicians

Telephone:	Free of charge. Physician verification only.
Written:	Annual subscription: $52.50 per roster; updated and sent to purchaser monthly. Mail requests and payment. Physician verification: $20 per request. Mail request and payment.
Electronic:	E-mail, Free of charge.

Idaho State Board of Medicine
PO Box 83720
Boise, IDAHO 83720-0058
Telephone: 208/327-7000
Fax: 208/327-7005
Web site: www.bom.state.id.us

Illinois

Illinois Department of Professional Regulation
Directory of licensed physicians

Telephone:	Free of charge. Call 217/782-0458.
Written:	Price changes at start of each month; call for current price. Specify sorting instructions. Mail requests and payment (money order or cashier's check payable to Dept. of Professional Regulation). Also accepts company checks.
Electronic:	Not provided.

Attention: Shirley Lanzotti
Request for Directory of Physicians and Surgeons
Data Processing Unit Department of Professional Regulation
320 W. Washington Street, Third Floor
Springfield, ILLINOIS 62786
Telephone: 217/785-0920
Fax: 217/557-8073
Web site: www.dpr.state.il.us

Illinois Department of Professional Regulation

Notes: Provides licensing certification to another state for $20 fee.

Verification of MD and DO licenses

Telephone:	Free of charge. Limit three verifications per call. Provide physician's name, license number, or Social Security number (if known).
Written:	First three verifications free; $20 for each additional verification. Mail requests, including physician names, license numbers (if known), and payment.
Electronic:	Automated verification system available at Web site.

Licensure Maintenance Unit
Department of Professional Regulation
320 W. Washington Street, Third Floor
Springfield, ILLINOIS 62786
Telephone: 217/782-0458   800/823-6100 (license renewal)
Fax: 217/557-8073
Web site: www.dpr.state.il.us

Licensure Maintenance Unit
Verification of licenses

Telephone:	Free of charge. Limit three verifications per call.
Written:	$20 per verification. Mail requests, including physician names and license numbers (if known), and payment.
Electronic:	Automated verification system available at Web site.

Department of Professional Regulation
Licensure Maintenance Unit
320 W. Washington Street, Third Floor
Springfield, ILLINOIS 62786
Telephone: 217/782-0458
Fax: 217/557-8073
Web site: www.dpr.state.il.us

Indiana

Indiana Medical Licensing Board
Listing of licensed physicians

Telephone: Free of charge via toll-free number listed.
Written: Fees differ per customized copy; call for more information. Mail requests and payment.
Electronic: Not provided.

> Medical Licensing Board
> Health Professions Bureau
> 402 W. Washington Street, Room 041
> Indianapolis, INDIANA 46204
> Telephone: 317/232-2960 (reception desk for Health Professions Bureau)   888/333-7515 (telephone verifications)   317/234-2060 (Medical Licensing Board)
> Fax: 317/233-4236
> Web site: www.in.gov/hpb

Medical Licensing Board
Verification of MD and DO licenses

Telephone: Free of charge. Provide physician's names or license numbers (if known).
Written: $10 per verification. Mail requests, including physician's name and license number (if known), and payment.
Electronic: Automated verification system available at Web site. Subscription required.

> Medical Licensing Board
> Health Professions Bureau
> 402 W. Washington Street, Room 041
> Indianapolis, INDIANA 46204
> Telephone: 888/333-7515   317/232-2960
> Fax: 317/233-4236
> Web site: www.in.gov/hpb

Iowa

Iowa Board of Medical Examiners
Verification of licenses

Telephone: Free of charge. Limit five verifications per day.
Written: $40 per verification. Mail requests, including physician's name and license number (if known), and payment.
Electronic: $3 fee for each verification; yearly subscription offered for $2,000.

> Iowa Board of Medical Examiners
> Board of Physician Assistant Examiners
> 400 S.W. Eighth Street, Suite C
> Des Moines, IOWA 50309-4686
> Telephone: 515/281-5171
> Fax: 515/242-5908
> Web site: www.docboard.org/ia

Iowa Board of Medical Examiners
Notes: $45 fee for copy of scores sent to another state. They also license acupuncturists and physician assistant supervisors.

Verification of MD and DO licenses

Telephone:	Not provided.
Written:	$15 per verifications for hospitals; $40 to another state. $2,000 per year for unlimited verifications. Mail requests, including physician names, license numbers (if known), and payment.
Electronic:	Information available on Web site.

Iowa Board of Medical Examiners
400 S.W. Eighth Street, Suite C
Des Moines, IOWA 50309-4686
Telephone: 515/281-5171 (IVR)   515/281-6641 (general information)
Fax: 515/242-5908
E-mail: ibme@ibme.state.ia.us
Web site: www.docboard.org

Kansas

Kansas Board of Healing Arts
Verification of MD and DO licenses

Telephone:	Free of charge. Limit three verifications per day.
Written:	$15 per verification with scores; free without scores. Mail or fax requests, including physician's name and license number (if known).
Electronic:	Not provided.

Kansas Board of Healing Arts
235 S.W. Topeka Boulevard
Topeka, KANSAS 66603
Telephone: 785/296-7413
Fax: 785/296-0852
E-mail: cabbott@ink.org
Web site: www.ksbha.org

Kentucky

Kentucky Board of Medical Licensure
Directory of licensed physicians

Telephone:	Not provided.
Written:	$15.90 per copy (plus $4 mailing and handling charge per directory). Mail requests and payment.
Electronic:	Information is available at our Web site.

Kentucky Board of Medical Licensure
310 Whittington Parkway, Suite 1B
Louisville, KENTUCKY 40222
Telephone: 502/429-8046   900/555-6500 (verifications)
Fax: 502/429-9923
E-mail: kbml@mail.state.ky.us
Web site: www.state.ky.us/agencies/kbml

Kentucky Board of Medical Licensure
Verification of MD and DO licenses
Telephone: Call automated verification number. Limit two verifications per call. $2.95 for first minute; $0.50 each additional minute. Provide physician's name and license number (if known). Verifications faxed upon request.
Written: $5 for 1–5 verifications; $7 for 6–10 verifications. Limit 10 verifications per query. Mail requests, including physician names and license numbers (if known), and payment.
Electronic: Not provided.

Kentucky Board of Medical Licensure
310 Whittington Parkway, Suite 1B
Louisville, KENTUCKY 40222
Telephone: 502/429-8046 (general information)   900/555-6500 (automated verification system)
Fax: 502/429-9923
E-mail: KBML@mail.state.ky.us
Web site: www.state.ky.us/agencies/KBML

Louisiana

Louisiana State Board of Medical Examiners
Directory of licensed physicians
Telephone: Not provided.
Written: Free of charge. $4 fee if forwarded to an organization other than the state board.
Electronic: Available on Web site.

Verifications Department
Louisiana State Board of Medical Examiners
PO Box 30250
New Orleans, LOUISIANA 70190-0250
Telephone: 504/568-6820
Fax: 504/568-8893
E-mail: lsbmever@lsbme.org
Web site: www.lsbme.org

Louisiana State Board of Medical Examiners
Verification of MD and DO licenses
Telephone: Free of charge. Limit three verifications per call.
Written: $5 per physician name. Mail requests, including physician names and license numbers (if known). Checks payable to LSBME.
Electronic: Free of charge at Web site.

Verifications Department
Louisiana State Board of Medical Examiners
PO Box 30250
New Orleans, LOUISIANA 70190-0250
Telephone: 504/568-6820, Ext. 252 (phone verifications)
504/568-6820, Ext. 260 (written verifications)
Web site: www.lsbme.org

Maine

Maine Board of Licensure in Medicine
Verification of MD licenses

Telephone:	Free of charge.
Written:	$15 per verification. Mail requests, including physician names and license numbers (if known), and payment.
Electronic:	Not provided.

> Maine Board of Licensure in Medicine
> Board of Licensure in Medicine
> 2 Bangor Street
> 137 State House Station
> Augusta, MAINE 04333
> Telephone: 207/287-3601
> Fax: 207/287-6590
> Web site: www.docboard.org/me_home.htm

Maine Board of Osteopathic Licensure
Directory of licensed physicians

Telephone:	Free of charge.
Written:	$15 per copy. Mail requests and payment.
Electronic:	Available free of charge on Web site.

> Maine Board of Osteopathic Licensure
> 142 State House Station
> Augusta, MAINE 04333-0142
> Telephone: 207/287-2480
> Fax: 207/287-3015
> E-mail: susan.e.strout@state.me.us
> Web site: www.docboard.org/me-osteo

Maine Board of Osteopathic Licensure
Verification of DO licenses

Telephone:	Free of charge.
Written:	$15 per verification. Mail requests, including physician names.
Electronic:	Automated verification system available at Web site.

> Maine Board of Osteopathic Licensure
> 142 State House Station
> Augusta, MAINE 04333-0142
> Telephone: 207/287-2480
> Fax: 207/287-3015
> E-mail: susan.e.strout@state.me.us
> Web site: www.docboard.org/me-osteo

Maryland

Maryland Board of Physician Quality Assurance
Verification of MD and DO licenses

Telephone: Free of charge. Limit 10 verifications per call (varies depending on call volume). Provide physician names and license numbers.

Written: $25 each. Mail requests, including physician names and license numbers.

Electronic: Not provided.

> Attention: Verifications
> Board of Physician Quality Assurance
> 4201 Patterson Avenue
> Baltimore, MARYLAND 21215-0095
> Telephone: 410/764-4777   410/764-4705   800/492-6836
> Fax: 410/358-2252
> Web site: www.docboard.org

Maryland Board of Physician Quality Assurance
Listing of licensed physicians

Telephone: Free verification.

Written: $25 verification fee. Mail request, including physician names and license numbers (if known).

Electronic: Automated verification system available at www.docboard.org.

> Board of Physician Quality Assurance
> 4201 Patterson Avenue
> PO Box 2571
> Baltimore, MARYLAND 21215-0095
> Telephone: 800/492-6836 (dial # key then Ext. 4705)   410/764-4705
> Fax: 410/358-2252
> E-mail: bpqa@erols.com
> Web site: www.docboard.org

Massachusetts

Massachusetts Board of Registration in Medicine
Verification of MD and DO licenses

Telephone: Free of charge. Limit four verifications per call.

Written: $10 per verification. Faxed upon request. Mail requests, including physician's name and license number (if known), self-addressed, stamped envelope, and check (payable to Commonwealth of Massachusetts). Waiver form available at Web site.

Electronic: Automatic verification system available at Web site.

> Attention: Verification request
> Board of Registration in Medicine
> Commonwealth of Massachusetts
> 10 West Street, Third Floor
> Boston, MASSACHUSETTS 02111
> Telephone: 617/727-3086   800/377-0550 (physician profiles)
> Fax: 617/357-8453
> Web site: www.massmedboard.org

Medical Licensing Agencies

Massachusetts Board of Registration in Medicine
Roster of licensed physicians

Telephone:	Free of charge.
Written:	$50 per copy; available in hard copy or CD-ROM format. Mail requests and payment to Public Information Division at the Board.
Electronic:	Not provided.

> Attention: Verification request
> Board of Registration in Medicine
> Commonwealth of Massachusetts
> 10 W. Street, Third Floor
> Boston, MASSACHUSETTS 02111
> Telephone: 617/727-3086   800/377-0550 (physician profiles)
> Fax: 617/357-8453
> Web site: www.massmedboard.org

Michigan

Department of Consumer and Industry Services
Verification of MD and DO licenses

Telephone:	Automated verification system: 900/555-8374; $1.50 per minute.
Written:	Verification to party other than U.S. state: $5. Written verification to another U.S. state: $15. Mail request, including licensee name and number, and payment to address below.
Electronic:	Automated verification system available at www.michigan.gov/bhser.

> Michigan Department of Consumer and Industry Services
> Bureau of Health Services
> Attention: Education Testing & Credentials Section
> PO Box 30670
> Lansing, MICHIGAN 48909
> Telephone: 517/335-0918   900/555-8374 (automated verification system)
> Fax: 517/373-2179
> E-mail: bhserinfo@michigan.gov
> Web site: www.michigan.gov/bhser

Michigan Department of Consumer & Industry Services
Listing of licensed physicians

Telephone:	Available at 900/555-8374; $1.50 per minute.
Written:	Fees differ per customized copy; call for more information. Mail request and payment.
Electronic:	Not provided.

> 525 W. Ottawa
> PO Box 30004
> Lansing, MICHIGAN 48909
> Telephone: 517/373-1820   900/555-8374 (verification number)   517/373-6873 (medical licensing)
> Web site: www.cis.state.mi.us

Minnesota

Minnesota Board of Medical Practice
Verification of MD and DO licenses
Telephone: Free of charge. Limit two verifications per call.
Written: $25 per verification. Mail requests, including physician names and license numbers (if known), and payment.
Electronic: Automated verification system available through Web site.

> Minnesota Board of Medical Practice
> 2829 University Avenue SE, Suite 400
> Minneapolis, MINNESOTA 55414-3246
> Telephone: 612/617-2130
> Fax: 612/617-2166
> Web site: www.bmp.state.mn.us

Minnesota Mailing List Service
Directory of licensed physicians
Telephone: Not provided.
Written: $60 for diskette; $50 for computer printout or labels. Dial License Line from computer modem for $2.50/min. Call for catalog, more information, and details about settings. Mail or phone request and payment.
Electronic: Not provided.

> State of Minnesota
> Mailing List Service
> 117 University Avenue
> Room 110A
> St. Paul, MINNESOTA 55155
> Telephone: 651/296-0930
> Fax: 651/297-8260
> E-mail: jean.hayes@state.mn.us
> Web site: www.minnesotabookstore.com

Mississippi

Mississippi State Board of Medical Licensure
Notes: Applications can be downloaded from the web site.
Verification of MD and DO licenses
Telephone: Not provided.
Written: $25 per verification. Mail requests, including physician names and license numbers (if known), date of original issue of license, expiration, and if there has been any disciplinary action taken by the board.
Electronic: Not provided.

> Mississippi State Board of Medical Licensure
> PO Box 9268
> Jackson, MISSISSIPPI 39286-9268
> Telephone: 601/987-3079
> Fax: 601/987-4159
> E-mail: mboard@msbml.state.ms.us
> Web site: www.msbml.state.ms.us

Mississippi State Board of Medical Licensure
Roster of licensed physicians
Telephone: Not provided.
Written: $125 per full list; $25 per verification. Mail requests and payment.
Electronic: Not provided.

> Mississippi State Board of Medical Licensure
> PO Box 9268
> Jackson, MISSISSIPPI 39286-9268
> Telephone: 601/987-3079
> Fax: 601/987-4159
> E-mail: mboard@msbml.state.ms.us
> Web site: www.msbml.state.ms.us

Mississippi State Board of Medical Licensure
Notes: State of Mississippi began licensing physician assistants in 2000. For information on regulations governing the practice of physician assistants, visit their Web site at www.msbml.state.ms.us/licensure_regulations.htm#PA%20scope.
Annual report of licensed physicians
Telephone: Not provided.
Written: $25 per verification. Mail requests, including physician assistant names and license numbers (if known), and payment.
Electronic: Not provided.

> State Medical Board of Licensure
> 1867 Crane Ridge Drive, Suite 200-B
> Jackson, MISSISSIPPI 39216
> Telephone: 601/987-3079
> Fax: 601/987-4159
> E-mail: mboard@msbml.state.ms.us
> Web site: www.msbml.state.ms.us

Missouri

Missouri Department of Health and Senior Services
Listing of licensed physicians
Telephone: Not provided.
Written: Listings available for a fee.
Electronic: Not provided.

> Missouri Department of Health and Senior Services
> CHIME
> PO Box 570
> Jefferson City, MISSOURI 65102
> Telephone: 573/751-6279
> Fax: 573/751-6280
> Web site: www.dhss.state.mo.us

Missouri State Board of Registration of the Healing Arts
Notes: $50 for certificate of scores.
Verification of MD and DO licenses

Telephone:	Free of charge. Limit five verifications per call. Provide physician's name and license number (if known).
Written:	Free of charge. Faxed upon request. Mail or fax requests, including physician names and license numbers (if known).
Electronic:	Automated verification system available at Web site.

State Board of Registration of the Healing Arts
PO Box 4
Jefferson City, MISSOURI 65102
Telephone: 573/751-0098
Fax: 573/751-3166
Web site: www.ecodev.state.mo.us/pr/healarts

Montana

Montana Board of Medical Examiners
Directory of licensed physicians

Telephone:	Not provided.
Written:	$20 per copy. Mail requests and payment.
Electronic:	Not provided.

Montana Medical Association
2021 11th Avenue
Helena, MONTANA 59601
Telephone: 406-443-4000
Fax: 406-443-4042
Web site: www.montanamedical.org

Montana Board of Medical Examiners
Verification of MD and DO licenses

Telephone:	Free of charge. Limit five verifications per call.
Written:	$20 per verification. Mail requests, including physician names and license numbers (if known), and payment.
Electronic:	Not provided.

Montana Board of Medical Examiners
PO Box 200513
301 S. Park Avenue (delivery only)
Helena, MONTANA 59620-0513
Telephone: 406/444-4284
Fax: 406/841-2363
Web site: www.discoveringmontana.com/dli/bsd

Nebraska

Department of Health and Human Services
Verification of MD and DO licenses

Telephone:	Free of charge. Limit three verifications per call. Provide physician's name and license number (if known).
Written:	$5 per verification to verify dates and license numbers; $25 fee for any further information. Mail requests, including physician names and license numbers (if known), and payment.
Electronic:	Automated verification system available at Web site.

Department of Health and Human Services
Regulation and Licensure
Credentialing Division
PO Box 94986
Lincoln, NEBRASKA 68509-4986
Telephone: 402/471-2118
Fax: 402/471-3577
E-mail: becky.wisell@hhss.state.ne.us
Web site: www.hhs.state.ne.us/lis/lis.asp

Department of Health and Human Services
Notes: Verification of disciplinary action is also $25.
Listing of licensed physicians
Telephone: Free of charge.
Written: $25 fee per name. Mail requests, including signed release form and payment.
Electronic: Information available at Web site.

Department of Health and Human Services
Regulation and Licensure
Credentialing Division
PO Box 94986
Lincoln, NEBRASKA 68509-4986
Telephone: 402/471-2118
Fax: 402/471-3577
E-mail: becky.wisell@hhss.state.ne.us
Web site: www.hhs.state.ne.us/lis/lis.asp

Nevada

Nevada State Board of Medical Examiners
Directory of licensed physicians
Telephone: 3 telephone verifications an hour.
Written: $25 per copy. Mail requests and payment.
Electronic: Not provided.

Nevada State Board of Medical Examiners
PO Box 7238
1105 Terminal Way, Suite 301
Reno, NEVADA 89510
Telephone: 775/688-2559
Fax: 775/688-2321
Web site: www.nsbme.govmail.state.nv.us

Nevada State Board of Medical Examiners
Verification of MD licenses
Telephone: Free of charge. Limit three verifications per call.
Written: $25 per verification. Mail requests, including physician names and license numbers (if known), and payment.
Electronic: Not provided.

Nevada State Board of Medical Examiners

PO Box 7238
Reno, NEVADA 89510
Telephone: 775/688-2559
Fax: 775/688-2321
Web site: www.state.nv.us/medical

Nevada State Board of Osteopathic Medicine
Directory of licensed physicians

Telephone:	Free of charge; limit five verifications per call.
Written:	Printout $10; diskette $25. Mail requests and payment.
Electronic:	Free list available via e-mail.

Nevada State Board of Osteopathic Medicine
2860 E. Flamingo Road, Suite G
Las Vegas, NEVADA 89121-5270
Telephone: 702/732-2147
Fax: 702/732-2079
E-mail: osteo@govmail.state.nv.us
Web site: www.osteo.state.nv.us

Nevada State Board of Osteopathic Medicine
Verification of DO licenses

Telephone:	Free of charge. Limit five verifications per call.
Written:	$10 per verification. Faxed upon request. Mail or fax requests, including physician's name and license number (if known).
Electronic:	Not provided.

Nevada State Board of Osteopathic Medicine
2860 E. Flamingo Road, Suite G
Las Vegas, NEVADA 89121
Telephone: 702/732-2147
Fax: 702/732-2079
E-mail: osteo@govmail.state.nv.us

New Hampshire

New Hampshire Board of Medicine
Verification of MD and DO licenses

Telephone:	Free of charge. Limit five verifications per call.
Written:	$20 per verification. Mail requests, including physician names and license numbers (if known), and payment.
Electronic:	Not provided.

New Hampshire Board of Medicine
2 Industrial Park Drive, Suite 8
Concord, NEW HAMPSHIRE 03301
Telephone: 603/271-1203 (option three)
Fax: 603/271-6702
Web site: www.state.nh.us/medicine

New Hampshire Board of Medicine
Listing of licensed physicians

Telephone: Free of charge. Limit five verifications per call.
Written: $200 per computer printout; $100 for listing on disk (must provide own disk). Mail requests and payment. $20 fee for individual verifications.
Electronic: Not provided.

New Hampshire Board of Medicine
2 Industrial Park Drive, Suite 8
Concord, NEW HAMPSHIRE 03301
Telephone: 603/271-6936 (verification)   603/271-6934 (renewals)
Fax: 603/271-6702
Web site: www.state.nh.us/medicine

New Jersey

New Jersey State Medical Board
Directory of licensed physicians

Telephone: Not available.
Written: Several formats available. $94, plus $0.02/name for lists and labels; $94, plus $0.005/name for magnetic tapes; $94, plus $0.015/name for diskettes. Call for information packet and order form. Mail order forms, requests, and payment.
Electronic: Not provided.

Centralized Licensing Division
New Jersey State Board of Medical Examiners
140 E. Front Street, Third Floor
Trenton, NEW JERSEY 08265
Telephone: 609/826-7100
Fax: 609/777-0956

New Jersey State Medical Board
Verification of MD and DO licenses

Telephone: Free of charge. Limit five verifications per call; unlimited verifications on automated verification system.
Written: Free of charge. Mail or fax requests, including physician names and license numbers (if known).
Electronic: Not provided.

Attention: License Verification Request
New Jersey State Board of Medical Examiners
PO Box 183
Trenton, NEW JERSEY 08265-0183
Telephone: 609/826-7100   973/273-8090 (automated verification system)
Fax: 609/826-7117
Web site: www.state.nj.us/lps/ca/bme/docdir.htm

New Mexico

New Mexico Board of Medical Examiners
Verification of licenses

Telephone: Free of charge.

Chapter 6

Written: $25 per name for letter of good standing; $5 per name ($15 minimum). To verify several names at once, send list. Mail requests, including physician assistant names and license numbers (if known), and payment.

Electronic: Free of charge via Web site, unless written confirmation is needed.

> New Mexico Board of Medical Examiners
> 491 Old Santa Fe Trail
> Lamy Building, Second Floor
> Santa Fe, NEW MEXICO 87501
> Telephone: 505/827-5022
> Fax: 505/827-7377
> E-mail: nmbme@state.nm.us
> Web site: www.nmbme.org

New Mexico Board of Medical Examiners
Verification of MD licenses

Telephone: Free of charge.

Written: $25 for letter of good standing; $5 per verification ($15 minimum). To verify several names at once, send list. Mail requests, including physician names and license numbers (if known), and payment.

Electronic: Information available on Web site.

> New Mexico Board of Medical Examiners
> 491 Old Santa Fe Trail
> Lamy Building, Second Floor
> Santa Fe, NEW MEXICO 87501
> Telephone: 505/827-5022
> Fax: 505/827-7377
> E-mail: nmbme@state.nm.us
> Web site: www.state.nm.us/nmbme

New Mexico Board of Osteopathic Medical Examiners
Verification of DO licenses

Telephone: Free of charge.

Written: $25 per verification. Mail requests, including physician names and license numbers (if known), and payment.

Electronic: Not provided.

> New Mexico Board of Osteopathic Medical Examiners
> PO Box 25101
> Santa Fe, NEW MEXICO 87504
> Telephone: 505/476-7120
> Fax: 505/476-7095
> E-mail: osteoboard@state.nm.us
> Web site: www.rld.state.nm.us

New York

Office of the Professions—Medical Licensing
Verification of licenses

Telephone: Free of charge. Limit two verifications per call if calling customer service automated attendant; limit five per call if calling customer service representative; unlimited if calling automated verification system. $1.50 for first minute; $1 for each additional minute.

Medical Licensing Agencies

Written: $20 per verification. Limit one verification. $10 per hundred names for multiple verifications. Mail requests, including physician's name, license number, date of birth, address, and payment (check or money order payable to NYS Education Dept).
Electronic: Automated verification system available at Web site.

Office of the Professions—Medical Licensing
New York State Education Department
89 Washington Avenue, Second Floor
Albany, NEW YORK 12234-1000
Telephone: 518/474-3817 (general information)   900/555-6978 (automated verification system)
Fax: 518/474-1449
E-mail: op4info@mail.nysed.gov
Web site: www.op.nysed.gov

Office of the Professions Medical Licensing
Notes: License fee for state to state verification is $20.
Verification of MD and DO licenses
Telephone: Free of charge. Limit two verifications per call if calling customer service automated attendant; limit five per call if calling customer service representative; unlimited if calling automated verification system. $1.50 for first minute, $1 for each additional minute.
Written: $20 per verification. Limit one verification. $10 per hundred names for multiple verifications. Mail requests, including physician's name, license number, date of birth, address and payment (check or money order payable to NYS Education Dept).
Electronic: Automatic verification system also available at Web site.

Office of the Professions—Medical Licensing
New York State Education Department
89 Washington Avenue, Second Floor
Albany, NEW YORK 12234-1000
Telephone: 518/474-3817 (general information, customer service automated attendant, customer service representative)   900/555-6978 (automated verification system)
Fax: 518/474-1449
E-mail: op4info@mail.nysed.gov
Web site: www.op.nysed.gov

North Carolina

North Carolina Medical Board
Verification of MD and DO licenses
Telephone: Internet verification.
Written: $15 for one verification. Mail requests, including physician's name and license number (if known), and payment.
Electronic: Automated verification system available at Web site.

North Carolina Medical Board
PO Box 20007
Raleigh, NORTH CAROLINA 27619
Telephone: 919/326-1100
Fax: 919/326-1130
Web site: www.ncmedboard.org

North Carolina Medical Board
Notes: Verification of MDs, DOs, nurse practitioners, and physician assistants.
Verification of licenses

Telephone: Free of charge. Limit three verifications per call.
Written: $25 for diskette copy. Datalink program also available. Call for more information. Mail requests and payment.
Electronic: Free of charge.

North Carolina Medical Board
1201 Front Street, Suite 100
Raleigh, NORTH CAROLINA 27609
Telephone: 919/326-1100
Fax: 919/326-1131
E-mail: info@ncmedboard.org
Web site: www.ncmedboard.org

North Dakota

North Dakota Medical Association
Directory of licensed physicians

Telephone: Directory can be ordered via telephone.
Written: $30 per copy, plus shipping and tax. Published annually in April. Mail requests and payment.
Electronic: Not provided.

North Dakota Medical Association
1025 N. Third Street
Bismarck, NORTH DAKOTA 58501
Telephone: 701/223-9475
Fax: 701/223-9476
E-mail: staff@ndmed.com
Web site: www.ndmed.org

North Dakota State Board of Medical Examiners
Verification of MD and DO licenses

Telephone: Free of charge. Limit two verifications per day.
Written: $15 per verification. Mail requests, including physician/physician assistant names and license numbers (if known), and payment.
Electronic: Free of charge.

North Dakota State Board of Medical Examiners
418 E. Broadway Avenue, Suite 12
Bismarck, NORTH DAKOTA 58501
Telephone: 701/328-6500
Fax: 701/328-6505
E-mail: bomex@tic.bisman.com
Web site: www.ndbomex.com

Ohio

Ohio State Medical Board
Roster of licensed physicians
Telephone: Not provided.
Written: Not provided.
Electronic: Free of charge.

> State Medical Board of Ohio
> 77 S. High Street, 17th Floor
> Columbus, OHIO 43215-6127
> Telephone: 614/466-3934
> Fax: 614/728-5946
> E-mail: med.recept@med.state.oh.us
> Web site: www.state.oh.us/med

State Medical Board of Ohio
Verification of MD and DO licenses
Telephone: Not provided.
Written: Not provided.
Electronic: Automated verification system available at Web site.

> State Medical Board of Ohio
> 77 S. High Street, 17th Floor
> Columbus, OHIO 43215-6127
> Telephone: 614/466-3934
> Fax: 614/728-5946
> Web site: www.state.oh.us/med

Oklahoma

Oklahoma State Board of Medical Licensure and Supervision
Verification of licenses
Telephone: Free of charge. Limit five verifications per call. Provide physician's name.
Written: $20 per verification. Mail requests, including names and license numbers (if known), and payment.
Electronic: Information available on Web site.

> Oklahoma State Board of Medical Licensure and Supervision
> PO Box 18256
> 5104 N. Francis, Suite C
> Oklahoma City, OKLAHOMA 73154
> Telephone: 405/848-6841, #1
> Fax: 405/848-8240
> E-mail: executive@osbmls.state.ok.us
> Web site: www.osbmls.state.ok.us

Oklahoma State Board of Medical Licensure and Supervision
Verification of licenses
Telephone: Free of charge.
Written: $20 per copy. Mail requests and payment.
Electronic: Free of charge.

Oklahoma State Board of Medical Licensure and Supervision
PO Box 18256
Oklahoma City, OKLAHOMA 73154
Telephone: 405/848-6841
Fax: 405/848-8240
E-mail: executive@osbmls.state.ok.us
Web site: www.osbmls.state.ok.us

Oklahoma State Board of Medical Licensure and Supervision
Verification of MD licenses
Telephone: Free of charge. Limit five verifications per call. Provide physician's name.
Written: $20 per verification. Mail requests, including physician names and license numbers (if known), and payment.
Electronic: Information available on Web site.

Oklahoma State Board of Medical Licensure and Supervision
PO Box 18256
Oklahoma City, OKLAHOMA 73154
Telephone: 405/848-6841
Fax: 405/848-8240
E-mail: executive@osbmls.state.ok.us
Web site: www.osbmls.state.ok.us

Oklahoma State Board of Osteopathic Examiners
Listing of licensed physicians
Telephone: Free of charge. Limit two verifications per day.
Written: $50 for computer printout; $50 for diskette. Mail or fax requests and mail payment.
Electronic: Available through Web site.

Oklahoma State Board of Osteopathic Examiners
4848 N. Lincoln Boulevard, Suite 100
Oklahoma City, OKLAHOMA 73105-3321
Telephone: 405/528-8625
Fax: 405/557-0653
Web site: www.docboard.org

Oklahoma State Board of Osteopathic Examiners
Verification of DO licenses
Telephone: Free of charge. Limit two verifications per call per day.
Written: $25 per verification. Mail requests, including physician names and license numbers (if known), and payment.
Electronic: Information available on Web site.

Oklahoma State Board of Osteopathic Examiners
4848 N. Lincoln Boulevard, Suite 100
Oklahoma City, OKLAHOMA 73105-3321
Telephone: 405/528-8625
Fax: 405/557-0653
Web site: www.docboard.org

Oregon

Oregon State Board of Medical Examiners
Directory of licensed physicians

Telephone: Provided free of charge.
Written: $10 fee per verification or five verifications at $7.50. $75 per copy; $300 for diskette version. Call or see Web site for more information. Mail requests and payment.
Electronic: Not provided.

Oregon State Board of Medical Examiners
1500 S.W. First Avenue, Suite 620
Portland, OREGON 97201-5826
Telephone: 503/229-5770
Fax: 503/229-6543
E-mail: bme.info@state.or.us
Web site: www.bme.state.or.us

Oregon State Board of Medical Examiners
Verification of MD and DO licenses

Telephone: Free of charge. Limit three verifications per call.
Written: $10 fee for 1–5 names; $7.50 for six or more. Mail requests, including physician's name and license number (if known), and payment.
Electronic: Not provided.

Oregon State Board of Medical Examiners
1500 S.W. First Avenue, Suite 620
Portland, OREGON 97201-5826
Telephone: 503/229-5770
Fax: 503/229-6543
E-mail: bme.info@state.or.us
Web site: www.bme.state.or.us

Pennsylvania

Bureau of Professional and Occupational Affairs
Listing of licensed physicians

Telephone: Not provided.
Written: Several options available. Call for order form, customized pricing, and format. Mail order form, requests, and payment.
Electronic: Not provided.

Bureau of Professional and Occupational Affairs
124 Pine Street
Harrisburg, PENNSYLVANIA 17101
Telephone: 717/787-8503
Fax: 717/783-2724

Pennsylvania State Board of Medicine
Verification of MD licenses

Telephone: Free of charge. Limit 10 verifications per day. Encouraged to go to Web site for verification.

Written: Free of charge. Faxed upon request (depending on quantity). Mail or fax requests, including physician names and license numbers (if known). Encouraged to go to Web site for verification.

Electronic: Verification via e-mail at medicine@dos.state.pa.us, or via Web site at www.licensepa.state.pa.us.

Pennsylvania State Board of Medicine
Bureau of Professional and Occupational Affairs
PO Box 2649
Harrisburg, PENNSYLVANIA 17105-2649
Telephone: 717/787-2381
Fax: 717/787-7769
E-mail: medicine@pados.dos.state.pa.us
Web site: www.dos.state.pa.us or www.licensepa.state.pa.us (for verification)

Pennsylvania State Board of Osteopathic Medicine
Notes: This organization only verifies licensure for osteopathic physicians.

Listing of licensed physicians

Telephone: Free of charge.

Written: Several options available. Call for order form, customized pricing, and format. Mail order form, requests, and payment.

Electronic: Verification available at www.licensepa.state.pa.us.

Pennsylvania State Board of Osteopathic Medicine
State Board of Medicine
PO Box 2649
Harrisburg, PENNSYLVANIA 17105-2649
Telephone: 717/783-4858
Fax: 717/787-7769
E-mail: osteopat@pados.dos.state.pa.us
Web site: www.dos.state.pa.us

Pennsylvania State Board of Osteopathic Medicine
Verification of DO licenses

Telephone: Free of charge. Limit 10 verifications per agency per call.

Written: Free of charge. Faxed upon request (depending on quantity). Mail or fax requests, including physician names and license numbers (if known).

Electronic: Verification available at www.licensepa.state.pa.us.

Pennsylvania State Board of Osteopathic Medicine
State Board of Medicine
PO Box 2649
124 Pine Street (courier address)
Harrisburg, PENNSYLVANIA 17105-2649
Telephone: 717/783-4858 (Osteopathic)   717/783-1400 or 717/787-2381 (Medical Board)
Fax: 717/787-7769
E-mail: osteopat@pados.dos.state.pa.us
Web site: www.dos.state.pa.us

Puerto Rico

Puerto Rico Board of Medical Examiners
Verification of MD and DO licenses

Telephone: Not provided.
Written: $25 per verification. Mail requests, including physician names and license numbers (if known), and payment (U.S. money order payable only to Secretary of Treasury).
Electronic: Not provided.

> Puerto Rico Board of Medical Examiners
> PO Box 13969
> San Juan, PUERTO RICO 00908
> Telephone: 787/782-8937   787/782-8949 (President's Office)
> Fax: 787/792-4436 or 787/706-0364

Puerto Rico Board of Medical Examiners
Listing of licensed physicians

Telephone: Not provided.
Written: Not provided.
Electronic: Not provided.

> Puerto Rico Board of Medical Examiners
> Call Box 13969
> San Juan, PUERTO RICO 00908
> Telephone: 787/782-8937   787/782-8949 (President's Office)
> Fax: 787/792-4436

Rhode Island

Rhode Island Board of Medical Licensure and Discipline
Verification of licenses

Telephone: Free of charge. Limit three verifications per call.
Written: Free of charge. Faxed upon request. Mail or fax requests, including physician names and license numbers (if known).
Electronic: Automated verification system available at Web site.

> Rhode Island Board of Medical Licensure and Discipline
> Rhode Island Department of Health
> 3 Capital Hill, Room 205
> Providence, RHODE ISLAND 02908
> Telephone: 401/222-3855
> Fax: 401/222-2158
> Web site: www.health.ri.org

Rhode Island Board of Medical Licensure and Discipline
Verification of MD and DO licenses

Telephone: Free of charge. Limit three verifications per call.
Written: Free of charge. Faxed upon request. Mail or fax requests, including physician names and license numbers (if known).
Electronic: Automated verification system available at Web site.

Attention: Verification request
Rhode Island Board of Medical Licensure and Discipline
Department of Health
3 Capitol Hill, Room 205
Providence, RHODE ISLAND 02908
Telephone: 401/222-3855
Fax: 401/222-2158
Web site: www.health.state.ri.us

Rhode Island Board of Medical Licensure and Discipline
Roster of licensed physicians

Telephone: Free of charge.
Written: Free of charge.
Electronic: Automated verification system available at Web site.

Attention: Verification request
Rhode Island Board of Medical Licensure and Discipline
Department of Health
3 Capitol Hill, Room 205
Providence, RHODE ISLAND 02908
Telephone: 401/222-3855
Fax: 401/222-2158
Web site: www.healthri.org

South Carolina

South Carolina Board of Medical Examiners
Verification of MD and DO licenses

Telephone: Not provided.
Written: Only if disciplinary history exists, all public information will be sent (research fee: $5, plus $0.15/page). Provide self-addressed, stamped envelope.
Electronic: Information available at Web site.

State Board of Medical Examiners of South Carolina
PO Box 11289
Columbia, SOUTH CAROLINA 29211-1289
Telephone: 803/896-4500
Fax: 803/896-4515
E-mail: medboard@mail.llr.state.sc.us
Web site: www.llr.state.sc.us/pol/medical

South Carolina Board of Medical Examiners
Roster of licensed physicians

Telephone: Not provided.
Written: $5 research fee (plus $0.15 per copied page).
Electronic: Free of charge. Provided on Web site.

State Board of Medical Examiners of South Carolina
PO Box 11289
Columbia, SOUTH CAROLINA 29211-1289
Telephone: 803/896-4500   803/896-4580 (automated application request line)

Medical Licensing Agencies

Fax: 803/896-4515
E-mail: medboard@mail.llr.state.sc.us
Web site: www.llr.state.sc.us/pol/medical

South Carolina Board of Medical Examiners
Notes: Verifies Physician Assistants, Respiratory Care Practitioners, DO licenses, and Acupuncturists.
Verification of licenses
Telephone: Not provided.
Written: Provided only if there is an action; in this case, send letter with self-addressed, stamped envelope. If disciplinary history exists, all public information will be sent (research fee: $5, plus $0.15/copy).
Electronic: Information available on Web site.

South Carolina Department Labor Licensing and Regulations
State Board of Medical Examiners of South Carolina
PO Box 11289
Columbia, SOUTH CAROLINA 29211-1289
Telephone: 803/896-4500
Fax: 803/896-4515
E-mail: medboard@mail.llr.state.sc.us
Web site: www.llr.state.sc.us/pol/medical

South Dakota

South Dakota State Board of Medical and Osteopathic Examiners
Verification of MD and DO licenses
Telephone: Not provided.
Written: $10 per verification. Faxed upon request. Mail requests, including physician's name and license number (if known), and payment (check or money order payable to SD Board of Medical Examiners).
Electronic: Not provided.

South Dakota State Board of Medical and Osteopathic Examiners
1323 S. Minnesota Avenue
Sioux Falls, SOUTH DAKOTA 57105
Telephone: 605/334-8343
Fax: 605/336-0270

South Dakota State Board of Medical and Osteopathic Examiners
Verification of licenses
Telephone: Not provided.
Written: Several customized options available. $40 per computer printout; $70 for labels; $75 for diskette. 6% in-state tax; no out-of-state tax. Mail requests and payment.
Electronic: Not provided.

South Dakota State Board of Medical and Osteopathic Examiners
1323 S. Minnesota Avenue
Sioux Falls, SOUTH DAKOTA 57105
Telephone: 605/334-8343
Fax: 605/336-0270

Tennessee

Tennessee Board of Dentistry
Verification of MD licenses

Telephone:	Free of charge. Call automated verification system.
Written:	Free of charge.
Electronic:	Automated verification available at Web site.

Tennessee Board of Dentistry
425 Fifth Avenue N
Cordell Hull Building, First Floor
Nashville, TENNESSEE 37247-1010
Telephone: 615/532-5073 (general information)   888/310-4650 (automated verification system)
Fax: 615/532-5369
Web site: www.state.tn.us/health

Tennessee Department of Health
Directory of licensed physicians

Telephone:	Not provided.
Written:	Not provided.
Electronic:	Not provided.

Health Statistics and Research
Cordell Hull Building, Fourth Floor
425 Fifth Avenue N
Nashville, TENNESSEE 37247-5262
Telephone: 615/741-1954
Web site: www.state.tn.us/health

Tennessee Department of Health
Directory of licensed physicians

Telephone:	Not provided.
Written:	Call for most up-to-date cost. Mail requests and payment.
Electronic:	Available at www.state.tn.us/health.

Tennessee Department of Health
Attention: Bonnie Harrah
Health Statistics and Research
Cordell Hull Building Fourth Floor
425-5th Avenue North
Nashville, TENNESSEE 37247-5262
Telephone: 615/741-4939
Fax: 615/532-7904
Web site: www.state.tn.us/health

Texas

Texas State Board of Medical Examiners, Acupuncture Examiners, and Physician Assistant Examiners
Verification of licenses

Telephone:	Free of charge. During high call volume, agents may limit verifications to three per call.
Written:	Free of charge. Mail or fax requests, including names and license numbers (if known).
Electronic:	Automated verification system available via computer modem. Access by dialing into TSBME computer (512/305-7035). User name: PV; password: TX. See TSBME Web site for more details.

Texas State Board of Medical Examiners
MC-240
PO Box 2018
Austin, TEXAS 78768-2018
Telephone: 512/305-7030 (Customer Information Center)   512/305-7035 (online verification system)
Fax: 512/463-9416
E-mail: veriscic@tsbme.state.tx.us
Web site: www.tsbme.state.tx.us

Texas State Board of Medical Examiners, Acupuncture Examiners, and Physician Assistant Examiners
Directory of licensed physicians

Telephone:	Free of charge. During high call volume, agents may limit verifications to three per call.
Written:	Free of charge. Mail or fax requests, including names and license numbers (if known).
Electronic:	Automated verification system available via computer modem. Access by dialing into TSBME computer (512/305-7035). User name: PV; password: TX. See TSBME Web site for more details.

Texas State Board of Medical Examiners
MC-240
PO Box 2018
Austin, TEXAS 78768-2018
Telephone: 512/305-7030 (Customer Information Center)   512/305-7035 (online verification system)
Fax: 512/463-9416
E-mail: verifcic@tsbme.state.tx.us
Web site: www.tsbme.state.tx.us

Utah

Utah Division of Occupational and Professional Licensing
Verification of MD and DO licenses

Telephone:	Free of charge. Limit three verifications per call.
Written:	$20 per verification. Mail or fax requests, including physicians' information.
Electronic:	Automated verification system available at Web site. Available for $5 per verification.

Utah Division of Occupational and Professional Licensing
PO Box 146741
Salt Lake City, UTAH 84114-6741
Telephone: 801/530-6628   866/275-3675 (toll-free in Utah only)
Fax: 801/530-6511
Web site: www.dopl.utah.gov

Utah Division of Occupational and Professional Licensure
Verification of licenses

Telephone: Free of charge. Limit three verifications per call.
Written: $20 fee. Mail or fax requests, including physician names, Social Security numbers, and license numbers (if known).
Electronic: Automated verification system available on Web site.

Utah Division of Occupational and Professional Licensure
160 E. 300 S
PO Box 146741
Salt Lake City, UTAH 84114-6741
Telephone: 801/530-6628
Fax: 801/530-6511
Web site: www.dopl.utah.gov

Vermont

Vermont Board of Medical Practice
Verification of MD licenses

Telephone: Free of charge. Limit two verifications per call.
Written: $20 per verification. Mail requests, including physician names and license numbers (if known), and payment.
Electronic: Automated verification system available at Web site.

Vermont Board of Medical Practice
109 State Street
Montpelier, VERMONT 05609-1106
Telephone: 802/828-2673
Fax: 802/828-5450
Web site: www.docboard.org

Vermont Board of Osteopathic Physicians and Surgeons
Annual report of licensed physicians

Telephone: Not provided.
Written: $20 per verification. Includes all professions licensed in-state. Mail request.
Electronic: Free of charge.

Vermont Board of Osteopathic Physicians and Surgeons
Office of the Secretary of State
26 Terrace Street, Drawer 9
Montpelier, VERMONT 05609-1106
Telephone: 802/828-2373
Fax: 802/828-2465
E-mail: patkins@sec.state.vt.us
Web site: www.sec.state.vt.us

Vermont Board of Osteopathic Physicians and Surgeons
Verification of DO licenses

Telephone: Free of charge. Limit five verifications per day.
Written: $20 per verification. Mail requests, including physician names and license numbers (if known), and payment.

Medical Licensing Agencies

Electronic: Automated verification system available at Web site.

Vermont Board of Osteopathic Physicians and Surgeons
Office of the Secretary of State
26 Terrace Street, Drawer 9
Montpelier, VERMONT 05609-1106
Telephone: 802/828-2373
Fax: 802/828-2465
E-mail: patkins@sec.state.vt.us
Web site: www.vtprofessionals.org

Virgin Islands

Virgin Islands Board of Medical Examiners
Directory of licensed physicians
Telephone: Not provided.
Written: Not provided.
Electronic: Not provided.

Virgin Islands Board of Medical Examiners
48 Sugar Estates
St. Thomas, VIRGIN ISLANDS 00802
Telephone: 340/774-0117
Fax: 340/777-4001

Virginia

Virginia Board of Medicine
Verification of MD and DO licenses
Telephone: Free of charge. Limit three verifications per day. Faxed upon request. Provide physician's name, license number, or Social Security number.
Written: Free of charge. Limit 10 verifications per day. Mail requests, including physician's name, license number, or Social Security number.
Electronic: Information available at Web site.

State Board of Medicine
Department of Health Professions
6606 W. Broad Street, Fourth Floor
Richmond, VIRGINIA 23230-1717
Telephone: 804/662-9388   804/662-7636 (automated verification system)
Fax: 804/662-9517
Web site: www.dhp.state.va.us

Washington

Washington Division of Professional Licensing
Directory of licensed physicians
Telephone: Call for most up-to-date prices and ordering information.
Written: Call for most up-to-date prices. Mail request and payment.
Electronic: Not provided.

Chapter 6

        Attn: Medical Quality Assurance Commission
        Division of Professional Licensing
        Department of Health
        PO Box 47866
        Olympia, WASHINGTON 98504-7866
        Telephone: 360/236-4700   360/664-4111 (automated verification system)
        Fax: 360/586-4573
        Web site: www.doh.wa.gov

Washington Division of Professional Licensing
Verification of MD licenses

Telephone: Free of charge. Limit three verifications per call via general information number; unlimited for automated verification line. Provide code MD and physician's license number.
Written: Free of charge. Mail or fax requests, including physician names and license numbers.
Electronic: Automated verification service available via computer modem. Dial 360/664-4144. For more information, call for brochure.

        Attn: Medical Quality Assurance Commission
        Division of Professional Licensing
        Department of Health
        PO Box 47866
        Olympia, WASHINGTON 98504-7866
        Telephone: 360/236-4700 (general information)   360/664-4111 (automated verification system)
        Fax: 360/586-4573
        Web site: www.doh.wa.gov or www.doh.wa.gov/medical

Washington State Board of Osteopathic Medicine and Surgery
Verification of licenses

Telephone: Verification provided at 360/236-4700.
Written: Call for most up-to-date fees. Mail request and payment.
Electronic: Not provided.

        Washington State Board of Osteopathic Medicine and Surgery
        Attn: Arlene Robertson
        Department of Health
        PO Box 47869
        Olympia, WASHINGTON 98504-7869
        Telephone: 360/236-4943
        Fax: 360/236-2406
        E-mail: jo.minor@doh.wa.gov
        Web site: www.doh.wa.gov

Washington State Board of Osteopathic Medicine and Surgery
Verification of DO licenses

Telephone: Free of charge. Limit three verifications per call. Provide physician's name and/or license number. For unlimited verifications, call automated verification system. Provide code OP and physician's license number.
Written: Free of charge. Mail or fax requests, including physician names and license numbers.
Electronic: Automated verification system available at Web site.

        Washington State Board of Osteopathic Medicine and Surgery
        Department of Health

PO Box 47869
Olympia, WASHINGTON 98504-7869
Telephone: 360/236-4943   360/664-4111 (automated verification system)   360/236-4700 (verification department)
Fax: 360/236-2406
Web site: www.doh.wa.gov

West Virginia

West Virginia Board of Medicine
Note: MD, Podiatrist, and Physician Assistant Licensing.
Verification of licenses
Telephone:	Free of charge. Limit three verifications per call.
Written:	$25 per verification. Mail requests, including physician names and license numbers (if known), and payment.
Electronic:	Not provided.

West Virginia Board of Medicine
101 Dee Drive
Charleston, WEST VIRGINIA 25311
Telephone: 304/558-2921
Fax: 304/558-2084
Web site: www.wvdhhr.org/wvbom

West Virginia Board of Medicine
Directory of licensed physicians
Telephone:	Free of charge. Limit three verifications per day.
Written:	$25 per copy. Mail requests and payment.
Electronic:	Not provided.

West Virginia Board of Medicine
101 Dee Drive
Charleston, WEST VIRGINIA 25311
Telephone: 304/558-2921
Fax: 304/558-2084
Web site: www.wvdhhr.org/wvbom

West Virginia Board of Medicine
Verification of MD licenses
Telephone:	Free of charge. Limit three verifications per call.
Written:	$25 per verification. Mail requests, including physician names, license numbers (if known), and payment.
Electronic:	Not provided.

West Virginia Board of Medicine
101 Dee Drive
Charleston, WEST VIRGINIA 25311
Telephone: 304/558-2921
Fax: 304/558-2084
Web site: www.wvdhhr.org/wvbom

West Virginia Board of Osteopathy
Listing of licensed physicians

Telephone: Not provided.
Written: $25 per physician.
Electronic: Not provided.

> West Virginia Board of Osteopathy
> 334 Penco Road
> Weirton, WEST VIRGINIA 26062
> Telephone: 304/723-4638
> Fax: 304/723-6723
> E-mail: bdosteo@mail.wvnet.edu
> Web site: www.state.wv.us/bdosteo

West Virginia Board of Osteopathy
Verification of DO licenses

Telephone: Not provided.
Written: $25 per verification; $10 for copy of exam scores. Mail requests, including physician names and license numbers (if known), and payment.
Electronic: Not provided.

> West Virginia Board of Osteopathy
> 334 Penco Road
> Weirton, WEST VIRGINIA 26062
> Telephone: 304/723-4638
> Fax: 304/723-6723
> E-mail: bdosteo@mail.wvnet.edu
> Web site: www.state.wv.us/bdosteo

Wisconsin

Wisconsin Medical Examining Board
Directory of licensed physicians

Telephone: Not provided.
Written: Fees differ per customized copy; call for price and order form. Mail requests, including order form and payment.
Electronic: Check Web site for more information.

> Medical Examining Board
> Department of Regulations and Licensing
> PO Box 8935
> Madison, WISCONSIN 53708
> Telephone: 608/261-7931
> Fax: 608/267-1803
> Web site: www.drl.state.wi.us

Wisconsin Medical Examining Board
Verification of MD and DO licenses

Telephone: Free of charge. Call 608/266-2811.
Written: Free of charge for local state; $10 per verification for other state boards.

Medical Licensing Agencies

Electronic: All verification requests must be accessed on agency's Web site (www.drl.state.wi.us). If you cannot access the Internet, submit your request in writing to address listed below.

> Medical Examining Board
> Department of Regulations and Licensing
> PO Box 8935
> Madison, WISCONSIN 53708-8935
> Telephone: 608/266-2811
> Fax: 608/261-7083
> E-mail: dorl@drl.state.wi.us
> Web site: www.drl.state.wi.us

Wyoming

Wyoming Board of Medicine
Notes: Verification of MD, DO, and PA licenses.
Directory of licensed physicians
Telephone: Free of charge. Limit one verification per call.
Written: $45 per directory; $25 per written verification; Mail requests and payment (business or company check payable to WY Board of Medicine).
Electronic: Not provided.

> Wyoming Board of Medicine
> 211 W. 19th Street, Second Floor
> Cheyenne, WYOMING 82002
> Telephone: 307/778-7053
> Fax: 307/778-2069
> E-mail: wyomedical@wyomedicalboard.org
> Web site: wyomedboard.state.wy.us

Wyoming Board of Medicine
Verification of MD and DO licenses
Telephone: Free of charge. Limit one verification per call.
Written: $25 per verification. Faxed upon request. Mail requests, including physician names and license numbers (if known), and payment.
Electronic: Free of charge on Web site.

> Wyoming Board of Medicine
> 211 W. 19th Street, Second Floor
> Cheyenne, WYOMING 82002
> Telephone: 307/778-7053
> Fax: 307/778-2069
> E-mail: wyomedical@wyomedicalboard.org
> Web site: www.wyomedboard.state.wy.us

Canadian College of Physicians and Surgeons Provincial Offices

Canadian College of Physicians and Surgeons Provincial Offices

Note: All fees are listed and payable in Canadian dollars only.

Alberta

College of Physicians and Surgeons of Alberta
Notes: Must be registered with Alberta College before practicing.
Verification of licenses
Telephone: Free of charge.
Written: $50 for Certificate of Good Standing for U.S. hospitals. Add $3.50 GST for Canadian hospitals. Mail requests, including physician names and license numbers (if known), signed release forms, and payment.
Electronic: Not provided.

College of Physicians and Surgeons of Alberta
10180-101 Street NW, Suite 900
Edmonton, ALBERTA T5J 4P8
CANADA
Telephone: 780/423-4764
Fax: 780/420-0651
E-mail: dharker@cpsa.ab.ca
Web site: www.cpsa.ab.ca

College of Physicians and Surgeons of Alberta
Notes: Medical directory shipped within Canada: $57.40. Outside Canada: $50.00 plus applicable postage; call for amount. Written verification of licensure within Canada: $53.50.
Directory of licensed physicians
Telephone: Not provided.
Written: $32.10 per copy (to ship in Canada). Call for updated price of shipment to U.S. Mail requests and payment.
Electronic: Not provided.

College of Physicians and Surgeons of Alberta
900 Manulife Place
10180-101 Street
Edmonton, ALBERTA T5J 4P8
CANADA
Telephone: 780/423-4764
Fax: 780/420-0651
Web site: www.cpsa.ab.ca

British Columbia

College of Physicians and Surgeons of British Columbia
Notes: All fees are listed and payable in Canadian dollars only.
Verification of licenses
Telephone: Free of charge. Limit three verifications per call.
Written: $50 per Certificate of Good Standing available only by physician's request. Mail requests, including physician names and license numbers (if known).
Electronic: Not provided.

Chapter 6

College of Physicians and Surgeons of British Columbia
1807 W. Tenth Avenue
Vancouver, BRITISH COLUMBIA V6J 2A9
CANADA
Telephone: 604/733-7758
Fax: 604/733-3503
Web site: www.cpsbc.ca

College of Physicians and Surgeons of British Columbia
Directory of licensed physicians

Telephone:	Not provided.
Written:	$50 per copy. Mail requests and payment.
Electronic:	Not provided.

College of Physicians and Surgeons of British Columbia
1807 W. Tenth Avenue
Vancouver, BRITISH COLUMBIA V6J 2A9
CANADA
Telephone: 604/733-7758   800/461-3008 (Only for B.C.)
Fax: 604/733-3503
E-mail: Questions@cpsbc.ca

Manitoba

College of Physicians and Surgeons of Manitoba
Verification of licenses

Telephone:	Free of charge. Limit five verifications per call.
Written:	Free of charge. Faxed upon request. Mail or fax requests, including physician names and license numbers (if known).
Electronic:	Information available on Web site.

College of Physicians and Surgeons of Manitoba
1000-1661 Portage Avenue
Winnipeg, MANITOBA R3J 3T7
CANADA
Telephone: 204/774-4344
Fax: 204/774-0750
E-mail: bpope@cpsm.mb.ca
Web site: www.cpsm.mb.ca

College of Physicians and Surgeons of Manitoba
Notes: Certificate of Good Standing requires a signature on consent form and fee of $53.50.
Directory of licensed physicians

Telephone:	Not provided.
Written:	$53.50 per copy, including GST. Mail requests and payment.
Electronic:	Free of charge via Web site. No information available regarding any type of disciplinary actions. Must submit those requests in writing.

College of Physicians and Surgeons of Manitoba
1661 Portage Avenue, Suite 1000

Winnipeg, MANITOBA R3J3T7
CANADA
Telephone: 204/774-4344
Fax: 204/774-0750
E-mail: bpope@cpsm.mb.ca
Web site: www.cpsm.mb.ca

New Brunswick

College of Physicians and Surgeons of New Brunswick
Verification of licenses

Telephone:	Free of charge. Limit 20 verifications per call.
Written:	$50 for letters of good standing. Verifications free of charge. Mail or fax requests, including physician names and license numbers (if known). Limit of six verifications per fax.
Electronic:	Not provided.

College of Physicians and Surgeons of New Brunswick
1 Hampton Road, Suite 300
Rothesay, NEW BRUNSWICK E2E 5K8
CANADA
Telephone: 506/849-5050   800/667-4641(verification line)
Fax: 506/849-5069
E-mail: info@cpsnb.org
Web site: www.cpsnb.org

College of Physicians and Surgeons of New Brunswick
Directory of licensed physicians

Telephone:	Verification for credentials only.
Written:	$50 per copy. Mail requests and payment.
Electronic:	Verification for credentials.

College of Physicians and Surgeons of New Brunswick
1 Hampton Road, Suite 300
Rothesay, NEW BRUNSWICK E2E 5K8
CANADA
Telephone: 506/849-5050   800/667-4641
Fax: 506/849-5069
E-mail: info@cpsnb.org
Web site: www.cpsnb.org

Newfoundland

Newfoundland Medical Board
Verification of licenses

Telephone:	Free of charge. Limit five verifications per call.
Written:	Free of charge. Faxed upon request. Mail or fax requests, including physician names and license numbers (if known). Certificate of Good Standing: $60
Electronic:	Not provided.

Newfoundland Medical Board
139 Water Street, Unit 6
Saint Johns, NEWFOUNDLAND A1C 1B2

Chapter 6

CANADA
Telephone: 709/726-8546
Fax: 709/726-4725
E-mail: nmb@thezone.net

Newfoundland Medical Board
Directory of licensed physicians

Telephone: Free of charge.
Written: Not provided.
Electronic: Not provided.

Newfoundland Medical Board
139 Water Street, Suite 603
Saint Johns, NEWFOUNDLAND A1C 1B2
CANADA
Telephone: 709/726-8546
Fax: 709/726-4725
E-mail: nmb@thezone.net

Northwest Territories

Health and Social Services
Directory of licensed physicians

Telephone: Free of charge.
Written: Free of charge. Certificate of Good Standing: $20 fee. Submit with physician's written consent form.
Electronic: Not provided.

Health and Social Services
Medical Profession
Registrar of Professional Licensing
Government of the Northwest Territories
Centre Square Tower, Eighth Floor, Box 1320
Yellowknife, NORTHWEST TERRITORIES X1A 2L9
CANADA
Telephone: 867/920-8058
Fax: 867/873-0484

Medical Profession, Health & Social Services
Verification of licenses

Telephone: Free of charge.
Written: Free of charge. Faxed upon request. Mail requests, including physician names and license numbers (if known).
Electronic: Not provided.

Medical Profession
Health and Social Services
Registrar of Professional Licensing
Government of the Northwest Territories
Box 1320
Yellowknife, NORTHWEST TERRITORIES X1A 2L9
CANADA

Canadian College of Physicians and Surgeons Provincial Offices

Telephone: 867/920-8058
Fax: 867/873-0484

Nova Scotia

College of Physicians and Surgeons of Nova Scotia
Verification of licenses

Telephone: Free of charge. Limit three verifications per call.
Written: Free of charge. Faxed upon request. Mail or fax requests, including physician names and license numbers (if known).
Electronic: Information available on Web site.

College of Physicians and Surgeons of Nova Scotia
1559 Brunswick Street, Suite 200
Halifax, NOVA SCOTIA B3J 2G1
CANADA
Telephone: 902/422-5823   877/282-7767
Fax: 902/422-5035
Web site: www.cpsns.ns.ca

College of Physicians and Surgeons of Nova Scotia
Directory of licensed physicians

Telephone: Free of charge.
Written: Not provided.
Electronic: Verification available on Web site.

College of Physicians and Surgeons of Nova Scotia
1559 Brunswick Street, Suite 200
Halifax, NOVA SCOTIA B3J 2G1
CANADA
Telephone: 902/422-5823
Fax: 902/422-5035
Web site: www.cpsns.ns.ca

Ontario

College of Physicians and Surgeons of Ontario
Verification of licenses

Telephone: Free of charge.
Written: Fee depends on number of verifications needed; call for exact amount. Mail requests, including physician names and license numbers (if known), and payment.
Electronic: Not provided.

College of Physicians and Surgeons of Ontario
80 College Street
Toronto, ONTARIO M5G 2E2
CANADA
Telephone: 416/967-2603   800/268-7096
Fax: 416/961-3330
Web site: www.cpso.on.ca

College of Physicians and Surgeons of Ontario
Directory of licensed physicians

Telephone: Not provided.
Written: Not provided.
Electronic: Not provided.

> College of Physicians and Surgeons of Ontario
> 80 College Street
> Toronto, ONTARIO M5G 2E2
> CANADA
> Telephone: 416/967-2600   800/268-7096
> Fax: 416/961-3330
> Web site: www.cpso.on.ca

Prince Edward Island

College of Physicians and Surgeons of Prince Edward Island
Verification of licenses

Telephone: Not provided.
Written: $50 for Certificate of Good Standing. For written requests, include physician names and license numbers, physician-signed release form, and payment.
Electronic: Not provided.

> College of Physicians and Surgeons of PEI
> 199 Grafton Street
> Charlottetown, PRINCE EDWARD ISLAND C1A 1L2
> CANADA
> Telephone: 902/566-3861
> Fax: 902/566-3861
> E-mail: mmacdonald@collegeofphysicians.pe.ca

College of Physicians and Surgeons of Prince Edward Island
Verification of licenses

Telephone: Not provided.
Written: $60 per copy. Mail requests and payment.
Electronic: Not provided.

> College of Physicians and Surgeons of PEI
> The Polyclinic Professional Centre
> 199 Grafton Street
> Charlottetown, PRINCE EDWARD ISLAND C1A 1L2
> CANADA
> Telephone: 902/566-3861
> Fax: 902/566-3861
> E-mail: mmacdonald@collegeofphysicians.pe.ca

Canadian College of Physicians and Surgeons Provincial Offices

Quebec

College des Medecines du Quebec
Verification of licenses

Telephone: Free of charge. Limit five verifications per call.
Written: $50 per verification. Mail requests, including physician names and license numbers (if known), and payment.
Electronic: Not provided.

> College des Medecines du Quebec
> 2170 Boulevard Rene-Levesque Ouest
> Montreal, QUEBEC H3H 2T8
> CANADA
> Telephone: 514/933-4441
> Fax: 514/933-3112
> E-mail: info@cmq.org
> Web site: www.cmq.org

College des Medecins du Quebec
Directory of licensed physicians

Telephone: Not provided.
Written: Fee subject to change; call for most up-to-date price. Mail requests and payment.
Electronic: Not provided.

> College des Medecins du Quebec
> 2170 Boul Rene, Levesque Ouest
> Montreal, QUEBEC H3H 2T8
> CANADA
> Telephone: 514/933-4441
> Fax: 514/933-3112
> E-mail: info@cmq.org
> Web site: www.cmq.org

Saskatchewan

College of Physicians and Surgeons of Saskatchewan
Verification of licenses

Telephone: Free of charge.
Written: $50 for Certificate of Good Standing for U.S. hospitals. Add $3.50 GST. Mail requests, including physician names and license numbers (if known), signed release forms, and payment.
Electronic: Not provided.

> College of Physicians and Surgeons of Saskatchewan
> 211 Fourth Avenue S
> Saskatoon, SASKATCHEWAN S7K 1N1
> CANADA
> Telephone: 306/244-7355
> Fax: 306/244-0090
> E-mail: cpss@quadrant.net
> Web site: www.quadrant.net/cpss

The 2003 Credentialing and Privileging Desk Reference

College of Physicians and Surgeons of Saskatchewan
Directory of licensed physicians

Telephone: Free of charge.
Written: $32.10 per copy of physicians mailing list (to ship in Canada). Call for updated price of shipment to U.S. Mail requests and payment. $53.50 for licensure verification.
Electronic: Not provided.

> College of Physicians and Surgeons of Saskatchewan
> 211 Fourth Avenue S
> Saskatoon, SASKATCHEWAN S7K 1N1
> CANADA
> Telephone: 306/244-7355
> Fax: 306/244-0090
> E-mail: cpss@quadrant.net
> Web site: www.quadrant.net/cpss

Yukon

Yukon Medical Council
Verification of licenses

Telephone: Free of charge.
Written: $5 for Certificate of Good Standing. Mail requests, including physician names and license numbers (if known), and payment.
Electronic: Free of charge. E-mail requests to carol.cameron@gov.yk.ca.

> Yukon Medical Council
> Consumer Services C5
> PO Box 2703
> Whitehorse, YUKON Y1A 2C6
> CANADA
> Telephone: 867/667-5111
> Fax: 867/667-3609
> E-mail: consumer@gov.yk.ca

Dental Licensing Agencies

Alabama

State Board of Dental Examiners of Alabama
Verification of licenses
Telephone: Free of charge. Limit three verifications per call.
Written: Free of charge. Mail, call, or fax requests, including dentist names and license numbers (if known). Faxed upon request.
Electronic: Not provided.

> State Board of Dental Examiners of Alabama
> 5346 Stadium Trace Parkway, Suite 112
> Hoover, ALABAMA 35244-4583
> Telephone: 205/985-7267
> Fax: 205/985-0674
> E-mail: bdeaal@bellsouth.net
> Web site: www.dentalboard.org

State Board of Dental Examiners of Alabama
Directory of licensed dentists
Telephone: Free of charge.
Written: $5 per copy. Mail requests and payment.
Electronic: Not provided.

> State Board of Dental Examiners of Alabama
> 5346 Stadium Trace Parkway, Suite 112
> Hoover, ALABAMA 35244-4583
> Telephone: 205/985-7267
> Fax: 205/985-0674
> E-mail: bdeaal@bellsouth.net
> Web site: www.dentalboard.org

Alaska

State of Alaska Board of Dental Examiners
Notes: General search Web site: www.dced.state.ak.us/occ.
Verification of licenses
Telephone: Free of charge. Limit 3–5 verifications per call.
Written: $20 per verification. Mail requests, including dentist names and license numbers (if known), and payment.
Electronic: Free of charge.

> State of Alaska Board of Dental Examiners
> Department of Community and Economic Development
> PO Box 110806
> Juneau, ALASKA 99811-0806
> Telephone: 907/465-2542
> Fax: 907/465-2974
> E-mail: wanda_fleming@dced.state.ak.us
> Web site: www.dced.state.ak.us/occ/pden.htm

State of Alaska Board of Dental Examiners
Directory of licensed dentists

Telephone: Free of charge. Limit three verifications per call.
Written: $20 per verification.
Electronic: Information available on Web site.

>State of Alaska Board of Dental Examiners
>Department of Community and Economic Development
>PO Box 110806
>Juneau, ALASKA 99811-0806
>Telephone: 907/465-2542
>Fax: 907/465-2974
>E-mail: wanda_fleming@dced.state.ak.us
>Web site: www.dced.state.ak.us/occ/pdem.htp

Arizona

Arizona State Board of Dental Examiners
Notes: Licensing requirements may be found at www.azleg.state.az.us. Click on Dental Practice Act Title 32-1201.
Verification of licenses

Telephone: Free of charge. Limit three verifications per call.
Written: $5 per verification. Mail requests, including dentist names and license numbers (if known), and payment.
Electronic: Not provided.

>Arizona State Board of Dental Examiners
>5060 N. 19th Avenue, Suite 406
>Phoenix, ARIZONA 85015-3214
>Telephone: 602/242-1492
>Fax: 602/242-1445
>Web site: www.azdentalboard.org

Arizona State Board of Dental Examiners
Notes: Also issue licenses for Dental Hygienists.
Directory of licensed dentists

Telephone: Free of charge.
Written: $5 per license (for dentists).
Electronic: Not provided.

>Arizona State Board of Dental Examiners
>5060 N. 19th Avenue, Suite 406
>Phoenix, ARIZONA 85015-3214
>Telephone: 602/242-1492
>Fax: 602/242-1445
>Web site: www.azdentalboard.org

Arkansas

Arkansas State Board of Dental Examiners
Verification of licenses

Telephone: Free of charge. Limit three verifications per call.
Written: Free of charge. Mail, call, or fax requests, including dentist names and license numbers. Faxed upon request.
Electronic: Free of charge. E-mail requests to asbde@mail.state.ar.us (include dentist names and license numbers).

Arkansas State Board of Dental Examiners
101 E. Capitol, Suite 111
Little Rock, ARKANSAS 72201
Telephone: 501/682-2085
Fax: 501/682-3543
E-mail: asbde@mail.state.ar.us
Web site: www.asbde.org

Arkansas State Board of Dental Examiners
Directory of licensed dentists

Telephone: Not provided.
Written: $50 per printed list; $50 per set of printed labels; $50 per list on diskette. Mail requests, including specific needs (e.g., names, addresses, license numbers, etc.) and sorting instructions.
Electronic: Not provided.

Arkansas State Board of Dental Examiners
101 E. Capitol, Suite 111
Little Rock, ARKANSAS 72201
Telephone: 501/682-2085
Fax: 501/682-3543
E-mail: asbde@mail.state.ar.us
Web site: www.asbde.org

California

Dental Board of California
Verification of licenses

Telephone: Free of charge. Limit three verifications per call.
Written: $2 fee. Mail or fax requests, including dentist names and license numbers.
Electronic: Electronic verification obtained via Department of Consumer Affairs page (dca.ca.gov). Check the license status, then scroll to Dental Board.

Dental Board of California
1432 Howe Avenue, Suite 85
Sacramento, CALIFORNIA 95825
Telephone: 916/263-2300
Fax: 916/263-2140
Web site: www.dbc.ca.gov

Dental Board of California
Directory of licensed dentists

Telephone: Free of charge.
Written: Free of charge unless certification is required.
Electronic: Free of charge. Available through Web site.

>Dental Board of California
>Department of Consumer Affairs
>1432 Howe Avenue, Suite 85
>Sacramento, CALIFORNIA 95825
>Telephone: 916/263-2300
>Fax: 916/263-2140
>Web site: www.dbc.ca.gov

Colorado

Colorado State Board of Dental Examiners
Directory of licensed dentists

Telephone: Call 303/894-7758 to purchase list.
Written: Not provided.
Electronic: Not provided.

>Colorado State Board of Dental Examiners
>1560 Broadway, Suite 1310
>Denver, COLORADO 80202
>Telephone: 303/894-7758   303/894-7890 (automated verification system)
>Fax: 303/894-7764
>Web site: www.dora.state.co.us/dental

Connecticut

Department of Public Health
Verification of licenses

Telephone: Free of charge. Limit 5–10 verifications per call (depending on call volume).
Written: Free of charge. Mail or fax requests, including dentist names, license numbers, and expiration dates. Faxed upon request.
Electronic: Not provided.

>Department of Public Health
>Dental Licensure
>410 Capitol Avenue, MS#12APP
>PO Box 340308
>Hartford, CONNECTICUT 06134-0308
>Telephone: 860/509-7651
>Fax: 860/509-5457
>Web site: www.dph.state.ct.us

Dental Licensing Agencies

Division of Health System Regulation
Directory of licensed dentists

Telephone: Not provided.
Written: $5.30 per standard file; $8 per custom file. Obtain a blank questionnaire by calling number listed. Mail completed questionnaire, Letter of Request, and check (payable to Treasurer, State of Connecticut).
Electronic: CD/ROM is $10.

Licensing and Registration
Division of Health System Regulation
State of Connecticut
410 Capitol Avenue MS#12MQA
PO Box 340308
Hartford, CONNECTICUT 06134-0308
Telephone: 860/509-7603
Fax: 860/509-7607
Web site: www.dph.state.ct.us

Delaware

Delaware State Board of Dental Examiners
Verification of licenses

Telephone: Free of charge.
Written: $15 per verification. Mail requests, including dentist names and license numbers (if known), and payment.
Electronic: Not provided.

Delaware State Board of Dental Examiners
861 Silver Lake Boulevard
Cannon Building, Suite 203
Dover, DELAWARE 19904
Telephone: 302/744-4522, Ext. 218   302/744-4520 (Gail Franzolino)
Fax: 302/739-2711
E-mail: gfranzolino@state.de.us

Delaware State Board of Dental Examiners
Directory of licensed dentists

Telephone: Not provided
Written: $25 per copy (available on paper or diskette). Mail requests and payment.
Electronic: Not provided.

Delaware State Board of Dental Examiners
861 Silver Lake Boulevard
Cannon Building, Suite 203
Dover, DELAWARE 19904
Telephone: 302/7444-4500, Ext. 520   302/744-4520 (Gail Franzolino)
Fax: 302/739-2711
E-mail: gfranzolino@state.de.us
Web site: www.professionallicensing.state.de.us

District of Columbia

Department of Health
Directory of licensed dentists

Telephone: Not provided.
Written: Provided. Call 202/442-9200 for current prices.
Electronic: Not provided.

>Department of Health
>Office of Professional Licensing
>825 N. Capital Street NE, Suite 2224
>Washington, DISTRICT OF COLUMBIA 20002
>Telephone: 202/442-9200
>Fax: 202/442-9431
>Web site: www.dchealth.com

United States Department of Health and Human Services
Verification of licenses

Telephone: Free of charge. Limit three verifications per call. Faxed upon request.
Written: $50 per verification. Mail requests, including dentist names and license numbers (if known), and payment.
Electronic: Not provided.

>Department of Health and Human Services
>200 Independence Avenue SW
>Washington, DISTRICT OF COLUMBIA 20201
>Telephone: 202/619-0257   877/696-6775
>Fax: 202/690-7203
>Web site: dhhs.gov

Florida

Division of Medical Quality Assurance Communications Services
Verification of licenses

Telephone: Free of charge. Limit three verifications per call.
Written: $25 per verification. Mail requests, including dentist names and license numbers (if known), and payment.
Electronic: Upon request. Will send written certification via fax.

>Division of Medical Quality Assurance Communications Services
>Client Services Unit
>CO1/Bin C99
>4052 Bald Cypress Way
>Tallahassee, FLORIDA 32399-3299
>Telephone: 850/488-0595
>Fax: 850/414-0864
>Web site: www.doh.state.fl.us/mqa

Dental Licensing Agencies

Georgia

Georgia Board of Dentistry
Verification of licenses

Telephone: Free of charge. Limit two verifications per call.
Written: $25 fee per request.
Electronic: Information available on Web site

Georgia Board of Dentistry
237 Coliseum Drive
Macon, GEORGIA 31217
Telephone: 478/207-1680
Fax: 478/207-1685
Web site: www.sos.state.ga.us/plb/dentistry

Georgia Board of Dentistry
Directory of licensed dentists

Telephone: Not provided.
Written: $25 per verification. Mail request and payment.
Electronic: Free of charge via Web site.

Georgia Board of Dentistry
237 Coliseum Drive
Macon, GEORGIA 31217-3858
Telephone: 478/207-1680
Fax: 478/207-1685
E-mail: rtmathis@sos.state.ga.us
Web site: www.sos.state.ga.us/plb/dentistry

Hawaii

Hawaii State Board of Dental Examiners
Verification of licenses

Telephone: Free of charge. Call 808/587-3295.
Written: $15 per verification. Mail requests, including dentist names and license numbers (if known), and payment.
Electronic: Not provided.

Hawaii State Board of Dental Examiners
Department of Commerce and Consumer Affairs
PO Box 3469
Honolulu, HAWAII 96801
Telephone: 808/586-3000
Web site: www.state.hi.us/dcca/pvl

Hawaii State Board of Dental Examiners
Directory of licensed dentists

Telephone: Free of charge. Call 808/586-3000.
Written: $15 fee for verification of Hawaii license.
Electronic: Not provided.

Hawaii State Board of Dental Examiners
Department of Commerce and Consumer Affairs
PO Box 3469
1010 Richards Street
Honolulu, HAWAII 96813
Telephone: 808/86-3000

Idaho

Idaho State Board of Dentistry
Verification of licenses

Telephone: Free of charge. Limit two verifications per call.
Written: Free of charge. Mail or fax requests, including dentist names and license numbers (if known).
Electronic: Automated verification system available at Web site.

Idaho State Board of Dentistry
PO Box 83720
Boise, IDAHO 83720-0021
Telephone: 208/334-2369
Fax: 208/334-3247
E-mail: smiller@isbd.state.id.us
Web site: www.state.id.us/isbd

Illinois

Licensure Maintenance Unit
Verification of licenses

Telephone: Free of charge. Limit three verifications per call.
Written: $20 per verification. Mail requests, including dentist names and license numbers (if known), and payment.
Electronic: Automated verification system available at Web site.

Department of Professional Regulation
Licensure Maintenance Unit
320 W. Washington Street, Third Floor
Springfield, ILLINOIS 62786
Telephone: 217/782-0458
Fax: 217/557-8073 (general inquiries should call first)
Web site: www.dpr.state.il.us

Licensure Maintenance Unit
Directory of licensed dentists

Telephone: Not provided.
Written: $20 fee. Must include dentist's name, license number (if known), and payment (cashier's check or money order made payable to Illinois Department of Professional Regulation).
Electronic: Not provided.

Illinois Department of Professional Regulation
Licensure Maintenance Unit
320 W. Washington Street, Third Floor
Springfield, ILLINOIS 62786
Telephone: 217/782-0458
Web site: www.dpr.state.il.us

Indiana

Indiana State Board of Dentistry
Verification of licenses
Telephone: Call 888/333-7515. Provide dentist's name or license number (if known).
Written: Free of charge in Indiana. $10 per verification to other states. Mail requests, including dentist's names and license numbers (if known).
Electronic: Automated verification system available at Web site. Call 800/236-5446 for more information.

Health Professions Bureau
Indiana State Board of Dentistry
402 W. Washington Street, Room 041
Indianapolis, INDIANA 46204
Telephone: 317/232-2960
Fax: 317/233-4236
Web site: www.in.gov/hpb

Indiana State Board of Dentistry
Directory of licensed dentists
Telephone: 888/333-7515.
Written: Provided only to other states. Practitioner pays $10 fee.
Electronic: Automated verification system available at Web site. Subscription or credit card required. Call 800/236-5446 for more information.

Health Professions Bureau
Indiana State Board of Dentistry
402 West Washington Street, Room 041
Indianapolis, INDIANA 46204
Telephone: 317-232-1129 317-232-2960
E-mail: koakley@hpb.state.in.us
Web site: www.state.in.us/hpb

Iowa

Iowa Board of Dental Examiners
Verification of licenses
Telephone: Free of charge. Limit three verifications per call.
Written: Free of charge. Mail or fax requests, including dentist names and license numbers. Faxed upon request.
Electronic: Not provided.

Iowa Board of Dental Examiners
400 S.W. Eighth Street, Suite D
Des Moines, IOWA 50309

Telephone: 515/281-5157
Fax: 515/281-7969
E-mail: ibde@bon.state.ia.us
Web site: www.state.ia.us/dentalboard

Iowa Board of Dental Examiners
Directory of licensed dentists
Telephone: Free of charge.
Written: Call for order form to order lists or labels.
Electronic: Not provided.

Iowa Board of Dental Examiners
400 S.W. Eighth Street, Suite D
Des Moines, IOWA 50309-4687
Telephone: 515/281-5157
Fax: 515/281-7969
E-mail: ibde@bon.state.ia.us
Web site: www.state.ia.us/dentalboard

Kansas

Kansas Dental Board
Verification of licenses
Telephone: Free of charge. Limit three verifications per call.
Written: Free of charge. Call, mail, or fax requests, including dentist names and license numbers. Faxed upon request.
Electronic: Information available on Web site.

Kansas Dental Board
3601 S.W. 29th Street, Suite 134
Topeka, KANSAS 66614-2062
Telephone: 785/273-0780
Fax: 785/273-7545
E-mail: dental@ink.org
Web site: www.accesskansas.org/kdb

Kansas Dental Board
Directory of licensed dentists
Telephone: Free of charge.
Written: Call for information.
Electronic: Not provided.

Kansas Dental Board
3601 S.W. 29th Street, Suite 134
Topeka, KANSAS 66614-2062
Telephone: 785/273-0780
Fax: 785/273-7545
E-mail: dental@ink.org
Web site: www.accesskansas.orgboard/kdb

Kentucky

Kentucky Board of Dentistry
Verification of licenses

Telephone: Free of charge. Limit three verifications per call.
Written: $10 per verification. Mail or fax requests, including dentist name and license number (if known), self-addressed, stamped envelope, and payment.
Electronic: Not provided.

Kentucky Board of Dentistry
10101 Linn Station Road, Suite 540
Louisville, KENTUCKY 40223
Telephone: 502/423-0573
Fax: 502/423-1239
Web site: dentistry.state.ky.us

Kentucky Board of Dentistry
Notes: Also issue licenses for dental hygienists, dental laboratories, and dental technicians.

Directory of licensed dentists

Telephone: Free of charge. No more than five requests at one time.
Written: $30 per disk. Mail requests and payment.
Electronic: Not provided.

Kentucky Board of Dentistry
10101 Linn Station Road, Suite 540
Louisville, KENTUCKY 40223
Telephone: 502/423-0573
Fax: 502/423-1239
Web site: dentistry.state.ky.us

Louisiana

Louisiana State Board of Dentistry
Verification of licenses

Telephone: Free of charge. Limit three verifications per call.
Written: Free of charge. Mail or fax requests, including dentist names and license numbers. Faxed upon request.
Electronic: Automated verification system available at Web site.

Louisiana State Board of Dentistry
1 Canal Place, Suite 2680
New Orleans, LOUISIANA 70130
Telephone: 504/568-8574
Fax: 504/568-8598
E-mail: bogden@bellsouth.net
Web site: www.lsbd.org

Chapter 6

Louisiana State Board of Dentistry
Notes: $25 fee for license verification to another state. Request in writing.
Directory of licensed dentists
Telephone: Free of charge. Limit three verifications per call.
Written: Free of charge.
Electronic: Available through Web site.

Louisiana State Board of Dentistry
365 Canal Street, Suite 2680
New Orleans, LOUISIANA 70130
Telephone: 504/568-8574
Fax: 504/568-8598
E-mail: bogden@bellsouth.net
Web site: www.lsbd.org

Maine

Maine Board of Dental Examiners
Verification of licenses
Telephone: Free of charge.
Written: $15 for up to 10 verifications; $1 each additional verification. Mail request, including dentist names and license numbers (if known), and payment.
Electronic: Free of charge.

Maine Board of Dental Examiners
2 Bangor Street
143 State House Station
Augusta, MAINE 04333-0143
Telephone: 207/287-3333
Fax: 207/287-8140
E-mail: anita.c.merrow@state.me.us
Web site: www.licenseverification.com/medental

Maryland

Maryland State Board of Dental Examiners
Verification of licenses
Telephone: Free of charge. Limit one verification per call.
Written: $10 per verification (free for hospitals). Mail requests, including dentist's name and license number, and payment.
Electronic: Not provided.

Maryland State Board of Dental Examiners
Spring Grove State Hospital
Benjamin Rush Building
55 Wade Avenue, Tulip Drive

Baltimore, MARYLAND 21228
Telephone: 410/402-8500
Fax: 410/402-8505
Web site: www.dhmh.state.md.us/dental

Maryland State Board of Dental Examiners
Directory of licensed dentists

Telephone:	Free of charge.
Written:	$125 per copy. Mail requests and payment.
Electronic:	Not provided.

Maryland State Board of Dental Examiners
Spring Grove State Hospital
Benjamin Rush Building
55 Wade Avenue
Baltimore, MARYLAND 21228
Telephone: 410/402-8500
Fax: 410/402-8505
Web site: www.dhmh.state.md.us/dental

Massachusetts

Massachusetts Board of Registration in Dentistry
Verification of licenses

Telephone:	Free of charge. Limit five verifications per call; available 9:00–5:00 p.m. EST.
Written:	$10 per verification. Mail requests, including dentist's name and license number, self-addressed, stamped envelope, and check (made payable to Commonwealth of Massachusetts).
Electronic:	Automated verification system available at Web site.

Massachusetts Board of Registration in Dentistry
239 Causeway Street, Fifth Floor
Boston, MASSACHUSETTS 02114
Telephone: 617/727-9928
Fax: 617/727-2366
Web site: www.state.ma.us/reg/boards/dn

Massachusetts Board of Registration in Dentistry
Directory of licensed dentists

Telephone:	Free of charge. Limit five verifications per call.
Written:	$10 charge. Accepts only checks or money orders.
Electronic:	Free of charge.

Massachusetts Board of Registration in Dentistry
239 Causeway Street, Fifth Floor
Boston, MASSACHUSETTS 02114
Telephone: 617/727-9928
Fax: 617/727-2366
Web site: www.state.ma.us/reg/boards/dn

Michigan

Michigan Bureau of Occupational and Professional Regulation
Verification of licenses

Telephone: Automated verification system. $1.50 per minute.
Written: Verifications to party other than U.S. state: $5 per verification. Written verifications to another U.S. state: $15 per verification. Mail request, including licensee name and number, and payment to address below.
Electronic: Automated verification available at Web site.

Michigan Department of Consumer & Industry Services
Bureau of Health Services
Education, Testing & Credentials Section
PO Box 30180
Lansing, MICHIGAN 48909
Telephone: 900/555-8374 (automated verification system)   517/335-0918 (general information)
Fax: 517/373-2179
Web site: www.cis.state.mi.us/bhser

Michigan Bureau of Occupational and Professional Regulation
Directory of licensed dentists

Telephone: Automated verification system: 900/555-8374. $1.50 per minute.
Written: Verifications to party other than U.S. state: $5 per verification. Written verifications to another U.S. state: $15 per verification. Mail request, including licensee name and number, and payment to address below.
Electronic: Available at Web site (www.cis.state.mi.uf/ohs).

Michigan Department of Consumer & Industry Services
Bureau of Health Services
Attn: Education, Testing & Credentials Section
PO Box 30180
Lansing, MICHIGAN 48909
Telephone: 517-335-0918 (general information)
Fax: 517-373-2179

Minnesota

Minnesota Board of Dentistry
Verification of licenses

Telephone: Not provided.
Written: $5 per verification. Mail requests, including dentist names and license numbers, and payment.
Electronic: Not provided to corporations or institutions.

Minnesota Board of Dentistry
2829 University Avenue SE, Suite 450
Minneapolis, MINNESOTA 55414
Telephone: 612/617-2250

Fax: 612/617-2260
Web site: www.dentalboard.state.mn.us

Mississippi

Mississippi State Board of Dental Examiners
Verification of licenses

Telephone: Free of charge.
Written: Free of charge. Mail or fax requests, including dentist names and license numbers (if known). If signature and seal of Board Director is required, fee is $20.
Electronic: Free of charge through Web site.

> Mississippi State Board of Dental Examiners
> 600 E. Amite Street, Suite 100
> Jackson, MISSISSIPPI 39201-2801
> Telephone: 601/944-9622
> Fax: 601/944-9624
> E-mail: dental@msbde.state.ms.us
> Web site: www.msbde.state.ms.us

Mississippi State Board of Dental Examiners
Directory of licensed dentists

Telephone: Free of charge.
Written: $125 per printed list or set of labels; $150 per list on diskette. Mail requests and payment.
Electronic: Information available on Web site.

> Mississippi State Board of Dental Examiners
> 600 E. Amite Street, Suite 100
> Jackson, MISSISSIPPI 39201-2801
> Telephone: 601/944-9622
> Fax: 601/944-9624
> E-mail: dental@msbde.state.ms.us
> Web site: www.msbde.state.ms.us

Missouri

Missouri Dental Board
Verification of licenses

Telephone: Free of charge. Limit three verifications per call.
Written: Free of charge. Mail requests, including dentist names and license numbers (if known), and signed release form (if requesting information regarding complaints or investigative action). $20 fee for out-of-state requests.
Electronic: Automated verification system available at Web site.

> Missouri Dental Board
> PO Box 1367
> 3605 Missouri Boulevard
> Jefferson City, MISSOURI 65102
> Telephone: 573/751-0040

Fax: 573/751-8216
E-mail: dental@mail.state.mo.us
Web site: www.ecodev.state.mo.us/pr/dental

Missouri Department of Health
Notes: File available from Missouri Dept. of Economic Development. Downloadable file from Internet (www.ecodev.state.mo.us/pr). Choose "Downloadable Profession Lists" and follow instructions. Call Steve Coller at 573/751-0033 with questions.

Directory of licensed dentists
Telephone: Not provided.
Written: $17.50 (plus $2.50 shipping and handling per copy). Mail requests and check made payable to Missouri Department of Health.
Electronic: Not provided.

Missouri Department of Health
CHIME
PO Box 570
Jefferson City, MISSOURI 65102

Montana

Montana Board of Dentistry
Verification of licenses
Telephone: Free of charge. Limited verifications.
Written: $20 per verification. Mail requests, including dentist name, license number (if known), city and state, and payment.
Electronic: Not provided.

Montana Board of Dentistry
301 S. Park, Fourth Floor
PO Box 200513
Helena, MONTANA 59620-0513
Telephone: 406/841-2390
Fax: 406/841-2305
E-mail: dlibsdden@state.mt.us
Web site: www.discoveringmontana.com/dli/den

Nebraska

Nebraska Department of Health and Human Services
Verification of licenses
Telephone: Free of charge. Limit five verifications per call.
Written: $5 per verification. $25 per verification if verification includes documentation of disciplinary action. Mail requests, including dentist names and license numbers (if known), and payment.
Electronic: Automated verification system available at Web site.

Dental Licensing Agencies

Department of Health and Human Services
Regulation and Licensure
Credentialing Division
PO Box 94986
Lincoln, NEBRASKA 68509-4986
Telephone: 402/471-2118
Fax: 402/471-3577
E-mail: bebacky.wisell@hhss.state.ne.us
Web site: www.hhs.state.ne.us/lis/lis.asp

Nebraska Department of Health and Human Services Regulation and Licensure
Verification of licenses

Telephone:	Provided.
Written:	Provided. Fees apply. Call department for specific cost.
Electronic:	Through Web site: www.hhs.state.ne.us/lis/lisasp.

Nebraska Department of Health and Human Services Regulation and Licensure
Credentialing Division
301 Centennial Mall South
PO Box 94986
Lincoln, NEBRASKA 68509-4986
Telephone: 402/471-2115
Fax: 402/471-3577
E-mail: marie.mcclatchey@hhss.state.ne.us
Web site: www.hhs.state.ne.us/crl/crlindex.htm

Nevada

Nevada State Board of Dental Examiners
Verification of licenses

Telephone:	Free of charge. Limit three verifications per call.
Written:	Free of charge. Mail or fax requests, including dentist names and license numbers (if known).
Electronic:	Not provided.

Nevada State Board of Dental Examiners
2295-B Renaissance Drive
Las Vegas, NEVADA 89119
Telephone: 702/486-7044
Fax: 702/486-7046
E-mail: nsbde@govmail.state.nv.us
Web site: www.nvdentalboard.org

Nevada State Board of Dental Examiners
Directory of licensed dentists

Telephone:	Free of charge. Limit three verifications per day.
Written:	$100 per copy of the full list.
Electronic:	Not provided.

Chapter 6

Nevada State Board of Dental Examiners
2295-B Renaissance Drive
Las Vegas, NEVADA 89119
Telephone: 702/486-7044
Fax: 702/486-7046
E-mail: nsbde@govmail.state.nv.us
Web site: www.nvdentalboard.org

New Hampshire

New Hampshire Board of Dental Examiners
Verification of licenses
Telephone: Free of charge. Limit four verifications per call.
Written: $5 per verification. Mail requests, including dentist names and license numbers (if known), and payment. Faxed upon request.
Electronic: Not provided.

New Hampshire Board of Dental Examiners
2 Industrial Park Drive
Concord, NEW HAMPSHIRE 03301-8520
Telephone: 603/271-4561
Fax: 603/271-6702
E-mail: dentalboard@nhsa.state.nh.us
Web site: www.state.nh.us/dental

New Hampshire Board of Dental Examiners
Notes: Copy of list of dentists/hygenists is $150. Available in print or disk form; please supply disk.
Directory of licensed dentists
Telephone: Free of charge. Limited to four per phone call.
Written: $5 fee per verification.
Electronic: Not provided.

New Hampshire Board of Dental Examiners
2 Industrial Park Drive
Concord, NEW HAMPSHIRE 03301-8520
Telephone: 603/271-4561
Fax: 603/271-6702
E-mail: dentalboard@nhsa.state.nh.us
Web site: www.state.nh.us./dental

New Jersey

New Jersey State Board of Dentistry
Verification of licenses
Telephone: Free of charge. Limit three verifications per call; unlimited verifications on automated verification system. Faxed upon request.
Written: Free of charge. Call, mail, or fax requests, including dentist names and license numbers (if known).
Electronic: Information available on Web site.

Dental Licensing Agencies

New Jersey State Board of Dentistry
124 Halsey Street
PO Box 45005
Newark, NEW JERSEY 07101
Telephone: 973/504-6405   973/273-8090 (automated verification system)
Fax: 973/273-8075
Web site: www.state.nj.us/lps/ca/medical.htm#den3

New Jersey State Board of Dentistry
Directory of licensed dentists
Telephone:	Not provided.
Written:	$94 plus $0.02/name per set of labels or printed list. $94 plus $0.15/name per list on diskette (supplied by customer).
Electronic:	Not provided.

New Jersey State Board of Dentistry
Licensing Agency/Directory of Licensed Dentists
PO Box 45005
Newark, NEW JERSEY 07101

New Mexico

New Mexico Board of Dental Health Care
Verification of licenses
Telephone:	Free of charge. Limit five verifications per call.
Written:	Free of charge. Mail or fax requests, including dentist names and license numbers (if known).
Electronic:	Information available on Web site.

New Mexico Board of Dental Health Care
PO Box 25101
2055 S. Pacheco, Suite 400
Santa Fe, NEW MEXICO 87504
Telephone: 505/476-7125
Fax: 505/476-7095
E-mail: dentalboard@state.nm.us
Web site: www.rld.state.nm.us/b&c/dental

New Mexico Board of Dental Health Care
Directory of licensed dentists
Telephone:	Free of charge.
Written:	$250 per copy. Mail requests and payment.
Electronic:	Free of charge.

New Mexico Board of Dental Health Care
PO Box 25101
2055 South Pacheco, Suite 400 87505
Santa Fe, NEW MEXICO 87504
Telephone: 505/476-7125

Fax: 505/476-7095
E-mail: dentalboard@state.nm.us
Web site: www.rld.state.nm.us/bnc/dental/index.htm

New York

Office of the Professions—Dental Licensing
Verification of licenses

Telephone: Free of charge. Limit two verifications per call if calling customer service automated attendant; limit five per call if calling customer service rep; unlimited if calling automated verification system. $1.50 for first minute; $1 for each additional minute.

Written: $20 per verification. Limit one verification. $10 per hundred names for multiple verifications. Mail requests, including dentist names, license numbers, date of birth, and address, and payment (check or money order payable to NYS Education Department).

Electronic: Verification available on Web site.

Office of the Professions—Dental Licensing
New York State Education Department
89 Washington Avenue, Second Floor
Albany, NEW YORK 12234-1000
Telephone: 518/474-3817 (general information)   900/555-6978 (automated verification system)
Fax: 518/474-1449
E-mail: op4info@mail.nysed.gov
Web site: www.op.nysed.gov/prof/profhome.htm

North Carolina

North Carolina State Board of Dental Examiners
Verification of licenses

Telephone: Free of charge. Limit three verifications per call.
Written: $15 per verification. Mail or fax requests, including dentist names and license numbers (if known).
Electronic: Free of charge.

North Carolina State Board of Dental Examiners
15100 Weston Parkway, Suite 101
Cary, NORTH CAROLINA 27513
Telephone: 919/678-8223
Fax: 919/678-8472
E-mail: info@ncdentalboard.org
Web site: www.ncdentalboard.org

North Carolina State Board of Dental Examiners
Directory of licensed dentists

Telephone: Not provided.
Written: $10 per name; $108 per report (includes name, license number, address, specialty, and county) or set of labels.
Electronic: Not provided.

Dental Licensing Agencies

North Carolina State Board of Dental Examiners
PO Box 32270
Raleigh, NORTH CAROLINA 27622-2270
Telephone: 919-571-4197
Fax: 919-571-8457
E-mail: spontello@ncdentalboard.org
Web site: www.ncdentalboard.org

North Dakota

North Dakota Board of Dentistry
Verification of licenses
Telephone: Free of charge.
Written: Free of charge. Mail or fax requests, including dentist names and license numbers (if known).
Electronic: Not provided.

North Dakota Board of Dentistry
PO Box 7246
Bismarck, NORTH DAKOTA 58507-7246
Telephone: 701/258-8600
Fax: 701/224-9824
E-mail: ndsbde@aptnd.com
Web site: www.nddentalboard.org

Ohio

Ohio State Dental Board
Verification of licenses
Telephone: Not provided.
Written: $1 per verification. Mail requests, including dentist's name and license number (if known), and payment. Faxed upon request.
Electronic: Information available on Web site.

Ohio State Dental Board
77 S. High Street, 18th Floor
Columbus, OHIO 43215-6135
Telephone: 614/466-2580
Fax: 614/752-8995
E-mail: tabion@mail.peps.state.oh.us
Web site: www.state.oh.us/den

Ohio State Dental Board
Directory of licensed dentists
Telephone: Not provided.
Written: $1 per copy. Mail requests and payment.
Electronic: Verification available at Web site.

Ohio State Dental Board
77 S. High Street, 18th Floor
Columbus, OHIO 43215-6135
Telephone: 614/466-2580
Fax: 614/752-8995
E-mail: tabion@mail.peps.state.oh.us
Web site: www.state.oh.us/den

Oklahoma

Board of Dentistry
Notes: Also provides licensing for dental hygienists.
Verification of licenses

Telephone:	Free of charge. Limit 10 verifications per call.
Written:	Free of charge. Call, fax, or mail requests, including dentist names and license numbers (if known). Faxed upon request.
Electronic:	Not provided.

Board of Dentistry
201 NE 38th Terrace, Suite Two
Oklahoma City, OKLAHOMA 73105
Telephone: 405/524-3592
Fax: 405/524-2223
E-mail: dentist@oklaosf.state.ok.us
Web site: www.dentist.state.ok.us

Board of Dentistry
Directory of licensed dentists

Telephone:	Free of charge. Limit 10 verifications per call.
Written:	Free of charge.
Electronic:	Free of charge.

Board of Dentistry
201 NE 38th Terrace, Suite Two
Oklahoma City, OKLAHOMA 73105
Telephone: 405/524-3592
Fax: 405/524-2223
E-mail: dentist@oklaosf.state.ok.us
Web site: www.dentist.state.ok.us

Oregon

Oregon Board of Dentistry
Verification of licenses

Telephone:	Free of charge. Limit five verifications per call.
Written:	$2.50 fee. Mail requests, including dentist names and license numbers (if known).
Electronic:	$50 for data processing order. No charge for e-mail of three orders or fewer.

Dental Licensing Agencies

Oregon Board of Dentistry
1515 S.W. Fifth Avenue, Suite 602
Portland, OREGON 97201
Telephone: 503/229-5520
Fax: 503/229-6606
E-mail: information@oregondentistry.org
Web site: www.oregondentistry.org

Oregon Board of Dentistry
Directory of licensed dentists

Telephone:	Free of charge. Limit four verifications per call.
Written:	$2.50 fee per name.
Electronic:	Not provided.

Oregon Board of Dentistry
1515 S.W. Fifth Avenue, Suite 602
Portland, OREGON 97201
Telephone: 503/229-5520
Fax: 503/229-6606
Web site: www.oregondentistry.org

Pennsylvania

Pennsylvania State Board of Dentistry
Verification of licenses

Telephone:	Free of charge. Limit three verifications per call.
Written:	Free of charge. Mail or fax requests, including dentist names and license numbers (if known).
Electronic:	Not provided.

Pennsylvania State Board of Dentistry
PO Box 2649
Harrisburg, PENNSYLVANIA 17105
Telephone: 717/783-7162
Fax: 717/787-7769
Web site: www.dos.state.pa.us

Pennsylvania State Board of Dentistry
Directory of licensed dentists

Telephone:	Free of charge.
Written:	$15 fee. Mail requests, including dentist's name and license number (if known), signed release form, and payment.
Electronic:	Information available at www.licensepa.state.pa.us.

Pennsylvania State Board of Dentistry
116 Pine Street, Fifth Floor
Harrisburg, PENNSYLVANIA 17101
Telephone: 717/783-7162

Fax: 717/787-7769
E-mail: dentistr@pados.dos.state.pa.us
Web site: www.dos.state.pa.us

Puerto Rico

Puerto Rico Board of Dental Examiners
Verification of licenses

Telephone: Free of charge. Specify profession.
Written: $20 per verification. Call for standardized forms (faxed upon request). Mail requests, including signed release forms, dentist names and license numbers, SASE, and payment (certified check or money order payable to Secretary of the Treasury of Puerto Rico).
Electronic: Not provided.

Puerto Rico Board of Dental Examiners
Department of Health
Office of Regulation and Certification of Health Care Professionals
PO Box 10200
Santurce, PUERTO RICO 00908-0020
Telephone: 787/725-8161
Fax: 787/725-7903

Puerto Rico Board of Dental Examiners
Directory of licensed dentists

Telephone: Not provided.
Written: Provided. $20 per verification.
Electronic: Not provided.

Puerto Rico Board of Dental Examiners
Department of Health
Office of Regulation and Certification of Health Care Professionals
PO Box 10200
Santurce, PUERTO RICO 00908-0020
Telephone: 787/725-8161 (receptionist)   787/725-8125 (administration)
787/725-8130
Fax: 787/725-7903

Rhode Island

Rhode Island State Board of Examiners in Dentistry
Verification of licenses

Telephone: Not provided.
Written: Free of charge. Mail requests, including dentist's name and license number (if known).
Electronic: Free of charge.

> Rhode Island State Board of Examiners in Dentistry
> Department of Health
> 3 Capitol Hill, Suite 104
> Providence, RHODE ISLAND 02908
> Telephone: 401/222-2827
> Fax: 401/222-1272
> E-mail: gailg@doh.state.ri.us
> Web site: www.health.state.ri.us

Rhode Island State Board of Examiners in Dentistry
Directory of licensed dentists

Telephone: Not provided.
Written: Available in printed list or on diskette. Call for more information.
Electronic: Information available on Web site.

> Rhode Island State Board of Examiners in Dentistry
> Department of Health
> 3 Capitol Hill, Suite 104
> Providence, RHODE ISLAND 02908
> Telephone: 401/222-2828
> Fax: 401/222-1272
> Web site: www.health.state.ri.us

South Carolina

South Carolina State Board of Dentistry
Verification of licenses

Telephone: Free of charge. Limit three verifications per call.
Written: Free of charge. Mail or fax requests, including dentist names and license numbers (if known).
Electronic: Not provided.

> South Carolina Department of LLR
> Board of Dentistry
> PO Box 11329
> Columbia, SOUTH CAROLINA 29211-1329
> Telephone: 803/896-4599
> Fax: 803/896-4596
> Web site: www.llr.state.sc.us

South Carolina State Board of Dentistry
Directory of licensed dentists

Telephone: Free of charge. Limit three verifications per call; more than three, request in writing.
Written: Free of charge.
Electronic: Not provided.

> South Carolina Department of LLR
> Board of Dentistry
> PO Box 11329
> Columbia, SOUTH CAROLINA 29211-1329
> Telephone: 803/896-4599
> Fax: 803/896-4596
> Web site: www.llr.state.sc.us

South Dakota

South Dakota State Board of Dentistry
Verification of licenses

Telephone: Free of charge. Limit one verification per call.
Written: Free of charge. Mail or fax requests, including dentist names and license numbers (if known). Faxed upon request.
Electronic: E-mail free of charge.

> South Dakota State Board of Dentistry
> PO Box 1037
> 106 W. Capitol
> Pierre, SOUTH DAKOTA 57501
> Telephone: 605/224-1282
> Fax: 605/224-7426
> E-mail: sdsbd@dtgnet.com
> Web site: www.state.sd.us/dcr/dentistry

South Dakota State Board of Dentistry
Directory of licensed dentists

Telephone: Free of charge.
Written: $85 per list.
Electronic: Information available through e-mail.

> South Dakota State Board of Dentistry
> PO Box 1037
> 106 W. Capitol
> Pierre, SOUTH DAKOTA 57501
> Telephone: 605/224-1282
> Fax: 605/224-7426
> E-mail: sdsbd@dtgnet.com
> Web site: www.state.sd.us/dcr/dentistry

Dental Licensing Agencies

Tennessee

Tennessee Board of Dentistry
Verification of licenses

Telephone: Free of charge. Call automatic verification number listed.
Written: Free of charge. Mail or fax requests, including dentist names and license numbers (if known). Faxed upon request.
Electronic: Free of charge at Web site.

Tennessee Board of Dentistry
Cordell Hull Building, First Floor
425 Fifth Avenue N
Nashville, TENNESSEE 37247-1010
Telephone: 800/310-4650   615/532-5073
Fax: 615/532-5369
Web site: www.state.tn.us/health

Texas

Texas State Board of Dental Examiners
Verification of licenses

Telephone: Free of charge. Limit one verification per day.
Written: $1.15 per verification; $5.75 per verification with official board seal. Mail requests, including dentist's name and license number (if known), and payment.
Electronic: Automated verification system available at Web site.

Texas State Board of Dental Examiners
333 Guadalupe
Tower Three, Suite 800
Austin, TEXAS 78701
Telephone: 512/463-6400
Fax: 512/463-7452
E-mail: webmaster@tsbde.state.tx.us
Web site: www.tsbde.state.tx.us

Texas State Board of Dental Examiners
Directory of licensed dentists

Telephone: Free of charge. Limit one verification per call.

Written: Price depends on needs. Mail request, including profession, license status, sorting instructions, desired list format, your name, and telephone number. Board will call with specific price after processing request.

Electronic: Automated verification system available at Web site.

Texas State Board of Dental Examiners
333 Guadalupe
Tower Three, Suite 800
Austin, TEXAS 78701
Telephone: 512/463-6400
Fax: 512/463-7452
E-mail: webmaster@tsbde.state.tx.us
Web site: www.tsbde.state.tx.us

Utah

Utah Board of Dentists and Dental Hygienists

Notes: Licensed professionals roster on CD/ROM; fee varies. Mail or phone request and payment to Utah Interactive; see Web site.

Verification of licenses

Telephone: Free of charge. Limit three verifications per call.

Written: $20 fee for more detailed information.

Electronic: Automated verification available at Web site. Convenience fee.

Utah Board of Dentists and Dental Hygienists
Division of Occupational and Professional Licensure
PO Box 146741
160 E. 300 S
Salt Lake City, UTAH 84114-6741
Telephone: 801/530-6628
Fax: 801/530-6511
Web site: www.dopl.utah.gov

Vermont

Vermont Board of Dental Examiners
Verification of licenses

Telephone: Free of charge.

Written: $20 per verification. Mail requests, including dentist names and license numbers (if known), and payment.

Electronic: Automated verification system available at Web site.

Vermont Board of Dental Examiners
Secretary of State's Office

Dental Licensing Agencies

26 Terrace Street, Drawer 09
Montpelier, VERMONT 05609-1106
Telephone: 802/828-2390
Fax: 802/828-2465
E-mail: dlafaill@sec.state.vt.us
Web site: www.sec.state.vt.us

Vermont Board of Dental Examiners
Directory of licensed dentists

Telephone: Free of charge.
Written: $20 fee.
Electronic: Visit Web site for more information.

Vermont Board of Dental Examiners
Office of the Secretary of State
26 Terrace Street, Drawer 09
Montpelier, VERMONT 05609-1106
Telephone: 802/828-2390
Fax: 802/828-2465
E-mail: dlapaill@sec.state.vt.us
Web site: www.sec.state.vt.us

Virginia

Virginia Board of Dentistry
Notes: Dental Hygienist licensing.
Verification of licenses

Telephone: Free of charge. Limit three verifications per day.
Written: Free of charge. Mail or fax requests, including dentist names and license numbers (if known).
Electronic: Automated verification system available at www.dhp.state.va.us/publicinformation.

Virginia Board of Dentistry
6606 W. Broad Street, Fourth Floor
Richmond, VIRGINIA 23230-1717
Telephone: 804/662-9906   804/662-7636 (automated verification number)
Fax: 804/662-7246
E-mail: deenbd@dhp.state.va.us
Web site: www.dhp.state.va.us

Virginia Board of Dentistry
Directory of licensed dentists

Telephone: Free of charge.
Written: Free of charge.
Electronic: Automated verification system available at Web site.

Virginia Board of Dentistry
Department of Health Professions
6606 W. Broad Street, Fourth Floor

Richmond, VIRGINIA 23230-1717
Telephone: 804/662-9906
Fax: 804/662-7246
E-mail: dendd@dhp.state.va.us
Web site: www.dhp.state.va.us

Washington

Department of Health Dental Quality Assurance Commission
Verification of licenses
Telephone: Free of charge.
Written: Free of charge. Mail or fax requests, including dentist names and license numbers (if known).
Electronic: Free of charge.

Department of Health Dental Quality Assurance Commission
PO Box 47867
Olympia, WASHINGTON 98504-7867
Telephone: 360/236-4861
Fax: 360/664-9077
E-mail: donna.johnson@doh.wa.gov
Web site: www.doh.wa.gov

Washington State Dental Quality Assurance Commission
Notes: $25 fee for transferring certification to another state. $25 fee for state seal applied to certification.
Directory of licensed dentists
Telephone: Free of charge.
Written: Unofficial certification requests and other written correspondence are free of charge.
Electronic: Unofficial certification requests are free of charge.

Washington State Dental Quality Assurance Commission
Department of Health
PO Box 47867
Olympia, WASHINGTON 98504-7867
Telephone: 360/236-4700   360/664-4111 (automated verification system)
Fax: 360/664-9077
E-mail: donna.johnson@doh.wa.gov
Web site: www.doh.wa.gov

West Virginia

West Virginia Board of Dental Examiners
Verification of licenses
Telephone: Free of charge. Limit three verifications per call.
Written: Free of charge. Mail or fax requests, including dentist names and license numbers (if known).
Electronic: Information available via e-mail.

West Virginia Board of Dental Examiners
PO Drawer 1459

Beckley, WEST VIRGINIA 25802-1459
Telephone: 304/252-8266
Fax: 304/252-2779
E-mail: apsa@citynet.net
Web site: www.wvdentalboard.org

West Virginia Board of Dental Examiners
Directory of licensed dentists
Telephone: Free of charge.
Written: Free of charge. Mail requests.
Electronic: Free of charge via e-mail.

West Virginia Board of Dental Examiners
PO Drawer 1459
Beckley, WEST VIRGINIA 25802-1459
Telephone: 304/252-8266
Fax: 304/252-2779
E-mail: apsa@citynet.net
Web site: www.wvdentalboard.org

Wisconsin

Wisconsin Dentistry Examining Board
Verification of licenses
Telephone: Not provided.
Written: $10 per verification to other boards.
Electronic: All verification requests must be accessed on agency's Web site (www.drl.state.wi.us). If you cannot access the Internet, submit your request in writing to Department of Regulation & Licensing, PO Box 8935, Madison, WI 53708-8935.

Wisconsin Dentistry Examining Board
PO Box 8935
Madison, WISCONSIN 53708-8935
Telephone: 608/266-2112
Fax: 608/261-7083
E-mail: dorl@drl.state.wi.us
Web site: www.drl.state.wi.us

Wisconsin Dentistry Examining Board
Notes: Recommended to call for certification or licensing information.
Verification of licenses
Telephone: Free of charge.
Written: Free of charge within Wisconsin; $10 fee for verification to another state regulatory board.
Electronic: Free of charge.

Wisconsin Dentistry Examining Board
PO Box 8935
Madison, WISCONSIN 53708-8935

Telephone: 608/266-2112
Fax: 608/261-7083
Web site: www.drl.state.wi.us

Wyoming

Wyoming Board of Dental Examiners
Directory of licensed dentists
Telephone: Free of charge.
Written: $15 per verification. Include signed release form. Payment with money order or cashier's check only.
Electronic: $1 per licensed dentist. Call main number first to request a release form.

Wyoming Board of Dental Examiners
2020 Carey Avenue, Suite 201
Cheyenne, WYOMING 82002
Telephone: 307/777-6529
Fax: 307/777-3508
E-mail: dbridg@state.wy.us
Web site: www.plboards.state.wy.us

Wyoming Professional Licensing Boards
Verification of licenses
Telephone: Free of charge. Limit five verifications per call.
Written: $20 per verification. Mail requests, including dentist names and license numbers (if known), and payment.
Electronic: Not provided.

Wyoming Professional Licensing Boards
Attention: Dental license verification request
2020 Carey Avenue, Suite 201
Cheyenne, WYOMING 82002
Telephone: 307/777-6529
Fax: 307/777-3508
E-mail: dbridg@state.wy.us
Web site: www.professionallicensing.state.wy.us

Podiatric Licensing Agencies

Alabama

Alabama State Board of Podiatry
Verification of licenses

Telephone: Not provided.
Written: Free of charge. Mail requests, including podiatrist names and license numbers (if known), and self-addressed, stamped envelope.
Electronic: Automated verification system available at Web site.

Alabama State Board of Podiatry
13 Innisbrook Lane
Birmingham, ALABAMA 35242
Telephone: 205/995-8537
Fax: 205/995-8537
Web site: www.alabamapodiatryboard.org

Alaska

Alaska State Medical Board
Verification of licenses

Telephone: Free of charge. Limit five verifications per call.
Written: $20 per verification. Mail requests, including podiatrist names and license numbers (if known), and payment, payable to State of Alaska.
Electronic: Automated verification system available at Web site. No disciplinary information.

Division of Occupational Licensing
Alaska State Medical Board
PO Box 110806
Juneau, ALASKA 99811-0806
Telephone: 907/465-2541   907/465-2695 (verification of licensure)   907/465-2756
Fax: 907/465-2974
E-mail: license@dced.state.ak.us
Web site: www.dced.state.ak.us/occ

Arizona

Arizona Board of Podiatry Examiners
Verification of licenses

Telephone: Free of charge. Limit one verification per call.
Written: Free of charge. Mail requests, including podiatrist names and license numbers (if known), and self-addressed, stamped envelope.
Electronic: Not provided.

Arizona Board of Podiatry Examiners
1400 W. Washington, Suite 230
Phoenix, ARIZONA 85007
Telephone: 602/542-3095
Fax: 602/542-3093
E-mail: linda.wells@podiatry.state.az.us

Arkansas

Arkansas Board of Podiatric Medicine
Verification of licenses
Telephone: Free of charge. Limit two verifications per call.
Written: Free of charge. Mail requests, including podiatrist names and license numbers (if known), and self-addressed, stamped envelope.
Electronic: Not provided.

> Arkansas Board of Podiatric Medicine
> 2001 Georgia Avenue
> Little Rock, ARKANSAS 72207-5014
> Telephone: 501/664-3668

Colorado

Colorado Podiatry Board
Verification of licenses
Telephone: Free of charge.
Written: Free of charge. Mail requests, including podiatrist names and license numbers (if known).
Electronic: Automated verification system available at Web site.

> Colorado Podiatry Board
> 1560 Broadway, Suite 1545
> Denver, COLORADO 80202-5140
> Telephone: 303/894-2464
> Fax: 303/894-7885
> E-mail: podiatrists@dora.state.co.us
> Web site: www.dora.state.co.us/podiatrists

Connecticut

Connecticut Department of Public Health
Notes: Verifications may also be done at www.ct-clic.com.
Verification of licenses
Telephone: Free of charge. Limit five verifications per call.
Written: Free of charge. Faxed upon request. Mail or fax requests, including podiatrist names, license numbers (if known), and Connecticut release forms (available upon request).
Electronic: Automated verification system available at www.state.ct.us/dph/scripts/hlthprof.asp.

> Division of Health Systems Regulation
> Department of Public Health
> 410 Capitol Avenue, MS 12 APP
> PO Box 340308
> Hartford, CONNECTICUT 06134-0308
> Telephone: 860/509-7603 (renewals)   860/509-7596 (CNA)
> Fax: 860/509-7607
> E-mail: webmaster.dph@po.state.ct.us
> Web site: www.dph.state.ct.us

Florida

Division of Medical Quality Assurance
Verification of licenses

Telephone: Free of charge. Limit three verifications per call.
Written: $25 per verification. Mail requests, including podiatrist names and license numbers (if known), and payment. Please include forwarding address. Faxed upon request.
Electronic: Upon request. Will send written certification via e-mail.

Division of Medical Quality Assurance
Client Services Unit
HMQAMS Bin C99
4052 Bald Cypress Way
Tallahassee, FLORIDA 32399-3299
Telephone: 850/488-0595
Fax: 850/414-0864
Web site: www.doh.state.fl.us/mqa

Georgia

Georgia State Board of Podiatry Examiners
Verification of licenses

Telephone: Free of charge. Limit three verifications per call.
Written: Free of charge if requested by another state board, otherwise fee of $25 imposed. Mail or fax requests, including podiatrist names and license numbers (if known).
Electronic: Information available on Web site free of charge. Form available on Web site.

Georgia State Board of Podiatry Examiners
237 Coliseum Drive
Macon, GEORGIA 31217
Telephone: 478/207-1686
Fax: 478/207-1699
E-mail: aomartin@sos.state.ga.us
Web site: www.sos.state.ga.us/plb/podiatry

Hawaii

Hawaii Board of Medical Examiners Department of Commerce and Consumer Affairs
Verification of licenses

Telephone: Free of charge. Provide podiatrist license numbers.
Written: $15 per verification. Mail requests, including podiatrist names and license numbers (if known), and payment.
Electronic: Not provided.

Consumer Resource Center
235 S. Beretania Street, Ninth Floor
Honolulu, HAWAII 96813
Telephone: 808/587-3295
Web site: www.hawaii.gov

Idaho

Bureau of Occupational Licensure
Verification of licenses

Telephone: Free of charge. Limit three verifications per call.
Written: $10 per verification. Mail requests, including podiatrist's name and license number (if known), and payment. $10 fee only if certifying signature is required.
Electronic: Free of charge for e-mail or fax verifications.

Idaho State Board of Podiatry
Bureau of Occupational Licensure
1109 Main Street, Suite 220
Boise, IDAHO 83702-5642
Telephone: 208/334-3233
Fax: 208/334-3945
E-mail: csimpson@ibol.state.id.us
Web site: www.state.id.us/ibol

Indiana

Indiana Board of Podiatric Medicine
Verification of licenses

Telephone: Free of charge. Unlimited verifications. Provide podiatrist names or license numbers (if known).
Written: $10 charge for out-of-state requests.
Electronic: Automated verification system available at Web site. Basic information free of charge. Detailed information is $2.50 per verification.

Health Professions Bureau
Indiana Board of Podiatric Medicine
402 W. Washington Street, Room W041
Indianapolis, INDIANA 46204
Telephone: 317/232-2960 (general information)   888/333-7515 (verifications only)
Fax: 317/233-4236
E-mail: hpb5@hpb.state.in.us
Web site: www.in.gov/hpb

Iowa

Professional Licensure Division
Notes: Automated verification number is 515/281-4031. Must have podiatrist's Social Security number to access information.

Verification of licenses

Telephone: Free of charge.
Written: $10 per verification. Mail requests, including podiatrists name and license number (if known).
Electronic: Not provided.

Iowa Board of Podiatry Examiners
Department of Public Health
Professional Licensure Division
Lucas Building, Fifth Floor
321 E. 12th Street
Des Moines, IOWA 50319-0075
Telephone: 515/281-4422
Fax: 515/281-3121
Web site: www.idph.state.ia.us/licensure

Kansas

Kansas Board of Healing Arts
Verification of licenses
Telephone: Free of charge. Limit three verifications per day.
Written: $15 for verifications with scores. Free without scores. Mail or fax requests, including podiatrist's name and license number (if known).
Electronic: Not provided.

Kansas State Board of Healing Arts
235 S.W. Topeka Boulevard
Topeka, KANSAS 66603
Telephone: 785/296-7413
Fax: 785/296-0852
E-mail: cabbott@ink.org
Web site: www.ink.org/public/boha

Kentucky

Kentucky State Board of Podiatry
Verification of licenses
Telephone: Free of charge.
Written: Free of charge. Mail requests, including podiatrist names and license numbers (if known), and self-addressed, stamped envelope.
Electronic: Not provided.

Kentucky Board of Podiatry
908B S. 12th Street
Murray, KENTUCKY 42071
Telephone: 270/759-0007
Fax: 270/753-0684

Louisiana

Louisiana State Board of Medical Examiners
Verification of licenses
Telephone: Free of charge. Limit three verifications per call.
Written: $5 per request. Mail requests, including podiatrist names and license numbers (if known).
Electronic: Information is available on Web site.

Chapter 6

    Louisiana State Board of Medical Examiners
    Verifications Department
    PO Box 30250
    New Orleans, LOUISIANA 70190-0250
    Telephone: 504/568-6820, Ext. 276 (Verification Department)
    Fax: 504/599-0503
    E-mail: lsbmever@lsmbe.org
    Web site: www.lsbme.org

Maine

Board of Licensure of Podiatric Medicine
Verification of licenses

Telephone: Free of charge. Limit two verifications per call.
Written: $15 per verification. Mail requests, including podiatrist names and license numbers (if known), and payment.
Electronic: Not provided.

    Board of Licensure of Podiatric Medicine
    35 State House Station
    Augusta, MAINE 04333
    Telephone: 207/624-8626
    Fax: 207/624-8637
    E-mail: diane.l.staples@state.me.us
    Web site: www.maineprofessionalreg.org

Maryland

Maryland Board of Podiatry
Verification of licenses

Telephone: Free of charge. Limit three verifications per call.
Written: $10 per verification. Mail requests, including podiatrist's name and license number (if known), and payment. Faxed upon request.
Electronic: Not provided.

    Maryland Board of Podiatry
    Department of Health & Mental Hygiene
    4201 Patterson Avenue
    Baltimore, MARYLAND 21215-2299
    Telephone: 410/764-4785
    Fax: 410/358-3083

Massachusetts

Board of Podiatry
Verification of licenses

Telephone: Free of charge. Limit three verifications per call.

Written: $10 per verification. Mail requests, including podiatrist names and license numbers (if known), and payment.
Electronic: Located on web: www.state.ma.us/reg/boards/pd.

>Division of Professional Licensure
>Board of Podiatry
>239 Causeway Street
>Boston, MASSACHUSETTS 02114
>Telephone: 617/727-1747
>Fax: 617/727-2669
>E-mail: heather.carnes@state.ma.us
>Web site: www.state.ma.us/reg/boards/pd

Michigan

Bureau of Health Services
Verification of licenses

Telephone: Call automated verification number at 900/555-8374. $1.50 per minute.
Written: Verifications to another party other than U.S. state: $5 per verification. Written verifications to another U.S. state: $15 per verification. Mail request, including licensee name and number, and payment to address below.
Electronic: Automated verification system available at Web site.

>Michigan Department of Consumer & Industry Services
>Bureau of Health Services
>Attn: Education, Testing & Credentials Section
>PO Box 30670
>Lansing, MICHIGAN 48909
>Telephone: 517/373-6873   900/555-8374 (automated verification system)   517/335-0918 (general information)
>Fax: 517/373-2179
>E-mail: bhserinfo@michigan.gov
>Web site: www.michigan.gov/bhser

Minnesota

Minnesota Board of Podiatric Medicine
Verification of licenses

Telephone: Not provided.
Written: Mail requests, including podiatrist names and license numbers (if known), and check for $30.
Electronic: Not provided.

>Minnesota Board of Podiatric Medicine
>2829 University Avenue SE, Suite 430
>Minneapolis, MINNESOTA 55414
>Telephone: 612/617-2200
>Fax: 612/617-2698
>E-mail: benesh.pod@state.mn.us

Mississippi

Mississippi State Board of Medical Licensure
Verification of licenses
Telephone: Not provided.
Written: $25 fee. Mail requests, including podiatrist names and license numbers (if known), and payment.
Electronic: Not provided.

> Mississippi State Board of Medical Licensure
> PO Box 9268
> Jackson, MISSISSIPPI 39286-9268
> Telephone: 601/987-3079
> Fax: 601/987-4159
> E-mail: mboard@msbml.state.ms.us
> Web site: www.msbml.state.ms.us

Montana

Montana Board of Medical Examiners
Verification of licenses
Telephone: Free of charge. Limit five verifications per call.
Written: $20 fee. Mail requests, including podiatrist names and license numbers (if known), and payment.
Electronic: Not provided.

> Montana Board of Medical Examiners
> PO Box 200513
> 301 S. Park Aveune
> Helena, MONTANA 59620-0513
> Telephone: 406/444-4284
> Fax: 406/841-2363
> E-mail: dlibsdmed@state.mt.us
> Web site: www.discoveringmontana.com/dli/med

Nebraska

Department of Health and Human Services
Verification of licenses
Telephone: Free of charge. Limit three verifications per call.
Written: $5 per verification to verify dates and license numbers. $25 per verification for any further information. Mail requests, including podiatrist names and license numbers (if known), and payment.
Electronic: Automated verification system available at Web site.

> Department of Health and Human Services
> Regulation and Licensure
> Credentialing Division
> PO Box 94986
> Lincoln, NEBRASKA 68509-4986
> Telephone: 402/471-2118

Fax: 402/471-3577
E-mail: becky.wisell@hhss.state.ne.us
Web site: www.hhs.state.ne.us/lis/lis.asp

Nevada

Nevada State Board of Podiatry
Notes: Call between 2:00 p.m. and 4:00 p.m. PST for verification information.
Verification of licenses
Telephone: Not provided.
Written: Free of charge. Mail requests, including podiatrist names and license numbers (if known).
Electronic: Not provided.

Nevada State Board of Podiatry
PO Box 12215
Reno, NEVADA 89501-2215
Telephone: 775/829-8066

New Hampshire

New Hampshire Board of Medicine
Verification of licenses
Telephone: Free of charge. Limit five verifications per call.
Written: $20 per verification. Mail requests, including podiatrist names and license numbers (if known), and payment.
Electronic: Not provided.

New Hampshire Board Medicine
2 Industrial Park Drive, Suite 8
Concord, NEW HAMPSHIRE 03301
Telephone: 603/271-1203
Fax: 603/271-6702
Web site: www.state.nh.us/medicine

New Jersey

New Jersey State Board of Medical Examiners
Verification of licenses
Telephone: Free of charge. Limit three verifications per call; unlimited verifications on automated verification system.
Written: Free of charge. Mail requests, including podiatrist names and license numbers (if known). Faxed upon request.
Electronic: Not provided.

New Jersey State Board of Medical Examiners
PO Box 183
Trenton, NEW JERSEY 08625-0183
Telephone: 609/292-4843
Fax: 609/826-7117

New Mexico

New Mexico Board of Podiatry
Verification of licenses

Telephone: Free of charge.
Written: $25 per. Mail requests, including podiatrist names and license numbers (if known).
Electronic: Not provided.

> New Mexico Board of Podiatry
> Regulation and Licensing Department
> PO Box 25101
> 2055 S. Pacheco, Suite 400
> Santa Fe, NEW MEXICO 87504
> Telephone: 505/476-7120
> Fax: 505/476-7095
> E-mail: podiatryboard@state.nm.us
> Web site: www.rld.state.nm.us

New York

Office of the Professions, Podiatric Licensing Agency
Verification of licenses

Telephone: Free of charge. Limit two verifications per call if calling customer service automated attendant; limit five per call if calling customer service representative; unlimited if calling automated verification system. $1.50 for first minute; $1 for each additional minute.
Written: $20 per verification. Limit one verification. $10 per hundred names for multiple verifications. Mail requests, including podiatrist's name, license number, date of birth, and address, and payment (check or money order payable to NYS Education Dept.).
Electronic: Automatic verification system available at Web site.

> Office of the Professions, Podiatric Licensing Agency
> New York State Education Department
> 89 Washington Avenue, Second Floor
> Albany, NEW YORK 12234-1000
> Telephone: 518/474-3817 (general information)   900/555-6978 (automated verification system)
> Fax: 518/474-3004
> E-mail: op4info@mail.nysed.gov
> Web site: www.op.nysed.gov

North Carolina

North Carolina Board of Podiatry Examiners
Verification of licenses

Telephone: Free of charge.
Written: Free of charge. Complete listing of all podiatrists: $100.
Electronic: Information available at Web site.

North Carolina Board of Podiatry Examiners
1500 Sunday Drive, Suite 102
Raleigh, NORTH CAROLINA 27607
Telephone: 919/787-5181 (main)
Fax: 919/787-4916
E-mail: info@ncbpe.com
Web site: www.ncbpe.org

North Dakota

North Dakota Board of Podiatric Medicine, Family Foot and Ankle Clinic
Verification of licenses
Telephone: Free of charge. Limit two verifications per call.
Written: Not provided.
Electronic: Not provided.

North Dakota Board of Podiatric Medicine
525 N Ninth Street
Bismarck, NORTH DAKOTA 58501
Telephone: 701/258-8120
Fax: 701/222-0229

Ohio

State Medical Board of Ohio
Verification of licenses
Telephone: Not provided.
Written: Not provided.
Electronic: Automated verification system available at Web site.

State Medical Board of Ohio
77 S. High Street, 17th Floor
Columbus, OHIO 43215-6127
Telephone: 614/466-3934
Fax: 614/728-5946
E-mail: med.recept@med.state.oh.us
Web site: www.state.oh.us/med

Oklahoma

Oklahoma State Board of Podiatry
Verification of licenses
Telephone: Free of charge. Limit five verifications per call.
Written: $10 per verification. Mail requests, including podiatrist names and license numbers (if known), and payment. Faxed upon request.
Electronic: Not provided.

Oklahoma State Board of Podiatry
PO Box 18256
Oklahoma City, OKLAHOMA 73154-0256
Telephone: 405/848-6841
Fax: 405/848-8240
E-mail: executive@osbmls.state.ok.us

Oregon

Oregon Board of Medical Examiners
Notes: Also license MDs, DOs and PAs.
Verification of licenses
Telephone: Free of charge. Limit three verifications per call.
Written: $10 fee for 1–4 names; $7.50 for five or more. Mail requests, including podiatrist's name and license number (if known), and payment.
Electronic: Not provided.

Oregon Board of Medical Examiners
1500 S.W. First Avenue, Suite 620
Portland, OREGON 97201-5826
Telephone: 503/229-5770
Fax: 503/229-6543
E-mail: bme.info@state.or.us
Web site: www.bme.state.or.us

Pennsylvania

Pennsylvania State Board of Podiatry
Verification of licenses
Telephone: Not provided.
Written: Provided only when there is no access to Web site.
Electronic: Available on www.licensepa.state.pa.us.

Pennsylvania State Board of Podiatry
Bureau of Professional and Occupational Affairs
PO Box 2649
Harrisburg, PENNSYLVANIA 17105-2649
Telephone: 717/783-4858
Fax: 717/787-7769
E-mail: podiatry@pados.dos.state.pa.us
Web site: www.dos.state.pa.us

Puerto Rico

Office of Regulation and Certification of Health Care Professionals
Verification of licenses
Telephone: Not provided.
Written: $20 per verification. Call or fax for standardized forms (faxed upon request). Mail requests, including

forms, podiatrist names and license numbers, self-addressed, stamped envelope, and payment (certified check or money order payable to Secretary of the Treasury of Puerto Rico).

Electronic: Not provided.

Department of Health
Office of Regulation and Certification of Health Care Professionals
PO Box 10200
Santurce, PUERTO RICO 00908-0020
Telephone: 787/725-8161 787/725-8125 787/725-8130
Fax: 787/725-7903

South Carolina

South Carolina Board of Podiatry Examiners
Verification of licenses

Telephone: Not provided.
Written: Free of charge. Mail requests, including podiatrist names and license numbers (if known) with return envelope.
Electronic: Free of charge.

South Carolina Board of Podiatry Examiners
PO Box 11289
110 Centerview Drive, Suite 202
Columbia, SOUTH CAROLINA 29211-1289
Telephone: 803/896-4685
Fax: 803/896-4515
E-mail: mail@llr.state.sc.us/pol.podiatry
Web site: www.llr.state.sc.us/podiatry

South Dakota

South Dakota Board of Podiatry Examiners
Verification of licenses

Telephone: Free of charge.
Written: Free of charge. Mail requests, including podiatrist names and license numbers (if known), and self-addressed, stamped envelope.
Electronic: Not provided.

South Dakota Board of Podiatry Examiners
135 E. Illinois, Suite 214
Spearfish, SOUTH DAKOTA 57783
Telephone: 605/642-1600
Fax: 605/642-1756
E-mail: proflic@rushmore.com
Web site: www.state.sd.us/dcr/podiatry

Tennessee

Tennessee Board of Registration in Podiatry
Verification of licenses
Telephone: Free of charge. Automated verification system.
Written: $20 fee.
Electronic: Automated verification system available at Web site.

Tennessee Board of Registration in Podiatry
Cordell Hull Building, First Floor
425 Fifth Avenue N
Nashville, TENNESSEE 37247-1010
Telephone: 615/532-5088 (general information)   888/310-4650 (automated verification system)
Fax: 615/532-5369
Web site: www.state.tn.us/health

Texas

Texas State Board of Podiatric Medical Examiners
Verification of licenses
Telephone: Free of charge. Limit three verifications per day.
Written: $2 per verification. Limit 15 verifications per week. Mail requests, including podiatrist's name and license number (if known), and self-addressed, stamped envelope.
Electronic: Licenses verified online at Web site. Licensed podiatrist list updated quarterly. Quarters begin 9/1 (Q1), 12/1 (Q2), 3/1 (Q3), and 6/1 (Q4). Contact Board via phone or e-mail for updated license information. No password needed to access list.

Texas State Board of Podiatric Medical Examiners
PO Box 12216
Austin, TEXAS 78711-2216
Telephone: 512/305-7000
Fax: 512/305-7003
E-mail: michele.wooldridge@foot.state.tx.us
Web site: www.foot.state.tx.us

Texas State Board of Podiatric Medical Examiners
Directory of licensed podiatrists
Telephone: Not provided.
Written: $100 per disk; $100 per printed list; $15 per any one city/county/zip code/etc. Provided on floppy disk or printed list. $2 per verification.
Electronic: Free of charge.

Texas State Board of Podiatric Medical Examiners
PO Box 12216
Austin, TEXAS 78711-2216
Telephone: 512/305-7000
Fax: 512/305-7003
E-mail: michele.wooldridge@foot.state.tx.us
Web site: www.foot.state.tx.us

Utah

Utah Division of Occupational and Professional Licensure
Verification of licenses

Telephone: Free of charge. Limit three verifications per call.
Written: $20 per verification.
Electronic: Automated verification system available at Web site.

> Utah Division of Occupational and Professional Licensure
> PO Box 146741
> 160 East 300 S
> Salt Lake City, UTAH 84114-6741
> Telephone: 801/530-6628
> Fax: 801/530-6511
> Web site: www.dopl.utah.gov

Vermont

Vermont Board of Medical Practice
Verification of licenses

Telephone: Free of charge. Limit two verifications per call.
Written: $20 per verification. Mail requests, including podiatrist names and license numbers (if known), and payment.
Electronic: Automated verification system available at Web site.

> Vermont Board of Medical Practice
> 109 State Street
> Montpelier, VERMONT 05609-1106
> Telephone: 802/828-2673
> Fax: 802/828-5450
> Web site: www.docboard.org

Virginia

Virginia Board of Medicine
Verification of licenses

Telephone: Free of charge. Limit three verifications per day. Provide podiatrist's name, license number, or Social Security number.
Written: Free of charge. Limit 10 verifications per day. Mail requests, including podiatrist's name, and license number or Social Security number.
Electronic: Visit Web site for more information.

> Virginia Board of Medicine
> 6606 W. Broad Street, Fourth Floor
> Richmond, VIRGINIA 23230
> Telephone: 804/662-9908
> Fax: 804/662-9517
> E-mail: medbd@state.va.us
> Web site: www.dhp.state.va.us

Washington

Washington State Podiatric Medical Board
Verification of licenses

Telephone: Free of charge. Limit three verifications; for unlimited verifications, call automated verification system. Provide podiatrist's name and license number; provide code PO and podiatrist's license number.

Written: Out-of-state fee: $50; businesses are free. Mail or fax requests, including podiatrist names and license numbers.

Electronic: Not provided.

> Washington State Podiatric Medical Board
> Department of Health
> PO Box 47869
> Olympia, WASHINGTON 98504-7869
> Telephone: 360/236-4943 360/664-4111 (automated verification system)
> Fax: 360/236-2406
> Web site: www.doh.wa.gov

Wisconsin

Wisconsin Medical Examining Board
Verification of licenses

Telephone: Not provided.

Written: $10 per verification for other state boards.

Electronic: All verification requests must be accessed on agency's Web site (www.drl.state.wi.us). If you cannot access the Internet, submit your request in writing to address below.

> Medical Examining Board
> Department of Regulations and Licensing
> PO Box 8935
> Madison, WISCONSIN 53708
> Telephone: 608/261-7931 608/261-7931
> Fax: 608/261-7083
> Web site: www.drl.state.wi.us/

Wyoming

Wyoming Board of Registration in Podiatry
Verification of licenses

Telephone: Free of charge.

Written: $25 per verification. Mail requests, including podiatrist names and license numbers (if known), and payment (certified check or money order).

Electronic: Not provided.

Wyoming Board of Registration in Podiatry
2020 Carey Avenue, Suite 201
Cheyenne, WYOMING 82002
Telephone: 307/777-3507
Fax: 307/777-3508
E-mail: nbrown@state.wy.us
Web site: www.plboards.state.wy.us

Chiropractic Licensing Agencies

Alabama

Alabama State Board of Chiropractic Examiners
Verification of licenses

Telephone: Not provided.
Written: $10 per verification. Mail requests, including chiropractor's name and license number (if known), and checklist of items needing verification (names, dates, disciplinary actions, etc.).
Electronic: Not provided.

Alabama State Board of Chiropractic Examiners
737 Logan Road
Clanton, ALABAMA 35045
Telephone: 205/755-8000
Fax: 205/755-0081
E-mail: sbolton@chiro.state.al.us
Web site: www.chiro.state.al.us

Alaska

Board of Chiropractic
Verification of licenses

Telephone: Free of charge. Limit three verifications per call.
Written: $20 per verification. Mail requests, including chiropractor names and license numbers (if known), and payment.
Electronic: Automated verification system available at Web site.

Alaska State Board of Chiropractic Examiners
Department of Community & Economic Development
Division of Occupational Licensing
PO Box 110806
Juneau, ALASKA 99811-0806
Telephone: 907/465-2589
Fax: 907/465-2974
E-mail: license@dced.state.ak.us
Web site: www.dced.state.ak.us/occ

Arizona

Arizona Board of Chiropractic Examiners
Verification of licenses

Telephone: Free of charge. Limit five verifications per call.
Written: $2 each. Faxed upon request. Mail or fax requests, including chiropractor names and license numbers (if known).
Electronic: Not provided.

Arizona Board of Chiropractic Examiners
5060 N. 19th Avenue, Suite 416
Phoenix, ARIZONA 85015
Telephone: 602/255-1444

Fax: 602/255-4289
E-mail: boy@goodnet.com
Web site: www.home.earthlink.net/^aimg1

Arkansas

Board of Chiropractic
Verification of licenses

Telephone: Free of charge. Limit six verifications per call.
Written: $5 per verification. Mail requests, including chiropractor names and license numbers (if known), and self-addressed, stamped envelope.
Electronic: Available on Web site.

Board of Chiropractic
101 E. Capital, Suite 209
Little Rock, ARKANSAS 72201
Telephone: 501/682-9015
Fax: 501/682-9016
E-mail: ann.gates@mail.state.ar.us
Web site: www.state.ar.us/asbce

California

Board of Chiropractic Examiners
Notes: Also verify certification of Good Standing of Licensure at $10 per verification to other states.
Verification of licenses

Telephone: Not provided.
Written: Mail requests, including chiropractor names and license numbers (if known), and payment ($3 per name). $5 for address verification; $10 for disciplinary information.
Electronic: Free of charge.

Board of Chiropractic Examiners
2525 Natomas Park Drive, Suite 260
Sacramento, CALIFORNIA 95833-4306
Telephone: 916/263-5355
Fax: 916/263-5369
Web site: www.chiro.ca.gov

Colorado

Board of Chiropractic Examiners
Verification of licenses

Telephone: Not provided.
Written: Not provided.
Electronic: Provided on Web site.

Board of Chiropractor Examiners
1560 Broadway, Suite 1310

Denver, COLORADO 80202
Telephone: 303/894-7758 (general information)
Fax: 303/894-7764
Web site: www.dora.state.co.us/chiropractic

Connecticut

Department of Public Health
Verification of licenses

Telephone: Free of charge. Limit three verifications per call.
Written: Free of charge. Limit 10 verifications per query. Faxed upon request. Mail or fax requests, including chiropractor names, license numbers (if known), and Connecticut release forms (available upon request).
Electronic: For verification of license, visit www.ct-clic.com.

Department of Public Health
Division of Health Systems Regulation
410 Capitol Avenue, MS 12 MQA
PO Box 340308
Hartford, CONNECTICUT 06134-0308
Telephone: 860/509-7603 860/509-7596
Fax: 860/509-7607
Web site: www.ct-clic.com

Delaware

Delaware Board of Chiropractic
Verification of licenses

Telephone: Not provided.
Written: $10 fee. Checks made payable to State of Delaware. Processing time: two weeks.
Electronic: Not provided.

Delaware Board of Chiropractic
Division of Professional Regulation
861 Silver Lake Boulevard
Cannon Building, Suite 203
Dover, DELAWARE 19904
Telephone: 302/744-4500
Fax: 302/739-2711

District of Columbia

Department of Health
Verification of licenses

Telephone: Not provided.
Written: $20 per verification. Mail requests, including chiropractor names and license numbers (if known), and payment made payable to D.C. Treasurer. Medical verifications for doctors is $50.
Electronic: Not provided.

Department of Health
Health Professional Licensing
825 N. Capital Street NE, Room 2224
Washington, DISTRICT OF COLUMBIA 20002
Telephone: 202/442-9200
Fax: 202/442-9431
Web site: www.dchealth.dc.gov

Florida

Board of Chiropractic
Verification of licenses

Telephone: Free of charge. Limit three verifications per call.
Written: $25 per verification. Mail requests, including chiropractor names and license numbers (if known), and payment.
Electronic: Upon request, will send written certification via e-mail or fax.

Division of Medical Quality Assurance
Client Services Unit
HMQAMS Bin C99
4052 Bald Cypress Way
Tallahassee, FLORIDA 32399-3299
Telephone: 850/488-0595
Fax: 850/414-0864
Web site: www.doh.state.fl.us/mqa

Georgia

Georgia Board of Chiropractic Examiners
Verification of licenses

Telephone: Free of charge. Limit three verifications per call.
Written: $25 fee. Faxed upon request. Mail or fax requests, including chiropractor names, license numbers (if known), and signed release forms.
Electronic: Not provided.

Georgia Board of Chiropractic Examiners
237 Coliseum Drive
Macon, GEORGIA 31217
Telephone: 478/207-1686
Fax: 478/207-1699
E-mail: aomartin@sos.state.ga.us
Web site: www.sos.state.ga.us/plb/chiro

Hawaii

Department of Commerce and Consumer Affairs Licensing Branch
Verification of licenses

Telephone: Consumer Resource Center: 808/587-3295. Provide chiropractor names and license numbers (if known).

Chiropractic Licensing Agencies

Written: $15 per verification. Mail requests, including chiropractor names, license numbers (if known), signed release forms, and payment.
Electronic: Not provided.

> Attention: Licensing Branch
> Department of Commerce and Consumer Affairs
> PO Box 3469
> 1010 Richards Street
> Honolulu, HAWAII 96801
> Telephone: 808/586-3000
> Fax: 808/586-3031
> Web site: www.state.hi.us/dcca/pvl

Idaho

Bureau of Occupational Licenses

Notes: Also issues licenses for medical counselors, doctors, chiropractors, optometrists, podiatrists, psychologists, and social workers.

Verification of licenses

Telephone: Free of charge.
Written: $10 per verification. Mail requests, including chiropractor's name and license number (if known), and payment. Verification without certifying signature is free.
Electronic: Free of charge for e-mail or fax verifications.

> Bureau of Occupational Licenses
> 1109 Main Street, Suite 220
> Boise, IDAHO 83702-5642
> Telephone: 208/334-3233
> Fax: 208/334-3945
> E-mail: anelson@ibol.state.id.us
> Web site: www.state.id.us/ibol

Illinois

Department of Professional Regulation Licensure Maintenance Unit

Verification of chiropractic licenses

Telephone: Free of charge. Limit three verifications per call. Provide chiropractor's name, license number (if known), or Social Security number.
Written: All requests are $20. Mail requests, including chiropractor names, license numbers (if known), and Social Security numbers, and payment.
Electronic: Automated verification system available at Web site.

> Licensure Maintenance Unit
> Department of Professional Regulation
> 320 W. Washington Street, Third Floor
> Springfield, ILLINOIS 62786
> Telephone: 217/782-0458
> Fax: 217/557-8073
> Web site: www.dpr.state.il.us

Indiana

Indiana Board of Chiropractic Examiners
Verification of licenses

Telephone: Free of charge. Limit one verification per call.
Written: $10 fee for verification to another state.
Electronic: Automated verification system available at Web site. Subscription required. Call 800/236-5446 for more information.

> Indiana Board of Chiropractic Examiners
> Health Professions Bureau
> 402 W. Washington Street, Room 041
> Indianapolis, INDIANA 46204
> Telephone: 317/232-2960 (general information)   888/333-7515 (verifications only)
> Fax: 317/233-4236
> E-mail: cvaught@hpb.state.in.us
> Web site: www.in.gov/hpb

Iowa

Board of Chiropractic Examiners
Verification of licenses

Telephone: Free of charge. Limit one verification per call.
Written: $10 per verification. Mail requests, including chiropractor's name and license number (if known), and payment.
Electronic: Not provided.

> Board of Chiropractic Examiners
> Department of Public Health
> Lucas Building, Fifth Floor
> 321 E. 12th Street
> Des Moines, IOWA 50319-0075
> Telephone: 515/281-4287
> Fax: 515/281-3121
> E-mail: khoover@idph.state.ia.us
> Web site: www.idph.state.ia.us/licensure

Kentucky

Kentucky Board of Chiropractic Examiners
Verification of licenses

Telephone: Free of charge. Limit 10 verifications per day.
Written: $3 per hard copy verification. Faxed upon request for $4.50. Mail or fax requests, including chiropractor names and license numbers (if known), and payment.
Electronic: Not provided.

> Kentucky Board of Chiropractic Examiners
> PO Box 183
> Glasgow, KENTUCKY 42142

Telephone: 270/651-2522
Fax: 270/651-8784
E-mail: kychiro@glasgow-ky.com

Louisiana

State Board of Examiners of Chiropractors
Verification of licenses

Telephone: Free of charge. Limited responses. Only to inquire if person is actively practicing.
Written: $25 per verification. Mail requests, including chiropractor names and license numbers (if known), and payment.
Electronic: Information available on Web site.

State Board of Examiners of Chiropractors
8621 Summa Avenue
Baton Rouge, LOUISIANA 70809
Telephone: 225/765-2322
Fax: 225/765-2640
E-mail: lsbce@eatel.net
Web site: www.lachiropracticboard.com

Maine

Board of Chiropractic Licensure
Verification of licenses

Telephone: Not provided.
Written: $10 per verification. Mail requests, including chiropractor names and license numbers (if known), and payment.
Electronic: Information available on Web site.

Department of Professional and Financial Regulation
Board of Chiropractic Licensure
35 State House Station
Augusta, MAINE 04333
Telephone: 207/624-8603
Fax: 207/624-8637
E-mail: linda.d.duffy@state.me.us
Web site: www.maineprofessionalreg.org

Maryland

Board of Chiropractic Examiners
Verification of licenses

Telephone: Not provided.
Written: $25 per verification. Mail requests, including chiropractor names and license numbers (if known), and payment.
Electronic: Not provided.

Board of Chiropractic Examiners
4201 Patterson Avenue
Baltimore, MARYLAND 21215-2299
Telephone: 410/764-4726
Fax: 410/358-1879
Web site: www.mdchiro.org

Massachusetts

Massachusetts Board of Registration of Chiropractors
Verification of licenses

Telephone: Free of charge. Limit three verifications per day.
Written: $10 per verification. Mail requests, including chiropractor's name and license number (if known), self-addressed, stamped envelope, and payment (check or money order payable to Commonwealth of Massachusetts).
Electronic: Visit Web site for more information.

Board of Registration of Chiropractors
239 Causeway Street, Fifth Floor
Boston, MASSACHUSETTS 02114
Telephone: 617/727-3069
Fax: 617/727-2669
Web site: www.state.ma.us/reg/boards/ch

Michigan

Department of Consumer and Industry Services
Verification of licenses

Telephone: Automated verification system: 900/555-8374. $1.50 per minute.
Written: Verifications to party other than U.S. state: $5 per verification. Written verifications to another U.S. state: $15 per verification. Mail request, including licensee name and number, and payment to address below.
Electronic: Automated verification system available at Web site.

Michigan Department of Consumer and Industry Services
Bureau of Health Services
Attn: Education, Testing & Credentials Section
PO Box 30180
Lansing, MICHIGAN 48909
Telephone: 517/335-0918 (general information)   900/555-8374 (automated verification system)
Fax: 517/373-2179
Web site: www.cis.state.mi.us/bhser

Minnesota

Minnesota Board of Chiropractic Examiners
Verification of licenses

Telephone: One name free of charge; send multiple name requests by mail with payment.
Written: $10 per verification. Mail requests, including chiropractor's name and license number (if known), and payment.
Electronic: Verification available through Web site.

Minnesota Board of Chiropractic Examiners
2829 University Avenue SE, Suite 300
Minneapolis, MINNESOTA 55414-3220
Telephone: 612/617-2222
Fax: 612/617-2224
Web site: www.mn-chiroboard.state.mn.us

Missouri

State Board of Chiropractic Examiners
Verification of licenses

Telephone: Free of charge. Limit three verifications per call.
Written: Free of charge. Faxed upon request. Mail or fax requests, including chiropractor names and license numbers (if known).
Electronic: Not provided.

State Board of Chiropractic Examiners
PO Box 672
3605 Missouri Boulevard
Jefferson City, MISSOURI 65102-0153
Telephone: 573/751-2104
Fax: 573/751-0735
E-mail: chiro@mail.state.mo.us
Web site: www.ecodev.state.mo.us/pr

Montana

Board of Chiropractors
Verification of licenses

Telephone: Free of charge.
Written: Free of charge. Mail or fax requests, including chiropractor names and license numbers (if known), and signed release forms.

Chapter 6

Electronic: Free of charge. E-mail requests to dlibsdchi@state.mt.us.

Board of Chiropractors
PO Box 200513
Helena, MONTANA 59620-0513
Telephone: 406/841-2393
Fax: 406/841-2305
E-mail: dlibsdchi@state.mt.us
Web site: www.discoveringmontana.com/dli/bsd

Nebraska

Regulations and Licensure, Credentials Division
Verification of licenses

Telephone: Free of charge.
Written: $25 per verification. Mail requests, including chiropractor names and license numbers (if known), and payment.
Electronic: Information available on our Web site.

Regulations and Licensure
Credentials Division
Health and Human Services
301 Centennial Mall S.
PO Box 94986
Lincoln, NEBRASKA 68509-4986
Telephone: 402/471-2115   402/471-2299 (chiropractic licensing)
Fax: 402/471-3577
Web site: www.hhs.state.ne.us/crl/profindex1.htm (licensing information)

New Hampshire

New Hampshire Board of Chiropractic Examiners
Verification of licenses

Telephone: Free of charge. Limit two verifications per call.
Written: Free of charge. Mail or fax requests, including chiropractor names and license numbers (if known).
Electronic: Not provided.

New Hampshire Board of Chiropractic Examiners
6 Hazen Drive
Concord, NEW HAMPSHIRE 03301-6527
Telephone: 603/271-4560
Fax: 603/271-4827

New Jersey

State Board of Chiropractic Examiners
Verification of licenses

Telephone: Free of charge. Limit three verifications per call; unlimited verifications on automated verification system. Faxed upon request.
Written: $40 per verification. Mail requests, including chiropractor names and license numbers (if known), and payment.
Electronic: Information available on Web site free of charge.

State Board of Chiropractic Examiners
124 Halsey Street, Sixth Floor
PO Box 45004
Newark, NEW JERSEY 07101
Telephone: 973/504-6395   973/273-8090 (automated verification system)
Fax: 973/273-8075
Web site: www.state.nj.us/lps/ca/medical.htm#chiro2

New Mexico

New Mexico Board of Chiropractic Examiners
Verification of licenses

Telephone: Free of charge.
Written: $25 per verification. Mail requests, including chiropractor names and license numbers (if known), and payment.
Electronic: Not provided.

New Mexico Board of Chiropractic Examiners
PO Box 25101
Santa Fe, NEW MEXICO 87504
Telephone: 505/476-7120
Fax: 505/476-7095
E-mail: ChiroBoard@state.nm.us
Web site: www.rld.state.nm.us

New York

Office of the Professions, Chiropractic Licensing
Verification of licenses

Telephone: Free of charge. Limit two verifications per call if calling customer service automated attendant; limit five per call if calling customer service representative; unlimited if calling automated verification system. $1.50 for first minute; $1 for each additional minute.
Written: $20 per verification. Limit one verification. $10 per hundred names for multiple verifications. Mail

requests, including chiropractor names, license numbers, date of birth and address, and payment (check or money order payable to NYS Education Department).

Electronic: Automated verification system also available at Web site.

> Office of Professions, Chiropractic Licensing
> New York State Education Department
> 89 Washington Avenue, Floor 2
> Albany, NEW YORK 12234-1000
> Telephone: 518/474-3817 (customer service)
> Fax: 518/474-1449
> E-mail: op4info@mail.nysed.gov
> Web site: www.op.nysed.gov

North Carolina

North Carolina Board of Chiropractic
Verification of licenses

Telephone: Free of charge.
Written: Free of charge. Faxed upon request. Mail or fax requests, including chiropractor names and license numbers (if known).
Electronic: Not provided.

> North Carolina Board of Chiropractic
> 174 Church Street N
> Concord, NORTH CAROLINA 28025
> Telephone: 704/793-1342
> Fax: 704/793-1385
> E-mail: ncchirobrd@juno.com
> Web site: www.ncchiroboard.org

Oregon

Oregon Board of Chiropractic Examiners
Verification of licenses

Telephone: Free of charge. Limit three verifications per call.
Written: $15 per hour plus $0.15 per page verification; fee includes approximately 10–12 names. Mail requests, including chiropractor's name and license number (if known), and payment.
Electronic: Not provided.

> Oregon Board of Chiropractic Examiners
> 3218 Pringle Road SE, Suite 150
> Salem, OREGON 97302-6311
> Telephone: 503/378-5816

Fax: 503/362-1260
E-mail: oregon.obce@state.or.us
Web site: www.obce.state.or.us

Pennsylvania

State Board of Chiropractic
Verification of licenses

Telephone:	Free of charge. Limit three verifications per call.
Written:	Free of charge. Faxed upon request. Mail or fax requests, including chiropractor names and license numbers (if known).
Electronic:	Verification available at Web site (www.licensepa.state.pa.us).

State Board of Chiropractic
PO Box 2649
Harrisburg, PENNSYLVANIA 17105
Telephone: 717/783-7155
Fax: 717/787-7769
E-mail: chiropra@pados.state.pa.us
Web site: www.dos.state.pa.us

Puerto Rico

Office of Regulation and Certification of Health Care Professionals
Verification of licenses

Telephone:	Not provided.
Written:	$20 per verification. Call or fax for standardized forms (faxed upon request). Mail requests, including forms, chiropractor names and license numbers, self-addressed, stamped envelope, and payment (certified check or money order payable to Secretary of the Treasury of Puerto Rico).
Electronic:	Not provided.

Office of Regulation and Certification of Health Care Professionals
Department of Health
PO Box 10200
Santurce, PUERTO RICO 00908-0020
Telephone: 787/725-8161 (switchboard)   787/725-8125 (administration)
787/725-8530 (continuing education)
Fax: 787/725-7903

Rhode Island

Division of Professional Regulation
Verification of licenses

Telephone:	Not provided.
Written:	Free of charge. Faxed upon request. Mail or fax requests, including chiropractor names and license

numbers (if known). $10 fee for license verification for their own licensure.
Electronic: Free of charge. Web site is the preferred route.

Division of Professional Regulation
Health Department
3 Capitol Hill, Room 104
Providence, RHODE ISLAND 02908
Telephone: 401/222-2828
Fax: 401/222-1272
Web site: www.health.state.ri.us

South Carolina

South Carolina Board of Chiropractic Examiners
Verification of licenses
Telephone: Free of charge. Limit three verifications per call.
Written: Free of charge. Faxed upon request. Mail or fax requests, including chiropractor names and license numbers (if known).
Electronic: Information is available on Web site.

Attention: Chiropractor license verification
South Carolina Board of Chiropractic Examiners
PO Box 11329
Columbia, SOUTH CAROLINA 29211-1329
Telephone: 803/896-4587
Fax: 803/896-4719
E-mail: homlesa@mail.llr.sc.us
Web site: www.llr.state.sc.us

South Dakota

Board of Chiropractic Examiners
Verification of licenses
Telephone: Free of charge. Limit two verifications per call.
Written: $10 per verification. Faxed upon request. Mail or fax requests, including chiropractor names and license numbers (if known).
Electronic: Not provided.

Board of Chiropractic Examiners
2603 Ella Lane
Yankton, SOUTH DAKOTA 57078
Telephone: 605/668-9017
Fax: 605/668-9017
Web site: www.state.sd.us/dcr/chiropractic

Chiropractic Licensing Agencies

Tennessee

Bureau of Health, Licensure & Regulations
Verification of licenses
Telephone: Free of charge. Call automated verification system.
Written: Not provided.
Electronic: Not provided.

Board of Chiropractic Examiners
First Floor, Cordell Hual Building
425 Fifth Avenue N
Nashville, TENNESSEE 37247-1010
Telephone: 615/532-5083 (general information)   888/310-4650 (automated verification system)
Fax: 615/532-5164
Web site: www.state.tn.us./health

Texas

Texas Board of Chiropractic Examiners
Verification of licenses
Telephone: Only to check if chiropractor is active.
Written: $1 per chiropractor name (plus $1 postage); postage is waived if self-addressed, stamped envelope is included. Limit 25 verifications per request. Faxed verifications upon request ($1 per sheet).
Electronic: Free of charge.

Texas Board of Chiropractic Examiners
333 Guadalupe, Suite 3-825
Austin, TEXAS 78701-3942
Telephone: 512/305-6700
Fax: 512/305-6705
E-mail: molly.vickers@tbce.state.tx.us
Web site: www.tbce.state.tx.us

Utah

Utah Division of Occupational and Professional Licensing
Verification of licenses
Telephone: Free of charge. Limit three verifications per call.
Written: $20 per in-house verification.
Electronic: Automated verification system available at Web site. $20 fee.

Utah Division of Occupational and Professional Licensing
PO Box 146741
Salt Lake City, UTAH 84114-6741
Telephone: 801/530-6628   866/275-3675 (in-state only)
Fax: 801/530-6511
Web site: www.dopl.utah.gov

Vermont

Office of the Secretary of State, License Verification Unit
Verification of licenses
Telephone: Free of charge.
Written: $20 per verification. Mail requests, including chiropractor names and license numbers (if known), and payment.
Electronic: Information available on Web site.

> Attention: Board of DC
> Office of the Secretary of State
> 26 Terrace Street, Drawer 09
> Montpelier, VERMONT 05609-1106
> Telephone: 802/828-2390
> Fax: 802/828-2465
> E-mail: dlafaill@sec.state.vt.us
> Web site: www.sec.state.vt.us

Virginia

Virginia State Board of Medicine
Verification of licenses
Telephone: Free of charge. Limit three verifications per day. Provide chiropractor's name, license number, or Social Security number. Please call 804/662-9908
Written: $10 fee to a state agency. Include chiropractor's name, and license number or Social Security number, and payment payable to Treasurer of Virginia. Include name and address where it should be sent.
Electronic: Not provided.

> State Board of Medicine
> Department of Health Professions
> 6606 W. Broad Street, Fourth Floor
> Richmond, VIRGINIA 23230-1717
> Telephone: 804/662-9908   804/662-7636 (automated verification number)
> Fax: 804/662-7281 (licensing board)   804/662-9517 (disciplinary board)
> Web site: www.dhp.state.va.us

Washington

Health Professions Quality Assurance
Verification of licenses
Telephone: Free of charge. Limit three verifications per call via general information number; unlimited for automated verification line. Provide code CH and chiropractor's license number.
Written: Free of charge. Faxed upon request. Mail or fax requests, including chiropractor names and license numbers (if known).
Electronic: Automated verification service available via computer modem. Dial 360/664-4871. For more information, call for brochure.

Chiropractic Licensing Agencies

Department of Health
Chiropractic Quality Assurance Commission
PO Box 47868
Olympia, WASHINGTON 98504-7868
Telephone: 360/236-4700 (customer service)
360/664-4700 (automated verification system)
Fax: 360/236-4922
E-mail: connie.glasgow@eoh.wa.gov or hpaa.csc@doh.wa.gov (customer service)
Web site: www.doh.wa.gov

Wisconsin

Department of Regulation and Licensing
Verification of licenses

Telephone: Free of charge.
Written: $10 per verification for other state boards.
Electronic: All verification requests must be accessed on agency's Web site (www.drl.state.wi.us). If you cannot access the Internet, submit your request in writing to address below.

Department of Regulation and Licensing
Bureau of Health Service Professions
PO Box 8935
Madison, WISCONSIN 53708-8935
Telephone: 608/261-2390   608/261-7931 (licensing)
Fax: 608/261-7083
E-mail: dorl@drl.state.wi.us
Web site: www.drl.state.wi.us

Wyoming

Professional Licensing Boards
Verification of licenses

Telephone: Free of charge. Limit three verifications per call.
Written: $25 per verification. Cashier's check or money order payable to State of Wyoming. Mail requests, including chiropractor names and license numbers (if known), and payment.
Electronic: Not provided.

Attention: Chiropractor license verification request
Professional Licensing Boards
2020 Carey Avenue, Suite 201
Cheyenne, WYOMING 82002
Telephone: 307/777-6529
Fax: 307/777-3508
E-mail: dbridg@state.wy.us
Web site: www.plboards.state.wy.us

Physician Assistant Licensing Agencies

Alaska

Alaska State Medical Board
Verification of licenses

Telephone: Free of charge. Limit five verifications per call.

Written: $20 per verification (made payable to State of Alaska). Mail requests, including physician assistant names and license numbers (if known), and payment. Mail to Alaska State Medical Board, PO Box 110806, Juneau, AK 99811-0806.

Electronic: Not provided.

Division of Occupational Licensing
Alaska State Medical Board
Leslie Gallant, Executive Administrator
550 W. Seventh Avenue, Suite 1500
Anchorage, ALASKA 99501
Telephone: 907/269-8163
Fax: 907/269-8196
Web site: www.dced.state.ak.us/occ/occstart.cfm

Arizona

Arizona State Board of Medical Examiners
Verification of licenses

Telephone: Free of charge. Limit two verifications per call.

Written: $5 per verification. Mail requests, including physician assistant names and license numbers (if known).

Electronic: Free of charge.

Arizona Board of Medical Examiners
9545 E. Doubletree Ranch Road
Scottsdale, ARIZONA 85258
Telephone: 480/551-2700
Fax: 480/551-2704
E-mail: questions@bomex.org
Web site: azdocinfo.com

Arkansas

Arkansas State Medical Board

Notes: Verifications of physicians, physician assistants, respiratory therapists, and occupational therapists.

Verification of licenses

Telephone: Not provided.

Written: $15 per verification. Mail requests, including physician assistant names and payment (check or money order).

Electronic: Modem verification service. Fax letter stating request for service.

Arkansas State Medical Board
2100 River Front Drive
Little Rock, ARKANSAS 72202-1793

Telephone: 501/296-1802
Fax: 501/603-3555
E-mail: office@armedicalboard.org
Web site: www.armedicalboard.org

California

Physician Assistant Committee
Verification of licenses

Telephone: Free of charge. Limit three verifications per call.
Written: Free of charge. Mail or fax requests, including physician assistant's full name, office address, city/town of practice, and license number (if known).
Electronic: Information available on the Web site.

Physician Assistant Committee
1424 Howe Avenue, Suite 35
Sacramento, CALIFORNIA 95825-3237
Telephone: 916/263-2670
Fax: 916/263-2671
E-mail: pacommittee@medbd.ca.gov
Web site: www.physicianassistant.ca.gov

Colorado

Colorado Board of Medical Examiners
Verification of licenses

Telephone: Free of charge. Limit four verifications per call.
Written: Free of charge. Mail requests, including physician assistant names and license numbers (if known).
Electronic: Free of charge.

Board of Medical Examiners
1560 Broadway, Suite 1300
Denver, COLORADO 80202-5140
Telephone: 303/894-7690   303/894-7434 (automated verification system)
Fax: 303/894-7692
E-mail: susan.miller@dora.state.co.us
Web site: www.dora.state.co.us/medical

Connecticut

Connecticut Department of Public Health
Verification of licenses

Telephone: Free of charge. Limit five verifications per call.
Written: Free of charge. Faxed upon request. Mail or fax requests, including physician assistant names, license numbers (if known), and Connecticut release forms (available upon request).
Electronic: Automated verification system available at www.state.ct.us/dph/scripts/hlthprof.asp.

Division of Health Systems Regulation
Department of Public Health
410 Capitol Avenue, MS12MQA
PO Box 340308
Hartford, CONNECTICUT 06134
Telephone: 860/509-7603   860/509-7596 (CNA calls only)
Fax: 860/509-7607
Web site: www.ct-clic.com

Delaware

Delaware Board of Medical Practice
Verification of licenses

Telephone: Free of charge.
Written: $10 per verification. Mail requests, including licensee's name, license number (if known), issue date and expiration date, and payment.
Electronic: Not provided.

Delaware Board of Medical Practice
861 Silver Lake Boulevard
Cannon Building, Suite 203
Dover, DELAWARE 19904
Telephone: 302/744-4500
Fax: 302/739-2711
Web site: www.professionallicensing.state.de.us

District of Columbia

Department of Health
Verification of licenses

Telephone: Free of charge. Limit three verifications per call. Three verifications per facility per day.
Written: $50 per verification for physicians; $20 per verification for other health professionals. Mail requests, including names and license numbers (if known), and payment. Make check payable to D.C. Treasurer.
Electronic: Not provided.

Department of Health
Health Professional Licensing
825 N. Capital Street, Suite 2224, Second Floor
Washington, DISTRICT OF COLUMBIA 20002
Telephone: 202/442-9200
Fax: 202/442-9431
Web site: www.dchealth.dc.gov

Florida

Division of Medical Quality Assurance
Verification of licenses

Telephone: Free of charge. Limit three verifications per call.
Written: $25 per verification. Mail requests, including physician assistant names and license numbers (if known), and payment.
Electronic: Information is available on Web site.

Division of Medical Quality Assurance
Client Services Unit
HMQAMS Bin C99
4052 Bald Cypress Way
Tallahassee, FLORIDA 32399-3299
Telephone: 850/488-0595
Fax: 850/414-0864
Web site: www.doh.state.fl.us/mqa

Georgia

Georgia Composite State Board of Medical Examiners
Verification of licenses

Telephone: Free of charge. Limit three verifications per call.
Written: Free of charge. Mail or fax requests, including physician assistant names and license numbers (if known).
Electronic: Verification available on Web site.

Composite State Board of Medical Examiners
2 Peachtree Street NW, 10th Floor
Atlanta, GEORGIA 30303
Telephone: 404/656-3913
Fax: 404/656-9723
Web site: www.medicalboard.state.ga.us

Illinois

Illinois Department of Professional Regulation
Verification of licenses

Telephone: Free of charge. Limit three verifications per call. Provide physician assistant's name, license number, or Social Security number (if known).

Physician Assistant Licensing Agencies

Written: First three verifications free; $20 for each additional verification. Mail requests, including physician assistant names, license numbers (if known), Social Security numbers, and payment.
Electronic: Automated verification system available at Web site.

>Licensure Maintenance Unit
>Department of Professional Regulation
>320 W. Washington Street, Third Floor
>Springfield, ILLINOIS 62786
>Telephone: 217/782-0458
>Fax: 217/557-8073
>Web site: www.dpr.state.il.us

Indiana

Indiana Medical Licensing Board
Verification of licenses
Telephone: Free of charge. Provide physician assistant names or license numbers (if known).
Written: $15 per verification. Mail requests, including physician assistant names and license numbers (if known), and payment.
Electronic: Automated verification system available at Web site. Subscription required. Call 800/236-5446 for more information.

>Health Professions Bureau
>Medical Licensing Board
>402 W. Washington Street, Room 041
>Indianapolis, INDIANA 46204
>Telephone: 888/333-7515   317/232-2960
>Fax: 317/233-4236
>Web site: www.ai.org/hpb

Kansas

Kansas Board of Healing Arts
Verification of licenses
Telephone: Free of charge. Limit three verifications per day.
Written: $15 for verifications with scores. Free without scores. Mail or fax requests, including physician assistant's name and license number (if known).
Electronic: Information available on Web site.

>Kansas State Board of Healing Arts
>235 S.W. Topeka Boulevard
>Topeka, KANSAS 66603
>Telephone: 785/296-7413
>Fax: 785/296-0852
>E-mail: cabbott@ink.org
>Web site: www.ksbha.org

Kentucky

Kentucky Board of Medical Licensure
Verification of licenses

Telephone: Call automated verification number. Limit two verifications per day. $2.95 for first minute; $0.50 for each additional minute. Provide physician's name and license number (if known). Verifications faxed upon request.

Written: $5 for 1–5 verifications; $7 for 6–10 verifications. Limit 10 verifications per query. Mail requests, including physician assistant names and license numbers (if known), and payment.

Electronic: Not provided.

Kentucky Board of Medical Licensure
310 Whittington Parkway, Suite 1B
Louisville, KENTUCKY 40222
Telephone: 502/429-8046 (general information) 900/555-6500 (automated verification system)
Fax: 502/429-9923
E-mail: kbml@mail.state.ky.us
Web site: www.state.ky.us/agencies/kbml

Louisiana

Louisiana State Board of Medical Examiners
Verification of licenses

Telephone: Free of charge. Limit three verifications per call.

Written: $4 per request. Mail requests, including physician assistant names and license numbers (if known).

Electronic: Information available on Web site.

Verifications Department
Louisiana State Board of Medical Examiners
PO Box 54403
New Orleans, LOUISIANA 70154-4403
Telephone: 504/568-6820
Fax: 504/568-8893
Web site: www.lsbme.org

Maine

Maine Board of Licensure in Medicine
Note: Web site is used only as a general information site, not for verification.

Verification of licenses

Telephone: Free of charge. Limit five verifications per call.

Written: $15 per verification. Mail requests, including physician assistant names and license numbers (if known), and payment.

Electronic: Not provided.

State of Maine
Board of Licensure in Medicine
137 State House Station

Physician Assistant Licensing Agencies

Augusta, MAINE 04333
Telephone: 207/287-3601
Fax: 207/287-6590
Web site: www.docboard.org/me_home.htm

Massachusetts

Massachusetts Board of Registration of Physician Assistants
Verification of licenses

Telephone: Free of charge. Limit three verifications per call.
Written: $10 per verification. Mail requests, including physician assistant's name and license number (if known). Faxed upon request.
Electronic: Automated verification system available.

Board of Registration of Physician Assistants
239 Causeway Street, Fifth Floor
Boston, MASSACHUSETTS 02114
Telephone: 617/727-3069
Fax: 617/727-2669
E-mail: gladys.m.clifton@state.ma.us/reg
Web site: www.state.ma.us/reg

Michigan

Bureau of Health Services
Verification of licenses

Telephone: Call automated verification number at 900/555-8374. $1.50 per minute.
Written: Verifications to party other than U.S. state: $5 per verification. Written verifications to another U.S. state: $15 per verification. Mail request, including licensee name and number, and payment.
Electronic: Automated verification system available at Web site.

Michigan Department of Consumer & Industry Services
Bureau of Health Services
Attention: Education Testing & Credentials Section
PO Box 30670
Lansing, MICHIGAN 48909
Telephone: 900/555-8374 (automated verification system)   517/335-0918 (general information)
Fax: 517/373-2179
Web site: www.cif.state.mi.us/free

Minnesota

Minnesota Board of Medical Practice
Verification of licenses

Telephone: Free of charge. Limit two verifications per call.
Written: $25 per verification. Mail requests, including physician assistant names and license numbers (if known), and payment.
Electronic: Automated verification system available through Web site.

Minnesota Board of Medical Practice
2829 University Avenue SE
Minneapolis, MINNESOTA 55414-3246
Telephone: 612/617-2130
Fax: 612/617-2166
Web site: www.bmp.state.mn.us

Missouri

Missouri State Board of Registration of the Healing Arts
Note: Physical therapists, speech pathologists, clinical audiologists, athletic trainers, and clinical perfusionists are also verified.

Verification of licenses

Telephone: Free of charge. Limit five verifications per call. Provide physician assistant's name and license number (if known).

Written: Free of charge. Faxed upon request. Mail or fax requests, including physician assistant's name and license number (if known).

Electronic: Automated verification system available at Web site.

State Board of Registration of the Healing Arts
PO Box 4
3605 Missouri Boulevard
Jefferson City, MISSOURI 65102
Telephone: 573/751-0098
Fax: 573/751-3166
E-mail: healarts@mail.state.mo.us
Web site: www.ecodev.state.mo.us/pr/healarts

Montana

Montana Board of Medical Examiners
Verification of licenses

Telephone: Free of charge. Limit five verifications per call.

Written: $20 per verification. Mail requests, including physician assistant names and license numbers (if known), and payment.

Electronic: Not provided.

Montana Board of Medical Examiners
PO Box 200513
301 S Park Avenue (delivery only)
Helena, MONTANA 59620-0513
Telephone: 406/4841-2359
Fax: 406/841-2363
Web site: www.decovering.com/dli/bsd

Nebraska

Department of Health and Human Services
Verification of licenses

Telephone: Free of charge. Limit three verifications per call. Provide physician assistant's name and license number (if known).

Written: $5 per verification to verify dates and license numbers; $25 per verification for any further information. Mail requests, including physician assistant's name and license number (if known), and payment.

Electronic: Automated verification system available at Web site.

Department of Health and Human Services
Regulation and Licensure
Credentialing Division
PO Box 94986
Lincoln, NEBRASKA 68509-4986
Telephone: 402/471-2115
Fax: 402/471-3577
E-mail: vicki.bumgarner@hhss.state.ne.us
Web site: www.hhs.state.ne.us/lis/lis.asp

Nevada

Nevada State Board of Medical Examiners
Verification of licenses

Telephone: Free of charge.

Written: $25 per verification. Mail requests, including physician assistant names and license numbers (if known), and payment.

Electronic: Not provided.

Nevada State Board of Medical Examiners
1105 Terminal Way, Suite 301
PO Box 7238
Reno, NEVADA 89510
Telephone: 775/688-2559
Fax: 775/688-2321
E-mail: nsbme@govmail.state.nv.us
Web site: www.state.nv.us/medical

New Hampshire

New Hampshire Board of Medicine
Verification of licenses

Telephone: Free of charge. Limit five verifications per call.

Written: $20 per verification. Mail requests, including physician assistant names and license numbers (if known), and payment.

Electronic: Not provided.

New Hampshire Board of Medicine
2 Industrial Park Drive, Suite 8

Concord, NEW HAMPSHIRE 03301
Telephone: 603/271-1203
Fax: 603/271-6702
Web site: www.state.nh.us/medicine

New Jersey

New Jersey State Board of Medical Examiners
Verification of licenses

Telephone: Free of charge. Limit five verifications per call; unlimited verifications on automated verification system.

Written: Free of charge. Mail or fax requests, including physician assistant names and license numbers (if known).

Electronic: Not provided.

New Jersey State Board of Medical Examiners
Attention: License verification request
140 E. Front Street, Second Floor
PO Box 183
Trenton, NEW JERSEY 08265
Telephone: 609/292-4843 (general information)   973/273-8090 (automated verification system)
Fax: 609/826-7117
Web site: www.state.nj.us/lps/ca/medical.htm

New York

Office of the Professions, Physician Assistant
Verification of licenses

Telephone: Free of charge. Limit two verifications per call if calling customer service automated attendant; limit five per call if calling customer service representative; unlimited if calling automated verification system. $1.50 for first minute; $1 for each additional minute.

Written: $20 per verification. Limit one verification. $10 per hundred names for multiple verifications. Mail requests, including physician assistant's name, license number, date of birth, and address, and payment (check or money order payable to NYS Education Dept.).

Electronic: Automated verification system available at Web site.

Office of the Professions, Physician Assistant
New York State Education Department
89 Washington Avenue, Second Floor
Albany, NEW YORK 12234-1000
Telephone: 518/474-3817 (customer service automated attendant, customer service representative)
900/555-6978 (automated verification system)
Fax: 518/474-1449
E-mail: op4info@mail.nysed.gov
Web site: www.op.nysed.gov

Physician Assistant Licensing Agencies

North Carolina

North Carolina Medical Board
Verification of licenses

Telephone: Not provided.
Written: $15 for single verification. Mail requests, including physician assistant's name, license number, Social Security number, and date of birth, and payment.
Electronic: Automated verification system available at Web site.

North Carolina Medical Board
1201 Front Street, Suite 100
Raleigh, NORTH CAROLINA 27609
Telephone: 919/326-1100
Fax: 919/326-1131
E-mail: info@ncmedboard.org
Web site: www.ncmedboard.org

North Dakota

North Dakota State Board of Medical Examiners
Note: $5 fee for verification requests to another state. Licensing of MDs, DOs, and PAs.
Verification of licenses

Telephone: Free of charge. Limit two verifications per call.
Written: $5 per verification. Mail requests, including physician assistant/physician names and license numbers (if known), and payment.
Electronic: Automated verification available at Web site.

North Dakota State Board of Medical Examiners
418 E. Broadway Avenue, Suite 12
Bismarck, NORTH DAKOTA 58501
Telephone: 701/328-6500
Fax: 701/328-6505
E-mail: bomex@tic.bisman.com
Web site: www.ndbomex.com

Ohio

State Medical Board of Ohio
Verification of licenses

Telephone: Not provided.
Written: Not provided.
Electronic: Automated verification system available at Web site.

State Medical Board of Ohio
77 S. High Street, 17th Floor
Columbus, OHIO 43215-6127
Telephone: 614/466-3934
Fax: 614/728-5946
E-mail: med.recept@med.state.oh.us
Web site: www.state.oh.us/med

Oregon

Oregon State Board of Medical Examiners
Verification of licenses

Telephone: Free of charge. Limit three verifications per call.
Written: $10 fee for 1–5 names; $7.50 fee for each additional name. Mail requests, including physician assistant's name and license number (if known), and payment.
Electronic: Not provided.

Oregon State Board of Medical Examiners
1500 SW First Avenue, Suite 620
Portland, OREGON 97201-5826
Telephone: 503/229-5770
Fax: 503/229-6543
E-mail: bme.info@state.or.us
Web site: www.bme.state.or.us

Pennsylvania

Pennsylvania State Board of Medicine
Verification of licenses

Telephone: Free of charge. Limit 10 verifications per day.
Written: Free of charge. Faxed upon request (depending on quantity). Mail or fax requests, including physician assistant names and license numbers (if known).
Electronic: Not provided.

Pennsylvania State Board of Medicine
Bureau of Professional and Occupational Affairs
PO Box 2649
Harrisburg, PENNSYLVANIA 17105-2649
Telephone: 717/787-2381
Fax: 717/787-7769

Rhode Island

Rhode Island Board of Medical Licensure and Discipline
Verification of licenses

Telephone: Free of charge. Limit three verifications per call.
Written: Free of charge. Faxed upon request. Mail or fax requests, including physician assistant names and license numbers (if known).
Electronic: Automated verification system available at Web site.

Attention: Verification request
Rhode Island Department of Health
Office of Health Professions Regulations
3 Capitol Hill, Room 104
Providence, RHODE ISLAND 02908-5097

Telephone: 401/222-2827
Fax: 401/222-1272
Web site: www.health.state.ri.us

South Carolina

South Carolina Board of Medical Examiners
Verification of licenses
Telephone: Not provided.
Written: $5 fee.
Electronic: Not provided.

South Carolina Board of Medical Examiners
PO Box 11289
Columbia, SOUTH CAROLINA 29211-1289
Telephone: 803/896-4500
Fax: 803/896-4515
Web site: www.llr.state.sc.us/pol/medical

South Dakota

South Dakota State Board of Medical and Osteopathic Examiners
Verification of licenses
Telephone: Not provided.
Written: $10 per verification. Faxed upon request. Mail requests, including physician assistant's name and license number (if known), and check (payable to South Dakota Board of Medical Examiners).
Electronic: Not provided.

South Dakota State Board of Medical and Osteopathic Examiners
1323 S. Minnesota Avenue
Sioux Falls, SOUTH DAKOTA 57105
Telephone: 605/334-8343
Fax: 605/336-0270

Tennessee

Committee for Physician Assistants
Verification of licenses
Telephone: Free of charge. Call automated verification system.
Written: Written verification available only on state-to-state. $10 fee.
Electronic: Automated verification system available at Web site.

Committee for Physician Assistants
425 Fifth Avenue N
Cordell Hull Building, First Floor
Nashville, TENNESSEE 37247-1010
Telephone: 615/532-4384 (general information)   888/310-4650 (automated verification system)
Fax: 615/253-4484
Web site: www.state.tn.us/health

Texas

Texas State Board of Medical Examiners, Acupuncture Examiners, and Physician Assistant Examiners
Verification of licenses

Telephone: Free of charge. During high call volume, agents may limit verifications to three per call.
Written: Free of charge. Mail or fax requests, including names and license numbers (if known).
Electronic: Automated verification system available via computer modem. Access by dialing into TSBME computer (512/305-7035). User name: PV; password: TX. See TSBME Web site for more details. Online verification at www.tsbme.state.tx.us

Texas State Board of Medical Examiners
MC-240
PO Box 2018
Austin, TEXAS 78768-2018
Telephone: 512/305-7030 (Customer Information Center)   512/305-7035 (online verification system)
Fax: 512/463-9416
E-mail: verifcic@tsbme.state.tx.us
Web site: www.tsbme.state.tx.us

Utah

Utah Division of Occupational and Professional Licensure
Verification of licenses

Telephone: Free of charge. Limit three verifications per call.
Written: $20 per verification.
Electronic: Automated verification system available on Web site. $5 fee.

Utah Division of Occupational and Professional Licensure
Division of Occupational and Professional Licensing
PO Box 146741
Salt Lake City, UTAH 84114-6741
Telephone: 801/530-6628
Fax: 801/530-6511
Web site: www.dopl.utah.gov

Vermont

Vermont Board of Medical Practice
Verification of licenses

Telephone: Free of charge. Limit two verifications per call.
Written: $20 per verification. Mail requests, including physician assistant names and license numbers (if known), and payment.
Electronic: Automated verification system available at Web site.

Vermont Board of Medical Practice
1 Prospect Street
Montpelier, VERMONT 05602-1106

Telephone: 802/828-2673
Fax: 802/828-5450
Web site: www.docboard.org

Virginia

Virginia Board of Medicine

Note: Out-of-state requests: Include name, license number or Social Security number, and fee ($10 made payable to Treasurer of Virginia). Also include complete name and address where verification should be sent.

Verification of licenses

Telephone: Free of charge. Limit three verifications per day. Provide physician assistant's name, license number, or Social Security number.
Written: Free of charge. Limit 10 verifications per day. Mail or phone requests, including physician assistant's name, and license number or Social Security number.
Electronic: Available at www.dhp.state.va.us.

State Board of Medicine
Department of Health Professions
6606 W. Broad Street, Fourth Floor
Richmond, VIRGINIA 23230-1717
Telephone: 804/662-9908   804/662-7636 (automated verification)
Fax: 804/662-7281
E-mail: med.board@dhp.va.us
Web site: www.dhp.state.va.us

Washington

Health Professions Quality Assurance Division

Verification of licenses

Telephone: Free of charge. Limit three verifications; unlimited for automated verification line. Provide physician assistant's name and license number; provide code PA and physician assistant's license number.
Written: Free of charge. Mail or fax requests, including physician assistant names and license numbers.
Electronic: Automated verification service through computer modem. Dial 360/664-4144. Call for brochure containing more information.

Health Professions Quality Assurance Division
Attn: Medical Quality Assurance Commission
Department of Health
1300 S.E. Quince
PO Box 47866
Olympia, WASHINGTON 98504-7866
Telephone: 360/236-4700 (general information)   360/664-4111 (automated verification system)
Fax: 360/586-4573
E-mail: lisa.pigott@doh.wa.gov
Web site: www.doh.wa.gov

West Virginia

West Virginia Board of Medicine
Verification of licenses
Telephone: Free of charge. Limit three verifications per call.
Written: $25 per verification. Mail requests, including physician assistant/physician names and license numbers (if known), and payment.
Electronic: Not provided.

West Virginia Board of Medicine
101 Dee Drive
Charleston, WEST VIRGINIA 25311
Telephone: 304/558-2921
Fax: 304/558-2084
Web site: www.wvdhhr.org/wvbom

Wisconsin

Wisconsin Medical Examining Board
Verification of licenses
Telephone: Free of charge.
Written: $10 per verification for other state boards.
Electronic: All verification requests must be accessed on agency's Web site (www.drl.state.wi.us). If you cannot access the Internet, submit your justification in writing to address below.

Medical Examining Board
Department of Regulation and Licensing
PO Box 8935
Madison, WISCONSIN 53708
Telephone: 608/266-2112
Fax: 608/261-7083
E-mail: dorl@drl.state.wi.us
Web site: www.drl.state.wi.us

Wyoming

Wyoming Board of Medicine
Note: $45 for list of physician assistant license numbers.
Verification of licenses
Telephone: Free of charge. Limit one verification per call.
Written: $25 per verification. Faxed upon request. Mail or fax requests, including physician assistant names and license numbers (if known).
Electronic: Not provided.

Wyoming Board of Medicine
211 W. 19th Street, Second Floor
Cheyenne, WYOMING 82002
Telephone: 307/778-7053
Fax: 307/778-2069
E-mail: wyomedical@wyomedicalboard.org
Web site: wyomedboard.state.wy.us

Nursing Licensing Agencies

Alabama

Alabama Board of Nursing
Verification of licenses

Telephone: Free of charge. Preferred use: automated verification system. Provide nurse's license number.
Written: $25 per verification. Call for a request form. Mail completed request forms, including nurse names and license numbers (if known), and payment.
Electronic: Not provided.

Alabama Board of Nursing
770 Washington Avenue, Suite 250
RSA Plaza
Montgomery, ALABAMA 36104
Telephone: 334/242-4060 (general information)   334/242-0767 (automated verification system)
Fax: 334/242-4360
Web site: www.abn.state.al.us

Alaska

Alaska Board of Nursing
Verification of licenses

Telephone: Free of charge. Limit five verifications per day; Internet verification strongly recommended.
Written: $20 per verification. Mail requests, including nurse names and license numbers (if known), and payment.
Electronic: Free of charge. Available on Web site (preferred method).

Alaska Board of Nursing
Department of Community and Economic Development
Division of Occupational Licensing
PO Box 110806
Juneau, ALASKA 99811-0806
Telephone: 907/465-2544 (last name A-K)   907/465-2648 (last name L-Z)
Fax: 907/465-2974
E-mail: licens@dced.state.ak.us
Web site: www.dced.state.ak.us/occ/pnur.htm

Arizona

Arizona State Board of Nursing
Verification of licenses

Telephone: Free of charge.
Written: $25 fee for RNs and LPNs; $10 fee for CNAs.
Electronic: Not provided.

Arizona State Board of Nursing
1651 E. Morten Avenue, Suite 210
Phoenix, ARIZONA 85020
Telephone: 602/331-8111

Fax: 602/906-9365
E-mail: arizona@azbn.org
Web site: www.azboardofnursing.org

Arkansas

Arkansas State Board of Nursing
Verification of licenses

Telephone:	Free of charge at 501/682-2200.
Written:	Not provided.
Electronic:	Automated verification system available at Web site. Subscription required.

Arkansas State Board of Nursing
University Tower Building, Suite 800
1123 S. University
Little Rock, ARKANSAS 72204
Telephone: 501/686-2700   501/682-2200 (phone verification)
Fax: 501/686-2714
Web site: www.arsbn.org

California

California Board of Registered Nursing
Verification of licenses

Telephone:	Free of charge. Callers with license numbers should call the toll-free automated system number listed; others should call the general information number listed.
Written:	$2 per verification. Mail requests, including nurse names and license numbers, and payment. $60 fee for out-of-state requests.
Electronic:	Not provided.

California Board of Registered Nursing
400 R Street, Suite 4030
Sacramento, CALIFORNIA 95814
Telephone: 916/322-3350 800/838-6828   (automated verification line—accessible only to calls originating within California)
Web site: www.rn.ca.gov

Fresno-UCSF School of Nursing
Notes: *Although UCSF no longer offers the Nurse Anesthesia (CRNA) Program, you may still verify degrees.*
Verification of degrees

Telephone:	Free of charge
Written:	Free of charge. Faxed upon request. Mail or fax requests, including signed release forms.
Electronic:	Not provided.

Office of Student Affairs, Room N-319X
Fresno-UCSF School of Nursing
Box 0602
2 Koret Way
San Francisco, CALIFORNIA 94143-0602

Telephone: 415/476-1435
Fax: 415/476-9707
Web site: nurseweb.ucsf.edu

Colorado

Colorado Board of Nursing
Verification of licenses
Telephone: Automated verification system at 303/894-7888.
Written: Not provided.
Electronic: Automated verification available on Web site.

Colorado Board of Nursing
1560 Broadway, Suite 880
Denver, COLORADO 80202
Telephone: 303/894-2430 (general information)   303/894-7888 (automated verification system)
Fax: 303/894-2821
Web site: www.dora.state.co.us/nursing

Connecticut

Connecticut Board of Examiners for Nursing
Verification of licenses
Telephone: Free of charge. Limit 5–10 verifications (depending on call volume).
Written: Free of charge. Mail or fax requests, including nurse names and license numbers (if known). Faxed upon request.
Electronic: Automated verification system available on Web site.

Department of Public Health
Board of Examiners for Nursing
410 Capitol Avenue
PO Box 340308
MS #12 MQA
Hartford, CONNECTICUT 06134-0308
Telephone: 860/509-7603
Fax: 860/509-7607
Web site: www.ct-clic.com

Delaware

Delaware Board of Nursing
Verification of licenses
Telephone: Not provided.
Written: $10 per verification. Mail requests, including nurse's name and license number (if known), and payment.
Electronic: Not provided.

Delaware Board of Nursing
Division of Professional Regulation
861 Silver Lake Boulevard

Canon Building, Suite 203
Dover, DELAWARE 19904
Telephone: 302/744-4516
Fax: 302/739-2711

District of Columbia

Department of Health
Verification of licenses

Telephone: Free of charge.
Written: $50 per verification from medical doctor; $20 for all others. Mail requests, including nurse names and license numbers (if known), and check or money order (payable to D.C. Treasurer).
Electronic: Not provided.

Department of Health
Health Professional Licensing Administration
825 N. Capitol Street NE, Room 2224
Washington, DISTRICT OF COLUMBIA 20002
Telephone: 202/442-9200
Fax: 202/442-9431
Web site: www.dchealth.dc.gov

Florida

Florida Board of Nursing
Verification of licenses

Telephone: Free of charge in emergency situations only (see telephone number listed).
Written: $25. Mail requests, including nurse names and license numbers (if known).
Electronic: Free of charge.

Florida Board of Nursing
4080 Woodcock Drive, Suite 202
Jacksonville, FLORIDA 32202
Telephone: 904/858-6940 (general information)   850/488-0595 (emergency telephone verifications only)
Web site: www.doh.state.fl.us/mqa

Georgia

Georgia Board of Nursing (RN)
Verification of licenses

Telephone: Not provided.
Written: Free of charge within United States.
Electronic: Automated verification system available at Web site.

Georgia Board of Nursing
237 Coliseum Drive
Macon, GEORGIA 31217
Telephone: 478/207-1640

Fax: 478/207-1660
E-mail: gabon@sos.state.ga.us
Web site: www.sos.state.ga.us/plb/rn

Hawaii

Hawaii Board of Nursing

Notes: Verification conducted via Consumer Resource Center at 808/587-3295 or www.ehawaiigov.org/serv/pvl. Must provide nurse's name and Social Security number or license number. For disciplinary information through Web site, visit www.ehawaiigov.org/serv/rico.

Verification of licenses

Telephone:	Free of charge.
Written:	$15 per verification. Mail requests, including nurse names and license numbers (if known), and check made payable to Commerce and Consumer Affairs.
Electronic:	Not provided.

Professional and Vocation Licensing Division
Hawaii Board of Nursing
PO Box 3469
Honolulu, HAWAII 96801
Telephone: 808/586-3000
Fax: 808/586-3031
Web site: www.state.hi.us/dcca/pvl

Idaho

Idaho Board of Nursing
Verification of licenses

Telephone:	Free of charge. Limit three verifications per call.
Written:	$0.50 per name if written verification is mailed back; add $1 per page if verification is faxed. Mail requests, including nurse names, Social Security numbers and license numbers (if known), and payment.
Electronic:	Not provided.

Idaho Board of Nursing
PO Box 83720
Boise, IDAHO 83720-0061
Telephone: 208/334-3110
Fax: 208/334-3262
E-mail: lcoley@ibn.state.id.us
Web site: www.state.id.us/ibn/ibnhome.htm

Illinois

Department of Professional Regulation
Verification of licenses

Telephone:	Free of charge. Limit three verifications per call.
Written:	$20 per verification. Mail requests, including nurse names and license numbers (if known), and payment.
Electronic:	Automated verification system available at Web site.

Department of Professional Regulation
Licensure Maintenance Unit
320 W. Washington Street, Third Floor
Springfield, ILLINOIS 62786
Telephone: 217/782-0458
Fax: 217/557-8073
Web site: www.dpr.state.il.us

Indiana

Indiana State Nursing Board
Verification of licenses

Telephone: Free of charge. Call 888/333-7515.
Written: $10 per verification. Mail requests, including nurse's name and license number (if known).
Electronic: Automated verification system available at Web site. Call 800/236-5446 for more information.

Indiana State Nursing Board
Health Professions Bureau
402 W. Washington Street, Room 041
Indianapolis, INDIANA 46204
Telephone: 317/234-2043
Fax: 317/233-4236
E-mail: hpb2@hpb.state.in.us
Web site: www.in.gov/hpb

Iowa

Iowa Board of Nursing
Verification of licenses

Telephone: Free of charge. Automated verification service.
Written: $3 for each verification. Mail requests, including nurse names and license numbers (if known).
Electronic: Information available on Web site.

Iowa Board of Nursing
River Point Business Park
400 S.W. Eighth Street, Suite B
Des Moines, IOWA 50309-4685
Telephone: 515/281-3255
Fax: 515/281-4825
E-mail: ibon@bon.state.ia.us
Web site: www.state.ia.us/nursing

Kansas

Kansas State Board of Nursing
Verification of licenses

Telephone: Not provided.
Written: Fewer than 6, $2; 6–10, $3; 11–15, $4; 16–20, $5; more than 20, additional $1 per five names. Faxed: Fewer than 6, $2.50; 6–10, $3.50; 11–15, $4.50; 16–20, $5.50, more than 20, additional $1.50 per

Nursing Licensing Agencies

	five names. Mail requests, names, license numbers, and payment.
Electronic:	Not provided.

Kansas State Board of Nursing
Landon State Office Building
900 S.W. Jackson, Suite 551-S
Topeka, KANSAS 66612-1230
Telephone: 785/296-4929   785/296-3928 (verifications)
Fax: 785/296-3929
E-mail: info@ksbn.ks.us
Web site: www.ksbn.org

Kentucky

Kentucky Board of Nursing
Verification of licenses

Telephone:	Call automated verification number listed. $2.95 for first minute; $0.50 for each additional minute.
Written:	$1 per name; minimum charge $10.
Electronic:	Electronic verification is provided at $0.70 per name.

Kentucky Board of Nursing
312 Wittington Parkway, Suite 300
Louisville, KENTUCKY 40222-5172
Telephone: 502/329-7000 (general information)   900/555-5700 (automated verification system)
Fax: 502/329-7011
E-mail: kbn@mail.state.ky.us
Web site: www.kdn.state.ky.us

Louisiana

Louisiana State Board of Nursing
Verification of licenses

Telephone:	Free of charge. Callers with license numbers or Social Security numbers should call the automated verification system. All other requests must be written.
Written:	Free of charge. Mail or fax requests, including nurse names and license numbers (if known). Faxed upon request.
Electronic:	Information and forms available at Web site.

Louisiana State Board of Nursing
3510 N. Causeway Boulevard, Suite 501
Metairie, LOUISIANA 70002
Telephone: 504/838-5332 (general information) 504/838-5430 (automated verification system)
Fax: 504/838-5349
E-mail: lsbn@lsbn.state.la.us
Web site: www.lsbn.state.la.us

Maine

Maine State Board of Nursing
Verification of licenses

Telephone: Free of charge. Limit five verifications per call.
Written: $2 per verification. Mail requests, including nurse names, license numbers or Social Security numbers, and payment.
Electronic: Free of charge online at www.state.me.us/boardofnursing.

Maine State Board of Nursing
158 State House Station
Augusta, MAINE 04333-0158
Telephone: 207/287-1133
Fax: 207/287-1149
Web site: www.state.me.us/boardofnursing

Maryland

Maryland Board of Nursing
Verification of licenses

Telephone: Free of charge. Call automated verification system.
Written: $10 per verification. Mail requests, including nurse's name and license number (if known), and payment. $100 annual subscription to have verifications faxed back.
Electronic: Not provided.

Maryland Board of Nursing
4140 Patterson Avenue
Baltimore, MARYLAND 21215-2254
Telephone: 410/585-1900   877/847-0624 (general information)   877/847-0626   410/585-1978 (automated verification system)
Fax: 410/358-3530
Web site: www.mbon.org

Massachusetts

Massachusetts Board of Registration in Nursing
Notes: Verifications conducted through the National Council.
Verification of licenses

Telephone: Free of charge.
Written: $30 for another state verification conducted through National Council.
Electronic: Not provided.

Massachusetts Board of Registration in Nursing
239 Causeway Street
Boston, MASSACHUSETTS 02114
Telephone: 617/727-9961
Fax: 617/727-1630
Web site: www.state.ma.us/reg/boards/rn

Michigan

Board of Nursing
Verification of licenses

Telephone: Call automated verification number. $1.50 per minute.

Written: Verifications to party other than U.S. state: $5 per verification. Written verifications to another U.S. state: $15 per verification. Mail request, including licensee name and number, and payment to address below.

Electronic: Information available on Web site.

Michigan Department of Consumer & Industry Services
Bureau of Health Services
Attention: Education Testing & Credentials Section
PO Box 30670
Lansing, MICHIGAN 48909
Telephone: 517/335-0918 (general information)   900/555-8374 (automated verification system)
Fax: 517/373-2179
Web site: www.cis.state.mi.us/free

Minnesota

Minnesota Board of Nursing
Verification of licenses

Telephone: Technical support for Minnesota list and license line: 612/296-0930 (Monday–Thursday 8:00 a.m. to 5:00 p.m.; Friday 8:00 a.m. to 3:00 p.m.)

Written: Free of charge. Mail or fax requests, including nurse's name, and license number or Social Security number.

Electronic: Minnesota License Line: 900/388-7888; information accessed by license number only. Charged per minute.

Minnesota Board of Nursing
2829 University Avenue SE, Suite 500
Minneapolis, MINNESOTA 55414-3253
Telephone: 612/617-2270 (general information)
Fax: 612/617-2190
E-mail: nursingboard@state.mn.us
Web site: www.nursingboard.state.mn.us

Mississippi

Mississippi Board of Nursing
Verification of licenses

Telephone: Free of charge. Callers with nurse's Social Security number or license number should call the automated verification number listed.

Written: $20 for out-of-state requests. Mail requests, including nurse names and license numbers (if known), and payment.

Electronic: Not provided.

Mississippi Board of Nursing
1935 Lakeland Drive, Suite B
Jackson, MISSISSIPPI 39216-5014

Telephone: 601/987-4188 (general information)   601/987-6858 (automated verification system)
Fax: 601/364-2352
Web site: www.msbn.state.ms.us

Missouri

Missouri State Board of Nursing
Verification of licenses

Telephone:	Free of charge. Limit four verifications per call.
Written:	Free of charge. Mail or fax requests, including nurse names and license numbers (if known). Faxed upon request.
Electronic:	Directory available through download at www.ecodev.state.mo.us/dr.

Missouri State Board of Nursing
PO Box 656
3605 Missouri Boulevard
Jefferson City, MISSOURI 65109
Telephone: 573/751-0681
Fax: 573/751-0075 or 573/751-6745
Web site: www.ecodev.state.mo.us/pr/nursing

Montana

Montana State Board of Nursing
Verification of licenses

Telephone:	Free of charge.
Written:	$25 per verification. Mail requests, including nurse names and license numbers (if known), and payment.
Electronic:	Not provided.

Montana State Board of Nursing
301 South Park
PO Box 200513
Helena, MONTANA 59620-0513
Telephone: 406/444-2071
Fax: 406/841-2343
E-mail: compolnur@state.mt.us
Web site: www.com.state.mt.us/license/pol/index.htm

Nebraska

Nebraska Department of Regulation and Licensure
Note: RN licenses must be renewed on October 31 (even years only). LPN licenses must be renewed on October 31 (odd years only).

Verification of licenses

Telephone:	Free of charge. Limit two verifications per call.
Written:	Not provided.
Electronic:	Not provided.

Nebraska Health and Human Services System
Department of Regulation and Licensure
Credentialing Division
PO Box 94986
Lincoln, NEBRASKA 68509-4986
Telephone: 402/471-4376
Fax: 402/471-1066
Web site: www.hhs.state.ne.us

Nevada

Nevada State Board of Nursing
Verification of licenses

Telephone: Free of charge.
Written: $25 per verification. Mail requests, including nurse names, license numbers (if known) or Social Security numbers, and payment.
Electronic: Information available on the Web site.

Nevada State Board of Nursing
PO Box 46886
Las Vegas, NEVADA 89114
Telephone: 702/486-5800
Fax: 702/486-5803
E-mail: lasvegas@nsbn.state.nv.us
Web site: www.nursingboard.state.nv.us

New Hampshire

New Hampshire Board of Nursing
Verification of licenses

Telephone: Free of charge. Callers with license numbers should call the toll-free automated system number listed; others should call the general information number listed.
Written: $25 per verification. Mail requests, including nurse names and license numbers (if known), and check payable to Treasurer of State of New Hampshire.
Electronic: Not provided.

New Hampshire Board of Nursing
PO Box 3898
78 Regional Drive
Concord, NEW HAMPSHIRE 03302-3898
Telephone: 603/271-2323 (general information)   603/271-6599 (automated verification system)
Fax: 603/271-6605
Web site: www.state.nh.us/nursing

New Jersey

New Jersey Board of Nursing
Verification of licenses

Telephone: Free of charge. Limit three verifications per day; unlimited verifications on automated verification system. Faxed upon request.

Chapter 6

Written: $25 per written verification. Mail requests, including nurse names, license numbers (if known), and payment. $30 verification fee for endorsement to another state (per state).
Electronic: Not provided.

New Jersey Board of Nursing
PO Box 45010
Newark, NEW JERSEY 07101
Telephone: 973/504-6430   973/273-8090 (automated verification system)
Fax: 973/648-3481
E-mail: polanskyp@smtp.lps.state.nj.us
Web site: www.state.nj.us/lps/ca/home.htm

New Mexico

New Mexico Board of Nursing
Verification of licenses

Telephone: Free of charge. Callers with nurse license numbers or Social Security numbers should use the 24-hour automated verification system; others should call the same number during business hours.
Written: Free of charge. Mail requests, including nurse names and license numbers (if known).
Electronic: Information available on Web site.

New Mexico Board of Nursing
4206 Louisiana NE, Suite A
Albuquerque, NEW MEXICO 87109
Telephone: 505/841-8340
Fax: 505/841-8347
E-mail: boardofnursing@state.nm.us
Web site: www.state.nm.us/nursing

North Carolina

North Carolina Board of Nursing
Verification of licenses

Telephone: Free of charge. Call automated verification number listed.
Written: Not provided.
Electronic: Available through Web site.

North Carolina Board of Nursing
PO Box 2129
Raleigh, NORTH CAROLINA 27602-2129
Telephone: 919/881-2272 (automated verification system)   919/782-3211 (general information)
Fax: 919/781-9461
Web site: www.ncbon.com

North Dakota

North Dakota Board of Nursing
Verification of licenses

Telephone: Free of charge.
Written: $5 for 1–5 verifications, $7 for 6–10, $9 for 11–15, $10 for 16–20, $20 for 21–50, and $35 for 51–100. Mail requests, including nurse names and license numbers (if known), and payment.
Electronic: Information at Web site.

North Dakota Board of Nursing
919 S. Seventh Street, Suite 504
Bismarck, NORTH DAKOTA 58504-5881
Telephone: 701/328-9777
Fax: 701/328-9785
E-mail: ckalanek@ndbon.org
Web site: www.ndbon.org

Ohio

Ohio Board of Nursing
Notes: We do not certify nurse's aides.
Verification of licenses

Telephone: Free of charge. Call automated verification number listed.
Written: $5 per verification. Mail requests, including nurse names and license numbers (if known), and payment (payable to Treasurer, State of Ohio).
Electronic: Automated verification system available at Web site. Requires license number or Social Security number.

Ohio Board of Nursing
17 S. High Street, Suite 400
Columbus, OHIO 43215
Telephone: 614/466-3947 (general information)   614/752-3980 (automated verification system)
Fax: 614/466-0388
Web site: www.state.oh.us/nur

Oklahoma

Oklahoma Board of Nursing
Verification of licenses

Telephone: Free of charge. Limit three verifications per call.
Written: Free of charge. Mail requests, including nurse names, license numbers, and expiration dates. (Please mail if requesting only one verification.) $30 fee per verification if from another board or out-of-state.
Electronic: Verification and renewal available at Web site.

Oklahoma Board of Nursing
2915 N. Classen Boulevard, Suite 524
Oklahoma City, OKLAHOMA 73106
Telephone: 405/962-1800
Fax: 405/962-1821
E-mail: oklahoma@osf.state.ok.us
Web site: www.youroklahoma.com/nursing

Oregon

Oregon State Board of Nursing
Note: Registered Nurses and LPNs are licensed.
Verification of licenses
Telephone: Free of charge. Call automated verification number listed.
Written: $12 per verification. Mail or fax requests, including nurse's name and license number (if known).
Electronic: Not provided.

Oregon State Board of Nursing
800 NE Oregon Street, Suite 465
Portland, OREGON 97232
Telephone: 503/731-4745 (general information)   503/731-3459 (automated verification system)
Fax: 503/731-4755
E-mail: oregon.bn.info@state.or.us
Web site: www.osbn.state.or.us

Pennsylvania

Pennsylvania State Board of Nursing
Verification of licenses
Telephone: Free of charge. Limit three verifications per call.
Written: $40 fee for verification of original licensure to another state.
Electronic: Information available on Web site (www.licensepa.state.pa.us).

Pennsylvania State Board of Nursing
PO Box 2649
Harrisburg, PENNSYLVANIA 17105-2649
Telephone: 717/783-7142
Fax: 717/783-0822
E-mail: nursing@pados.dos.state.pa.us
Web site: www.dos.state.pa.us

Puerto Rico

Office of Regulation and Certification of Health Care Professionals
Verification of licenses
Telephone: Not provided.
Written: $20 per verification. Call or fax for standardized forms (faxed upon request). Mail requests, including forms, nurse names and license numbers, self-addressed, stamped envelope, and payment (certified check or money order payable to Secretary of the Treasury of Puerto Rico).
Electronic: Not provided.

Department of Health
Office of Regulation and Certification of Health Care Professionals
PO Box 10200
Santurce, PUERTO RICO 00908-0020

Telephone: 787/725-8161   787/725-7904   787/725-8125
Fax: 787/725-7903

Rhode Island

Rhode Island Board of Nurse Registration & Nursing Education
Verification of licenses

Telephone: Encouraged to use Web site for verification.
Written: Free of charge. Mail requests, including nurse names and license numbers (if known). Encouraged to use Web site for verification.
Electronic: Information available on Web site.

Rhode Island Board of Nurse Registration & Nursing Education
Department of Health
3 Capitol Hill, Room 105
Providence, RHODE ISLAND 02908-5097
Telephone: 401/222-5700
Fax: 401/222-3352
Web site: www.healthri.org

South Carolina

South Carolina State Board of Nursing
Verification of licenses

Telephone: Free of charge. Limit three verifications per call.
Written: Free of charge. Mail or fax requests, including nurse names, dates of birth, and license numbers (if known) or Social Security numbers.
Electronic: Information available at www.llr.state.sc.us.

South Carolina State Board of Nursing
PO Box 12367
Columbia, SOUTH CAROLINA 29211-2367
Telephone: 803/896-4550
Fax: 803/896-4525
Web site: www.llr.state.sc.us/pol/nursing

South Dakota

South Dakota Board of Nursing
Verification of licenses

Telephone: Free of charge.
Written: Free of charge. Call, mail, or fax requests, including nurse names and license numbers (if known).
Electronic: Not provided.

South Dakota Board of Nursing
4300 S. Louise Avenue, Suite C1
Sioux Falls, SOUTH DAKOTA 57106-3124
Telephone: 605/362-2760
Fax: 605/362-2768
Web site: www.state.sd.us/dcr/nursing

Tennessee

Tennessee Board of Nursing
Verification of licenses

Telephone: Free of charge.
Written: $15 per verification. Mail requests, including nurse names and license numbers (if known), signed release form, and payment.
Electronic: Automated verification system available at Web site.

Tennessee Board of Nursing
Department of Health
Cordell Hull Building, First Floor
Nashville, TENNESSEE 37247-1010
Telephone: 888/310-4650
Web site: www.state.tn.us/health

Texas

Texas Board of Nurse Examiners
Verification of licenses

Telephone: Free of charge. Provide nurse's license number or Social Security number.
Written: $20 fee for written information; no state-to-state verification.
Electronic: Verification available through e-mail free of charge.

Texas Board of Nurse Examiners
333 Guadalupe, Suite 3-460
PO Box 430
Austin, TEXAS 78701
Telephone: 512/305-7400
Fax: 512/305-7401
E-mail: webmaster@bne.state.tx.us
Web site: www.bne.state.tx.us

Vermont

Vermont State Board of Nursing
Verification of licenses

Telephone: Free of charge.
Written: $20 per verification. Mail requests, including nurse names and license numbers (if known), and payment. Faxed upon request.
Electronic: Not provided.

Vermont State Board of Nursing
81 River Street
Montpelier, VERMONT 05609-1106
Telephone: 802/828-2453
Fax: 802/828-2484
E-mail: bashford@sec.state.vt.us
Web site: www.vtprofessionals.org/nurses

Virginia

Virginia Board of Nursing
Verification of licenses
Telephone: Free of charge. Call automated verification number 804/662-7636.
Written: Free of charge. Mail or fax requests, including nurse names, and license numbers (if known) or Social Security numbers.
Electronic: Information is available on Web site.

Virginia Board of Nursing
6606 W. Broad Street, Fourth Floor
Richmond, VIRGINIA 23230-1717
Telephone: 804/662-9909 (general information)   804/662-7636 (automated verification system)
Fax: 804/662-9512
E-mail: nursebd@dhp.state.va.us
Web site: www.dhp.state.va.us/nurse/choose.htm

Washington

Washington State Nursing Care Quality Assurance Commission
Verification of licenses
Telephone: Free of charge. Call automated license verification system at 360/664-4111 or fax 360/236-4818.
Written: Free of charge. Mail requests, including nurse names and license numbers (if known). Or fax to 360/236-4818.
Electronic: Available by e-mail.

Washington State Nursing Care Quality Assurance Commission
Department of Health
PO Box 47864
Olympia, WASHINGTON 98504-7864
Telephone: 360/236-4700 (office)   360/664-4111 (automated verification system)
Fax: 360/236-4818
E-mail: hpqa.csc@doh.wa.gov
Web site: www.doh.wa.gov/nursing

West Virginia

West Virginia Board of Examiners for Registered Professional Nurses
Verification of licenses
Telephone: Free of charge.
Written: Free of charge in-state (with self-addressed stamped envelope); $30 to verify to another state. Will complete agency form. Mail requests, including nurse names and license numbers (if known), and payment.
Electronic: Not provided.

West Virginia Board of Examiners for Registered Professional Nurses
101 Dee Drive
Charleston, WEST VIRGINIA 25311-1620

Telephone: 304/558-3596
Fax: 304/558-3666
E-mail: westvirginiarn@ncsbn.org
Web site: www.state.wv.us/nurses/rn

Wisconsin

State of Wisconsin Department of Regulation & Licensing Board of Nursing
Verification of licenses

Telephone: Free of charge.
Written: Free of charge. Used only for endorsements to other states for a $10 fee. Web site verification strongly recommended.
Electronic: Information available on Web site.

State of Wisconsin Department of Regulation & Licensing Board of Nursing
PO Box 8935
Madison, WISCONSIN 53708-8935
Telephone: 608/266-2112
Fax: 608/261-7083
E-mail: dorl@drl.state.wi.us
Web site: www.drl.state.wi.us

Wyoming

Wyoming State Board of Nursing
Verification of licenses

Telephone: Free of charge.
Written: $40 per verification if a seal is required. Mail requests, including nurse names and license numbers (if known), and payment. Faxed upon request (free of charge).
Electronic: Not provided.

Wyoming State Board of Nursing
2020 Carey Avenue, Suite 110
Cheyenne, WYOMING 82002
Telephone: 307/777-7601
Fax: 307/777-3519
E-mail: ckoski@state.wy.us
Web site: nursing.state.wy.us

Psychology Licensing Agencies

Alabama

Alabama Board of Examiners in Psychology
Verification of licenses

Telephone: Free of charge. Limit two verifications per call.
Written: Free of charge. Mail requests, including psychologist names and license numbers (if known).
Electronic: Not provided.

> Alabama Board of Examiners in Psychology
> 660 Adams Avenue, Suite 360
> Montgomery, ALABAMA 36104
> Telephone: 334/242-4127
> Web site: psychology.state.al.us

Alaska

Alaska Board of Psychologist and Psychological Associate Examiners
Verification of licenses

Telephone: Free of charge.
Written: $20 per verification. Mail requests, including psychologist names and license numbers (if known), and payment.
Electronic: Not provided.

> State of Alaska
> Department of Community & Economic Development
> Division of Occupational Licensing
> PO Box 110806
> Juneau, ALASKA 99811-0806
> Telephone: 907/465-3811
> Fax: 907/465-2974
> E-mail: ginger_morton@dced.state.ak.us
> Web site: www.dced.state.ak.us/occ/ppsy.htm

Arizona

Arizona Board of Psychologist Examiners
Verification of licenses

Telephone: Free of charge. Limit 15 verifications per day.
Written: $2 per verification. Mail requests, including psychologist names and license numbers (if known), and payment.
Electronic: Free of charge.

> Arizona Board of Psychologist Examiners
> 1400 W. Washington, Room 235
> Phoenix, ARIZONA 85007
> Telephone: 602/542-8162
> Fax: 602/542-8279
> E-mail: info@psychboard.az.gov
> Web site: www.psychboard.az.gov

Chapter 6

Arkansas

Board of Examiners in Psychology
Verification of licenses

Telephone: Not provided.
Written: $10 per verification. Mail requests, including psychologist's name and license number (if known), signed release form, and self-addressed, stamped envelopes.
Electronic: Not provided.

Board of Examiners in Psychology
101 E. Capitol, Suite 415
Little Rock, ARKANSAS 72201
Telephone: 501/682-6168
Fax: 501/682-6165
E-mail: ginger.wages@mail.state.ar.us
Web site: www.accessarkansas.org/abep

California

California Board of Psychology
Verification of licenses

Telephone: Free of charge. Limit three verifications per call.
Written: Free of charge. Call for order form 07M-106. Mail requests, order form, and self-addressed, stamped envelope.
Electronic: Information available on Web site.

License Verification
1422 Howe Avenue, Suite 22
Sacramento, CALIFORNIA 95825-3200
Telephone: 916/263-2696
Fax: 916/263-2944
E-mail: bopmail@dca.ca.gov
Web site: www.psychboard.ca.gov

Colorado

Board of Psychologist Examiners
Verification of licenses

Telephone: Free of charge. Limit three verifications per call.
Written: Free of charge. Mail requests, including psychologist names and license numbers (if known).
Electronic: Automated verification at Web site.

Board of Psychologist Examiners
1560 Broadway, Suite 1370
Denver, COLORADO 80202
Telephone: 303/894-7767
Fax: 303/894-7747
Web site: www.dora.state.co.us/mental-health/psyboard.htm

Connecticut

Department of Public Health
Verification of licenses

Telephone: Free of charge. Limit three verifications per call. When calling customer service (860/509-7603), you may receive a busy signal due to high call volume. In this case, fax the verification request.

Written: Free of charge. Limit 10 verifications per query. Faxed upon request. Mail or fax requests, including psychologist names and license numbers (if known), and Connecticut release forms (upon request). If faxing, specify Attention: Frank.

Electronic: Automated verification system available at www.state.ct.us/dph/scripts/hlthprof.asp.

Connecticut Board of Examiners of Psychologists
Department of Public Health
410 Capitol Avenue, MS #12MQA
PO Box 340308
Hartford, CONNECTICUT 06134-0308
Telephone: 860/509-7603
Fax: 860/509-7607 or 860/509-8457
Web site: www.ct-clic.com

Delaware

Board of Examiners of Psychology
Verification of licenses

Telephone: Not provided.

Written: $10 per verification. Mail requests, including psychologist's name and license number (if known), and payment.

Electronic: Not provided.

Board of Examiners of Psychology
Division of Professional Regulation
861 Silver Lake Boulevard
Cannon Building, Suite 203
Dover, DELAWARE 19904
Telephone: 302/739-4507 302/744-4507 (Victoria L. Gingrich)
Fax: 302/739-2711
Web site: www.professionallicensing.state.de.us/boards/psychology

District of Columbia

District of Columbia Board of Psychology
Verification of licenses

Telephone: Free of charge.

Written: $20 per verification; check made payable to D.C. Treasurer. Mail requests, including psychologist names and license numbers (if known), and payment.

Electronic: Not provided.

Board of Psychology
825 North Capitol Street NE
Suite 2224
Washington, DISTRICT OF COLUMBIA 20002

Telephone: 202/442-4764
Fax: 202/442-9431
Web site: http://dchealth.dc.gov

Florida

Florida Board of Psychology
Verification of licenses

Telephone: Free of charge. Limit three verifications per call.
Written: $25 per verification. Mail requests, including physician names and license numbers (if known), and payment.
Electronic: Upon request, will send written certification via e-mail or fax.

Division of Medical Quality Assurance
Client Services Unit
HMQAMS/Bin C99
4050 Bald Cypress Way, Bin C05
Tallahassee, FLORIDA 32399-3255
Telephone: 850/245-4373
Fax: 850/487-9626
E-mail: health@doh.state.fl.us
Web site: www.doh.state.fl.us/mqa

Georgia

Georgia State Board of Examiners of Psychologists
Verification of licenses

Telephone: Free of charge. Limit three verifications per call.
Written: $25. Faxed upon request. Mail or fax requests, including psychologist names and license numbers (if known), and signed release forms.
Electronic: Not provided.

Georgia State Board of Examiners of Psychologists
237 Coliseum Drive
Macon, GEORGIA 31217-3858
Telephone: 912/207-1670
Fax: 912/207-1676
E-mail: sosweb@sos.state.ga.us
Web site: www.sos.state.ga.us

Hawaii

Board of Psychology
Verification of licenses

Telephone: Free of charge. Provide psychologist's license number.
Written: $15 per verification. Mail requests, including psychologist's name and license number.
Electronic: Online verification available at www.ehawaiigov.org/serv/pvl.

Psychology Licensing Agencies

Board of Psychology
Department of Commerce and Consumer Affairs
PO Box 3469
Honolulu, HAWAII 96801
Telephone: 808/586-3000 (licensing information) 808/586-2693 (Board) 808/587-3295 (verifications and complaints)
Fax: 808/586-3031
E-mail: psychology@dcca.state.hi.us
Web site: www.state.hi.us/dcca/pvl

Idaho

Board of Psychologist Examiners
Verification of licenses

Telephone: Free of charge.
Written: Free of charge; $10 for verifications signed and sealed by bureau chief. Mail or fax requests, including psychologist names and license numbers (if known), and payment (if applicable).
Electronic: Not provided.

Idaho Board of Psychologist Examiners
1109 Main Street, Suite 220
Boise, IDAHO 83702-5642
Telephone: 208/334-3233
Fax: 208/334-3945
E-mail: ibol@ibol.state.id.us
Web site: www.state.id.us/ibol/psy.htm

Illinois

Clinical Psychologists Licensing & Disciplinary Committee
Verification of licenses

Telephone: Free of charge. Limit three verifications per call. Provide psychologist's name, license number, and Social Security number (if known).
Written: First three verifications free of charge.
Electronic: Automated verification system available at Web site.

Licensure Maintenance Unit
Clinical Psychologists Licensing & Disciplinary Committee
320 W. Washington Street, Third Floor
Springfield, ILLINOIS 62786
Telephone: 217/524-2167
Fax: 217/557-8073
Web site: www.dpr.state.il.us/who/psych.asp

Indiana

Indiana State Psychology Board
Verification of licenses

Telephone: Call 888/333-7515. Give psychologist's name or license number (if known).
Written: Not provided.
Electronic: Automated verification system available at Web site. No fee for simple verification. Subscription or credit card required for further information. Call 800/236-5446 for more information.

> Indiana State Psychology Board
> Health Professions Bureau
> 402 W. Washington Street, Room 041
> Indianapolis, INDIANA 46204
> Telephone: 317/234-2057 (receptionist)   317/234-2057 (Psychology Board)
> Fax: 317/233-4236
> E-mail: hpb7@hpb.state.in.us
> Web site: www.in.gov/hpb

Iowa

Board of Psychology Examiners
Verification of licenses

Telephone: Free of charge.
Written: $10 per verification. Mail requests, including psychologist's name and license number (if known), and payment.
Electronic: Automated verification at 515/281-4031.

> Board of Psychology Examiners
> Department of Public Health
> Lucas State Office Building, Fifth Floor
> 321 E. 12th Street
> Des Moines, IOWA 50319-0075
> Telephone: 515/281-4401
> Fax: 515/281-3121
> E-mail: jscheffe@idph.state.ia.us
> Web site: www.idph.state.ia.us/licensure

Kansas

Behavioral Sciences Regulatory Board
Verification of licenses

Telephone: Not provided.
Written: $5 per verification. Mail requests, including psychologist names and license numbers (if known), signed release forms, and payment.
Electronic: Available at Web site, if INK subscription is current. Online verifications: $2.

> Behavioral Sciences Regulatory Board
> 712 S. Kansas Avenue
> Topeka, KANSAS 66603-3817

Telephone: 785/296-3240
Fax: 785/296-3112
E-mail: lallen@ink.org
Web site: www.ksbsrb.org/psychologists.html

Kentucky

Kentucky Board of Examiners of Psychology
Verification of licenses

Telephone: Free of charge. Limit two per day.
Written: $15 per verification. Mail requests, including psychologist names and license numbers (if known), signed release forms, and payment.
Electronic: Verifications available on Web site.

Kentucky Board of Examiners of Psychology
PO Box 1360
Frankfort, KENTUCKY 40602
Telephone: 502/564-3296, Ext. 225
Fax: 502/564-4818
E-mail: wendy.satterly@mail.state.ky.us
Web site: www.state.ky.us/agencies/finance/boards/psychology

Louisiana

State Board of Examiners of Psychologists
Verification of licenses

Telephone: Free of charge.
Written: $5 per verification. Mail requests, including psychologist names and license numbers (if known), and payment.
Electronic: Free of charge.

State Board of Examiners of Psychologists
8280 YMCA Plaza Drive
Building 8B
Baton Rouge, LOUISIANA 70810
Telephone: 225/763-3935
Fax: 225/763-3968
E-mail: lsbep@earthlink.net
Web site: www.lsbep.org

Maine

Board of Examiners of Psychologists
Verification of licenses

Telephone: Not provided.
Written: $10 per verification. Mail requests, including psychologist names and license numbers (if known), and payment.
Electronic: Free of charge. Disciplinary actions also available.

Chapter 6

> Board of Examiners of Psychologists
> 35 State House Station
> Augusta, MAINE 04333-0035
> Telephone: 207/624-8603
> Fax: 207/624-8637
> Web site: www.maineprofessionalreg.org

Maryland

Board of Examiners of Psychologists
Verification of licenses

Telephone:	Free of charge. Limit three verifications per day.
Written:	$20 per verification. Mail requests, including psychologist names and license numbers (if known), and payment.
Electronic:	Not provided.

> Board of Examiners of Psychologists
> 4201 Patterson Avenue
> Baltimore, MARYLAND 21215
> Telephone: 410/764-4787
> Fax: 410/358-7896
> E-mail: brownju@dhmh.state.md.us

Massachusetts

Division of Professional Licensure
Verification of licenses

Telephone:	No longer available.
Written:	$10 per verification, made payable to Commonwealth of Massachusetts. Mail requests, including psychologist's name and license numbers (if known), self-addressed, stamped envelope, and payment.
Electronic:	Automated verification system available at Web site.

> Board of Registration of Psychologists
> 239 Causeway Street
> Boston, MASSACHUSETTS 02114
> Telephone: 617/727-9925
> Fax: 617/727-1627
> E-mail: karen.schwartz@state.ma.us
> Web site: www.state.ma.us/reg

Michigan

Board of Psychology
Verification of licenses

Telephone:	Automated verification system: 900/555-8374. $1.50 per minute.
Written:	Verifications to party other than U.S. state: $5 per verification. Written verifications to another U.S. state: $15 per verification. Mail request, including licensee name and number, and payment to address below.
Electronic:	Automated verification system available at Web site.

Psychology Licensing Agencies

Michigan Board of Psychology
Bureau of Health Services
Attn: Education Testing & Credentials Section
611 West Ottawa
Lansing, MICHIGAN 48909
Telephone: 517/373-9102 (general information)   900/555-8374 (automated verification system)
Fax: 517/241-2895
Web site: www.cis.state.mi.us

Minnesota

Minnesota Board of Psychology
Verification of licenses

Telephone: Not provided.
Written: $20 per verification. Mail requests, including psychologist names and license numbers (if known), and payment.
Electronic: Not provided.

Minnesota Board of Psychology
2829 University Avenue SE, Suite 320
St. Paul, MINNESOTA 55414-3237
Telephone: 612/617-2230
Fax: 612/617-2240
E-mail: psychology.board@state.mn.us

Mississippi

Mississippi State Board of Psychological Examiners
Verification of licenses

Telephone: Free of charge. Limit five verifications per call.
Written: Free of charge. Mail requests, including psychologist names and license numbers (if known), self-addressed, stamped envelopes, and payment.
Electronic: Fax psychologist names to number listed.

Mississippi State Board of Psychological Examiners
4273 I-55N
Suite 104
Jackson, MISSISSIPPI 39202
Telephone: 601/321-0616
Fax: 662/751-4628
E-mail: hedwards@maminc.net

Missouri

State Committee of Psychologists
Verification of licenses

Telephone: Free of charge.
Written: Free of charge. Mail requests, including psychologist names and license numbers (if known), signed release forms, and payment. Verification to another state (state agency only): $25.
Electronic: Not provided.

State Committee of Psychologists
PO Box 1335
3605 Missouri Boulevard
Jefferson City, MISSOURI 65102-0153
Telephone: 573/751-0099
Fax: 573/526-3489
E-mail: scop@mail.state.mo.us
Web site: www.ded.state.mo.us/regulatorylicensing/professionalregistration/psych

Montana

Board of Psychologists
Verification of licenses

Telephone:	Free of charge.
Written:	Free of charge. Mail requests, including psychologist names and license numbers (if known), signed release forms.
Electronic:	Free of charge.

Board of Psychologists
301 S. Park Avenue, Fourth Floor
PO Box 200513
Helena, MONTANA 59620-0513
Telephone: 406/841-2394
Fax: 406/841-2305
E-mail: dlibsdpsy@state.mt.us
Web site: www.discoveringmontana.com/dli/psy

Nebraska

Nebraska Board of Examiners of Psychologists
Verification of licenses

Telephone:	Free of charge. Limit three verifications per call. Provide psychologist's name and license number (if known).
Written:	$5 per verification to verify dates and license numbers. $25 per verification for any further information. Mail requests, including psychologist names and license numbers (if known), and payment.
Electronic:	Automated verification system available at Web site.

Nebraska Health and Human Services System
Department of Regulation and Licensure
Credentialing Division
301 Centennial Mall South, PO Box 94986
Lincoln, NEBRASKA 68509-4986
Telephone: 402/471-2117
Fax: 402/471-3577
E-mail: kris.chiles@hhss.state.ne.us
Web site: www.hhs.state.ne.us/lis/lis.asp

Nevada

State of Nevada Board of Psychological Examiners
Verification of licenses

Telephone: Free of charge. Limit five verifications per call. Open Monday–Thursday, 9:00 a.m. to 12:00 p.m.
Written: $15 per verification. Mail requests, including psychologist names and license numbers (if known).
Electronic: Not provided.

> State of Nevada Board of Psychological Examiners
> PO Box 2286
> Reno, NEVADA 89505-2286
> Telephone: 702/688-1268
> Fax: 775/688-1272
> E-mail: nbop@govmail.state.nv.us

New Hampshire

Board of Mental Health Practice
Notes: Also social worker and mental health worker licensing.
Verification of licenses

Telephone: Free of charge. Limit five verifications per day.
Written: Free of charge. Mail requests, including psychologist names and license numbers (if known).
Electronic: Not provided.

> Board of Mental Health Practice
> 49 Donovan Street
> Concord, NEW HAMPSHIRE 03301
> Telephone: 603/271-6762
> Fax: 603/271-3950
> Web site: webster.state.nh.us/mhpb

New Jersey

New Jersey State Board of Psychological Examiners
Verification of licenses

Telephone: Free of charge. Limit three verifications per call. 973/273-8090 (24 hours a day).
Written: Free of charge.
Electronic: Available on Web site.

> New Jersey State Board of Psychological Examiners
> PO Box 45017
> Newark, NEW JERSEY 07101
> Telephone: 973/504-6460
> Fax: 973/273-8020
> Web site: www.state.nj.us/lps/ca/medical.htm#psy13

New Mexico

New Mexico Board of Psychologist Examiners
Verification of licenses

Telephone: Free of charge.
Written: Free of charge. Faxed upon request. Mail or fax requests, including psychologist names and license numbers (if known).
Electronic: Web page verifications (www.rld.state.nm.us).

New Mexico Board of Psychologist Examiners
2055 S. Pacheco Street, Suite 400
PO Box 25101
Santa Fe, NEW MEXICO 87504-25101
Telephone: 505/476-7077
Fax: 505/476-7087
E-mail: gloria.carrillo@state.nm.us
Web site: www.rld.state.nm.us/b&c/psychology

New York

State Board for Psychology
Notes: Additional e-mail address for Psychology Board: opunit3@mail.nysed.gov.
Verification of licenses

Telephone: Free of charge. Limit two verifications per call if calling customer service automated attendant; limit five per call if calling customer service representative; unlimited if calling automated verification system. $1.50 for first minute; $1 for each additional minute.
Written: $20 per verification. Limit one verification. $10 per hundred names for multiple verifications. Mail requests, including licensee's name, license number, date of birth, and address, and payment (check or money order payable to NYS Education Dept.).
Electronic: Automated verification system also available at Web site.

New York State Board for Psychology
NYS Education Department
89 Washington Avenue, Second Floor
Albany, NEW YORK 12230-1000
Telephone: 518/474-3817, Ext. 150 (general information)   900/555-6978 (automated verification system)
Fax: 518/486-2981
E-mail: op4info@mail.nysed.gov or psychbd@mail.nysed.gov
Web site: www.op.nysed.gov

North Carolina

North Carolina Psychology Board
Notes: License to practice psychology granted every two years.
Verification of licenses

Telephone: Free of charge. Limit five verifications per call.
Written: $10 per verification. Mail requests, including psychologist names and license numbers (if known), and payment.
Electronic: Information available on Web site.

North Carolina Psychology Board
895 State Farm Road, Suite 101
Boone, NORTH CAROLINA 28607
Telephone: 828/262-2258
Fax: 828/265-8611
E-mail: ncpsybd@helicon.net
Web site: www.ncpsychologyboard.org

North Dakota

State Board of Psychologist Examiners
Verification of licenses

Telephone: Free of charge. Limit four verifications per call.
Written: $10 per request. Faxed upon request. Mail or fax requests, including psychologist names and license numbers (if known), and payment.
Electronic: Available on Web site.

State Board of Psychologist Examiners
PO Box 8380
Grand Forks, NORTH DAKOTA 58202
Telephone: 701/777-2044
Fax: 701/777-3454

Ohio

State Board of Psychology
Verification of licenses

Telephone: Free of charge.
Written: Free of charge. Faxed upon request. Mail or fax requests, including psychologist names and license numbers (if known), and self-addressed, stamped envelope. Provide names and items needing verification. Do not use fax cover sheet.
Electronic: Free of charge.

State Board of Psychology
77 S. High Street, Suite 1830
Columbus, OHIO 43215-6108
Telephone: 614/466-8808
Fax: 614/728-7081
E-mail: psy.license@exchange.state.oh.us
Web site: www.state.oh.us/psy

Oklahoma

State Board of Examiners of Psychologists
Verification of licenses

Telephone: Free of charge. Limit two verifications per call.
Written: Free of charge. Faxed upon request. Mail or fax requests, including psychologist names and license numbers (if known), and self-addressed, stamped envelopes.
Electronic: Not provided.

State Board of Examiners of Psychologists
201 N.E. 38th Terrace, Suite 3
Oklahoma City, OKLAHOMA 73105
Telephone: 405/524-9094
Fax: 405/271-6137

Oregon

Board of Psychologist Examiners
Verification of licenses

Telephone: Not provided.
Written: $5 per verification. Mail requests, including psychologist names and payment.
Electronic: Automated verification system available at Web site.

Board of Psychologist Examiners
3218 Pringle Road SE, Suite 130
Salem, OREGON 97302-6309
Telephone: 503/378-4154
Fax: 503/378-3575
E-mail: oregon.bpe@state.or.us
Web site: www.obpe.state.or.us

Pennsylvania

State Board of Psychology
Verification of licenses

Telephone: Free of charge. Limit three verifications per call.
Written: Free of charge. Faxed upon request. Mail or fax requests, including psychologist names and license numbers (if known).
Electronic: Free of charge at www.licensepa.state.pa.us.

State Board of Psychology
PO Box 2649
Harrisburg, PENNSYLVANIA 17105-2649
Telephone: 717/783-7155
Fax: 717/787-7769
E-mail: psycholo@pados.dos.state.pa.us
Web site: www.dos.state.pa.us/bpoa.site

Puerto Rico

Office of Regulation and Certification of Health Care Professionals
Verification of licenses

Telephone: Free of charge. Specify profession.
Written: $20 per verification. Call or fax for standardized forms (faxed upon request). Mail requests, including forms, psychologist names and license numbers, self-addressed, stamped envelope, and payment (certified check or money order payable to Secretary of the Treasury of Puerto Rico).
Electronic: Not provided.

Office of Regulation and Certification of Health Care Professionals
Department of Health
PO Box 10200
Santurce, PUERTO RICO 00908-0020
Telephone: 787-725-8161 (general information)   787-725-8121 (administration)
787-725-8130 (director)
Fax: 787-725-7903

Rhode Island

Rhode Island Board of Psychology
Notes: *Due to volume of incoming calls, it is preferable to access Web site for any information.*
Verification of licenses
Telephone: Free of charge. Limit two verifications per call. Preferred method: Web site.
Written: Faxed upon request. Mail or fax requests, including psychologist's name and license number (if known).
Electronic: Free of charge.

Board of Psychology
Health Department
3 Capitol Hill, Room 104
Providence, RHODE ISLAND 02908-5097
Telephone: 401/222-2827
Fax: 401/222-1272
Web site: www.healthri.org/hsr/professions/license.htm

South Carolina

South Carolina Board of Examiners in Psychology
Verification of licenses
Telephone: Free of charge.
Written: Free of charge. Faxed upon request. Mail or fax requests, including psychologist names and license numbers (if known).
Electronic: Available through Web site.

South Carolina Board of Examiners in Psychology
110 Centerview Drive, Kingstreet Building
PO Box 11329
Columbia, SOUTH CAROLINA 29211-1329
Telephone: 803/896-4664
Fax: 803/896-4687
E-mail: mckittrk@mail.llr.stste.sc.us
Web site: www.llr.state.sc.us

South Dakota

Board of Examiners of Psychologists
Verification of licenses
Telephone: Free of charge. Limit 10 verifications per call.

Written: Free of charge. Mail requests, including psychologist names and license numbers (if known), and self-addressed, stamped envelope.
Electronic: Not provided.

> Board of Examiners of Psychologists
> Department of Commerce & Regulation
> 135 E. Illinois, Suite 214
> Spearfish, SOUTH DAKOTA 57783
> Telephone: 605/642-1600
> Fax: 605/642-1756
> E-mail: proflic@rushmore.com
> Web site: www.state.sd.us/dcr/psychologists

Tennessee

Board of Examiners in Psychology
Verification of licenses

Telephone: Not provided.
Written: $15 per verification. Faxed upon request only after payment is received. Mail requests, including psychologist's name and license number (if known), and payment.
Electronic: Not provided.

> Board of Examiners in Psychology
> Health-Related Boards
> Cordell Hull Building, First Floor
> 425 Fifth Avenue N
> Nashville, TENNESSEE 37247-1010
> Telephone: 888/310-4650   615/532-5127
> Fax: 615/532-5369
> Web site: www.state.tn.us/health

Texas

State Board of Examiners of Psychologists
Verification of licenses

Telephone: Free of charge. Limit three verifications per call per day.
Written: $20 per verification. Mail requests, including psychologist names and license numbers (if known), and payment.
Electronic: Not provided.

> State Board of Examiners of Psychologists
> 333 Guadalupe, Suite 2-450
> Austin, TEXAS 78701
> Telephone: 512/305-7700
> Fax: 512/305-7701
> Web site: www.tsbep.state.tx.us

Utah

Division of Occupational and Professional Licensing
Verification of licenses

Telephone: Free of charge. Limit three verifications per call.
Written: Free of charge. Mail requests, including psychologist names, Social Security numbers, and license numbers (if known).
Electronic: Automated verification system available at Web site.

Division of Occupational and Professional Licensing
PO Box 146741
Heber and Wells Building
160 East 300 South
Salt Lake City, UTAH 84114-6741
Telephone: 801/530-6628
Fax: 801/530-6511
Web site: www.dopl.utah.gov

Vermont

Board of Psychological Examiners
Verification of licenses

Telephone: Free of charge. Limit four verifications per call.
Written: $20 per verification. Mail requests, including psychologist names and license numbers (if known), and payment.
Electronic: Automated verification system available at Web site.

Office of Professional Regulation
Board of Psychological Examiners
26 Terrace Street
Montpelier, VERMONT 05609-1106
Telephone: 802/828-2373
Fax: 802/828-2465
E-mail: patkins@sec.state.vt.us
Web site: www.vtprofessionals.org

Virginia

Board of Psychology
Verification of licenses

Telephone: Free of charge. Call 804/662-7636.
Written: Free of charge.
Electronic: Automated verification system available at Web site.

Board of Psychology
6606 W. Broad Street, Fourth Floor
Richmond, VIRGINIA 23230-1717
Telephone: 804/662-9913
Fax: 804/662-7250

E-mail: psy@dhp.state.va.us
Web site: www.dhp.state.va.us/psychology

Washington

State Examining Board of Psychology
Verification of licenses

Telephone:	Free of charge. Limit three verifications per call via general information number; unlimited for automated verification line. Provide code PY and psychologist's license number.
Written:	Free of charge. Mail requests, including psychologist names and license numbers (if known).
Electronic:	Not provided.

>State Examining Board of Psychology
>Department of Health
>PO Box 47869
>Olympia, WASHINGTON 98504-7869
>Telephone: 360/236-4910 (general information)   360/664-4111 (automated verification system)
>Fax: 360/236-4909
>E-mail: janice.boden@doh.wa.gov
>Web site: www.wa.gov/doh/hpqa-licensing/hps7/psychology

West Virginia

Board of Examiners of Psychologists
Verification of licenses

Telephone:	Free of charge.
Written:	Free of charge. Faxed upon request. Mail or fax requests, including psychologist names and license numbers (if known).
Electronic:	Free of charge.

>Board of Examiners of Psychologists
>PO Box 3955
>1205 Quarrier Street, Room 200
>Charleston, WEST VIRGINIA 25339-3955
>Telephone: 304/558-0604   304/558-3040 (credentialing)
>Fax: 304/558-0608
>E-mail: wvpsychologybd@mail.state.wv.us

Wisconsin

Wisconsin Psychology Examining Board
Verification of licenses

Telephone:	Not provided.
Written:	$10 per verification for other state boards. Free of charge to hospitals for verification for initial appointment. Mail requests, including each psychologist's name, license number, and a self-addressed, stamped envelope.
Electronic:	Online verifications available at Web site (go to Credential Holder Query and enter a name and profession).

Bureau of Health Service Professions
PO Box 8935
Madison, WISCONSIN 53708-8935
Telephone: 608/267-7223
E-mail: web@drl.state.wi.us
Web site: www.drl.state.wi.us

Wyoming

State Board of Psychology
Verification of licenses

Telephone: Free of charge. Limit three verifications per call.
Written: $15 per verification. Must be cashier's check or money order made payable to State of Wyoming. Mail requests, including psychologist name and license numbers (if known), and payment.
Electronic: Not provided.

Professional Licensing Boards
Attention: Psychologist license verification request
2020 Carey Avenue, Suite 201
Cheyenne, WYOMING 82002
Telephone: 307/777-6529
Fax: 307/777-3508
E-mail: dbridg@state.wy.us
Web site: soswy.state.wy.us/director/ag-bd/psych.htm

CHAPTER 7

Board Certification

Chapter 7
Board Certification

In addition to verifying education, training, and other credentials, hospitals should investigate whether a physician is board-certified. Since the early 20th century, groups of individuals working in specialty areas have banded together to form specialty boards, which establish requirements for achieving a certificate or diploma in specialties and influence the content of training programs. Practitioners who meet all of the requirements these specialty boards establish—most certifying boards review applicants' training records and ethical qualifications and require applicants to pass examinations before awarding certificates—are referred to as *board certified* or as *diplomates*.

The American Board of Medical Specialties (ABMS) notes that the fundamental objective of its member boards is to act in the public interest by improving medical care through established qualifications for candidates, and by evaluating those who apply for certification. There are 24 member boards offering 37 general and 89 subspecialty certificates. Each specialty board acts independently in determining its requirements and policies for certification. All member boards require a written exam and most also require an oral exam. ABMS does not certify podiatrists, dentists, oral surgeons, chiropractors or non-physician practitioners. More than 85 percent of physicians licensed in the United States are certified by at least one ABMS member board.

However, there are more than 180 self-designated medical boards in the United States that are not ABMS members. These boards were established essentially in the same way as the ABMS boards: A group of specialists decided that a board was needed, incorporated themselves as a board, and saw to it that the board established rigorous certification requirements. Some self-designated boards, however, might not demand the same extent of training, practice quality, and ethics. For this reason, in some states (New Jersey, for example), individuals who are certified by non-ABMS boards are not permitted to advertise as board-certified practitioners. The AMA recognizes only diplomates of ABMS boards as board-certified. The ABMS member boards are subject to extensive requirements and careful review in connection with achieving ABMS recognition; but because there is not an outside agency to review the requirements and procedures of self-designated boards and to attest to the quality of their certification requirements, self-designated boards are extremely variable in quality and purpose. If in doubt about whether a doctor has ABMS-recognized certification, the ABMS offers a verification service called The Certified Doctor *(www.abms.org)*, which provides a simple way to check. When setting criteria for appointment and privileges, medical staffs must give careful consideration to specifying which certifying boards are considered acceptable.

The Joint Commission on Accreditation of Healthcare Organizations (JCAHO) does not require board certification for appointment or privileges, but Standard MS.5.15.2 states that board certification is an excellent benchmark and should be considered when delineating clinical privileges.

Understanding specialization

Today, many physicians and other health care professionals are specialists. Specialization is an important issue in hospitals and managed care organizations. Before authorizing a practitioner to undertake advanced clinical procedures, a hospital must investigate the individual's specialized training and experience. Most managed care organizations make a distinction between specialists and generalist physicians (often called primary care practitioners [PCPs]). But even PCPs are commonly required to be board certified either in family practice or one of the small number of specialties considered to be broad enough to permit their diplomates to perform generalist care (for example, pediatrics or internal medicine).

Because the traditional route to specialization is advanced or graduate training/education—essentially what medicine and some other fields call residencies—verifying whether a practitioner has completed a residency program is an important part of credentialing and privileging (see **Chapter 3: Schools, Colleges, and Educational Programs** for more information on residency verification).

Osteopathic specialists

In the medical profession, some physicians are trained as osteopaths and receive the Doctor of Osteopathy (DO) degree rather than the MD degree. Both DOs and MDs are licensed to perform surgery and prescribe medication in all 50 states, although in some states, DOs are licensed by a different agency than MDs. Osteopaths can essentially be considered in training to be equal to MDs (allopathic physicians). Osteopathic training includes additional training in the musculoskeletal system and manipulative treatment. DOs are trained to practice a "whole person" approach to medicine, meaning that they assess the overall health of their patients, including home and work environments, in addition to treating specific symptoms or illnesses. Many osteopathic physicians are members of the American Osteopathic Association (AOA). The AOA has 18 approved specialty boards, each of which has jurisdiction over the examination leading to certification in its particular specialty/subspecialty. In addition, ABMS member boards certify both MDs and DOs who meet their requirements. Many DOs are board certified by an ABMS member board.

Although MDs rarely, if ever, apply to osteopathic boards, osteopathic physicians in many specialty fields actually have a choice as to whether to apply to an ABMS or an AOA board, or both.

Board certification for practitioners other than MDs and DOs

Many specialty boards exist for nonphysician health care professions. Specifically, there are specialty boards for dentists, podiatrists, chiropractors, physician assistants, and nurses. Like the ABMS and AOA, the major certifying bodies for these professions—for example, the American Dental Association—recognize specific boards. Hospitals can assume that diplomates of boards that are recognized by the main umbrella organization of a profession have the level of training and qualifications typically associated with board certification. For some professions—for example, physician assistants, nurse anesthetists, and nurse-midwives—the national specialty organization itself is the certifying agent. As with self-designated boards for physicians, some boards for nonphysician practitioners that are not recognized by the national specialty organization may be worthy of recognition for credentialing purposes. As with self-designated boards for physicians, organizations must determine for themselves which self-designated boards they will recognize.

Subspecialty and added qualifications certification

Subspecialties are areas of further specialization within a specialty area. Pediatric surgery, for example, is a subspecialty of surgery. Many specialty boards offer subspecialty certificates or "certificates of added qualifications" to qualified practitioners. Eligibility for a subspecialty certificate typically requires training beyond what is required for a general specialty certificate, so subspecialty certification signifies a level of training beyond the general board certificate. In many fields, subspecialization is considered desirable for academicians and those practicing in large, highly specialized, tertiary-care hospitals. Practitioners who have general certificates only (i.e., they have been certified in a specialty but not in a subspecialty) are considered trained and competent in their general specialty area. They have had "basic training" that covers the whole specialty area but have not had the extensive emphasis in the subspecialty area. Subspecialists often handle the most difficult or rare cases and tend to be found in major academic medical centers in large cities.

Recertification

An increasing number of boards now offer time-limited certificates only—as opposed to the traditional lifetime certificates—and require competence assessments/examinations for certificate renewal. Most AMA member boards require recertification after 10 years, with the exception of family practice (seven years), obstetrics/gynecology (seven years), and pediatrics (seven years). Starting in 2004, AOA will require its member boards to limit certification to 10 years or fewer. This move is in recognition of the fact that recent board certification implies—but, of course does not guarantee—a high level of professional competence, and that after a period of time, skills and knowledge might diminish. Time-limited certificates encourage specialists to maintain a high competence level and offer the public more meaningful evidence of current competence. This trend toward recertification means that organizations must stay up-to-date with the recertification practices of each of the specialty boards. When an individual's board certificate expires, organizations must verify the renewal through the primary source if board certification is a requirement of medical staff appointment or privileges.

ABMS recently approved replacing its recertification program with a Maintenance of Certification (MOC) program. This program focuses on physician practice assessment based on performance rather than just success on a written exam. The MOC includes assessment of six "general competencies": patient care, interpersonal and communication skills, professionalism, medical knowledge, practice-based learning and improvement, and systems-based practice. It contains four basic components: evidence of professional training, lifelong learning with involvement in periodic self-assessment, cognitive expertise, and evaluation of performance in practice. ABMS now requires all of its member boards to transition their recertification programs into MOC programs.

On its Web site, the ABMS publishes tables that show certification and recertification requirements *(www.abms.org/ GeneralReq.asp)*. Use these tables as a quick reference to determine whether a physician is still board-eligible based on time limits for certification.

Understanding the terms board certified, board eligible, board admissible, and board qualified

Medical specialty boards require high standards of training and performance and ensure them through the administration of rigid examinations. Sometimes, however, practitioners who are not specifically certified by the ABMS or AOA, but who have taken additional training or completed all requirements for certification except the examination, may describe themselves as board eligible, board admissible, or board qualified to distinguish themselves from those without any specialty training. Unfortunately, many of these physicians completed training years ago and are, in fact, no longer eligible to sit for the exam. Although widely used in the past, most boards no longer use the term "board eligible." AMBS discourages the use of "board eligible" by its member boards, preferring instead to note an individual's precise position in the certification process.

Board exams are typically offered on an annual basis and coincide with completion of the training program for the specialty. Some board certification exams are a two-step process consisting of a written exam and an oral exam. For some specialties, such as obstetrics and gynecology, the certification process cannot be completed until the applicant has accumulated and submitted patient case profiles for patients treated in the private practice setting. Thus, it may take one or more years after completion of training to complete the entire certification process. In addition, boards set a minimum amount of time after the physician has completed training or part one of the exam in which to complete the certification process. Failure to complete the process within the required time will result in ineligibility to sit for the exam.

Unlike ABMS member boards, the AOA continues to use the term "board eligible" and grants that status to candidates who

- document satisfactory completion of an AOA-approved residency or preceptorship program if applicable
- document the satisfactory completion of an AOA-approved internship and the completion of the practice requirement
- are and remain members in good standing of the AOA or the Canadian Osteopathic Association
- meet all the requirements established by the appropriate specialty board
- have applied to and been accepted as a registrant by the appropriate specialty board

Some specialty boards will not respond to requests for information about where individuals stand in the certification process, so it is not always possible for credentialing organizations to obtain verification of individual practitioners' status. We have, however, indicated in the following specialty board listings whether each board recognizes and will verify any terms other than "board certified."

Chiropractic boards
The Federation of Chiropractic Licensing Boards defines a "diplomate" as a practitioner who has taken all the extensive extra education and passed the certification examinations. "Board qualified" means the education is complete, but not the final examination.

Chapter overview

The remainder of this chapter is organized into eight sections—one for each of the following groups of health care professionals:

- Allopathic physicians
- Osteopathic physicians
- Dentists
- Podiatrists
- Chiropractors
- Physician assistants
- Nurse anesthetists
- Nurse-midwives

Each section describes the recognized umbrella organization for the profession and contains separate alphabetical entries on each of the specialty boards recognized by the umbrella organization.

Each board entry in this chapter includes the following key information:

- The board's use of the terms "board eligible," "board admissible," and "board qualified"
- A listing of the subspecialty and/or added qualifications certificates that the board offers
- Whether the board grants time-limited certificates and, if so, the limit and date on which time-limited certification was implemented
- The board's process for verifying certification of its diplomates
- The board's contact information

As mentioned above, nurse anesthetists, nurse-midwives, and physician assistants are examined and certified by their main professional organizations, not separate specialty boards; therefore, the sections for these professionals discuss these professional organizations only.

Guidelines for querying specialty boards

Although the entries in this chapter include any specific policies and requirements each board has for processing verifications, there are some general procedures that might help to expedite the verification process and ensure that verifications are sent to the appropriate person. Consider the following when requesting a telephone and/or written verification:

- Identify yourself clearly and state the purpose for your query when requesting telephone verifications
- Include self-addressed, stamped envelopes when requesting written verifications
- Provide any useful information—such as the name (and maiden name, if applicable), certification date, birth date, and Social Security number of a diplomate in question—to help an office retrieve the records and information more quickly and easily
- Include some sort of direction on the envelope or fax cover sheet of a verification request (e.g., Attention: Board diplomate certification verification request enclosed)
- Include clear and specific instructions as to where and to whom a board should mail or fax back written verifications (giving a department name, contact name, and/or title can help to ensure that the verification reaches the correct person)
- Include a photograph of the diplomate in question to reduce the possibility of someone successfully adopting the identity of the diplomate

The above guidelines and the specific information contained in the following sections will help ensure timely and accurate verifications of board certification. Please note that, although each board listed was contacted individually, board policies and procedures sometimes change. We appreciate receiving any updates, suggestions, and/or information you encounter regarding any of the boards described in this chapter.

Guidelines to board certification time limits

For your convenience, we've created a table that lists the recertification requirements and the month and year in which the recertification requirements were instated. This table is located in this book's Appendix.

American Board of Medical Specialties (ABMS)

American Academy of Clinical Toxicology
Note: There are four types of physician members: Active Members, International Members, Associate Members (all of whom focus in medical toxicology), and Resident Members. Active Members are certified. Please contact the Board for more information.

Certification time limits:
Recertification every four years.

Verification of membership
Telephone: Not provided.
Written: Not provided.
Electronic: Not provided.

> 777 E. Park Drive
> PO Box 8820
> Harrisburg, PENNSYLVANIA 17105-8820
> Telephone: 717/558-7847
> Fax: 717/558-7841
> E-mail: aact@pamedsoc.org
> Web site: www.clintox.org

American Board of Allergy and Immunology

General certificates:
- Allergy and immunology.

Subspecialty certificates:
- Clinical and laboratory immunology.

Certification time limits:
Allergy and immunology–Prior to 1989: lifetime certification. As of January 1, 1989: 10 years.
Clinical and laboratory immunology–Prior to 1994: lifetime certification. As of January 1, 1994: 10 years.

Verification of certificates
Telephone: Not provided.
Written: $35 per verification. Mail requests, including physician names, date of birth or Social Security number, and payment.
Electronic: Free of charge at www.abms.org

> American Board of Allergy and Immunology
> 510 Walnut Street, Suite 1701
> Philadelphia, PENNSYLVANIA 19106-3699
> Telephone: 215/592-9466
> Fax: 215/592-9411
> E-mail: abai@abai.org
> Web site: www.abai.org

American Board of Anesthesiology

Are *board eligible*, *board admissible*, and *board qualified* recognized terms?
Uses *"board eligible"* to describe applicants who have been approved to take the board's examination.

General certificates:
- Anesthesiology

Subspecialty certificates:
- Critical care medicine and pain medicine.

Certification time limits:
Prior to 2000: lifetime certification. As of 2000: 10 years.

Verification of certificates
Telephone: Free of charge. Provide name and Social Security number.
Written: $10 per verification. Mail requests, including physicians names, Social Security numbers, and payment. Faxed upon request.
Electronic: Verification available through www.certifacts.org.

> American Board of Anesthesiology
> 4101 Lake Boone Trail
> The Summit, Suite 510
> Raleigh, NORTH CAROLINA 27607-7506
> Telephone: 919/881-2570
> Fax: 919/881-2575
> Web site: www.abanes.org

American Board of Colon and Rectal Surgery

General certificates:
- Colon and rectal surgery.

Certification time limits:
Prior to 1990: lifetime certification. As of January 1, 1990: renewable every 10 years.

Verification of certificates
Telephone: Not provided.
Written: $35 per verification. Mail requests, including physician name, signed release form, and payment. Faxed upon request.
Electronic: Verification available by request.

> American Board of Colon and Rectal Surgery
> 20600 Eureka Road, Suite 600
> Taylor, MICHIGAN 48180
> Telephone: 734/282-9400
> Fax: 734/282-9402
> E-mail: admin@abcrs.org
> Web site: www.abcrs.org

American Board of Dermatology

General certificates:
- Dermatology.

Subspecialty certificates:
- Dermatopathology, Clinical and laboratory dermatological immunology.

Certification time limits:
Dermatology: 10 years.

Verification of certificates

Telephone:	Not provided.
Written:	$25 per verification. Mail requests, including physician names and payment.
Electronic:	Not provided.

American Board of Dermatology
Henry Ford Hospital
1 Ford Place
Detroit, MICHIGAN 48202
Telephone: 313/874-1088
Fax: 313/872-3221
E-mail: abdermc@hfhs.org
Web site: www.abderm.org

American Board of Emergency Medicine

General certificates:
- Emergency medicine.

Subspecialty certificates:
- Medical toxicology, pediatric emergency medicine, sports medicine, and undersea and hyperbaric medicine.

Certification time limits: 10 years.

Verification of certificates

Telephone:	Free of charge. Limited information only.
Written:	$25 per verification. Mail requests, including physician name, signed release form, and payment.
Electronic:	Not provided.

American Board of Emergency Medicine
3000 Coolidge Road
East Lansing, MICHIGAN 48823
Telephone: 517/332-4800
Fax: 517/332-2234
E-mail: abem@abem.org
Web site: www.abem.org

Chapter 7

American Board of Family Practice

General certificates:
- Family practice.

Certificates of added qualifications:
- Geriatric medicine, Sports medicine, Adolescent medicine.

Certification time limits:
General certificates: Seven years. Subspecialty certificates: 10 years.

Verification of certificates

Telephone: Not provided.
Written: $25 per verification. Mail requests, including physician names and payment.
Electronic: Verification available at www.abfp.org/verifications at no charge.

> American Board of Family Practice
> c/o Verifications Department
> 2228 Young Drive
> Lexington, KENTUCKY 40505-4294
> Telephone: 859/269-5626   888/995-5700 (toll-free)
> Fax: 859/335-7509
> E-mail: general@abfp.org
> Web site: www.abfp.org

American Board of Internal Medicine

General certificates:
- Internal medicine.

Subspecialty certificates:
- Cardiovascular disease, Endocrinology, diabetes, and metabolism, Gastroenterology, Hematology, Infectious disease, Medical oncology, Nephrology, Pulmonary disease, Rheumatology.

Certificates of added qualifications:
- Adolescent medicine, Clinical and laboratory immunology (with American Board of Allergy and Immunology), Clinical cardiac electrophysiology, Critical care medicine, Geriatric medicine, Interventional cardiology, Sports medicine.

Certification time limits:
Critical-care medicine. As of January 1, 1987: 10 years.
Geriatric medicine: as of January 1, 1988: 10 years.
All others: prior to 1990: lifetime certification. As of January 1, 1990: 10 years.

Verification of certificates

Telephone: Free of charge. Provide physician's name and Social Security number or certificate number.
Written: Free of charge. Mail requests, including physician names, and Social Security numbers or certificate numbers.
Electronic: www.certifacts.org.

Specialty Boards

American Board of Internal Medicine
510 Walnut Street, Suite 1700
Philadelphia, PENNSYLVANIA 19106-3699
Telephone: 215/446-3500 800/441-2246
Fax: 215/446-3470
E-mail: request@abim.org
Web site: www.abim.org

American Board of Medical Genetics, Inc.

General certificates:
- Clinical biochemical genetics; Clinical biochemical/Molecular genetics (offered only in 1990 and 1993), Clinical cytogenetics; Clinical genetics; Clinical molecular genetics; Specialty exam in molecular genetic pathology.

Certification time limits:
Prior to 1993: lifetime certification. As of January 1, 1993: 10 years.

Verification of certificates
Telephone: Not provided.
Written: $35 per verification. Mail requests, including physician names and payment.
Electronic: Not provided.

American Board of Medical Genetics, Inc.
9650 Rockville Pike
Bethesda, MARYLAND 20814-3998
Telephone: 301/571-1825
Fax: 301/571-1895
E-mail: srobinson@genetics.faseb.org
Web site: www.abmg.org

American Board of Medical Specialties (ABMS)

Verification of certificates
Telephone: Consumers only call 866/275-2267. Companies call 800/521-8110 for information on Official ABMS Directory of Board Certified Medical Specialists (also on CD/ROM). Available through publisher only.
Written: Not provided.
Electronic: Not provided.

American Board of Medical Specialties
1007 Church Street
Suite 404
Evanston, ILLINOIS 60201
Telephone: 847/491-9091
Fax: 847/328-3596
Web site: www.abms.org

American Board of Neurological Surgery

Note: National certifying agency for neurosurgery.

General certificates:
- Neurological surgery.

Certification time limits: Lifetime certification prior to 1999. After 1999: 10 years.

Verification of certificates

Telephone: Free of charge; prefer written request.
Written: Free of charge. Mail or fax requests, including physician names and signed release forms.
Electronic: Not provided.

> American Board of Neurological Surgery
> Smith Tower, Suite 2139
> 6550 Fannin Street
> Houston, TEXAS 77030
> Telephone: 713/790-6015
> Fax: 713/794-0207
> E-mail: abns@tmh.tmc.edu
> Web site: www.abns.org

American Board of Nuclear Medicine

General certificates:
- Primary certification for nuclear medicine.

Certification time limits:
Prior to 1992: lifetime certification. As of January 1, 1992: 10 years.

Verification of certificates

Telephone: Not provided.
Written: $25 per verification. Mail requests, including physician names and payment. Faxed upon request.
Electronic: Not provided.

> American Board of Nuclear Medicine
> 900 Veteran Avenue
> Los Angeles, CALIFORNIA 90024-1786
> Telephone: 310/825-6787
> Fax: 310/794-4821
> Web site: www.abnm.org

American Board of Obstetrics and Gynecology

General certificates:
- Obstetrics and Gynecology.

Subspecialty certificates:
- Critical care medicine, Gynecologic oncology, Maternal and Fetal medicine, Reproductive endocrinology.

Certification time limits:
As of 2001, certificates are limited to six years for all certification.

Verification of certificates

Telephone: Not provided.
Written: $25 per verification. Mail requests, including physician names and payment. Faxed upon request for an additional $15.
Electronic: Not provided.

> American Board of Obstetrics and Gynecology
> 2915 Vine Street
> Dallas, TEXAS 75204
> Telephone: 214/871-1619
> Fax: 214/871-1943
> Web site: www.abog.org

American Board of Ophthalmology

General certificates:
- Ophthalmology.

Certification time limits:
Prior to 1992: lifetime certification. As of July 1, 1992: 10 years.

Verification of certificates

Telephone: Not provided.
Written: $35 per certification. Mail requests, including physician names and payment.
Electronic: Not provided.

> American Board of Ophthalmology
> 111 Presidential Boulevard, Suite 241
> Bala Cynwyd, PENNSYLVANIA 19004
> Telephone: 610/664-1175
> Fax: 610/664-6503
> E-mail: mrladden@abop.org
> Web site: www.abop.org

American Board of Orthopaedic Surgery

General certificates:
- Orthopedic surgery.

Subspecialty certificates:
- Hand surgery.

Certification time limits: Prior to 1986: lifetime certification. As of January 1, 1986: 10 years.

Verification of certificates

Telephone: Free of charge. Limited information only.
Written: $25 per verification. Mail requests, including physician names, signed release forms, and payment.
Electronic: Not provided.

> American Board of Orthopaedic Surgery
> 400 Silver Cedar Court
> Chapel Hill, NORTH CAROLINA 27514
> Telephone: 919/929-7103
> Fax: 919/942-8988
> Web site: www.abos.org

American Board of Otolaryngology

General certificates:
- Otolaryngology.

Certification time limits: Prior to 2002: lifetime certification. Beginning 2002: renewal every 10 years.

Verification of certificates

Telephone: Free of charge.
Written: $20 per verification. Mail requests, including physician names and payment.
Electronic: Not provided.

> American Board of Otolaryngology
> 3050 Post Oak Boulevard, Suite 1700
> Houston, TEXAS 77056-6579
> Telephone: 713/850-0399
> Fax: 713/850-1104
> Web site: www.aboto.org

American Board of Pathology

Are *board eligible,* *board admissible,* and *board qualified* recognized terms?
Does not recognize above terms.

General certificates:
- Anatomic & clinical pathology, Anatomic pathology, Clinical pathology.

Subspecialty certificates:
- Blood banking/transfusion medicine, Chemical pathology, Cytopathology, Dermatopathology (with the American Board of Dermatology), Forensic pathology, Hematology, Immunopathology (ended 1999), Medical microbiology, Neuropathology, Pediatric pathology.

Certification time limits:
Lifetime certification. As of January 1, 1996: voluntary recertification. Time-limited certificates take effect January 1, 2006.

Verification of certificates

Telephone:	Not provided.
Written:	$25 per verification. Mail requests, including physician names and payment.
Electronic:	Not provided.

American Board of Pathology
PO Box 25915
Tampa, FLORIDA 33622-5915
Telephone: 813/286-2444
Fax: 813/289-5279
Web site: www.abpath.org

American Board of Pediatrics

Are *board eligible*, *board admissible*, and *board qualified* recognized terms?
Does not recognize above terms.

General certificates:
- Pediatrics.

Subspecialty certificates:
- Adolescent medicine, Clinical & laboratory immunology, Medical toxicology, Neonatal-perinatal medicine, Pediatric cardiology, Pediatric critical care medicine, Pediatric emergency medicine, Pediatric endocrinology, Pediatric gastroenterology, Pediatric hematology-oncology, Pediatric infectious disease, Pediatric nephrology, Pediatric pulmonology, Pediatric rheumatology, Sports medicine.

Certification time limits: Prior to May 1988: lifetime certification. As of May 1, 1988: 7 years.

Verification of certificates

Telephone:	Free of charge. Limit three verifications per day. Provide physician's Social Security number.
Written:	$25 per verification. Mail requests, including physician names, Social Security numbers, and maiden names (if applicable), and payment.
Electronic:	www.abp.org.

American Board of Pediatrics
111 Silver Cedar Court
Chapel Hill, NORTH CAROLINA 27514
Telephone: 919/929-0461
Fax: 919/929-9255
E-mail: abpeds@abpeds.org
Web site: www.abp.org

Chapter 7

American Board of Physical Medicine and Rehabilitation

Are *board eligible*, *board admissible*, and *board qualified* recognized terms?
Uses the term "board admissible" to describe applicants whose applications have been reviewed and who are approved to take the examination for the current year.

General certificates:
- Physical medicine and rehabilitation.

Subspecialty certificates:
- Spinal cord injury medicine, Pain medicine.

Certification time limits:
Prior to May 1993: lifetime certification. As of May 1, 1993: 10 years for both general and subspecialty certificates.

Verification of certificates
Telephone: Free of charge.
Written: $35 per verification. Mail requests, including physician names and payment.
Electronic: Not provided.

> American Board of Physical Medicine and Rehabilitation
> 21 First Street SW, Suite 674
> Rochester, MINNESOTA 55902
> Telephone: 507/282-1776
> Fax: 507/282-9242
> E-mail: office@abpmr.org
> Web site: www.abpmr.org

American Board of Plastic Surgery, Inc.

General certificates:
- Plastic surgery.

Subspecialty certificates:
- Hand surgery.

Certification time limits:
General certification: Prior to November 1995: lifetime certification. As of November 1, 1995: 10 years. Hand surgery: 10 years.

Verification of certificates
Telephone: Free of charge. Limit three verifications per call.
Written: Free of charge. Limit three per month. $25 for each additional verification. Mail requests, including physician names and payment.
Electronic: Not provided.

> American Board of Plastic Surgery, Inc.
> 7 Penn Center, Suite 400
> 1635 Market Street
> Philadelphia, PENNSYLVANIA 19103-2204

Telephone: 215/587-9322
Fax: 215/587-9622
E-mail: info@abplsurg.org
Web site: www.abplsurg.org

American Board of Preventive Medicine

General certificates:
- Aerospace medicine, Occupational medicine, Public health/general preventive medicine.

Subspecialty certificates:
- Medical toxicology, Undersea medicine.

Certification time limits:
Prior to 1997: lifetime certification. As of January 1, 1997: 10 years

Verification of certificates
Telephone: Free of charge.
Written: $25 per certification. Mail requests, including physician names and payment.
Electronic: Available on www.certifacts.org.

American Board of Preventive Medicine
330 S. Wells Street, Suite 1018
Chicago, ILLINOIS 60606
Telephone: 312/939-2276
Fax: 312/939-2218
E-mail: abpm@abprevmed.org
Web site: www.abprevmed.org

American Board of Psychiatry and Neurology

General certificates:
- Psychiatry, Neurology, Neurology with special qualifications in child neurology.

Subspecialty certificates:
- Addiction psychiatry, Child and adolescent psychiatry, Forensic psychiatry, Geriatric psychiatry, Clinical neurophysiology, Pain management, Neurodevelopmental disabilities.

Certification time limits:
Prior to October 1994: lifetime certification. As of October 1, 1994: 10 years.

Verification of certificates
Telephone: Not provided.
Written: $25 per verification. Mail requests, including physician names, dates of birth, and Social Security numbers, signed release forms, and payment.
Electronic: www.certifacts.org

American Board of Psychiatry and Neurology
500 Lake Cook Road, Suite 335
Deerfield, ILLINOIS 60015
Telephone: 847/945-7900
Web site: www.abpn.com

American Board of Radiology

General certificates:
- Radiology (last offered in 1979), Diagnostic radiology, Radiation oncology, Radiological physics.

Certificates of added qualifications:
- Neuroradiology, Pediatric radiology, Vascular & interventional radiology, Special Competence in Nuclear radiology.

Certification time limits:
Prior to November 1995: lifetime certification. As of November 1, 1995: 10 years. Radiation oncology and CAOs only.

Verification of certificates
Telephone: Not provided.
Written: $25 per verification. Mail requests, including physician names and payment.
Electronic: www.abms.org.

American Board of Radiology
4541 E. Williams Boulevard, Suite 200
Tucson, ARIZONA 85711
Telephone: 520/790-2900
Fax: 520/790-3200
E-mail: info@theabr.org
Web site: www.theabr.org

American Board of Surgery

General certificates:
- Surgery.

Subspecialty certificates:
Hand surgery, Pediatric surgery, Surgical critical care, Vascular surgery.

Certification time limits:
Prior to 1976: lifetime certification. As of January 1, 1976: 10 years.

Verification of certificates
Telephone: Free of charge.
Written: Free of charge. Mail requests, including physician names.
Electronic: Provided at www.certifacts.org.

American Board of Surgery
1617 John F. Kennedy Boulevard, Suite 860
Philadelphia, PENNSYLVANIA 19103-1847

Telephone: 215/568-4000
Fax: 215/563-5718
Web site: www.absurgery.org

American Board of Thoracic Surgery

General certificates:
- Thoracic surgery.

Certification time limits:
Prior to May 1976: lifetime certification. As of May 1, 1976: 10 years.

Verification of certificates
Telephone: Not provided.
Written: $50 per verification. Mail requests, including physician names and payment.
Electronic: Not provided.

American Board of Thoracic Surgery
1 Rotary Center, Suite 803
Evanston, ILLINOIS 60201
Telephone: 847/475-1520
Fax: 847/475-6240
E-mail: abts_evanston@msn.com
Web site: www.abts.org

American Board of Urology, Inc.

General certificates:
- Urology.

Certification time limits:
Prior to February 1985: lifetime certification. As of February 1, 1985: 10 years.

Verification of certificates
Telephone: Not provided.
Written: $35 per verification. Mail requests, including physician names, signed release forms, and payment.
Electronic: Not provided.

American Board of Urology, Inc.
2216 Ivy Road, Suite 210
Charlottesville, VIRGINIA 22903
Telephone: 434/979-0059
Fax: 434/979-0266
Web site: www.abu.org

American College of Medical Toxicology

Note: There are four types of physician members: Active Members, International Members, Associate Members (all of whom focus on medical toxicology), and Resident Members. Active Members are certified. Please contact the Board for more information.

Verification of membership
Telephone: Not provided.
Written: Not provided.
Electronic: Information available on Web site.

> American College of Medical Toxicology
> 777 E. Park Drive
> PO Box 8820
> Harrisburg, PENNSYLVANIA 17105-8820
> Telephone: 717/558-7846
> Fax: 717/558-7841
> E-mail: ashambaugh@pamedsoc.org
> Web site: www.acmt.net

American Osteopathic Association (AOA) Boards

Are *board eligible*, *board admissible*, and *board qualified* recognized terms?
The AOA and all its member boards use the term *board eligible* to describe the status of applicants who have satisfactorily completed an AOA-approved residency or preceptorship program.

General certificates:
- Diagnostic radiology.
- Radiation oncology.

Certificates of added qualifications:
- Vascular and interventional radiology.
- Body imaging.
- Neuroradiology.
- Nuclear radiology.
- Pediatric radiology.

Certification time limits:
Lifetime certification.

Verification of certificates
Telephone: Not provided.
Written: Not provided.
Electronic: $20 per AOA Osteopathic Physician Profile Report ordered over Internet at www.aoa-net.org.

> American Osteopathic Association
> 142 E. Ontario Street
> Chicago, ILLINOIS 60611

Telephone: 312/202-8000
Fax: 312/202-8200
Web site: www.aoa-net.org

American Osteopathic Board of Anesthesiology

General certificate:
- Anesthesiology.

Certificates of added qualifications:
- Critical care medicine.
- Pain management.

Certification time limits:
Prior to 2000: lifetime certification. As of January 1, 2000: 10 years.

Verification of certificates
Telephone: Not provided.
Written: Not provided; contact the AOA.
Electronic: $15 per AOA Osteopathic Physician Profile Report ordered over Internet (www.aoa-net.org).

American Osteopathic Board of Anesthesiology
17201 E. US Highway 40, Suite 204
Independence, MISSOURI 64055-6427
Telephone: 816/373-4700
Fax: 816/373-1529

American Osteopathic Board of Dermatology

Are *board eligible*, *board admissible*, and *board qualified* recognized terms?
See AOA policy above.

General certificates:
- Dermatology.

Certificates of added qualifications:
- MOHS-micrographic surgery.
- Dermatopathology.

Certification time limits:
Lifetime certification in dermatology. Every 10 years for certificates of added qualifications.

Verification of certificates
Telephone: AOA Profile Department: 800/621-1773, Ext. 8145.
Written: $20 for AOA Profile Report. Call 800/621-1773, Ext. 8145.
Electronic: $15 per AOA Osteopathic Physician Profile Report ordered over Internet (www.aoa-net.org).

American Osteopathic Board of Dermatology
5426 N. Academy Boulevard, Suite 205
Colorado Springs, COLORADO 80918
Telephone: 719/531-5400
Fax: 719/531-9545
Web site: www.aoa-net.org

American Osteopathic Board of Emergency Medicine

Are *board eligible*, *board admissible*, and *board qualified* recognized terms?
See AOA policy above.

General certificates:
- Emergency medicine.

Certificates of added qualifications:
- Emergency medical services.
- Medical toxicology.

Certification time limits:
Prior to 1994: lifetime certification. As of January 1, 1994: 10 years.

Verification of certificates
Telephone: Not provided.
Written: Not provided; contact the AOA.
Electronic: $15 per AOA Osteopathic Physician Profile Report ordered over Internet (www.aoa-net.org).

American Osteopathic Board of Emergency Medicine
142 E. Ontario Street, Eighth Floor
Chicago, ILLINOIS 60611
Telephone: 312/335-1065
Fax: 312/335-5489

American Osteopathic Board of Family Physicians

General certificates:
- Family practice.

Certificates of added qualifications:
- Geriatric medicine.
- Sports medicine.
- Addiction medicine.

Certification time limits:
Prior to March 1997: lifetime certification. As of March 1997: eight years.

Verification of certificates
Telephone: Not provided; contact the AOA. Board will verify board eligibility.
Written: Not provided.
Electronic: $15 per AOA Osteopathic Physician Profile Report ordered over Internet (www.aoa-net.org).

American Osteopathic Board of Family Physicians
330 E. Algonquin Road, Suite 6
Arlington Heights, ILLINOIS 60005
Telephone: 847/640-8477 800/390-5801 (recorded information line)
Web site: www.aobfp.org

American Osteopathic Board of Internal Medicine

Are *board eligible*, *board admissible*, and *board qualified* recognized terms?
See AOA policy above.

General certificates:
- Internal Medicine, Allergy/immunology, Cardiology, Endocrinology, Gastroenterology, Hematology, Infectious disease, Pulmonary diseases, Nephrology, Oncology, Rheumatology.

Certificates of added qualifications:
- Critical care medicine, Electrophysiology, Geriatric medicine, Sports medicine, Addiction medicine.

Certification time limits:
Prior to 1993: lifetime certification. As of January 1, 1993: 10 years.

Verification of certificates
Telephone: Not provided.
Written: Submit to AOBIM in writing (via letter or e-mail). $15 verification fee.
Electronic: $15 per AOA Osteopathic Physician Profile Report ordered over Internet (www.aoa-net.org).

American Osteopathic Board of Internal Medicine
Attn: Gary Slick
20201 S Crawford Ave.
Olympia Fields, ILLINOIS 60461
Telephone: 708/747-4000, Ext. 1909
E-mail: gls_aobim@ameritch.net

American Osteopathic Board of Neurology and Psychiatry

Are *board eligible*, *board admissible*, and *board qualified* recognized terms?
See AOA policy above.

General certificates:
- Neurology, Psychiatry, Child/adolescent psychiatry, Child/adolescent neurology.

Certificates of added qualifications:
- Addiction medicine.

Certification time limits:
Prior to 1996: lifetime certification. As of January 1, 1996: 10 years.

Verification of certificates

Telephone: Not provided; contact the AOA.
Written: Not provided; contact the AOA.
Electronic: $15 per AOA Osteopathic Physician Profile Report ordered over Internet (www.aoa-net.org).

American Osteopathic Board of Neurology and Psychiatry
2250 Chapel Avenue
Cherry Hill, NEW JERSEY 08002
Telephone: 609/601-1225

American Osteopathic Board of Neuromusculoskeletal Medicine

Note: Organization AOA/BMM.

Are *board eligible*, *board admissible*, and *board qualified* recognized terms?
See AOA policy above.

Certificates:
- Neuromusculoskeletal medicine.
- Osteopathic manipulative medicine.

Certification time limits:
Prior to 1995: lifetime certification. As of January 1, 1995: 10 years.

Verification of certificates

Telephone: Free of charge.
Written: Free of charge. Faxed upon request. Mail or fax requests, including signed release forms and payment.
Electronic: $15 per AOA Osteopathic Physician Profile Report ordered over Internet (www.aoa-net.org).

American Osteopathic Board of Neuromusculoskeletal Medicine
3500 DePauw Boulevard, Suite 1080
Indianapolis, INDIANA 46268
Telephone: 317/879-1881
Fax: 317/879-0563
Web site: www.academyofosteopathy.org

American Osteopathic Board of Nuclear Medicine

Verification of certificates

Telephone: $25 per AOA Osteopathic Physician Profile Report ordered via phone number listed.
Written: Not provided.
Electronic: $25 per AOA Osteopathic Physician Profile Report ordered over Internet (www.aoa-net.org).

American Osteopathic Board of Nuclear Medicine
Attention: Robbin McClary
142 E. Ontario Street
Chicago, ILLINOIS 60611
Telephone: 312/202-8266

Fax: 312/202-8202
Web site: www.aoa-net.org/certification/miclear.htm

American Osteopathic Board of Ophthalmology and Otorhinolaryngology

General certificates:
- Facial plastic surgery, Ophthalmology, Otorhinolaryngology, Otorhinolaryngology and facial plastic surgery.

Certification time limits:
Ophthalmologists: Prior to 2000: lifetime certification. As of January 1, 2000: 10 years.
Otorhinolaryngologists: Prior to 2002: lifetime certification. As of January 1, 2002: 10 years

Verification of certificates
Telephone: Not provided.
Written: Free of charge.
Electronic: Not provided.

> American Osteopathic Board of Ophthalmology and Otorhinolaryngology
> 3 MacKoil Avenue
> Dayton, OHIO 45403
> Telephone: 937/252-0868
> Fax: 937/252-0968

American Osteopathic Board of Orthopedic Surgery

Are *board eligible, board admissible,* and *board qualified* recognized terms?
See AOA policy above.

General certificates:
- Orthopedic surgery.

Certification time limits:
Prior to 1994: lifetime certification. As of January 1, 1994: 10 years.

Verification of certificates
Telephone: Not provided; contact the AOA. Board will verify board eligibility.
Written: Not provided; contact the AOA.
Electronic: $15 per AOA Osteopathic Physician Profile Report ordered over Internet (www.aoa-net.org).

> American Osteopathic Board of Orthopedic Surgery
> PO Box 707
> Hershey, PENNSYLVANIA 17033-0707
> Telephone: 877/98-AOBOS (toll-free)
> Fax: 717/534-0624
> E-mail: aobos@aobos.org
> Web site: aobos.org

American Osteopathic Board of Preventive Medicine

Are *board eligible*, *board admissible*, and *board qualified* recognized terms?
See AOA position above.

General certificates:
- Preventive medicine/aerospace medicine, Preventive medicine/occupational-environmental medicine, Preventive medicine/public health.

Certificates of added qualifications:
- Occupational medicine.

Certification time limits:
Prior to 1994: lifetime certification. As of January 1, 1994: 10 years.

Verification of certificates
Telephone: Not provided.
Written: Not provided; contact the AOA.
Electronic: $15 per AOA Osteopathic Physician Profile Report ordered over Internet (www.aoa-net.org).

> American Osteopathic Board of Preventive Medicine
> 12535 Lt. Nichols Road
> Fairfax, VIRGINIA 22033-2433
> Telephone: 623/910-9424
> Fax: 623/776-7965

American Osteopathic Board of Proctology

Are *board eligible*, *board admissible*, and *board qualified* recognized terms?
See AOA policy above.

General certificates:
- Proctology.

Certification time limits:
Lifetime certification.

Verification of certificates
Telephone: Not provided.
Written: Not provided; contact the AOA.
Electronic: $15 per AOA Osteopathic Physician Profile Report ordered over Internet (www.aoa-net.org).

> American Osteopathic Board of Proctology
> 300 Forest Avenue
> Dayton, OHIO 45405
> Telephone: 937/222-2096
> Fax: 937/222-2946

Specialty Boards

American Osteopathic Board of Surgery

Are *board eligible*, *board admissible*, and *board qualified* recognized terms?
See AOA policy above.

General certificates:
- General vascular surgery, Neurological surgery, Plastic and reconstructive surgery, Surgery, Thoracic cardiovascular surgery, Urological surgery.

Certification time limits:
Lifetime certification.

Verification of certificates
Telephone: Not provided.
Written: Not provided; contact the AOA.
Electronic: $15 per AOA Osteopathic Physician Profile Report ordered over Internet (www.aoa-net.org).

> American Osteopathic Board of Surgery
> 3 MacKoil Avenue
> Dayton, OHIO 45403
> Telephone: 800/782-5355 937/252-0868
> Fax: 937/252-0968
> E-mail: info@aobs.org   Web site: www.aobs.org

American Dental Association (ADA) Boards

American Board of Dental Public Health

Are *board eligible*, *board admissible*, and *board qualified* recognized terms?
Uses the term *"board eligible"* to describe applicants whose applications have been reviewed and who are approved to take the board's examination. Candidates may remain board eligible for five years.

General certificates:
- Dental public health.

Certification time limits:
Prior to 2000: lifetime certification. As of January 1, 2000: 10 years.

Verification of certificates
Telephone: Free of charge.
Written: Free of charge. Mail requests, including signed release forms and self-addressed, stamped envelope.
Electronic: Not provided.

> American Board of Dental Public Health
> 1321 N.W. 47th Terrace
> Gainesville, FLORIDA 32605
> Telephone: 352/378-6301
> Fax: 352/367-8430
> E-mail: slotzkar@yahoo.com

Chapter 7

American Board of Endodontics

Are *board eligible*, *board admissible*, and *board qualified* recognized terms?
Uses the term *"board eligible"* to describe applicants whose applications have been reviewed and who are approved to take the board's examination.

General certificates:
- Endodontics.

Certification time limits:
Prior to 1997: lifetime certification. As of January 1, 1997: 10 years.

Verification of certificates
Telephone: Not provided.
Written: $10 per verification. Mail requests, including signed release form.
Electronic: www.aae.org

> American Board of Endodontics
> 211 E. Chicago Avenue, Suite 1100
> Chicago, ILLINOIS 60611
> Telephone: 312/266-7310
> Fax: 312/266-9982
> E-mail: abe@aae.org
> Web site: www.aae.org

American Board of Oral and Maxillofacial Pathology

General certificates:
- Oral pathology.

Certification time limits:
Lifetime certification.

Verification of certificates
Telephone: Not provided.
Written: $25 per verification. Mail requests, including signed release forms and payment.
Electronic: Not provided.

> American Board of Oral and Maxillofacial Pathology
> 4830 W. Kennedy Boulevard, Suite 690
> Tampa, FLORIDA 33609
> Telephone: 813/286-2444
> Fax: 813/289-5279

American Board of Oral and Maxillofacial Surgery

Are *board eligible*, *board admissible*, and *board qualified* recognized terms?
Uses the term *"board eligible"* to describe applicants whose applications have been reviewed and who are in the process of taking the board's examination.

General certificates:
- Oral and maxillofacial surgery.

Certification time limits:
Prior to 1988: lifetime certification. As of January 1, 1988: 10 years.

Verification of certificates
Telephone: Not provided.
Written: $25 per verification. Mail requests, including signed release forms and payment.
Electronic: Provided. Visit Web site listed.

> American Board of Oral and Maxillofacial Surgery
> 625 N. Michigan Avenue, Suite 1820
> Chicago, ILLINOIS 60611
> Telephone: 312/642-0070
> Fax: 312/642-8584
> Web site: www.aboms.org

The American Board of Orthodontics

Are *board eligible*, *board admissible*, and *board qualified* recognized terms?
Board eligible describes applicants who have completed the application (Phase I) and written (Phase II) portions of the board's examination. Once board eligible candidates have taken the oral/clinical portion (Phase III), they become board certified.

General certificates:
- Orthodontics.

Certification time limits:
Lifetime certification. 15-year certificates (as of 1998).

Verification of certificates
Telephone: Not provided.
Written: $20 per verification. Faxed upon request. Mail or fax requests, including signed release forms.
Electronic: Not provided.

> The American Board of Orthodontics
> 401 N. Lindbergh Boulevard, Suite 308
> St. Louis, MISSOURI 63141
> Telephone: 314/432-6130
> Fax: 314/432-8170
> E-mail: info@americanboardortho.com

American Board of Pediatric Dentistry

Are *board eligible, board admissible,* and *board qualified* recognized terms?
Uses the term "board eligible" to describe applicants whose applications have been reviewed and who are approved to take the board's examination.

General certificates:
- Pediatric dentistry.

Certification time limits:
Prior to September 6, 1991: lifetime certification. As of September 6, 1991: 10 years.

Verification of certificates
Telephone: Not provided.
Written: Free of charge. Faxed upon request. Mail or fax requests, including signed release forms.
Electronic: Not provided.

> American Board of Pediatric Dentistry
> 1193 Woodgate Drive
> Carmel, INDIANA 46033-9232
> Telephone: 317/573-0877
> Fax: 317/846-7235
> E-mail: drjrroche@cs.com
> Web site: www.abpd.org

American Board of Periodontology

Are *board eligible, board admissible,* and *board qualified* recognized terms?
Uses the term *board eligible* to describe applicants who have completed the written portion (Part I) of its examination. Board eligible applicants have six years to take the oral portion (Part II) of the examination.

General certificates:
- Periodontology.

Certification time limits:
Lifetime certification, with the obligation to complete certain continuing education requirements every three years.

Verification of certificates
Telephone: Not provided.
Written: $10 per verification. Mail requests, including signed release form.
Electronic: Not provided.

> American Board of Periodontology
> 4157 Mountain Road, PBN 249
> Pasadena, MARYLAND 21122
> Telephone: 410/437-3749
> Fax: 410/437-4021

E-mail: abperio@msn.com
Web site: www.perio.org

American Board of Prosthodontics

Are *board eligible*, *board admissible*, and *board qualified* recognized terms?
Board eligible means applicant has a reviewed application and is approved to take the board's examination. Board eligible status is limited to six years. The written examination must be taken within two years of establishing board eligibility.

General certificates:
- Prosthodontics.

Certification time limits:
As of January 1, 1996: Eight years (applies to all active diplomates). No grandfathering.

Verification of certificates
Telephone: Not provided.
Written: $25 per verification. Faxed upon request. Mail or fax requests, including signed release forms.
Electronic: Not provided.

American Board of Prosthodontics
PO Box 271894
West Hartford, CONNECTICUT 6127
Telephone: 860/679-2649
Fax: 860/679-1370

American Dental Association

Are *board eligible*, *board admissible*, and *board qualified* recognized terms?
Does not recognize above terms.

Verification of membership
Telephone: Not provided.
Written: Not provided.
Electronic: Not provided.

American Dental Association
211 E. Chicago Avenue
Chicago, ILLINOIS 60611-2678
Telephone: 312/440-2500
Fax: 312/440-2883
Web site: www.ada.org

Chapter 7

American Podiatric Medical Association Boards

American Board of Podiatric Orthopedics & Primary Podiatric Medicine
Note: Web site subscription available for $300.

Are *board eligible*, *board admissible*, and *board qualified* recognized terms?
Does not recognize above terms.

General certificates:
- Diplomate.

Certification time limits:
Prior to 1993: lifetime certification. As of January 1, 1993: 10 years.

Verification of certificates
Telephone: Not provided.
Written: $25 per verification. Mail requests, including signed release forms and payment (check, MC, Visa, or AMEX). Directory also available. $300 for CD/ROM; $300 for yearly Web site usage.
Electronic: Not provided.

> American Board of Podiatric Orthopedics & Primary Podiatric Medicine
> 22910 Crenshaw Boulevard, Suite B
> Torrance, CALIFORNIA 90505
> Telephone: 310/891-0100   310/891-6036
> Fax: 310/891-0500
> E-mail: admin@abpoppm.org
> Web site: www.abpoppm.org

American Board of Podiatric Surgery

Are *board eligible*, *board admissible*, and *board qualified* recognized terms?
Board qualified means a podiatrist has passed the written examination for certification in foot surgery and has demonstrated capability to diagnose general medical problems, such as surgical management of foot and ankle diseases, deformities, or traumas.

General certificates:
Foot and ankle surgery (pre-1991); Foot Surgery, reconstruction/rear-foot ankle surgery. Foot and ankle surgery (after January 1, 1991).

Certification time limits:
Prior to 1991: lifetime certification. As of January 1, 1991: every 10 years.

Verification of certificates
Telephone: Not provided.
Written: $25 for up to four verifications; $15 for five to 10 verifications; $10 for more than 10 verifications. Mail or fax requests, including podiatrist-signed release forms and payment (check, American Express, MC, Visa).
Electronic: Check Web site for more information.

American Board of Podiatric Surgery
3330 Mission Street
San Francisco, CALIFORNIA 94110-5009
Telephone: 415/826-3200
Fax: 415/826-4640
E-mail: info@abps.org
Web site: www.abps.org

Nursing Boards

American Association of Nurse Anesthetists (AANA)

General certificates:
- Certified Registered Nurse Anesthetist.

Certification time limits:
Lifetime certification. Voluntary recertification every two years through Council on Recertification.

Verification of certificates
Telephone: Free of charge. Limit three verifications per call. Provide AANA ID numbers.
Written: Free of charge. Faxed upon request. Mail or fax requests, including signed release forms.
Electronic: www.aana.com

American Association of Nurse Anesthetists
222 S. Prospect Avenue
Park Ridge, ILLINOIS 60068-4001
Telephone: 847/692-7050, Ext. 3096 or Ext. 3091
Fax: 847/692-7082
E-mail: banderson@aana.com
Web site: www.aana.com

ACNM Certification Council, Inc.

General certificates:
- Nurse-midwifery (ACNM is the only organization to certify nurse mid-wives).

Certification time limits:
Prior to 1996: lifetime certification. As of January 1, 1996: eight years.

Verification of certificates
Telephone: Free of charge.
Written: $20 fee. Faxed upon request. Mail requests.
Electronic: www.accmidwife.org

ACNM Certification Council Inc
8201 Corporate Drive, Suite 550
Landover, MARYLAND 20785
Telephone: 301/459-1321
Fax: 301/731-7825
E-mail: acnmcertcn@accmidwife.org
Web site: www.accmidwife.org

American Nurses Credentialing Center

Note: American Nurses Credentialing Center is a subsidiary of the American Nurses Association. Certifies nurses in five categories: generalist, clinical specialist, modular, administration, and nurse practitioner.

General certificates:
- Cardiac rehabilitation nurse, Community health nurse, College health nurse, General nurse, Gerontological nurse, Home health nurse, Informatics nurse, Medical-surgical nurse, Pediatric nurse, Perinatal nurse, Psychiatric and mental health nurse, School nurse, Nursing continuing education/Staff development.

Clinical Specialist certificates (Advanced practice):
- Adult psychiatric and mental health nursing clinical specialist, Child and adolescent psychiatric and mental health nursing clinical specialist, Community health nursing clinical specialist, Gerontological nursing clinical specialist, Home health nursing clinical specialist, Medical-surgical nursing clinical specialist.

Modular exam certification:
- Nursing case management, Ambulatory care.

Administration certificates:
- Advanced nursing administration, Nursing administration.

Nurse Practitioner certificates (Advanced practice):
- Acute care nurse practitioner, Adult nurse practitioner, Family care nurse practitioner, Gerontological nurse practitioner, Pediatric nurse practitioner, School nurse practitioner.

Certification time limits:
Five years.

Verification of certificates
Written: $10 per verification. Mail requests, including signed release form and payment.
Electronic: www.nursingworld.org

American Nurses Credentialing Center
600 Maryland Avenue SW, Suite 100 W
Washington, DISTRICT OF COLUMBIA 20024-2571
Telephone: 800/284-CERT   202/651-7000 (American Nurses Association)
Fax: 202/651-7001
E-mail: ancc@ana.org
Web site: www.nursingworld.org

Psychology Boards

American Board of Professional Psychology

Subspecialty certificates:
- Behavioral psychology, Clinical psychology, Clinical neuropsychology, Counseling psychology, Family psychology, Forensic psychology, Group psychology, Health psychology, School psychology, Psychoanalysis, Rehabilitational psychology.

Certification time limits:
Lifetime certification.

Verification of certificates

Telephone: Free of charge.
Written: Free of charge. Faxed upon request. Mail, phone, or fax requests, including signed release forms.
Electronic: Free of charge.

> American Board of Professional Psychology
> 514 E. Capital Avenue
> Jefferson Ciy, MISSOURI 65101
> Telephone: 573/634-5607
> Fax: 573/634-7157
> E-mail: office@abpp.org
> Web site: www.abpp.org

American Psychological Association

Certificate of proficiency:
- Treatment of alcohol and other psychoactive substance abuse disorders.

Certification time limits:
Three years.

Verification of certificates

Telephone: Free of charge.
Written: Free of charge. Faxed upon request. Mail or fax requests.
Electronic: Information available on Web site: www.apa.org.

> American Psychological Association
> College of Professional Psychology
> 750 First Street NE
> Washington, DISTRICT OF COLUMBIA 20002-4242
> Telephone: 202/336-6100
> Fax: 202/336-5797
> E-mail: apacollege@apa.org
> Web site: www.apa.org/college

Chapter 7

Other Boards

National Commission on Certification of Physician Assistants

General certificates:
- Physician assistant.

Certification time limits:
Two years.

Verification of certificates

Telephone: Free of charge. Provide physician assistant's name and Social Security number.
Written: Free of charge. Faxed upon request. Mail or fax requests, including signed release forms.
Electronic: Not provided.

> National Commission on Certification of Physician Assistants
> 157 Technology Parkway, Suite 800
> Norcross, GEORGIA 30092
> Telephone: 770/734-4500
> Fax: 770/734-4535
> Web site: www.nccpa.net

Certification Board for Nutrition Specialists

Telephone: Not provided.
Written: Not provided.
Electronic: Not provided.

> Certification Board for Nutrition Specialists
> Hospital for Joint Diseases
> 301 E. 17th Street
> New York, NEW YORK 10003
> Telephone: 212-777-1037 212-777-1103
> E-mail: office@cert-nutrition.org
> Web site: cert-nutrition.org

Specialty Boards

National Board for Certification of Orthopedic Technicians

Telephone: Not provided.
Written: Not provided.
Electronic: Not provided.

Certification time limits:
Six years.

Verification of certificates

> National Board for Certification of Orthopedic Technicians
> c/o Columbia Assessment Services
> 120 First Flight Lane
> Morrisville, NORTH CAROLINA 27560
> Telephone: 919/572-6880
> Fax: 919/61-2426
> E-mail: srustin@castlelearning.com

National Board of Medical Examiners

Are *board eligible*, *board admissible*, and *board qualified* recognized terms?
Certify that applicant is a diplomate of the National Board of Examiners.

Annual report of licensed physicians
Telephone: Free of charge.
Written: Free of charge.
Electronic: Not provided.

> National Board of Medical Examiners
> 3750 Market Street
> Philadelphia, PENNSYLVANIA 19104
> Telephone: 215/590-9500
> Fax: 215/590-9555
> Web site: www.nbme.org or www.usmle.org

CHAPTER 8

How to Use Practitioner Data Banks

Chapter 8
How to Use Practitioner Data Banks

This chapter contains information about the data banks hospitals may consult when credentialing physicians and other health care professionals. Each section includes a data bank's history, purpose, services, requirements, and querying policies and procedures. The following data banks are covered:

- The National Practitioner Data Bank (NPDB)
- The Healthcare Integrity and Protection Data Bank (HIPDB)
- The Federation Physician Data Center of the Federation of State Medical Boards (FSMB) (formerly known as the Board Action Data Bank)
- The American Medical Association (AMA) Physician Masterfile
- The Federation Credentials Verification Service of the FSMB
- The National Register of Health Service Providers in Psychology
- The Chiropractic Information Network/Board Action Databank (CIN-BAD) of the Federation of Chiropractic Licensing Boards
- The American Osteopathic Association (AOA) Official Osteopathic Physician Profile Report
- The Department of Health and Human Services Office of Inspector General (OIG) List of Excluded Individuals/Entities
- The Controlled Substances Act (CSA) Registration Database

NPDB

Background information
The NPDB, a national register of physicians, dentists, and other health care practitioners, was established by the federal government in response to provisions of the Health Care Quality Improvement Act of 1986 (HCQIA) as amended (Title IV). It began operations in 1990 and operates under a contract on behalf of the federal Department of Health and Human Services (HHS) and is managed by its Division of Quality Assurance (DQA).

The NPDB was developed in response to the "malpractice crisis" of the 1980s. Its primary objective is "to improve the quality of health care by encouraging state licensing boards, hospitals, professional societies, and other health care entities to identify and discipline those who engage in unprofessional behavior; and to restrict the ability of incompetent physicians, dentists, and other health care practitioners to move from state to state without disclosure or discovery of previous medical malpractice payment and adverse action history. Adverse action can involve licensure, clinical privileges, and professional society memberships."[1] It also contains information about medical malpractice payments by or on behalf of practitioners. On March 3, 1997, the NPDB added a new category—Medicare and Medicaid Exclusion Reports—which gives information about practitioners who are denied participation in or payment from Medicare or Medicaid programs.

---

[1] NPDB Web site

Currently, like the HIPDB, the Health Resources and Services Administration (HRSA), Bureau of Health Professions (BHPr), and DQA manage the data bank. HRSA is an agency of HHS. The data bank operations are accessible online through the Integrated Query and Reporting Service (IQRS), which is conducted through a secure Web site.

Reporting to the NPDB

Federal law requires any organization that evaluates and monitors the work of health care professionals to report final adverse actions relating to clinical competence or professional misconduct involving a physician (Doctor of Medicine [MD], Doctor of Osteopathic Medicine [DO]) or dentist (Doctor of Dental Science [DDS] or Doctor of Dental Medicine [DMD]) to the NPDB and appropriate state licensing agency within 15 days of the action. For example, a hospital must report actions relating to inadequate clinical competence or misconduct that adversely affected the privileges of physicians and dentists. A professional society that conducts professional reviews of its members must report adverse membership actions that relate to professional competence or misconduct within 30 days of the action. Organizations have the option of reporting actions against health care practitioners other than physicians and dentists, but are not required to do so. Malpractice insurers, including self-insured health care organizations, must report payments made on behalf of all health care practitioners—not just physicians and dentists—as a result of malpractice judgments or settlements. The NPDB requires insurers to report payments to both the state licensing agency and the NPDB within 30 days of the date on which payments are made.

Which events must be reported, and which are not required to be reported?

The nature of NPDB report-triggering events varies, depending on the type of reporting organization.

According to the *NPDB Guidebook*, hospitals must report "professional review action, based on reasons related to professional competence or conduct, adversely affecting clinical privileges for a period longer than 30 days; or voluntary surrender or restriction of clinical privileges while under, or to avoid, investigation."

The *NPDB Guidebook* defines a professional review action as "an activity of a health care entity with respect to an individual physician, dentist, or other health care practitioner: (1) to determine whether the physician, dentist, or other health care practitioner may have clinical privileges with respect to, or membership in, the entity; (2) to determine the scope or conditions of such privileges or membership; or (3) to change or modify such privileges or membership."

Many hospitals do not consider a letter of reprimand or a requirement to take continuing education necessary to report. Similarly, an investigation may be defined narrowly in medical staff bylaws; thus, informally checking into a questionable incident may not be considered an investigation. Many hospitals have deliberately fashioned some corrective actions to provide them with the option of handling an errant practitioner without having to file an NPDB report. Hospitals and their attorneys must make their own decisions about the ethical implications of extremely narrow definitions.

Some actions taken by state licensing agencies and professional associations are not reportable. For example, dropping someone from appointment or membership for failure to pay dues or revoking licensure for failure to pay fees are actions not related to incompetence or misconduct and, therefore, need not be reported. State licensure boards do not have to report denials of initial applications for licensure or settlement agreements that impose monitoring of a practitioner for a specific period of time, unless the monitoring constitutes a restriction or reprimand of the license. Similarly, it is not required that hospitals report a voluntary resignation from a medical staff or relinquishment of privileges because of a change in professional activities or interests. However, hospitals are required to report the adverse action if a physician resigns or relinquishes privileges during or in lieu of an investigation.

Sometimes determining whether a situation must be reported is less clear-cut. For example, suspending a hospital medical staff appointee from appointment and all privileges for failure to complete charts might or might not relate to professional incompetence or misconduct. It depends on the reason the charts are not completed (for example, work overload versus alcoholism) and on the structure of the decision-making process (for example, suspension of privileges via decision of the medical staff's peer review system versus an administrative action by the chief of staff). Because failure to report an adverse action and, conversely, inappropriately reporting an action that is not adverse might subject a hospital to legal penalties, the hospital's legal counsel should review any unclear situations.

On behalf of a licensed practitioner, insurers must report any payment that is limited to exchanges of money and that results from a written claim or judgment. This requirement applies to any individual or organization making payment—even those that might not consider themselves insurers—including any physician or health care organization that pays a patient to settle a claim (unless such payment is made before a written claim is submitted). Insurers need not report payments made as a result of suits against health care organizations, such as clinics or group practices that do not name individual practitioners. (Exception: If the named defendant is a sole practitioner identified as a "professional corporation," a payment made for the professional corporation must be reported for the practitioner.)

How the NPDB processes a report
When the NPDB receives a report, it sends a practitioner-notification document to both the practitioner involved and the reporting entity. With this method, a practitioner has the opportunity to dispute the contents of a report or correct the report if he or she successfully establishes that the report is incorrect.

If a practitioner wishes to correct a report, his or her first step is to discuss the issue with the reporting entity to see whether an agreement about any corrections can be arranged. If the parties can reach an agreement, then the reporting entity makes the necessary corrections. If they do not reach an agreement, the secretary of the federal HHS has the authority to review the issue and make any appropriate corrections. Any corrections to the report verification document must be sent back to the NPDB within 30 days. The NPDB will notify the practitioner once the corrections have been made.

Querying the NPDB
Note: For a bonus quick checklist guide to registering and querying the NPDB, turn to p. 537 in this chapter.

Hospitals are the only organizations required by law to obtain the NPDB records of applicants (frequently referred to as "querying"). Hospitals must query the NPDB for information about all types of health care professionals—not just physicians and dentists—who are applying for medical staff appointment or initial, additional, or expanded privileges. Additionally, hospitals must obtain records from the NPDB files for individuals who are being considered for privileges only and not for appointment.

Every two years, each hospital must query the NPDB about practitioners at the hospital who have medical staff appointment or clinical privileges. Hospitals that reappoint and reprivilege annually need not query annually (although they may, if they choose).

Every hospital should query the NPDB not just to satisfy the law, but also as good risk management and patient protection practice to uncover any undisclosed practitioner problems. Because hospitals and other health care organizations must report significant disciplinary actions against physicians and dentists, NPDB reports are one mechanism by which to identify all major disciplinary and malpractice problems that have occurred since 1989. And because some organizations also report actions against other types of health care practitioners, NPDB reports about such practitioners often provide valuable information.

The NPDB has a provision by which health care organizations may authorize other organizations—called "authorized

Chapter 8

agents"—to query on their behalf. These authorized agents are typically companies or organizations that provide credentials
verification services (CVOs). However, authorized agents may query only on behalf of their contracted organizations and cannot query on their own behalf. Also, to comply with federal law, a separate query must be made for each hospital that an authorized agent represents, even if one professional is being checked on behalf of several hospitals. (In other words, a CVO cannot share information it obtains on behalf of one hospital with another.)

Individual practitioners have the right to "self-query" the NPDB at any time regarding the content of their own files. If a practitioner has never received notice from the NPDB of an adverse action report, no negative information should be in his or her file. Even so, a practitioner might be interested in querying in order to ensure that no incorrect information has been entered into his or her file or to obtain a copy of his or her NPDB report for a prospective employer or other organization or person.

Hospitals and other authorized agencies sometimes ask practitioners to obtain and provide them with free self-query copies of NPDB reports to avoid paying the fee. These organizations should note, however, that practitioner copies are not considered primary source verification by the Joint Commission on Accreditation of Healthcare Organizations (JCAHO), nor does this meet the hospital's obligations for querying under the HCQIA. Unauthorized agencies—such as a physician search and recruiting company—will also sometimes ask practitioners to request NPDB self-reports for their files. Practitioners should be aware that, when they give copies of their self-reports to such agencies, they relinquish the confidentiality protection that a direct relationship with the NPDB provides. In theory, any report given outside the confidentiality protection could be passed on to others without limitation. Also in theory, anyone providing NPDB information or an NPDB report to an unauthorized person is committing a crime. Persons and organizations receiving confidential information from the NPDB-HIPDB either directly or indirectly from another party must use it solely with respect to the purpose for which it was provided. Any person who violates these confidentiality provisions is subject to a civil money penalty of up to $11,000 for each violation. Individual health care practitioners who obtain information about themselves from the NPDB-HIPDB are permitted to share that information with anyone they choose. The *NPDB Guidebook* states that an organization can provide a copy of the data bank report to the practitioner but recommends that the hospital's Entity Identification Number be removed or obliterated from the report.

State licensing agencies may query the NPDB at any time. Professional societies may query when screening membership or affiliation, or when carrying out professional review activities. An attorney for a plaintiff who is suing a hospital that did not query the NPDB (as required by law) is authorized under the law to obtain information regarding a practitioner named in the lawsuit. Malpractice insurers may not query, although they are required to report adverse actions. Interested members of the public, such as prospective patients or employers, may not query the NPDB.

Mechanics of querying the NPDB

Before the entitled entities may query the NPDB, hospitals and other eligible organizations must first register to receive information and authorization. To facilitate registration, the NPDB contacts organizations it knows are eligible. Organizations that have not been contacted but believe they are eligible should contact the NPDB themselves. A hospital that has not been contacted by the NPDB or been given an identification number is not excused from the required querying and reporting obligations. The following table identifies the querying requirements:

Entity	Requirement
Hospitals[2] Screening applicants for medical staff appointment or granting of clinical privileges; every two years for physicians, dentists, or other health care practitioners on the medical staff or granted clinical privileges. Hospitals are not required to query more than once every two years on a practitioner who is continuously on staff.	Must query
At other times as they deem necessary	May query
Other health care entities Screening applicants for membership or affiliation; supporting profession review activities	May query
Physicians, dentists, and other health care practitioners Regarding their own files	May query

To query the NPDB, entities must use the Integrated Query Reporting Service (IQRS), an electronic, Web-based system for querying and reporting. The NPDB does not accept written requests for information from hospitals and other health care entities. At the time of publication, the cost of an electronic query and response was $5 per name, which must be paid by credit card or electronic funds transfer. Practitioners who wish to self-query also must do so online for a $10 fee. Please note that fees are subject to change.

Failure to report or query: How does the federal law encourage use of the NPDB?
NPDB operation is facilitated by a system of rewards and penalties for reporting or failing to report to the NPDB and for querying or failing to query the NPDB. These rewards and penalties are established under Health Care Quality Improvement Act of 1986. Specifically, hospitals that query the NPDB benefit in two ways. First, hospitals that query the NPDB (as they are required to do) are protected from release of information to attorneys engaged in suing the hospital over a professional liability claim. Negative information about a hospital's medical staff appointee, which is on file with the NPDB, is kept confidential and cannot be used as evidence in a trial. The other reward is immunity from certain lawsuits, such as antitrust violation suits by practitioners who were denied privileges through the peer review process. When a hospital refuses to award privileges to a practitioner as a result of information from an NPDB report, the hospital and its individual peer review participants are protected from any resulting antitrust suits. This protection might significantly facilitate a hospital's peer review activities, because fear of lawsuits often discourages physicians from participating in peer review and medical staff governance.

NPDB-related penalties might result from a number of possible actions or failures to act. A hospital's failure to submit a report on a reportable professional review action to the NPDB might lead to loss of the hospital's confidentiality protection for three years. A hospital's failure to query the NPDB, as required by law, might lead to release of NPDB information to a plaintiff's attorney and also to a presumption in court that the hospital possessed but ignored NPDB information. In addition, the name of the offending hospital will be published in the *Federal Register*. Such penalties could be damaging to a hospital's defense in liability lawsuits as well as to its public image.

---

[2] NPDB Web site

A state licensing agency's failure to report might lead to loss of the agency's designation as a source of information for the NPDB. Failure by an insurer to report payment on behalf of a practitioner can lead to a fine of up to $10,000. Finally, because information reported to or received from the NPDB is considered confidential, release of information to an unauthorized person or agency can result in a $10,000 fine.

Should the public have access to NPDB information?
Since its inception, a movement has developed demanding public access to the NPDB. Some members of the general public, and consumer groups, complain that the NPDB contains information about practitioners that should be made available to anyone who wishes to obtain it. These proponents of public access say patients should be able to use this information in making informed health care decisions. Access would allow them to refuse the services of a practitioner whom they otherwise would not choose if they knew the details of his or her record. They argue that the government is protecting practitioners to the detriment of the public's safety. Their claim is that a publicly funded agency should release its information to members of the public. (In fact, while tax dollars indeed funded the start-up phase of the NPDB, it is now funded entirely by users' fees.)

Practitioners—mainly physicians—have expressed concerns that much of the NPDB information would be misunderstood if it were released to the public. The American Medical Association has lobbied intensely to disallow public access. In their defense, studies have demonstrated that most low-quality care does not lead to malpractice liability, and many malpractice payments result from settlements of nuisance lawsuits or from scientifically insupportable jury decisions. Furthermore, liability exposure is heavily related to particular medical specialties in which high-risk clinical care is frequently needed.

Thus, even when a practitioner's NPDB record shows many liability payments, which suggests to a member of the public that the practitioner is not competent, the reality might be completely different. For example, currently any medical malpractice settlement requiring a payment must be reported to the NPDB, even "nuisance settlements" (generally, around $100, thus many practitioners would have to admit that they had been reported to the NPDB. However, as the AMA states, malpractice data is a poor indication of quality. Defenders of the current system believe the information should be available only to those who are knowledgeable enough to use it properly, such as medical staff peer reviewers and state licensing authorities. These experts can and do protect the public without unfairly and improperly penalizing competent practitioners.

The practitioners' position on public access to NPDB information was supported the day Congress passed the Health Care Quality Improvement Act of 1986 (HCQIA). The HCQIA states that no NPDB information shall be made available, except in the case that a hospital fails to query the NPDB about a practitioner who later is sued. In that case, the plaintiff's attorney may obtain the practitioner's NPDB record.

The House Commerce Oversight and Investigation Subcommittee held hearings in March 2002 to discuss opening the NPDB to the general public. Participants expressed concern regarding the inconsistent, incomplete format of the data. It was brought to the attention of the Committee that no distinction is made between physicians in high-risk or low-risk specialties, for instance. And sometimes the best physicians take on the sickest patients, thus incurring the most risk. Malpractice awards don't necessarily indicate incompetent physicians, because insurance companies often settle lawsuits (occasionally without the physician's consent) to avoid costly court proceedings.

Common questions regarding the NPDB
- *How long do adverse action reports remain in an NPDB record?*
  NPDB files are permanent. Once adverse action reports are entered into NPDB files, they are never removed

(unless a practitioner can establish that a report was made in error).

- *How much credit should be given to NPDB adverse reports?*
Neither the HCQIA nor JCAHO specify the importance of NPDB reports in relation to other pieces of credentialing information. The NPDB was created not to replace traditional means of credentialing, but to supplement them. It is another resource that hospitals, state licensing boards, and other health care entities can use to conduct a thorough check on the qualifications of practitioners. At the previously mentioned hearing of the House Commerce Oversight and Investigation Subcommittee, one person testified regarding a practitioner with multiple malpractice reports because he failed to send employees home from a factory that experienced a chemical explosion. Although from the NPDB reports you could not tell whether the practitioner did anything wrong, there were about 177 reports as a result of this one incident. Clearly hospitals and other organizations should carefully examine the NPDB reports, and practitioners should be given the opportunity to furnish explanations about any questionable or adverse reports. Consider this information in context with all of the physician's other pertinent credentials. In late November 2000, the General Accounting Office (GAO) issued a report that questioned the integrity of the information in the NPDB. More specifically, the report questioned the accuracy and completeness of the information submitted to the NPDB and cited erroneous and misleading information about malpractice, privilege restriction, and licensure reports in the data bank. The GAO also requested that HHS improve its oversight of the practitioner data bank. Industry experts advise credentialing professionals not to rely solely on the data bank when verifying physicians' credentials.

- *What about interns, residents, and other trainees who are subject to discipline?*
Physicians in training programs are not subject to NPDB reporting when the clinical actions in question were under the auspices of the training program and were not covered by privileges. However, if a reportable adverse professional action occurs with a physician trainee who works outside the scope of his or her training program (for example, moonlights), an NPDB report is required.

Other sources of NPDB-related information

Before the NPDB existed, no single agency collected the same information that the NPDB does, but some organizations did monitor some of the information the NPDB currently tracks. Hospitals and health care organizations seeking information prior to 1990 should consider using other sources for such information.

For example, individual state licensing agencies might provide information about licensure actions against licensees upon request. Obtaining complete information from these sources, however, requires asking applicants to list all of the states in which they have ever had licenses and then individually contacting each agency. Some applicants have had licenses in so many states that they might not even remember all of them. Furthermore, an individual who has been disciplined in another state might not provide that information to the hospital, gambling that the hospital will not learn about it elsewhere.

The Federation of State Medical Boards (FSMB) provides information about licensure discipline of physicians in all states dating back to the early 20th century. Hospitals must contract in advance to receive this service from the Physician Board Action Data Bank.

Many health care organizations provide information to other hospitals and organizations about practitioners who have been staff members in past years. An organization should always ask for information from other organizations in connection with every application for appointment or privileges. However, because they fear litigation, hospitals are usually extremely cautious in offering information that could be seen as negative. Even when an applicant has been subject to disciplinary action, a hospital might report simply that the applicant was on staff and departed in good standing. Hospitals may agree to not reveal the details of actions as part of a contractual arrangement with physicians. Also, if a practitioner served many years before, the information is likely to be less detailed and less useful, and details of his or her privileges and quality record are usually not available. In fact, information might establish nothing more than whether the practitioner was an appointee in good standing of the medical or professional staff. Thus, hospitals and other organizations should query a practitioner's prior affiliations but should not base credentialing decisions solely on problem-free reports.

Generally, liability insurers will provide claims information, with the consent of the insured party. The information provided varies widely between insurers. Some will provide only basic information, such as number of claims filed and settlements made, and some will provide detailed information concerning the alleged acts. Medical staffs should determine exactly what information needs to come from the insurer and place the burden on the applicant to make sure the required information is provided. If a lawsuit has been adjudicated, the trial record (and appeal record, if the suit has been appealed) is usually public information. However, obtaining the record and reading it is so complicated that, except in the most serious cases, the effort is not likely to be worth the information obtained.

NPDB contact information

Health care organizations and practitioners may obtain more information by contacting the NPDB directly.

National Practitioner Data Bank—Healthcare Integrity and Protection Data Bank
P.O. Box 10832
Chantilly, VIRGINIA 20153-0832
NPDB Helpline: 800/767-6732
Web site: www.npdb-hipdb.com

HIPDB

Background Information

The Health Insurance Portability and Accountability Act of 1996 instructed the Secretary of HHS to create the Health Integrity and Protection Data Bank (HIPDB). The HIPDB is a data collection program for reporting and disclosure of certain final adverse actions taken against health care practitioners, providers, and suppliers.

The HIPDB collects information about

- licensure and certification actions
- exclusions from participation in federal and state health care programs
- criminal convictions
- civil judgments related to health care
- other adjudicated actions or decisions

Like the NPDB, the Health Resources and Services Administration (HRSA), Bureau of Health Professions (BHPr), and Division of Quality Assurance (DQA) manage the data bank. HRSA is an agency of the HHS. The data bank operations are accessible online through the IQRS, which is conducted through a secure Web site.

Accessing the HIPDB

Health plans and federal and state government agencies are defined as entities entitled to query the HIPDB. Hospitals providing a self-insurance plan to their employees would be considered a "health plan" and are required to query and report to the HIPDB. Queries and reports must be made thorough use the IQRS, an electronic, Web-based system for querying and reporting. At the time of publication, the cost of an electronic query and response is $5 per name and must be paid by credit card or electronic funds transfer. However, fees are subject to change. Health care practitioners, providers, and suppliers may self-query the HIPDB at any time. This must be done online and a $10 fee is required.

NPDB-HIPDB information is not available to the general public. However, people and entities may request data that does not identify any particular entity or subject.[3]

HIPDB contact information
Health care organizations and practitioners may obtain more information by contacting the HIPDB.

National Practitioner Data Bank—Healthcare Integrity and Protection Data Bank
P.O. Box 10832
Chantilly, VIRGINIA 20153-0832
NPDB Helpline: 800/767-6732
Web site: www.npdb-hipdb.com

The Federation Physician Data Center of the FSMB

Background information on the FSMB
The membership of the FSMB consists of the medical boards of all states, the District of Columbia, Guam, Puerto Rico, the Virgin Islands, and 13 of the 16 osteopathic boards in the United States. The Canadian provincial medical licensing authorities are affiliate members.

Founded in 1912, the FSMB is a parent organization of the Accreditation Council for Continuing Medical Education and the Educational Commission for Foreign Medical Graduates (ECFMG). It is also a member of the National Board of Medical Examiners (NBME). The FSMB was a founding member of what is now the American Board of Medical Specialties (ABMS) and is an associate member of that body.

The FSMB functions as a representative for its member medical boards. On behalf of these boards, the FSMB develops medical regulation policies, facilitates communication between states on legislative issues, drafts statutory language and legislative testimony, and assists with legislative strategies.

To help facilitate the licensure process by endorsement among the states, the FSMB maintains a complete computer record of FLEX, Special Purpose Examination (SPEX) and USMLE scores, and biographical information about examinees. In addition to its involvement in medical evaluation and examination (see Chapter 4: Licensing Agencies for more information about physician examinations), the FSMB publishes materials to inform its members of medical, regulatory, and disciplinary issues. Publications issued by the FSMB include the quarterly *Journal of Medical Licensure and Discipline*, the monthly FSMB *NewsLine*, the biennial *Exchange*, the annual *FSMB Handbook, A Model for the Preparation of a Guidebook on Medical Discipline*, and *A Guide to the Essentials of a Modern Medical Practice Act* and its companion document, *The Elements of a Modern State Medical Board*. These publications are available on FSMB's Web site listed below.

History of the Federation Physician Data Center (formerly called the Board Action Data Bank)
Since its founding, the FSMB has performed the critical function of collecting, maintaining, and reporting actions taken against physicians as reported by its member licensing agencies and other governmental authorities. Until the 1960s, the FSMB reported actions against physicians by publishing them in its monthly *Federation Bulletin*. But as physician licensing became more complex and the number of physicians and reported actions increased, the FSMB realized it had to systematize its board action data files. So in the 1960s and 1970s, the FSMB created the Board Action Data

---

[3] NPDB Web site

Bank (using an index card filing system) and began a separate monthly publication exclusively for reporting board actions, the *Board Action Report*.

In response to advances in technology—specifically, computer systems—the FSMB began planning and developing the computerized Board Action Data Bank in the early 1980s. Due in large part to financial contributions from several governmental organizations, including the Division of Medicine, the Bureau of Health Professions, the HRSA, and the United States HHS, the Board Action Data Bank became significantly more sophisticated and inclusive. The Federation implemented its current system in 1998.

Today, the Board Action Data Bank is known as the Federation Physician Data Center. It is the predominant source of information on the licensure and disciplinary histories of physicians and is consulted regularly by military, government, and private organizations involved in the employment/regulation of physicians.

Contents of the Federation Physician Data Center

The Federation Physician Data Center currently contains more than 117,00 reports of actions related to more than 35,000 physicians. Individual state and provincial licensing agencies and disciplinary boards as well as other authorities report these actions to the FSMB. As physician review and disciplinary agencies continue to increase activity and improve the timeliness and thoroughness of reports, the number of reports in the Board Action Data Bank will continue to increase significantly.

For an action to be reported in the Federation Physician Data Center, it must be public information and legally releasable to state licensing agencies and other organizations with the recognized authority to review physicians. Two types of actions are taken against physicians: prejudicial and nonprejudicial. Typical prejudicial, or disciplinary, actions contained in the data bank include revocations, probations, suspensions, consent orders, and Medicare sanctions. Nonprejudicial actions are actions that do not relate to discipline—such as reinstatement of licensure, replacement of lost or destroyed licenses, or license denials—but are reported to ensure that records are complete and to prevent misrepresentation or the fraudulent use of lost or stolen credentials. For example, data bank files contain biographic data on each physician to ensure proper identification.

Actions reported to the FSMB are permanently stored in the Federation Physician Data Center, as are subsequent actions, such as license reinstatements. To ensure the accuracy of information contained in the Federation Physician Data Center, however, all actions reported to the FSMB are reviewed before being recorded. The FSMB verifies all actions in writing and obtains supporting documentation, such as copies of board orders, court findings, final decrees, and stipulations for all actions. The FSMB maintains hard copies of such supporting documentation for all actions in its files.

As another quality control measure, the FSMB also periodically conducts random audits of Federation Physician Data Center files. These audits involve reviewing and verifying the contents of data bank files to ensure accuracy.

In addition to reviewing actions itself, the FSMB uses other means to ensure that files contained in the Federation Physician Data Center are accurate and complete. It publishes annual reports containing summaries of all actions reported each year and sends these reports to the individual reporting authorities for their review. When necessary, the individual reporting authorities clarify or offer additional information to improve data bank action reports.

Querying the Federation Physician Data Center

The FSMB maintains specific policies for accessing information contained in the Federation Physician Data Center. The amount of information provided and fee depend on the type of organization requesting information.

Two different methods are offered:

• The online Board Action Data Search is accessible via a secure Web site that allows on-screen verification of those names that have immediately been assigned the status of "Clean." A brief description of disciplinary actions will appear in the Board Action Report, which can be viewed online. The customer must contact the reporting agency in order to learn the details of each action. Online submissions are invoiced on a monthly basis at the fee of $7 for each name entered. The Board Action Data Search can also be accessed via file transfer protocol (FTP). This method allows downloading of the physician biographic information from your computer and importing it directly into the FSMB's computer, allowing you to bypass the need for data entry into their database.

• The Disciplinary Alert Service provides subscribers the ability to submit identifying data on MDs, DOs, and physician assistants to the Federation Physician Data Center for retention in a subscriber, specific data table. Any reports to the Federation will be cross-referenced against the subscriber's identifying data table. If a report matches one of the providers in the subscriber's data table, the subscriber is notified via email that an action has been reported. The subscriber will then have the opportunity to download the disciplinary information that pertains to the provider for review. Fees for the Disciplinary Alert Service are based on an annual subscription rate.

Organizations may request reports on a maximum of 200 physicians at one time if using a paper listing. Requests may also be submitted on a variety of electronic media (formatted to FSMB specifications) and must be alphabetized by physicians' last names and include the following information for each physician in question: full name (last, first, and middle), date of birth, the name of the physician's medical school and year of graduation, and Social Security number (if available).

Public access to data

In January 2001, FSMB opened DocInfo to the public (www.docinfo.org). Consumers can search for physicians by name, address, and medical specialty for $9.95 per physician search. Reports include the type of disciplinary action taken against a physician by state medical boards, the date of the action, the state medical board or licensing agency that initiated the action, and the reason the action was taken, as well as actions taken by a federal regulatory board and sanctions taken by the military. Online searches (using a credit card) provide immediate results.

Requests are also accepted by mail by downloading the Disciplinary Search Request Form. Mailed requests take about five to seven business days to process.

FSMB contact information

For more information about the FSMB's Federation Physician Data Center, eligible organizations may contact the Board Action Services Federation Physician Data Center department of the FSMB.

Attention: Board Action Services
Federation of State Medical Boards of the United States, Inc.
400 Fuller Wiser Road, Suite 300
Euless, TEXAS 76039-3855
Telephone: 817/868-4000
Fax: 817/868-4098
Web site: www.fsmb.org

Chapter 8

Federation Credentials Verification Service

Background information
In 1996, the FSMB began its Federation Credentials Verification Service (FCVS). Physicians may fill out an application, and the FCVS will then verify the information through primary sources, noting any problems or discrepancies between information provided by the physician and that obtained from primary sources. The FCVS will then provide the primary-source verification to organizations per the physician's wish. Not all state licensing boards accept FCVS information as primary-source verification. At the time of publication, the base fee for this service (paid by the physician) is $250. Additional surcharges may be charged to cover expenses incurred to collect examination transcripts, ECFMG certification, etc. Subsequent profiles (called subsequent requests) cost $50 each, plus applicable surcharges.

The FCVS conducts primary-source verification of the following information for each physician and physician assistant:

- Identity
- Medical education
- Postgraduate training
- Licensure
- ECFMG certification
- Board action history

The FCVS permanently stores the physician's verified information and submits the complete application and findings, for a fee, to the entities designated by the physician.

FSMB contact information
For more information about FCVS, eligible organizations may contact the FSMB.

Attention: Board Action Services
Federation of State Medical Boards of the United States, Inc.
400 Fuller Wiser Road, Suite 300
Euless, TEXAS 76039-3855
Telephone: 817/868-4000
Fax: 817/868-4098
Web site: www.fsmb.org

AMA Physician Masterfile

Background information
The American Medical Association (AMA) Physician Masterfile database was established in 1906 as a source of biographic data of all United States physicians. In its initial years, the Masterfile included the full name, date of birth, medical college attended, year of graduation, year of licensure, and office address of each physician. All Masterfile data elements were verified with primary sources, and were manually recorded in an index card filing system. In the late 1950s, the AMA converted its index card Masterfile to a computerized system. The newly computerized Masterfile also expanded to include national board (National Board of Medical Examiners or NBME) certification, specialty board certification, primary and secondary self-designated specialties, location and type of practice, sources of income, principal employer, specialty society memberships, and professorial appointments of each physician. These data elements were also verified with primary sources, except for the items related to practice, which were gathered from physicians.

Today's AMA Physician Masterfile is a comprehensive source of demographic, educational, and practice information on all United States physicians with MD degrees—including both AMA members and nonmembers, physicians who were trained in the United States and are temporarily located overseas, and foreign medical graduates residing in the United States. The Masterfile also contains information on DOs who are AMA members, are enrolled in or have completed residency training programs approved by the Accreditation Council for Graduate Medical Education (ACGME), have had disciplinary actions taken against them by state licensing agencies, or have specifically requested to be included in the Masterfile.

Contents of the AMA Physician Masterfile

Physician records contained in the Masterfile are created once a student enters an accredited United States medical school. (Records for foreign medical graduates are initiated when the physician enters an ACGME-accredited residency program.) As a physician's training and career progress, relevant information is added to his or her record.

All Masterfile records contain the following information on each physician:

- Full name, address, and telephone number
- Date and place of birth
- Major professional activity (patient care or non-patient care)
- Self-designated practice area
- Medical or osteopathic school name and year of graduation
- State licensure—year(s), state(s), status, expiration date(s), type(s) (e.g., temporary, limited, or unlimited), and final disciplinary actions
- Year of NBME and ECFMG certification
- Specialty board certification and subcertification year(s) and expiration date(s) by ABMS member boards; current and prior medical training (hospital name, dates of training, and specialty)
- Federal Drug Enforcement Administration (DEA) registration status and disciplinary actions
- Medicare/Medicaid sanctions
- AMA Physician's Recognition Award (PRA) if applicable

All physician information on the Profile is from a primary source except demographic information provided by the physician (e.g., self-designated practice specialty, current address, etc.) These sources—what the AMA calls "data providers"—include medical schools, hospitals, state licensing agencies, the NBME, the ABMS, the Surgeons General of the United States Government, the ECFMG, the Federation Physician Data Center of the FSMB, the DEA, and medical societies.

With help from its affiliates and data providers, the AMA's Department of Data Services continually updates the information contained within the Masterfile.

Obtaining information from the AMA Physician Masterfile

The AMA's Physician Profile service is the most common source of information for hospitals and others seeking Masterfile data for credentialing purposes. The Physician Profile service, coordinated through the AMA's Department of Physician Data Services, provides computerized printouts of information on individual physicians. All printouts include the information contained in the Masterfile record of the physician in question.

Organizations verifying physician credentials directly must set up a Physician Profile account. Set up an account either online or by mail/fax by obtaining and completing a Physician Profile Data Agreement and Order Form from the AMA's Department of Physician Data Services (see number and address below, or download a copy from the AMA's Web site below. Credentials verification organizations (CVOs)—organizations that verify physician credentials for a third party—must sign a Credentials Verification Organization Agreement with the AMA.

The AMA charges a fee of $26 per profile request.

Chapter 8

The AMA Physician Masterfile as primary-source verification

The National Committee for Quality Assurance (NCQA) recognizes the AMA Physician Masterfile as a primary source to verify medical education, residency training, and specialty board certification. The American Accreditation Health Care Commission (formerly the Utilization Review Accreditation Commission [URAC]) also considers the Physician Masterfile a primary source of information for verifying licensure, medical education, residency training, board certification, DEA registration status, and state and federal disciplinary sanctions.

In the fall of 1995, the AMA established to the JCAHO's satisfaction that it was prepared to meet all JCAHO requirements for CVOs. As a result, the JCAHO officially recognized the AMA Physician Masterfile as a "designated equivalent source . . . [of] specific items . . . identical to the information at the primary source."

The significance of this designation is that organizations can regard information from the AMA Physician Masterfile as being just as authoritative as information obtained directly from primary sources. JCAHO standards specifically reference the AMA Masterfile as a designated equivalent source for two specific items: graduation and completion of residency. The physician profiles from the AMA Physician Masterfile also include other primary source-reported information that is similar to primary source-verified information provided by a CVO. In order for the additional information on the AMA profile to be used by the hospital as primary source verification, the organization must be able to achieve a level of confidence in the information provided by the Masterfile. JCAHO guidelines contain nine specific elements that must be evaluated by the hospital in order to achieve this level of confidence. The AMA has published a document titled "Response to The JCAHO Principles for Users of External Credentialing Agencies and Sources (Such as the AMA Physician Masterfile)." Individual organizations should review this document to determine whether it is confident that all nine of the JCAHO's elements are addressed.

Many organizations that use the designated Masterfile information will still want to contact primary sources to inquire about the quality and content of the work applicants did during training. For example, even though the Masterfile might state that a physician completed a residency in surgery, the organization to which the physician is applying will still want to know what was included in the training and what the physician's supervisors thought of the quality of his or her work. This information can be obtained only from the residency program.

American Medical Association Directory of Physicians in the United States

For those who prefer to use printed materials, the AMA publishes the *American Medical Association Directory of Physicians* in the United States. This four-volume directory lists all United States physicians—including those who are temporarily practicing overseas—alphabetically and by geographic region. It includes each physician's professional mailing address, medical school of graduation, initial year of license in the state where the current professional address is located, self-designated primary and secondary specialties, type of practice, ABMS board certification, and AMA Physician's Recognition Award status. The directory is a good resource to assist in credentials verification activities. It is also available on CD/ROM.

AMA Physician Masterfile contact information

For additional information about the AMA Physician Masterfile, AMA Physician Profiles service, or the accreditation agencies that accept the AMA Physician Masterfile as primary-source information on physician credentials, contact the AMA:

AMA Department of Credentialing Products
Attention: Patrick McDonald
American Medical Association
515 N. State Street
Chicago, ILLINOIS 60610
Telephone: 312/464-4972
E-mail: patrick_mcdonald@ama-assn.org
Web site: www.ama-assn.org

National Register of Health Service Providers in Psychology

Background information

To be eligible for the "Health Service Providers in Psychology" credential of the National Register of Health Service Providers in Psychology (also known as the National Register), psychologists must have a doctoral degree in psychology, have at least two years (3,000 hours) of supervised experience in health services in psychology (including 1,500 hours internship or organized training program and 1500 hours of supervised postdoctoral experience), and be currently licensed or certified by a state, provincial, or territorial board of examiners of psychology to practice at the independent practice level. In order to continue to be listed in the National Register, the psychologist must maintain at least one active, unrestricted psychology license at the independent practice level, and submit a yearly renewal fee and ethics attestation form. The National Register conducts primary source verification of the doctoral degree, experience, licensure, and areas of expertise. Ethical violations, expired licenses, additions, deletions, or changes are included in the database.

The National Register monitors official actions and reports regarding psychologists' professional and ethical conduct on an ongoing basis for over 14,000 registrants. The Online Searchable Database contains information on psychologists' education, training, licensure, and practice histories. Health care organizations and insurance providers may use the National Register for several purposes, including verifying psychologists' credentials or screening psychologists. Although neither the Joint Commission on Accreditation of Healthcare Organizations (JCAHO) nor the National Committee for Quality Assurance (NCQA) has made a statement specifically recognizing the National Register as a primary source verification, presumably the National Register could be used as a CVO by organizations processing psychologist applications. The rules applicable to use of any CVO would apply.

Accessing National Register information

The National Register is an annual directory containing detailed information on psychologists who have met or exceeded established national standards of excellence. The cost is $299 per copy. Cost includes a subscription to the Register Report, which is published biannually and contains updates to the directory.

A subscription to the Online Searchable Data Base costs $399 for one year and includes a one-year subscription to the Register Report. The general public can receive immediate access to an account that provides a limited number of queries for personal use.

National Register contact information

National Register of Health Service Providers in Psychology
1120 G Street NW, Suite 330
Washington, DISTRICT OF COLUMBIA 20005
Telephone: 202/783-7663   Fax: 202/347-0550
Web site: www.nationalregister.com

Chiropractic Information Network-Board Action Databank (CIN-BAD) of the Federation of Chiropractic Licensing Boards

Background information

Chiropractic Information Network-Board Action Databank (CIN-BAD) is an online service of the Federation of Chiropractic Licensing Boards (FCLB). FCLB members include chiropractic-licensing boards in all U.S. states, all Canadian provinces, Puerto Rico, the U.S. Virgin Islands, and the Australian states of New South Wales and Victoria.

The Official Actions Databank (OAD) contains information on chiropractors, including actions taken by chiropractic regulatory licensing boards and/or exclusions from Medicare/Medicaid reimbursement by the HHS. Member boards from chiropractic licensing bodies in all U.S. states, Washington, DC, Puerto Rico, Virgin Islands and Guam, plus some Canadian provinces and Australian states, voluntarily report some or all board actions to the CIN-BAD system. Public actions by the licensing boards include revocation/suspension/removal of license, probation or limitations on practice (and the removal of such actions), and fines. Medicare/Medicaid exclusions reported by HHS is included. The database allows for generation of dated verification reports for confirming that a name search was unsuccessful and allows users to place a document into their files that confirms the search was completed. Reports also list birth date, addresses, education, and license status. You may view a sample report on the FCLB Web site.

FCLB has plans for an additional online database called ALLDoCS (All Legally Licensed Doctors of Chiropractic). This database will contain primary-source information on chiropractors' licensure, education, board actions/sanctions, and Medicare/Medicaid exclusion. This database is expected to be operational in early 2003.

CIN-BAD is an NCQA-approved verification source for chiropractic board actions; FCLB will seek NCQA approval as a primary verification source for education and licensure once it has completed ALLDoCS.

Accessing CIN-BAD information

Subscribers pay an annual access fee, which covers account set-up, user training, and unlimited queries utilizing metered usage. CIN-BAD measures data bank usage and charges a $10 fee only to print reports on doctors with public actions. There are two annual subscriptions available:

1. $500 per year for those who query the data bank for their own, internal use; for example, a managed care organization
2. $1,500 per year for those who, operating in a for-profit capacity, query the data bank on behalf of another organization; for example, a credentials verification organization

Contact the FCLB for more information about accessing CIN-BAD as a subscriber.

Non-subscribers may request searches of the Official Actions Databank. There is a $20 fee per name for this search. To request a search, from the FCLB Web site, print a copy of the query form, and mail or fax the form to the FCLB office (see CIN-BAD contact information). If you do not have Internet access, you may call the FCLB office to request a copy of the query form.

CIN-BAD contact information
Federation of Chiropractic Licensing Boards
901 54th Avenue, Suite 101
Greeley, COLORADO 80634-4400
Telephone: 970/356-3500   Fax: 970/356-3599
E-mail: fclb@fclb.org
Web site: www.fclb.org

AOA Official Osteopathic Physician Profile Report

Background of the AOA Official Osteopathic Physician Profile Report
The AOA introduced the Official Osteopathic Physician Profile Report in 1999. The AOA Osteopathic Physician Profile Report is the official source for osteopathic physician information, combining the AOA's board certification verification letter, the AOA physician profile, and AOA Directory information.

Contents of the AOA Official Osteopathic Physician Profile Report
The profile report contains up-to-date, primary-source information, including the following:

- AOA pre- and postdoctoral education and training, including dates of attendance and completion
- all state licenses with expiration dates
- osteopathic specialty board certification and expiration dates
- AOA-accredited continuing medical education
- DEA status
- state and federal sanction alerts
- former name(s) and former addresses (city/state)

The AOA Official Osteopathic Physician Profile Report as primary-source verification
The AOA report meets primary-source requirements for osteopathic medical education, osteopathic postdoctoral training and osteopathic specialty board certification for the AOA Healthcare Facilities Accreditation Program, the JCAHO, the NCQA, the American Accreditation Healthcare Commission, Inc/URAC, and the National Association of Insurance Commissioners.

Obtaining an AOA Official Osteopathic Physician Profile Report
The AOA provides several means for obtaining its Profile Report. The AOA charges $15 for orders via its Web site and fulfills these orders instantly. For organizations that prefer the paper form, the AOA will mail Profile Reports within five days, or fax reports within 24 hours, for $20 per report.

Profile Report contact information
American Osteopathic Association
142 E. Ontario Street
Chicago, ILLINOIS 60611
Telephone: 800/621-1773, Ext. 8145 (toll-free)
Fax: 312/202-8200
E-mail: info@aoa-net.org
Web site: www.aoa-net.org

Office of Inspector General (OIG) List of Excluded Individuals/Entities

The OIG maintains a Web site that includes a database of individuals and entities excluded from federal programs, including Medicare and Medicaid. This database is available free of charge to anyone, including the public at http://exclusions.oig.hhs.gov/. It can be searched by name, state, classification, and exclusion type. Corporate compliance requires health care organizations to allow only providers not excluded by the OIG to treat federal patients. A health care organization can be fined up to $10,000 for each service billed by an excluded provider. In addition, no Medicare or Medicaid payment(s) will be made to a facility for services provided by an excluded party. Although most physicians sign a consent form stating that they have not been sanctioned or excluded from a state or federal program, they do not always provide information concerning sanctions or exclusions that occur after appointment. Federal law states that any entity or individual who is responsible for a sanctioned entity or individual may also be subject to "permissive" exclusion if they know or should know of the actions leading to sanction and do not exclude that individual from performing services. This "permissive" exclusion allows the agency to use its discretion in deciding whether or not to impose an exclusion from participation in the federal programs. In addition, cumulative reports can be downloaded and imported into database or spreadsheet software.

Contact Information
Office of Inspector General Department of Health and Human Services
Room 5541, Cohen Building
330 Independence Avenue SW
Washington, DC 20201
Telephone: 202/619-1343
Fax: 202/260-8512
E-mail: paffairs@oig.hhs.gov
Web site: www.oig.hhs.gov

Controlled Substances Act Registration Database (official DEA authorized database)

The Controlled Substances Act (CSA) Registration Database is maintained by the National Technical Information Service of the U.S. Department of Commerce. It consists of records of more than one million individuals registered under the act, including registrants doing business under their individual names rather than a business name. The database, which is updated twice monthly, can be used to certify a practitioner's DEA status.

Each DEA record contains the following information:

- DEA registration number
- Business activity code (pharmacy, practitioner, hospitals, etc.)
- Drug schedules
- Expiration date
- Name of company or individual
- Street address
- City, state, and ZIP code

Obtaining information from the CSA Database
Subscriptions range in price from $1,750 for a single user to $22,000 for an unlimited number of concurrent users. A sample search is available on the Web site. The database is also available in a CD/ROM for $900 with quarterly updates or $1,920 with monthly updates.

Note: You can call the DEA at 800/882-9539 for a verbal verification of a DEA registration number at no charge. You can view a listing of DEA actions by year at www.deadiversion.usdoj.gov/fed_regs/index.html.

Contact information
National Technical Information Service
U.S. Department of Commerce
Springfield, VA 22161
Telephone: 800/363-2068
E-mail: subscriptions@ntis.fedworld.gov
Web site: http://deanumber.com

Bonus! Quick Checklist Guide to the NPDB

Registering with the NPDB
Before they can obtain information from the data bank, health care entities and individual practitioners must register with the NPDB.

Step 1: Obtain registration form and related information at *www.npdb-hipdb.com/register.html*.
Step 2: Determine eligibility for accessing the data bank by following the guideline information provided on that Web page.
Step 3: Complete and submit registration forms.
Step 4: Receive registration confirmation by mail. A unique data bank identification (DBID) number and password will be enclosed. (Note: The DBID and password are required for reporting and/or querying.)

Querying the NPDB
Health care entities must follow the steps below when conducting a query:

1. Visit the NPDB's Integrated Querying and Reporting Service page at *www.npdb-hipdb.com/welcome.html* and enter your DBID and password

2. Enter query data and submit request

3. Pay by credit card or electronic funds transfer (fee is $5 per practitioner name)

4. Receive a separate confirmation number for each request submitted at the time of your query

5. Retrieve query results electronically within four to six hours of receipt by data bank

Bonus! Quick Checklist Guide to the NPDB *cont.*

Practitioners conducting self-queries must follow the steps listed below:

1. Download a self-query form at *www.npdb-hipdb.com/sqinstr-i.html* or obtain a copy by calling 800/767-6732

2. Submit notarized form to the data bank by mail with credit card information

3. Receive query results by mail within two weeks of receipt by data bank (self-queries are $10 each)

Contacting the NPDB
For further information about the NPDB, use the following resources:

- Help line: 800/767-6732 (operates Monday through Friday, 8:30 am to 6:00 pm, Eastern Standard Time)
- Web site: www.npdb-hipdb.com (information about the data bank's history, purpose, and querying/reporting instructions)

Source: Rena Cutchin, editor, Briefings on Credentialing, *an Opus Communications publication.*

CHAPTER 9
Specialty Associations, Societies, Colleges, and Academies

Chapter 9
Specialty Associations, Societies, Colleges, and Academies

In addition to forming specialty boards, many specialists have organized themselves into other types of groups devoted to furthering the public's access to high-quality care and scientific progress. Such organizations—typically called specialty associations, societies, colleges, or academies—provide many valuable services for those concerned with health care. (Note: The medical colleges discussed in this chapter are not the same medical colleges that a student would attend to earn a medical degree.) For example, many organizations

- provide detailed information about the scope of their specialties
- offer sample criteria for hospital medical staffs to use in privileging
- represent the interests of their members in lobbying efforts with various government agencies
- work with related certification boards to develop board requirements
- provide teaching material to residency programs

Additionally, many specialty organizations enact codes of ethics, monitor the quality of care provided by their members, participate in task forces and investigations to settle professional issues, and sponsor public education programs. In fact, one specialty organization, the American College of Surgeons, started a hospital inspection program as a public service, which evolved into the Joint Commission on Accreditation of Healthcare Organizations (JCAHO). Medical specialty organizations maintain educational materials for their members, including peer review journals and other periodicals that physicians can use as resources on which to base medical activities and decisions. Many medical societies and colleges have close connections with government agencies (e.g., the Centers for Medicare & Medicaid Services, U.S. Congress, the Medicare Payment Advisory Commission, the Agency for Health Care Policy and Research, and the Food and Drug Administration) and spend time lobbying for pertinent medical and consumer issues.

Levels of membership differ by organization. Most societies include a category for "active" members—typically reserved for practitioners who meet the full requirements for membership—and an "associate" or "candidate" category—designed to encourage younger physicians and residents to participate in society activities. Medical colleges may break their membership into categories such as Medical Student or Candidate, Associate, Fellow, and Master. Membership in these organizations is an expression of dedication to the highest standards of medical practice. Fellowship is an honor reserved for those recognized by their peers for personal integrity, superior competence, professional accomplishment, and demonstrated scholarship. Masters generally comprise a small group of highly distinguished physicians who achieve recognition by being forerunners in the practice of medicine or medical research, or have made significant contributions to medical science or the art of medicine. Most specialty organizations are quite restrictive in their membership. Typically, members must meet training, experience, and academic requirements far beyond those of the related certification board.

Letters of recommendation or nomination by other members are often required. Such organizations make a continuous and strenuous effort to maintain ethical standards—even revoking membership for those who do not continue to meet the membership requirements. Therefore, membership in such exclusive specialty organizations can sometimes signify an additional level of professional achievement that reaches above board certification. (Some specialty organizations award members the right to use their membership status as a credential to appear after their names. For example, "FACS" signifies a fellowship in the American College of Surgeons, and "FACP" signifies fellowship in the American College of Physicians.

It is not always easy to distinguish such highly selective specialty organizations from those that are open to anyone willing to pay dues. Even those organizations with restrictive membership requirements might be concerned more with research or academic achievements than with clinical competence. Thus, membership in a specialty association, society, college, or academy should not be assumed to signify anything in particular, until the specific membership requirements of that particular organization are known.

The following section contains a listing of specialty associations, societies, colleges, and academies organized by specialty area. All organizations included in this list were contacted individually to ensure that all contact information is current upon publication. Readers might benefit from referring to this listing when seeking information about a particular area or privilege idea, or to verify membership. Please note that the following organizations have different purposes, policies, services, and requirements, so the level of assistance and information they provide will likely vary.

Addictionology

American Academy of Addiction Psychiatry
7301 Mission Road, Suite 252
Prairie Village, KANSAS 66208
Telephone: 913/262-6161   Fax: 913/262-4311
E-mail: info@aaap.org
Web site: www.aaap.org

American Osteopathic Academy of Addiction Medicine
5550 Friendship Boulevard, Suite 310
Chevy Chase, MARYLAND 20815-7231
Telephone: 301/968-4170   Fax: 301/968-4199
E-mail: aoaam@osteohdq.org

American Society of Addiction Medicine
4601 N. Park Avenue Arcade, Suite 101
Chevy Chase, MARYLAND 20815
Telephone: 301/656-3920   Fax: 301/656-3815
E-mail: E-mail@asam.org
Web site: www.asam.org

International Society of Addiction Medicine
Foothills Hospital
1403 29th Street, NW
Calgary, ALBERTA T2N 2T9
CANADA
Telephone: 403/670-2025   Fax: 403/670-2056
E-mail: nady.el-guebaly@calgaryhealthregion.ca
Web site: www.3.sympatico.ca/pmdoc/isam

International Society of Addiction Medicine
PO Box 1873
Kingston, ONTARIO K7L 5J7
CANADA
Telephone: 613/541-3951   Fax: 613/541-0175
E-mail: csam@kingston.net
Web site: www.csam.org

Chapter 9

Allergy, asthma, and immunology

American Academy of Allergy, Asthma, and Immunology
611 E. Wells Street
Milwaukee, WISCONSIN 53202-9939
Telephone: 414/272-6071   Fax: 414/272-6070
E-mail: info@aaaai.org
Web site: www.aaaai.org

American Academy of Otolaryngic Allergy
1990 M Street NW, Suite 680
Washington, DISTRICT OF COLUMBIA 20036
Telephone: 202/955-5010   Fax: 202/955-5016
E-mail: aaoaf@aaoaf.org
Web site: www.aaoaf.org

American Association of Immunologists
9650 Rockville Pike
Bethesda, MARYLAND 20814-3994
Telephone: 301/530-7178   Fax: 301/571-1816
E-mail: infoaai@aai.faseb.org
Web site: www.aai.org

American College of Allergy, Asthma, and Immunology
85 W. Algonquin Road, Suite 550
Arlington Heights, ILLINOIS 60005
Telephone: 847/427-1200   Fax: 847/427-1294
Web site: www.allergy.mcg.edu

American In-vitro Allergy and Immunology Society
Note: Annual scientific meetings.
PO Box 341461
Bethesda, MARYLAND 20827-1461
Telephone: 301/263-0703   Fax: 301/263-0776
E-mail: aiais@erols.com
Web site: www.invitroallergy.org

American Osteopathic College of Allergy and Immunology
9535 East Doubletree Ranch Road
Scottsdale, ARKANSAS 85258
Telephone: 480/657-7703   Fax: 480/657-7715
Web site: www.goodnet.com/~osteo/-index.html

Asthma and Allergy Foundation of America
1233 20th Street NW, Suite 402
Washington, DISTRICT OF COLUMBIA 20036
Telephone: 202/466-7643   800/727-8462   Fax: 202/466-8940
E-mail: info@aafa.org
Web site: www.aafa.org

Specialty Associations, Societies, Colleges, and Academies

Joint Council of Allergy, Asthma, and Immunology
50 N. Brockway Street, Suite 3-3
Palatine, ILLINOIS 60067
Telephone: 847/934-1918   Fax: 847/934-1820
E-mail: jcaai@aol.com
Web site: www.jcaai.org

Allied health—general

American Association of Bioanalysts
917 Locust Street, Suite 1100
St. Louis, MISSOURI 63101-1419
Telephone: 314/241-1445   Fax: 314/241-1449
E-mail: aab@aab.org
Web site: www.aab.org

American Board of Electrodiagnostic Medicine
Note: American Board of Electrodiagnostic Medicine (ABEM) is an independent credentialing body, operating as a committee of the American Association of Electrodiagnostic Medicine (AAEM). Autonomous for purposes of credentialing criteria and procedures.

421 First Avenue SW, Suite 300E
Rochester, MINNESOTA 55902
Telephone: 507/288-0100   Fax: 507/288-1225
E-mail: abem@aaem.net
Web site: www.aaem.net/abem.html

American Clinical Neurophysiology Society (formerly American Electroencephalographic Society)
1 Regency Drive
PO Box 30
Bloomfield, CONNECTICUT 06002
Telephone: 860/243-3977   Fax: 860/286-0787
E-mail: acns@ssmgt.com
Web site: www.acns.org

American Society for Cytotechnology
1500 Sunday Drive, Suite 102
Raleigh, NORTH CAROLINA 27607
Telephone: 919/787-5181   800/948-3947 (toll-free)   Fax: 919/787-4916
E-mail: knorris@olsonmgmt.com
Web site: www.asct.com

American Society of Cytopathology
400 W. Ninth Street, Suite 201
Wilmington, DELAWARE 19801
Telephone: 302/429-8802   Fax: 302/429-8807
E-mail: asc@cytopathology.org
Web site: www.cytopathology.org

Chapter 9

American Society of Radiologic Technologists
15000 Central Avenue SE
Albuquerque, NEW MEXICO 87123-3917
Telephone: 505/298-4500   Fax: 505/298-5063
Web site: www.asrt.org

Association of Schools of Allied Health Professions
1730 M Street NW, Suite 500
Washington, DISTRICT OF COLUMBIA 20036
Telephone: 202/293-4848   Fax: 202/293-4852
E-mail: asahp1@asahp.org
Web site: www.asahp.org

Canadian Society for Medical Laboratory Science
PO Box 2830, LCD 1
Hamilton, ONTARIO L8N3N8
CANADA
Telephone: 905/528-8642   Fax: 905/528-4968
E-mail: khdavis@csmls.org
Web site: www.csmls.org

Department of Health
Office of Professional Licensing
825 N. Capital Street NE, Second Floor
Washington, DISTRICT OF COLUMBIA 20002
Telephone: 202/442-9200   Fax: 202/442-9431
Web site: www.dchealth.com

Maryland Board of Physician Quality Assurance
Attention: Verifications
4201 Patterson Avenue
PO Box 2571
Baltimore, MARYLAND 21215-0095
Telephone: 800-492-6836 (dial # key), Ext. 4705   410/764-4777   Fax: 410/358-2252
E-mail: bpqa@erols.com
Web site: www.docboard.org

National Association Medical Staff Services
PO Box 140647
Austin, TEXAS 78714-0647
Telephone: 512/454-7928   Fax: 512/454-3036
E-mail: namss@namss.org
Web site: www.namss.org

National Registry of Emergency Medical Technicians
6610 Busch Boulevard
PO Box 29233
Columbus, OHIO 43229
Telephone: 614/888-4484
Web site: www.nremt.org

Anesthesiology

American Academy of Anesthesiologist Assistants
PO Box 81362
Wellesley, MASSACHUSETTS 02481-0004
Telephone: 800/757-5858   Fax: 781/239-3259
Web site: www.anesthetist.org

American Association of Nurse Anesthetists
222 S. Prospect Avenue
Park Ridge, ILLINOIS 60068-4001
Telephone: 847/692-7050   Fax: 847/692-6968
E-mail: info@aana.com
Web site: www.aana.com

American Dental Society of Anesthesiology, Inc.
211 E. Chicago Avenue, Suite 780
Chicago, ILLINOIS 60611
Telephone: 312/664-8270   Fax: 312/642-9713
E-mail: adsa@compuserve.com
Web site: www.adsahome.org

American Osteopathic College of Anesthesiologists
17201 E. US Highway 40, Suite 204
Independence, MISSOURI 64055-6427
Telephone: 816/373-4700   Fax: 816/373-1529
E-mail: osteoanest@aol.com
Web site: members.aol.com/osteoanest/aoca.htm

American Society for the Advancement of Anesthesia and Sedation in Dentistry
6 E. Union Avenue
PO Box 551
Bound Brook, NEW JERSEY 8805
Telephone: 732/469-9050   Fax: 732/271-1985
Web site: www.sedation4dentist.com

American Society of Anesthesiologists
520 N. Northwest Highway
Park Ridge, ILLINOIS 60068-2573
Telephone: 847/825-5586   Fax: 847/825-1692
E-mail: mail@asahq.org
Web site: www.asahq.org

American Society of Critical Care Anesthesiologists
520 N. Northwest Highway
Park Ridge, ILLINOIS 60068-2573
Telephone: 847/825-5586   Fax: 847/825-5658
E-mail: ascca@asahq.org
Web site: www.ascca.org

Chapter 9

American Society of Regional Anesthesia and Pain Medicine
Note: Offers educational programs for the ACCME.
PO Box 11086
2209 Dickens Road
Richmond, VIRGINIA 23230-1086
Telephone: 804/282-0010   Fax: 804/282-0090
E-mail: asra@societyhq.com
Web site: www.asra.com

Canadian Anesthesiologists Society
1 Eglinton Avenue E, Suite 208
Toronto, ONTARIO M4P 3A1
CANADA
Telephone: 416/480-0602   Fax: 416/480-0320
E-mail: anesthesia@cas.ca
Web site: www.cas.ca

National Board of Anesthesiology, Inc.
11817 Summit
Kansas City, KANSAS 64114
Telephone: 785/842-7067   Fax: 816/836-8953

Society for Obstetric Anesthesia and Perinatology
2209 Dickens Road
PO Box 11086
Richmond, VIRGINIA 23230-1086
Telephone: 804/282-5051   Fax: 804/282-0090
E-mail: soap@societyhq.com
Web site: www.soap.org

Society for Pediatric Anesthesia
2209 Dickens Road
PO Box 11086
Richmond, VIRGINIA 23230-1086
Telephone: 804/282-9780   Fax: 804/282-0090
E-mail: spa@societyhq.com
Web site: www.pedsanesthesia.org

Specialty Associations, Societies, Colleges, and Academies

Society of Neurological Anesthesia and Critical Care
2209 Dickens Road
PO Box 11086
Richmond, VIRGINIA 23230-1086
Telephone: 804/673-9037   Fax: 804/282-0090
E-mail: snacc@societyhq.com
Web site: www.snacc.org

Cardiology

American College of Cardiology
9111 Old Georgetown Road
Bethesda, MARYLAND 20814-1699
Telephone: 301/897-5400 800/253-4636
Fax: 301/897-9745
Web site: www.acc.org

American College of Cardiovascular Administrators
701 Lee Street, Suite 600
Des Plaines, ILLINOIS 60016
Telephone: 847/759-8601   Fax: 847/759-8602
E-mail: info@aameda.org
Web site: www.aameda.org

Chiropractic

American Chiropractic Association
1701 Clarendon Boulevard
Arlington, VIRGINIA 22209
Telephone: 703/276-8800   800/986-INFO (4636)   Fax: 703/243-2593
E-mail: memberinfo@americanchiro.org
Web site: www.acatoday.com

Canadian Chiropractic Association
1396 Eglinton Avenue West
Toronto, ONTARIO M6C 2E4
CANADA
Telephone: 800-668-2076 416-781-5656 Fax: 416-781-7344
E-mail: ccachiro@ccachiro.org
Web site: www.ccachiro.org

International Chiropractic Pediatric Association
5295 Highway 78, Suite D362
Stone Mountain, GEORGIA 30087-3414
Telephone: 770/982-9037   Fax: 770/736-1651
E-mail: info@4icpa.org
Web site: www.4icpa.org

Chapter 9

Colon and rectal surgery

American Society of Colon and Rectal Surgeons
85 W. Algonquin Road, Suite 550
Arlington Heights, ILLINOIS 60005-4425
Telephone: 847/290-9184   Fax: 847/290-9203
E-mail: ascrs@execadmin.com
Web site: www.fascrs.org

Counseling

American Mental Health Counselors Association
801 N. Fairfax Street, Suite 304
Alexandria, VIRGINIA 22314
Telephone: 703/548-6002   800/326-2642   Fax: 703/548-4775
E-mail: vmoore@amhca.org
Web site: www.amhca.org

National Board for Certified Counselors Incorporated and Affiliates
3 Terrace Way, Suite D
Greensboro, NORTH CAROLINA 27403-3660
Telephone: 336/547-0607   Fax: 336/547-0017
E-mail: nbcc@nbcc.org
Web site: www.nbcc.org

Critical care/trauma medicine

American Association of Critical Care Nurses
101 Columbia, Suite 200
Aliso Viejo, CALIFORNIA 92656
Telephone: 949/362-2000   Fax: 949/362-2020
E-mail: aacn.info@aacn.org
Web site: www.aacn.org

American Burn Association
625 N. Michigan Avenue, Suite 1530
Chicago, ILLINOIS 60611
Telephone: 312/642-9260   Fax: 312/642-9130
E-mail: info@ameriburn.org
Web site: www.ameriburn.org

American Trauma Society
8903 Presidential Parkway, Suite 512

Specialty Associations, Societies, Colleges, and Academies

Upper Marlboro, MARYLAND 20772-2656
Telephone: 800-556-7890   Fax: 301-420-0617
E-mail: atstrauma@aol.com
Web site: www.amtrauma.org

Canadian Critical Care Society
Nine EN242
200 Elizabeth Street
Toronto, ONTARIO M5G 1L7
CANADA
Telephone: 416/340-3573   Fax: 416/595-9486

Dentistry

Academy for Implants and Transplants
PO Box 223
Springfield, VIRGINIA 22150
Telephone: 703/451-0001   Fax: 703/451-0004

Academy of General Dentistry
211 E. Chicago Avenue, Suite 900
Chicago, ILLINOIS 60611-1999
Telephone: 312/440-4300   Fax: 312/440-0559
Web site: www.agd.org

Academy of Oral Dynamics
8919 Sudley Road
Manassas, VIRGINIA 20111
Telephone: 703/368-1166   Fax: 703/361-4666

American Academy of Pediatric Dentistry
211 E. Chicago Avenue, Suite 700
Chicago, ILLINOIS 60611
Telephone: 312/337-2169   Fax: 312/337-6329
E-mail: aapdinfo@aapd.org
Web site: www.aapd.org

American Academy of Periodontology
737 N. Michigan Avenue, Suite 800
Chicago, ILLINOIS 60611
Telephone: 312/787-5518   Fax: 312/787-3670
Web site: www.perio.org

American Association of Endodontists
211 E. Chicago Avenue, Suite 1100
Chicago, ILLINOIS 60611
Telephone: 312/266-7255   Fax: 312/266-9867
E-mail: info@aae.org
Web site: www.aae.org

Chapter 9

American Association of Hospital Dentists Inc.
211 E. Chicago Avenue
Chicago, ILLINOIS 60611
Telephone: 312/440-2660   Fax: 312/440-2824
E-mail: specialdentcare@yahoo.com
Web site: www.foscod.org

American Association of Orthodontists
401 N. Lindbergh Boulevard
St. Louis, MISSOURI 63141-7816
Telephone: 314/993-1700   Fax: 314/997-1745
Web site: www.aaortho.org

American Association of Public Health Dentistry
3760 SW Lyle Court
Portland, OREGON 97221
Telephone: 503/242-0712   Fax: 503/242-0721
E-mail: natoff@aol.com
Web site: www.pitt.edu/~aaphd

American College of Dentists
839J Quince Orchard Boulevard
Gaithersburg, MARYLAND 20878-1603
Telephone: 301/977-3223   Fax: 301/977-3330
E-mail: info@facd.org
Web site: www.facd.org

American College of Prosthodontists
211 E. Chicago Avenue, Suite 1000
Chicago, ILLINOIS 60611
Telephone: 312/573-1260   Fax: 312/573-1257
E-mail: acp@prosthodontics.org
Web site: www.prosthodontics.org

American Dental Assistants Association
203 N. LaSalle, Suite 1320
Chicago, ILLINOIS 60601-1225
Telephone: 312/541-1550   Fax: 312/541-1496
Web site: www.dentalassistant.org

American Dental Association
211 E. Chicago Avenue
Chicago, ILLINOIS 60611-2678
Telephone: 312/440-2500   Fax: 312/440-2883
Web site: www.ada.org

American Dental Education Association
1625 Massachusetts Avenue NW, Suite 600
Washington, DISTRICT OF COLUMBIA 20036-2212
Telephone: 202/667-9433   Fax: 202/667-0642

E-mail: membership@adea.org
Web site: www.adea.org

American Dental Society of Anesthesiology, Inc.
211 E. Chicago Avenue, Suite 780
Chicago, ILLINOIS 60611
Telephone: 312/664-8270   Fax: 312/642-9713
E-mail: adsaHome@cs.com
Web site: www.adsaHome.org

American Society for the Advancement of Anesthesia Sedation in Dentistry
6 E. Union Avenue
Bound Brook, NEW JERSEY 8805
Telephone: 732/469-9050   Fax: 732/271-1985
Web site: www.sedation4dentist.com

American Society of Dentistry for Children
211 E. Chicago Avenue
Suite 710
Chicago, ILLINOIS 60611
Telephone: 312/943-1244   Fax: 312/943-5341
E-mail: asdckids@aol.com
Web site: www.asdckids.org

Canadian Dental Association
1815 Alta Vista Drive
Ottawa, ONTARIO K1G3Y6
CANADA
Telephone: 613/523-1770   Fax: 613/523-7736
E-mail: receptionist@cda-adc.ca
Web site: www.cda-adc.ca

National Association of Dental Assistants
900 S. Washington, Suite G13
Falls Church, VIRGINIA 22046
Telephone: 703/237-8616   Fax: 703/533-1153

National Dental Association
3517 16th Street NW
Washington, DISTRICT OF COLUMBIA 20010
Telephone: 202/588-1697   Fax: 202/588-1244
E-mail: admin@ndaonline.org
Web site: www.ndaonline.org

Dermatology

American Osteopathic College of Dermatology
1501 E. Illinois Street
PO Box 7525

Kirksville, MISSOURI 63501
Telephone: 660/665-2184   800/449-2623   Fax: 660/627-2623
E-mail: execdirector@aocd.org
Web site: www.aocd.org

American Society for Dermatologic Surgery
5550 Meadowbrook Drive, Suite 120
Rolling Meadows, ILLINOIS 60008
Telephone: 847/956-0900   Fax: 847/956-0999
E-mail: asds@neton-line
Web site: www.aboutskinsurgery.com

Canadian Dermatology Association
521-774 Echo Drive
Ottawa, ONTARIO K1S 5N8
CANADA
Telephone: 613/730-6262   Fax: 613/730-8262
E-mail: contact.cda@dermatology.ca
Web site: www.dermatology.ca

Dermatology Foundation
1560 Sherman Avenue, Suite 870
Evanston, ILLINOIS 60201-4808
Telephone: 847/328-2256   Fax: 847/328-0509
E-mail: dfgen@dermatologyfoundation.org
Web site: www.dermatologyfoundation.org

Emergency medicine

American College of Emergency Physicians
1125 Executive Circle
Irving, TEXAS 75038-2522
Telephone: 972/550-0911   Fax: 972/580-2816
Web site: www.acep.org

American College of Osteopathic Emergency Physicians
142 E. Ontario Street, Suite 550
Chicago, ILLINOIS 60611
Telephone: 800/521-3709   312/587-3709   Fax: 312/587-9951
Web site: www.acoep.org

Canadian Association of Emergency Physicians
104-1785 Alta Vista Drive
Ottawa, ONTARIO K1G 3Y6
CANADA
Telephone: 613/523-3343   Fax: 613/523-0190
E-mail: admin@caep.ca
Web site: www.caep.ca

Specialty Associations, Societies, Colleges, and Academies

National Registry of Emergency Medical Technicians
6610 Busch Boulevard
PO Box 29233
Columbus, OHIO 43229
Telephone: 614/888-4484   Fax: 614/888-8920
E-mail: billb@nremt.org
Web site: www.nremt.org

Society for Academic Emergency Medicine
901 N. Washington Avenue
Lansing, MICHIGAN 48906
Telephone: 517/485-5484   Fax: 517/485-0801
E-mail: saem@saem.org
Web site: www.saem.org

Endocrinology

American Association of Clinical Endocrinologists
1000 Riverside Avenue, Suite 205
Jacksonville, FLORIDA 32204
Telephone: 904/353-7878   Fax: 904/353-8185
Web site: www.aace.com

The Endocrine Society
Note: Provides verification of educational credits.
4350 E. West Highway, Suite 500
Bethesda, MARYLAND 20814
Telephone: 301/941-0200   Fax: 301/941-0259
Web site: www.endo-society.org

Women in Endocrinology
c/o N. Weigel
Dept. of Molecular and Cellular Biology
1 Baylor Plaza
Baylor College of Medicine
Houston, TEXAS 77030
Web site: www.women-in-endo.org

Endoscopy

American Society for Gastrointestinal Endoscopy
13 Elm Street
Manchester, MASSACHUSETTS 01944
Telephone: 978/526-8330   Fax: 978/526-4018
E-mail: asge@shore.net
Web site: www.asge.org

Society of American Gastrointestinal Endoscopic Surgeons
2716 Ocean Park Boulevard, Suite 3000

Santa Monica, CALIFORNIA 90405
Telephone: 310/314-2404   Fax: 310/314-2585
E-mail: sagesweb@sages.org
Web site: www.sages.org

Environmental medicine

American Academy of Environmental Medicine
Medical Specialty Association
7701 E. Kellogg, Suite 625
Wichita, KANSAS 67207
Telephone: 316/684-5500   Fax: 316/684-5709
E-mail: centraloffice@aaem.com
Web site: www.aaem.com

American College of Occupational and Environmental Medicine
1114 N. Arlington Heights Road
Arlington Heights, ILLINOIS 60004-4770
Telephone: 847/818-1800   Fax: 847/818-9266
Web site: www.acoem.org

National Environmental Health Association
720 S. Colorado Boulevard
South Tower, Suite 970
Denver, COLORADO 80246-1925
Telephone: 303/756-9090   Fax: 303/691-9490
E-mail: staff@neha.org
Web site: www.neha.org

Occupational and Environmental Medical Association of Canada
54 Forward Avenue
London, ONTARIO N6H 1B7
CANADA
Fax: 519-439-8840
E-mail: oemac@oemac.org
Web site: www.oemac.org

Family medicine

American Academy of Family Physicians
11400 Tomahawk Creek Parkway
Leawood, KANSAS 66211-2672
Telephone: 913/906-6000   Fax: 913/906-6075
E-mail: fp@aafp.org   Web site: www.aafp.org

American College of Osteopathic Family Physicians
330 E. Algonquin Road, Suite One
Arlington Heights, ILLINOIS 60005
Telephone: 847/228-6090   800/323-0794 (toll-free)   Fax: 847/228-9755
Web site: www.acofp.org

Specialty Associations, Societies, Colleges, and Academies

American Osteopathic Association
142 E. Ontario Street
Chicago, ILLINOIS 60611
Telephone: 800/621-1773, Ext. 8285   312/202-8285   Fax: 312/202-8445
Web site: www.aoa-net.org

College of Family Physicians of Canada
2630 Skymark Avenue
Mississauga, ONTARIO L4W 5A4
CANADA
Telephone: 905/629-0900   800/387-6197   Fax: 905/629-0893
E-mail: info@cfpc.ca
Web site: www.cfpc.ca

Gastroenterology

American College of Gastroenterology
4900B S. 31st Street
Arlington, VIRGINIA 22206
Telephone: 703/820-7400   Fax: 703/931-4520
E-mail: cd005258@mindspring.com
Web site: www.acg.gi.org

American Gastroenterological Association
7910 Woodmont Avenue, Suite 700
Bethesda, MARYLAND 20814
Telephone: 301/654-2055   Fax: 301/654-5920
E-mail: member@gastro.org
Web site: www.gastro.org

American Society for Gastrointestinal Endoscopy
13 Elm Street
Manchester, MASSACHUSETTS 01944-1314
Telephone: 978/526-8330   Fax: 978/526-4018
E-mail: asge@shore.net
Web site: www.asge.org

North American Society for Pediatric Gastroenterology, Hepatology, and Nutrition
PO Box 6
Flourtown, PENNSYLVANIA 19031
Telephone: 215/233-0808   Fax: 215/233-3939
E-mail: naspghan@naspghan.org
Web site: www.naspghan.org

Society of American Gastrointestinal Endoscopic Surgeons
2716 Ocean Park Boulevard, Suite 3000
Santa Monica, CALIFORNIA 90405

Telephone: 310/314-2404   Fax: 310/314-2585
E-mail: sagesweb@sages.org
Web site: www.sages.org

General medicine

Accreditation Council for Graduate Medical Education
Note: Also provides accreditation of Medical Residency Programs.
515 N. State Street, Suite 2000
Chicago, ILLINOIS 60610-4322
Telephone: 312/464-4920   Fax: 312/464-4098
Web site: www.acgme.org

Aerospace Medical Association
Note: Annual seminar provides credits for CME and CUE requirements.
320 S. Henry Street
Alexandria, VIRGINIA 22314-3579
Telephone: 703/739-2240   Fax: 703/739-9652
Web site: www.asma.org

American Academy of Pain Management
Note: Multidisciplinary membership. Offers board certification in pain management.
13947 Mono Way #A
Sonora, CALIFORNIA 95370
Telephone: 209/533-9744   Fax: 209/533-9750
E-mail: aapm@aapainmanage.org
Web site: www.aapainmanage.org

American Association of Physician Specialists, Inc.
2296 Henderson Mill Road, Suite 206
Atlanta, GEORGIA 30345
Telephone: 770/939-8555   Fax: 770/939-8559
Web site: www.aapsga.org

American College of Medicine
820 N. Orleans, Suite 208
Chicago, ILLINOIS 60610
Telephone: 312/440-0699   Fax: 312/440-0580
E-mail: iaos@aol.com
Web site: www.ascmso.com

American College of Physicians/American Society of Internal Medicine (ACP-ASIM)
2011 Pennsylvania Avenue, NW
Philadelphia, PENNSYLVANIA 19106
Telephone: 800/523-1546 (general office)   Fax: 215/351-2799
Web site: www.acponline.org

American Holistic Medical Association
6728 McLean Village Drive

Specialty Associations, Societies, Colleges, and Academies

McLean, VIRGINIA 22101
Telephone: 703/556-9245   Fax: 703/556-8729
E-mail: info@holisticmedicine.org
Web site: www.holisticmedicine.org

American Medical Association
515 N. State Street
Chicago, ILLINOIS 60610
Telephone: 800/665-2882   Fax: 312/464-5801
Web site: www.ama-assn.org/amaprofiles

American Physiological Society
9650 Rockfield Pike
Bethesda, MARYLAND 20814-3991
Telephone: 301/530-7164   Fax: 301/571-8305
E-mail: info@the-aps.org
Web site: www.the-aps.org

American Society of Bariatric Physicians
5453 E. Evans Place
Denver, COLORADO 80222-5234
Telephone: 303/770-2526   Fax: 303/779-4834
E-mail: info@asbp.org
Web site: www.asbp.org

American Society of Contemporary Medicine and Surgery
820 N. Orleans, Suite 208
Chicago, ILLINOIS 60610
Telephone: 312/440-0699   Fax: 312/440-0580
E-mail: iaos@aol.com
Web site: www.ascmso.com

Association for Hospital Medical Education
Note: Association for Graduate, Continuing, and Undergraduate Medical Education.
419 Beulah Road
Pittsburgh, PENNSYLVANIA 15235
Telephone: 412/244-9302   Fax: 412/243-4693
E-mail: ahmeinpgh@aol.com
Web site: www.ahme.med.edu

Association for the Advancement of Wound Care
HMP Communications
950 W. Valley Road, Suite 2800
Wayne, PENNSYLVANIA 19087
Telephone: 800/237-7285   610/688-8220   Fax: 610/688-1060
E-mail: aawchelp@voicenet.com
Web site: www.hmpcommunications.com

Association of American Medical Colleges
2450 N. Street NW

Washington, DISTRICT OF COLUMBIA 20037-1127
Telephone: 202/828-0400   Fax: 202/828-1125
Web site: www.aamc.org

Association of American Physicians and Surgeons, Inc.
1601 N. Tucson Boulevard, Suite 9
Tucson, ARIZONA 85716
Telephone: 520/327-4885   Fax: 520/326-3529
Web site: www.aapsonline.org

Association of Military Surgeons of the United States
9320 Old Georgetown Road
Bethesda, MARYLAND 20814
Telephone: 301/897-8800   Fax: 301/530-5446
E-mail: amsus@amsus.org
Web site: www.amsus.org

Canadian Medical Association
1867 Alta Vista Drive
Ottawa, ONTARIO K1G 3Y6
CANADA
Telephone: 613/731-9331   800/267-9703 (toll-free)   Fax: 613/731-7314
Web site: www.cma.ca

Committee of Interns and Residents
386 Park Avenue S., Room 1502
New York, NEW YORK 10016
Telephone: 212/725-5500   Fax: 212/779-2413
E-mail: info@cirdoc.org
Web site: www.cirseiu.org

Council of Medical Specialty Societies
51 Sherwood Terrace, Suite M
Lake Bluff, ILLINOIS 60044
Telephone: 847/295-3456   Fax: 847/295-3759
E-mail: mailbox@cmss.org
Web site: www.cmss.org

Mississippi State Board of Medical Licensure
Note: A computerized list will be provided to hospitals and credentialing agencies for a $125 fee, to be utilized for verification purposes only. One free update may be requested within the Board's fiscal year during the months of August through April.
1867 Crane Ridge Drive, Suite 200-B
Jackson, MISSISSIPPI 39216
Telephone: 601/987-3079   Fax: 601/987-4159
Web site: www.msbml.stste.ms.us

National Health Council, Inc.
1730 M Street NW, Suite 500

Washington, DISTRICT OF COLUMBIA 20036-4505
Telephone: 202/785-3910   Fax: 202/785-5923
E-mail: info@nhcouncil.org
Web site: www.nationalhealthcouncil.org

National Medical Association
1012 Tenth Street NW
Washington, DISTRICT OF COLUMBIA 20001
Telephone: 202/347-1895   Fax: 202/842-3293
Web site: www.nma.net.org

National Resident Matching Program
2501 M Street NW, Suite 1
2450 N Street NW (mailing address)
Washington, DISTRICT OF COLUMBIA 20037
Telephone: 202/828-0676   Fax: 202/828-1121
E-mail: nrmp@aamc.org
Web site: www.nrmp.org

Royal College of Physicians and Surgeons of Canada
774 Echo Drive
Ottawa, ONTARIO K1S 5N8
CANADA
Telephone: 800/668-3740   613/730-8177   Fax: 613/730-8830
Web site: rcpsc.medical.org

Society for Ambulatory Care Professionals
One N. Franklin, 28th Floor
Chicago, ILLINOIS 60606
Telephone: 312/422-3900   Fax: 312/422-4577
Web site: www.atta.org

The Wound Healing Society
1550 S. Coast Highway, Suite 201
Laguna Beach, CALIFORNIA 92651
Telephone: 888/434-4234   Fax: 949/376-3456
E-mail: membership@woundheal.org
Web site: www.woundhealsoc.org

Tulsa County Medical Society
2021 S. Lewis, Suite 560
Tulsa, OKLAHOMA 74104
Telephone: 918/743-6184

Chapter 9

Geriatric medicine

American Aging Association
The Sally Balin Medical Center
110 Chesley Drive
Media, PENNSYLVANIA 19063
Telephone: 610/627-2626   Fax: 610/565-9747
E-mail: ameraging@aol.com
Web site: www.americanaging.org

American Association of Homes and Services for the Aging
2519 Connecticut Avenue NW
Washington, DISTRICT OF COLUMBIA 20008-1520
Telephone: 202/783-2242   Fax: 202/783-2255
E-mail: member@aahsa.org
Web site: www.aahsa.org

American Geriatrics Society
350 Fifth Avenue, Suite 801
New York, NEW YORK 10118
Telephone: 212/308-1414   Fax: 212/832-8646
E-mail: info.amger@americangeriatrics.org
Web site: www.americangeriatrics.org

National Council on the Aging, Inc.
409 Third Street SW
Washington, DISTRICT OF COLUMBIA 20024
Telephone: 202/479-1200   Fax: 202/479-0735
E-mail: info@ncoa.org
Web site: www.ncoa.org

New England Gerontological Association
1 Cutts Road
Durham, NEW HAMPSHIRE 03824-3102
Telephone: 603/868-5757
E-mail: genetsr@mediaone.net
Web site: www.negaonline.org

The Gerontological Society of America
1030 15th Street NW, Suite 250
Washington, DISTRICT OF COLUMBIA 20005-1503
Telephone: 202/842-1275   Fax: 202/842-1150
E-mail: geron@geron.org
Web site: www.geron.org

Head and neck surgery

American Academy of Otolaryngology, Head and Neck Surgery
1 Prince Street
Alexandria, VIRGINIA 22314-3357
Telephone: 703/836-4444   Fax: 703/683-5100

E-mail: info@entnet.org
Web site: www.entnet.org

American Head and Neck Society
601 N. Caroline Street
Baltimore, MARYLAND 21287
Telephone: 410/955-4446   Fax: 410/955-7766
E-mail: dwalla@jhmi.edu
Web site: www.headandneckcancer.org

American Head and Neck Society
200 Lothrop Street, Suite 519
Pittsburgh, PENNSYLVANIA 15213
Telephone: 412/647-2227   412/647-2209 (main)   Fax: 412/647-8944
E-mail: rwagner@pitt.edu
Web site: www.headandneckcancer.org

Hematology

American Society of Hematology
1900 M Street NW, Suite 200
Washington, DISTRICT OF COLUMBIA 20036
Telephone: 202/776-0544   Fax: 202/776-0545
E-mail: ash@hematology.org
Web site: www.hematology.org

Hospice care

American Academy of Hospice and Palliative Medicine
Note: Individuals seeking certification in a specific medical field can call 301/439-8001 for details.
4700 W. Lake Avenue
Glenview, ILLINOIS 60025-1485
Telephone: 847/375-4712   Fax: 847/375-6312
E-mail: aahpm@aahpm.org
Web site: www.aahpm.org

Hospice and Palliative Nurses Association National Board for Certification of Hospice and Palliative Nurses
Penn Center W. One, Suite 229
Pittsburgh, PENNSYLVANIA 15276
Telephone: 412/787-9301   Fax: 412/787-9305
E-mail: hpna@hpna.org
Web site: www.hpna.org

Chapter 9

Hospital-related organizations

Academy for Healthcare and Management
1129 20th Street, Suite 600
Washington, DISTRICT OF COLUMBIA 20036-3421
Telephone: 202/778-3200   Fax: 202/778-8506
Web site: webmaster@aahp.org

American Academy of Hospice and Palliative Medicine
4700 W. Lake Avenue
Glenview, ILLINOIS 60025-1485
Telephone: 847/375-4712   Fax: 847/734-8671
E-mail: aahpm@aahpm.org
Web site: www.aahpm.org

American Academy of Medical Administrators
701 Lee Street, Suite 600
Des Plaines, ILLINOIS 60016
Telephone: 847/759-8600   Fax: 847/759-8602
E-mail: info@aameda.org
Web site: www.aameda.org

American Baptist Homes and Hospitals Association
PO Box 851
Valley Forge, PENNSYLVANIA 19482-0851
Telephone: 610/768-2411   Fax: 610/768-2453
Web site: www.nationalministries.org

American College of Health Care Administrators
300 N. Lee Street, Suite 301
Alexandria, VIRGINIA 22314
Telephone: 703/739-7900   Fax: 703/739-7901
E-mail: info@achca.org
Web site: www.achca.org

American College of Healthcare Executives
1 N. Franklin Street, Suite 1700
Chicago, ILLINOIS 60606
Telephone: 312/424-2800   Fax: 312/424-0023
E-mail: ache@ache.org
Web site: www.ache.org

American Health Care Association
1201 L Street NW
Washington, DISTRICT OF COLUMBIA 20005
Telephone: 202/842-4444   Fax: 202/842-3860
Web site: www.ahca.org

American Health Lawyers Association
1025 Connecticut Avenue NW, Suite 600

Washington, DISTRICT OF COLUMBIA 20036-5405
Telephone: 202/833-1100   Fax: 202/833-1105
E-mail: info@healthlawyers.org
Web site: www.healthlawyers.org

American Hospital Association
1 N. Franklin, 32nd Floor
Chicago, ILLINOIS 60606-3401
Telephone: 312/422-3000   Fax: 312/422-4796
Web site: www.aha.org

American Medical Rehabilitation Providers Association
1606 20th Street NW, Third Floor
Washington, DISTRICT OF COLUMBIA 20009
Telephone: 888-346-4624   202-265-4404   Fax: 202-833-9168
Web site: amrpa.firminc.com

American Society of Law Medicine and Ethics
Note: Membership includes attorneys, hospital CEOs, and other executives.
765 Commonwealth Avenue, Suite 1634
Boston, MASSACHUSETTS 02215
Telephone: 617/262-4990   Fax: 617/437-7596
E-mail: info@aslme.org
Web site: www.aslme.org

Association of University Programs in Health Administration
730 11th Street NW, Fourth Floor
Washington, DISTRICT OF COLUMBIA 20001
Telephone: 202/638-1448   Fax: 202/638-3429
E-mail: aupha@aupha.org
Web site: www.aupha.org

Boston Medical Center
Medical Staff Services
One Boston Medical Center Place
Mallory 410
Medical Staff Office
Boston, MASSACHUSETTS 02118
Telephone: 617/414-5423   Fax: 617/414-3506
E-mail: bobdemayo@bmc.org
Web site: www.bmc.org

Federation of American Health Systems
801 Pennsylvania Avenue NW, Suite 245
Washington, DISTRICT OF COLUMBIA 20004-2604

Chapter 9

Telephone: 202/624-1500   Fax: 202/737-6462
E-mail: info@fahs.com
Web site: www.americashospitals.com

Jacobi Medical Center
Note: Jacobi Medical Center formerly known as Bronx Medical Center. Send verification requests to Jacobi Medical Center for residencies that took place at Jacobi Medical Center only.
Attention: Residency verification request
Staff House, Room 103
1400 Pelham Parkway
Bronx, NEW YORK 10461
Telephone: 718/918-3230   Fax: 718/918-5235

National Association of Psychiatric Health Systems
325 Seventh Street NW, Suite 625
Washington, DISTRICT OF COLUMBIA 20004-2802
Telephone: 202/393-6700   Fax: 202/783-6041
E-mail: naphs@naphs.org
Web site: www.naphs.org

National Association of Public Hospitals
1301 Pennsylvania Avenue NW, Suite 950
Washington, DISTRICT OF COLUMBIA 20004
Telephone: 202/585-0100   Fax: 202/585-0101
E-mail: naph@naph.org
Web site: www.naph.org

National Council and Association for Community Behavioral Health Care
12300 Twinbrooke Parkway, Suite 320
Rockville, MARYLAND 20852
Telephone: 301/984-6200   Fax: 301/881-7159
Web site: www.nccbh.org

National Rural Health Association
1320 19th Street NW, Suite 350
Washington, DISTRICT OF COLUMBIA 20036
Telephone: 202/232-6200   Fax: 202/232-1133
E-mail: dc@nrharural.org
Web site: www.nrharural.org

University of Chicago Hospitals
Office of House Staff Affairs
5841 S. Maryland Avenue
MC 1052
Chicago, ILLINOIS 60637
Telephone: 773/702-6760   Fax: 773/702-0861

University of Wisconsin Hospital & Clinics
House Staff Office
600 Highland Avenue H4/831 8320
Madison, WISCONSIN 53792-8310
Telephone: 608/263-0572   Fax: 608/263-9830

Internal medicine

American College of Osteopathic Internists
3 Bethesda Metro Center, Suite 508
Bethesda, MARYLAND 20814
Telephone: 800/327-5183   301/656-8877   Fax: 301/656-7133
E-mail: acoi@acoi.org
Web site: www.acoi.org

American College of Physicians/American Society of Internal Medicine (ACP-ASIM)
2011 Pennsylvania Avenue NW, Suite 800
Washington, DISTRICT OF COLUMBIA 20066-1837
Telephone: 202/261-4500   800/523-1546, Ext. 2600   Fax: 202/835-0443
Web site: www.acponline.org

American College of Physicians/American Society of Internal Medicine (ACP-ASIM)
190 N. Independence Mall West
Philadelphia, PENNSYLVANIA 19106-1572
Telephone: 800-523-1546   215-351-2400   Fax: 215-351-2799
Web site: www.acponline.org

Canadian Society of Internal Medicine
774 Echo Drive
Ottawa, ONTARIO K1S 5N8
CANADA
Telephone: 613/730-6244   Fax: 613/730-1116
E-mail: csim@rcpsc.edu
Web site: csim.medical.org

Society of General Internal Medicine
2501 M Street NW, Suite 575
Washington, DISTRICT OF COLUMBIA 20037
Telephone: 202/887-5150   Fax: 202/887-5405
E-mail: info@sgim.org
Web site: www.sgim.org

Laser medicine

American Society for Laser Medicine and Surgery, Inc.
2404 Stewart Square
Wausau, WISCONSIN 54401
Telephone: 715/845-9283   Fax: 715/848-2493
E-mail: information@aslms.org
Web site: www.aslms.org

Managed care

Academy for Healthcare and Management
1129 20th Street, Suite 600
Washington, DISTRICT OF COLUMBIA 20036-3421
Telephone: 202/778-3200
E-mail: webmaster@aahp.org
Web site: www.aahp.org

American Association of Managed Care Nurses
4435 Waterfront Drive, Suite 101
PO Box 4913
Glen Allen, VIRGINIA 23058-4913
Telephone: 804/747-9698   Fax: 804/747-5316
E-mail: rbailey@aamcn.org
Web site: www.aamcn.org

American College of Managed Care Medicine
4435 Waterfront Drive, Suite 101
Glen Allen, VIRGINIA 23060
Telephone: 804/527-1906   Fax: 804/747-5316
E-mail: sreed@acmcm.org
Web site: www.acmcm.org

National Association of Managed Care Physicians, Inc.
4435 Waterfront Drive, Suite 101
PO Box 4765
Glen Allen, VIRGINIA 23060
Telephone: 804/527-1905   Fax: 804/747-5316
E-mail: sreed@namcp.com
Web site: www.namcp.com

Maxillofacial surgery

American Association of Oral and Maxillofacial Surgeons
9700 W. Bryn Mawr Avenue
Rosemont, ILLINOIS 60018-5701
Telephone: 847/678-6200   Fax: 847/678-4619
E-mail: inquires@aaoms.org
Web site: www.aaoms.org

American Cleft Palate Craniofacial Association
Note: Nonprofit organization.
104 S. Estes Drive, Suite 204
Chapel Hill, NORTH CAROLINA 27514
Telephone: 919/933-9044   Fax: 919/933-9604
E-mail: cleftline@aol.com
Web site: www.cleftline.org

Nephrology

Renal Physicians Association
4701 Randolph Road, Suite 102
Rockville, MARYLAND 20852
Telephone: 301/468-3515   Fax: 301/468-3511
E-mail: rpa@renalmd.org
Web site: www.renalmd.org

Neurological surgery

American Association of Neurological Surgeons
5550 Meadowbrook Drive
Rolling Meadows, ILLINOIS 60008
Telephone: 847/378-0500   Fax: 847/378-0600
E-mail: info@aans.org
Web site: www.aans.org

The Society of Neurological Surgeons
University of Michigan
University Hospital TC 2128
1500 E. Medical Center Drive
Ann Arbor, MICHIGAN 48109-0338
Telephone: 734/936-5015   Fax: 734/936-9294
Web site: www.med.umich.edu

UCLA Medical Center
Division of Neurosurgery
PO Box 957039
Los Angeles, CALIFORNIA 90095-7039
Telephone: 310/825-3998   Fax: 310/825-7245
E-mail: neurosur@medsch.ucla.edu

Neurology

American Academy of Neurology
1080 Montreal Avenue
St. Paul, MINNESOTA 55116-2311
Telephone: 651/695-1940   Fax: 651/695-2791
E-mail: membership@aan.com
Web site: www.aan.com

American Association of Neuroscience Nurses
4700 W. Lake Avenue
Glenview, ILLINOIS 60025
Telephone: 888/557-2266   Fax: 847/375-6333
E-mail: aann@aann.org
Web site: www.aann.org

American College of Neuropsychiatrists
28595 Orchard Lake Road, Suite 200
Farmington Hills, MICHIGAN 48334
Telephone: 248/553-0010, Ext. 295   Fax: 248/553-0818
E-mail: acn-aconp@msn.com

American Society of Electroneurodiagnostic Technologists, Inc.
204 W. 7th Street
Carroll, IOWA 51401-2317
Telephone: 712/792-2978   Fax: 712/792-6962
E-mail: info@aset.org
Web site: www.aset.org

American Society of Pediatric Neuroradiology
2210 Midwest Road, Suite 207
Oak Brook, ILLINOIS 60523-8205
Telephone: 630/574-0220, Ext. 226   Fax: 630/574-0661
E-mail: kcammarata@asnr.org
Web site: www.asnr.org/aspnr

Nuclear medicine

Canadian Association of Nuclear Medicine
774 Echo Drive
Ottawa, ONTARIO K1S 5N8
CANADA
Telephone: 613/730-6254   Fax: 613/730-1116
E-mail: canm@rcpsc.edu
Web site: www.canm.medical.org

Specialty Associations, Societies, Colleges, and Academies

Society of Nuclear Medicine
1850 Samuel Morse Drive
Reston, VIRGINIA 20190-5316
Telephone: 703/708-9000   Fax: 703/708-9015
Web site: www.snm.org

Washington Hospital School of Radiography
155 Wilson Avenue
Washington, PENNSYLVANIA 15301
Telephone: 724/223-3134 (School of x-ray)   Fax: 724/228-2019
E-mail: kwilliams@thewashingtonhospital.org
Web site: www.welnet.org

Nursing

Air & Surface Transport Nurses Association (formerly National Flight Nurses Association)
915 Lee Street
Denver, COLORADO 60016-6569
Telephone: 800/897-6362
E-mail: dmalcolm@ena.org
Web site: www.astna.org

American Academy of Ambulatory Care Nursing
E. Holly Avenue, Box 56
Pittman, NEW JERSEY 08071
Telephone: 856/256-2350   Fax: 856/589-7463
E-mail: aaacn@ajj.com
Web site: www.aaacn.inurse.com

American Academy of Nurse Practitioners
National Administrative Office
PO Box 12846
Austin, TEXAS 78711
Telephone: 512/442-4262   Fax: 512/442-6469
E-mail: admin@aanp.org
Web site: www.aanp.org

American Academy of Nursing
600 Maryland Avenue SW, Suite 100 W.
Washington, DISTRICT OF COLUMBIA 20024-2571
Telephone: 202/651-7000   Fax: 202/651-7001
E-mail: tgaffney@ana.org
Web site: www.nursingworld.org

American Association of Colleges of Nursing
Note: Verification of membership in association.
1 Dupont Circle, Suite 530

Washington, DISTRICT OF COLUMBIA 20036
Telephone: 202/463-6930   Fax: 202/785-8320
Web site: www.aacn.nche.edu

American Association of Critical Care Nurses Certification Corporation
101 Columbia
Aliso Viejo, CALIFORNIA 92656
Telephone: 949/362-2000   Fax: 949/362-2020
E-mail: certcorp@aacn.org
Web site: www.certcorp.org

American Association of Legal Nurse Consultants
4700 W. Lake Avenue
Glenview, ILLINOIS 60025-1485
Telephone: 847/375-4713   Fax: 877/734-8668
E-mail: info@aalnc.org
Web site: www.aalnc.org

American Association of Managed Care Nurses
4435 Waterfront Drive, Suite 101
Glen Allen, VIRGINIA 23060
Telephone: 804/747-9698   Fax: 804/747-5316
E-mail: amason@aamcn.org
Web site: www.aamcn.org

American Association of Neuroscience Nurses
4700 W. Lake Avenue
Glenview, ILLINOIS 60025
Telephone: 888-557-2266   Fax: 847-375-6333
E-mail: aann@aann.org
Web site: www.aann.org

American Association of Nurse Anesthetists
222 S. Prospect Avenue
Park Ridge, ILLINOIS 60068-4001
Telephone: 847/692-7050   Fax: 847/692-6968
Web site: www.aana.com

American Association of Nurse Attorneys
Note: Verification of nurse attorneys membership.
7794 Grow Drive
Pensacola, FLORIDA 32514
Telephone: 850/474-3646   Fax: 850/484-8762
E-mail: taana@puetzamc.com
Web site: www.taana.org

American Association of Occupational Health Nurses
2920 Brandywine Road, Suite 100
Atlanta, GEORGIA 30341
Telephone: 770/455-7757   Fax: 770/455-7271

Specialty Associations, Societies, Colleges, and Academies

E-mail: aaohn@aaohn.org
Web site: www.aaohn.org

American Association of Spinal Cord Injury Nurses
75-20 Astoria Boulevard
Jackson Heights, NEW YORK 11370-1177
Telephone: 718/803-3782   Fax: 718/803-0414
Web site: www.aascin.org

American College of Nurse-Midwives
818 Connecticut Avenue NW, Suite 900
Washington, DISTRICT OF COLUMBIA 20006
Telephone: 202/728-9860   Fax: 202/728-9897
E-mail: info@acnm.org
Web site: www.midwife.org

American Holistic Nurses' Association
PO Box 2130
Flagstaff, ARIZONA 86003-2130
Telephone: 800/278-2462 (toll-free)   Fax: 520/526-2752
E-mail: ahna-flag@flaglink.com
Web site: www.ahna.org

American Nephrology Nurses Association
E. Holly Avenue, Box 56
Pitman, NEW JERSEY 08071-0056
Telephone: 856/256-2320   888/600-2662 (toll-free)   Fax: 856/589-7463
E-mail: anna@ajj.com
Web site: www.annanurse.org

American Nurses Credentialing Center
600 Maryland Avenue SW, Suite 100 West
Washington, DISTRICT OF COLUMBIA 20024-2571
Telephone: 202/651-7000   Fax: 202/651-7001
E-mail: ancc@ana.org
Web site: www.nursingworld.org

American Nurses Credentialing Center
600 Maryland Avenue SW, Suite 100 W.
Washington, DISTRICT OF COLUMBIA 20024-2571
Telephone: 202/651-7000   Fax: 202/651-7004
E-mail: phamm@ana.org
Web site: www.nursecredentialing.org

American Nurses Foundation
600 Maryland Avenue SW, Suite 100 W.
Washington, DISTRICT OF COLUMBIA 20024
Telephone: 202/651-7227   Fax: 202/651-7354

E-mail: anf@ana.org
Web site: www.nursingworld.org/anf

American Organization of Nurse Executives
1 N. Franklin Street
Chicago, ILLINOIS 60606
Telephone: 312/422-2800   Fax: 312/422-4504
Web site: www.aone.org

Arizona State University, College of Nursing
Registrar Records Department
PO Box 872602
Tempe, ARIZONA 85287
Telephone: 480/965-2987   Fax: 480/965-8468
E-mail: nursing@asu.edu
Web site: www.nursing.asu.edu

Association of Pediatric Oncology Nurses
4700 W. Lake Avenue
Glenview, ILLINOIS 60025
Telephone: 847/375-4724   Fax: 847/375-6324
E-mail: info@apon.org
Web site: www.apon.org

Association of Peri Operative Registered Nurses, Inc.
Association of Operating Room Nurses, Inc.
2170 S. Parker Road, Suite 300
Denver, COLORADO 80231-5711
Telephone: 303/755-6300   800/755-2676   Fax: 303/750-2927
Web site: www.aorn.org

Association of Rehabilitation Nurses
4700 W. Lake Avenue
Glenview, ILLINOIS 60025
Telephone: 847/375-4710   800/229-7530   Fax: 877/734-9384
E-mail: info@rehabnurse.org
Web site: www.rehabnurse.org

Baromedical Nurses Association
PO Box 24113
Baltimore, MARYLAND 21227
Telephone: 410-789-5690   Fax: 410-512-8918
E-mail: pgbatz@aol.com
Web site: www.hyperbaricnurses.org

Board of Certification for Emergency Nursing
915 Lee Street
Des Plaines, ILLINOIS 60016
Telephone: 847/460-2630   Fax: 847/460-2631
E-mail: bcen@ena.org   Web site: www.ena.org/bcen

Specialty Associations, Societies, Colleges, and Academies

Boston College School of Nursing
Office of Student Services
Lyons Hall
140 Commonwealth Avenue
Chestnut Hill, MASSACHUSETTS 02467
Telephone: 617/552-3300   800/294-0294 (student services)   617/552-2230 (nursing)   Fax: 617/552-0745
E-mail: soninfo@bc.edu
Web site: www.bc.edu/studentservices

Canadian Nurses Association
50 Driveway
Ottawa, ONTARIO K2P1E2
CANADA
Telephone: 613/237-2133   Fax: 613/237-3520
Web site: www.cna-nurses.ca

Columbia University School of Nursing
Office of the Registrar
Mail Code 9202
1150 Amsterdam Avenue
New York, NEW YORK 10027
Telephone: 212/854-7375
Web site: www.columbia.edu/cu/registrar/certification

Duke University
Office of the University Registrar
Attention: Certification
103 Allen Building, Box 90054
Durham, NORTH CAROLINA 27708-0054
Telephone: 919/684-2813   Fax: 919/684-4500
E-mail: fenne007@mc.duke.edu
Web site: registrarduke.edu

Emergency Nurses Association
915 Lee Street
Des Plaines, ILLINOIS 60016
Telephone: 847/460-4000   Fax: 847/460-4001
E-mail: enainfo@ena.org
Web site: www.ena.org

Emory University, Nell Hodgson Woodruff School of Nursing
1520 Clifton Road
Atlanta, GEORGIA 30322
Telephone: 404/727-3500   Fax: 404/727-9668
Web site: www.nurse.emory.edu

Emory University, Nell Hodgson Woodruff School of Nursing, Nurse-Midwifery Program
Attention: Director
Student Affairs Office

1520 Clifton Road
Atlanta, GEORGIA 30322
Telephone: 404/727-3500   Fax: 404/727-9668
E-mail: nhallor@nurse.emory.edu
Web site: www.nursing.emory.edu

Frontier School of Midwifery and Family Nursing, Inc.
Office of the Registrar
PO Box 528
195 School Street
Hyden, KENTUCKY 41749
Telephone: 606/672-2312   Fax: 606/672-3776
E-mail: jlwoods@midwives.org
Web site: www.midwives.org   www.frontierfnp.org

Georgetown University School of Nursing & Health Studies
3700 Reservoir Road NW
Washington, DISTRICT OF COLUMBIA 20057
Telephone: 202/687-3118   Fax: 202/687-5553
Web site: www.snhs.georgetown.edu

Hospice and Palliative Nurses Association/National Board for Certification of Hospice and Palliative Nurses
National Office
Penn Center West One, Suite 229
Pittsburgh, PENNSYLVANIA 15276
Telephone: 412/787-9301   Fax: 412/787-9305
E-mail: hpna@hpna.org
Web site: www.hpna.org

Idaho State University
Note: University provides Nursing, Dentistry, and Pharmacy degrees.
Office of Registration and Records
Campus Box 8196
Pocatello, IDAHO 83209-8196
Telephone: 208/282-2661   Fax: 208/282-4231
Web site: www.isu.edu

Indiana University Bloomington School of Nursing
Office of the Registrar
Franklin Hall 100
601 E. Kirkwood
Bloomington, INDIANA 47405-1223
Telephone: 812/855-0121   812/855-7505 (transcript)   812/855-1736 (nursing)   Fax: 812/855-6986
E-mail: registrar@indiana.edu
Web site: www.registrar.indiana.edu

Specialty Associations, Societies, Colleges, and Academies

Infusion Nurses Society, Inc.
Infusion Nurses Certication Corporation
220 Norwood Park S
Norwood, MASSACHUSETTS 02062
Telephone: 781/440-9408   Fax: 781/440-9409
E-mail: melissa.scull@ins1.org
Web site: www.ins1.org

Johns Hopkins University School of Nursing
Business Office
Room 338
525 N. Wolfe Street
Baltimore, MARYLAND 21205-2110
Telephone: 410/955-1243   410/955-7548 (nursing)   Fax: 410/955-9177
Web site: son.jhmi.edu

Loyola University Chicago, Niehoff School of Nursing
Note: Degree verifications now handled by Credentials, Inc. Telephone: 800/646-1858; Web site: www.degreechk.com.
6525 North Sheridan Road
Chicago, ILLINOIS 60626
Telephone: 773/508-3000
Web site: www.luc.edu/depts/regrec/degreechk.

Marycrest International University—Nursing Department
Registrar's Office
1607 W. 12th Street
Davenport, IOWA 52804
Telephone: 319/326-9278
E-mail: registrar@mcrest.edu
Web site: nursing@mcrest.edu

Michigan State University
Note: Verifications available through clearing house.
Registrar's Office
Administration Building, Room 150
East Lansing, MICHIGAN 48824-1317
Telephone: 517/353-4678   800/496-4678 (Registrar main)   800/605-6424 (nursing)   Fax: 517/432-3347
E-mail: reg@msu.edu
Web site: www.msu.edu

Montana State University, Bozeman
101 Montana Hall
Bozeman, MONTANA 59717-2660
Telephone: 406/994-6650   Fax: 406/994-1972
E-mail: registrar@montana.edu   Web site: www.montana.edu/registrar

National Association for Practical Nurse Education and Service
8607 Second Avenue #404A
Silver Spring, MARYLAND 20910-2745

Telephone: 301/588-2491   Fax: 301/588-2839
E-mail: napnes@bellatlantic.net
Web site: www.napnes.org

National Association of Hispanic Nurses
1501 16th Street NW
Washington, DISTRICT OF COLUMBIA 20036
Telephone: 202/387-2477   Fax: 202/483-7183
E-mail: thehispanic@earthlink.net
Web site: www.thehispanicnurses.org

National Association of Pediatric Nurse Practitioners
20 Brace Road, Suite 200
Cherry Hill, NEW JERSEY 08034
Telephone: 856/857-9700   Fax: 856/857-1600
E-mail: info@napnap.org
Web site: www.napnap.org

National Association of Physician Nurses
900 S. Washington Street, Suite G13
Falls Church, VIRGINIA 22046
Telephone: 703/237-8616   Fax: 703/533-1153
E-mail: naesaa@starpower.net

National Association of Registered Nurses
11512 Allecingie Parkway, Suite D
Richmond, VIRGINIA 23235
Telephone: 804/794-6513   Fax: 804/379-7698
Web site: www.associationusa.org

National Black Nurses Association, Inc.
Note: Also provides verification of degrees and certification. Membership open to all nurses.
8630 Fenton Street, Suite 330
Silver Spring, MARYLAND 20910
Telephone: 301/589-3200   Fax: 301/589-3223
E-mail: nbna@erols.com
Web site: www.nbna.org

National Federation of Licensed Practical Nurses
605 Poole Drive
Garner, NORTH CAROLINA 27529
Telephone: 919/779-0046   800/948-2511 (toll-free)   Fax: 919/779-5642
Web site: www.nflpn.org

National League for Nursing
61 Broadway, 33rd Floor
New York, NEW YORK 10006-2701
Telephone: 800-669-9656 212-363-5555 Fax: 607-723-8408
Web site: www.nln.org

Specialty Associations, Societies, Colleges, and Academies

National Student Nurses Association, Inc.
45 Main Street, Suite 606
Brooklyn, NEW YORK 11201
Telephone: 718/210-0705   Fax: 718/210-0710
E-mail: nsna@nsna.org
Web site: www.nsna.org

New Mexico State University
Note: For Institutional Research, contact Miriam Mayer.
Department of the Registrar
Box 30001, Dept. MSC 3AR
Las Cruces, NEW MEXICO 88003-8001
Telephone: 505/646-3411   Fax: 505/646-1579
E-mail: registrar@nmsu.edu
Web site: www.nmsu.edu

Oncology Nursing Certification Corporation
501 Holiday Drive
Pittsburgh, PENNSYLVANIA 15220
Telephone: 412/921-7373   Fax: 412/921-6565
E-mail: oncc@ons.org
Web site: www.ons.org

Rutgers College of Nursing
Office of the Registrar
The State University of Rutgers
Blumenthal Hall, Room 309
249 University Avenue
Newark, NEW JERSEY 07102
Telephone: 973/353-5324   Fax: 973/353-1357
Web site: www.registrar.rutgers.edu

Society of Otorhinolaryngology and Head-Neck Nurses
116 Canal Street, Suite A
New Smyrna Beach, FLORIDA 32168
Telephone: 904/428-1695   Fax: 904/423-7566
E-mail: sohnnet@aol.com
Web site: www.sohnnurse.com

Southeastern Louisiana University, College of Nursing & Health Sciences, Hammond Campus
Enrollment Services
SLU Box 10835
Hammond, LOUISIANA 70402
Telephone: 985/549-2156   Fax: 985/549-2869
Web site: www.selu.edu

Southwestern Adventist University, Department of Nursing
100 Hillcrest Drive
Keene, TX 76059
Telephone: 800/433-2240   Fax: 817/556-4744
E-mail: buncht@swau.edu   Web site: www.swau.edu

The Association of Women's Health, Obstetric and Neonatal Nurses
2000 L Street NW, Suite 740
Attention: Maxine Haliburton
Washington, DISTRICT OF COLUMBIA 20036
Telephone: 202/261-2400   Fax: 202/728-0575
Web site: www.awhonn.org

The University of Mississippi Medical Center, School of Nursing
2500 N. State Street
Jackson, MISSISSIPPI 39216
Telephone: 601/984-6200   601/984-1080 (division of student services and records)
Web site: www.umc.edu

The University of Texas, Houston School of Nursing
Office of the Registrar
PO Box 20036
Houston, TEXAS 77225
Telephone: 713/500-3333   Fax: 713/500-3356
Web site: www.registrar.uth.tmc.edu

UCLA School of Nursing
PO Box 951702
Los Angeles, CALIFORNIA 90095-1702
Telephone: 310/825-7181   Fax: 310/206-7433
Web site: www.nursing.ucla.edu

Union College Division of Health Sciences, Nursing Program
Note: Also provides accreditation for Physician Assistant Program.
3800 S. 48th Street
Lincoln, NEBRASKA 68506
Telephone: 402/486-2524 (School of Nursing)   402/486-2527 (Physician Assistant Program)   Fax: 402/486-2559
E-mail: nrsgprog@ucollege.edu
Web site: www.ucollege.edu/hlthsci

University at Buffalo School of Nursing, Nurse Practitioner
Note: They also verify Adult Health Nurse Practitioner, Pediatrics Nurse Practitioner, Family Nurse Practitioner, and Maternal and Women's Health Nurse Practitioner degrees.
Student Affairs Office
1040 Kimball Tower
3435 Main Street
Buffalo, NEW YORK 14214
Telephone: 716/829-2537   Fax: 716/829-2021
Web site: www.nursing.buffalo.edu

University of Alabama at Birmingham
Office of Student Affairs
1530 Third Avenue South
Birmingham, ALABAMA 35294-1210
Telephone: 205/ 975-7529
Web site: www.uab.edu

Specialty Associations, Societies, Colleges, and Academies

University of Arkansas for Medical Sciences, College of Nursing
Registrar's Office
4301 W. Markham Slot 529
Little Rock, ARKANSAS 72205
Telephone: 501/686-5224 (Registrar)   501/686-5374 (general)   Fax: 501/686-8350
Web site: www.nursing.uams.edu

University of Colorado Health Sciences Center, School of Nursing
4200 E. Ninth Avenue
Campus Box C-288-6
Denver, COLORADO 80262
Telephone: 303/315-5592   Fax: 303/315-8660
E-mail: son.oasis@uchsc.edu
Web site: www.uchsc.edu

University of Delaware, Department of Nursing
McDowell Hall
Newark, DELAWARE 19716
Telephone: 302/831-2193   Fax: 302/831-2382
E-mail: ud-nursing@udel.edu
Web site: www.uddl.edu/nursing

University of Hawaii, School of Nursing and Dental Hygiene
Office of the Dean
2528 McCarthy Mall
Webster Hall 402
Honolulu, HAWAII 96822
Telephone: 808/956-8522   Fax: 808/956-3257
Web site: www.nursing.hawaii.edu

University of Kentucky, College of Nursing
Registrar's Office
Ten Funkhouser Building
Lexington, KENTUCKY 40506-0054
Telephone: 859/257-3161   859/323-5108 (College of Nursing)   Fax: 859/257-7160
Web site: www.uky.edu

University of Las Vegas, Department of Nursing
Office of the Registrar
4505 S. Maryland Parkway, Box 453018
Las Vegas, NEVADA 89154-3018
Telephone: 702/895-3360   Fax: 702/895-4807
Web site: www.unlv.edu

University of Memphis
Office of the Registrar
119 Administration Building
Memphis, TENNESSEE 38152
Telephone: 901/678-2000   901/678-2810 (student information)   Fax: 901/678-1425
Web site: www.memphis.edu

University of Miami, School of Nursing
5801 Red Road
PO Box 248153
Coral Gables, FLORIDA 33124-3850
Telephone: 305/284-3666 (general information)   305/284-4325 (student services)   Fax: 305/284-4827
Web site: www.miami.edu/nur

University of Minnesota, School of Nursing
Student Services Center
200 Fraser Hall
Minneapolis, MINNESOTA 55455
Telephone: 612/625-5333   612/624-4454 (nursing)   Fax: 612/625-4351
E-mail: helpingu@umn.edu
Web site: www.umn.edu

University of New Hampshire, Department of Nursing
Registrar's Office
11 Garrison Avenue
Stoke Hall
Durham, NEW HAMPSHIRE 03824-3511
Telephone: 603/862-1500   Fax: 603/862-0655
E-mail: registrars.office@unh.edu
Web site: www.unh.edu/registrar

University of South Carolina, College of Nursing
Office of the University Registrar
1521 Greene Street
Columbia, SOUTH CAROLINA 29208
Telephone: 803/777-5555   803/777-5555 (degree verifications)   Fax: 803/777-6349
E-mail: registrar@sc.edu
Web site: www.sc.edu.

University of South Florida, College of Nursing
MDC Box 22
12901 Bruce B. Downs Boulevard
Tampa, FLORIDA 33612-4766
Telephone: 813/974-9305   Fax: 813/974-5418
E-mail: pmartini@hsc.usf.edu
Web site: hsc.usf.edu/nursing

University of Wyoming
Note: All verifications now handled through clearinghouse at 703/742-4200
Office of Registration and Records
PO Box 3964
Laramie, WYOMING 82071-3964
Telephone: 307/766-5272 (general information)   703/742-4200 (verification)   Fax: 307/766-3960
Web site: www.uwyo.edu/reg/trans

Yale School of Nursing
Office of Admisssions
100 Church Street S
New Haven, CONNECTICUT 06536
Telephone: 203/785-2389   Fax: 203/737-5409
Web site: www.nursing.yale.edu

Obstetrics and gynecology

American College of Nurse-Midwives
818 Connecticut Avenue NW, Suite 900
Washington, DISTRICT OF COLUMBIA 20006
Telephone: 202/728-9860   Fax: 202/728-9897
E-mail: info@acnm.org
Web site: www.midwife.org

American College of Obstetricians and Gynecologists
PO Box 96920
Washington, DISTRICT OF COLUMBIA 20090-6920
Telephone: 202/638-5577   Fax: 202/863-4994
E-mail: membership@acog.org
Web site: www.acog.org

American College of Osteopathic Obstetricians and Gynecologists
900 Auburn Road
Pontiac, MICHIGAN 48342-3365
Telephone: 248/332-6360   Fax: 248/332-4607
E-mail: acoog@acoog.com
Web site: www.acoog.com

Association of Reproductive Health Professionals
Note: Accredited by ACCME.
2401 Pennsylvania Avenue NW, Suite 350
Washington, DISTRICT OF COLUMBIA 20037-1718
Telephone: 202/466-3825   Fax: 202/466-3826
E-mail: arhp@arhp.org
Web site: www.arhp.org

International Childbirth Education Association, Inc.
PO Box 20048
Minneapolis, MINNESOTA 55420
Telephone: 612/854-8660   Fax: 612/854-8772
E-Mail: info@icea.org
Web site: www.icea.org

National Perinatal Association
3500 E. Fletcher Avenue, Suite 205
Tampa, FLORIDA 33613-4712
Telephone: 813/971-1008   Fax: 813/971-9306

E-mail: npa@nationalperinatal.org
Web site: www.nationalperinatal.org

Society of Obstetricians and Gynecologists of Canada
780 Echo Drive
Ottawa, ONTARIO K1S 5R7
CANADA
Telephone: 613/730-4192   Fax: 613/730-4314
E-mail: alalonde@sogc.com
Web site: www.sogc.org

The Association of Women's Health, Obstetric, and Neonatal Nurses
2000 L Street NW, Suite 740
Washington, DISTRICT OF COLUMBIA 20036
Telephone: 202/261-2400   Fax: 202/728-0575
Web site: www.awhonn.org

Occupational medicine

American Association of Occupational Health Nurses, Inc.
2920 Brandywine Road, Suite100
Atlanta, GEORGIA 30341
Telephone: 770/455-7757   Fax: 770/455-7271
E-mail: aaohn@aaohn.org
Web site: www.aaohn.org

American Osteopathic College of Occupational and Preventive Medicine
PO Box 2606
Leesburg, VIRGINIA 20177
Telephone: 703/443-8869   800/558-8686 (toll-free)   Fax: 703/443-0576
Web site: aocopm.org

Occupational and Environmental Medical Association of Canada
54 Forward Avenue
London, ONTARIO N6H 1B7
CANADA
Telephone: Fax: 519-439-8840
E-mail: oemac@oemac.org
Web site: www.oemac.org

Occupational therapy

American Occupational Therapy Association, Inc.
4720 Montgomery Lane
PO Box 31220
Bethesda, MARYLAND 20824-1220
Telephone: 301/652-2682   Fax: 301/652-7711
Web site: www.aota.org

Oncology

American College of Mohs Micrographic Surgery and Cutaneous Oncology
930 N. Meacham Road
Schaumburg, ILLINOIS 60173
Telephone: 847/330-9830   Fax: 847/330-1135
E-mail: info@mohscollege.org
Web site: www.mohscollege.org

American Society for Therapeutic Radiology and Oncology
12500 Fair Lakes Circle, Suite 375
Fairfax, VIRGINIA 22033
Telephone: 800/962-7876   Fax: 703/502-7852
E-mail: meetings@astro.org
Web site: www.astro.org

American Society of Clinical Oncology
1900 Duke Street, Suite200
Alexandria, VIRGINIA 22314
Telephone: 703/299-0150   Fax: 703/299-1044
E-mail: info@asco.org
Web site: www.asco.org

Oncology Nursing Certification Corporation
501 Holiday Drive
Pittsburgh, PENNSYLVANIA 15220-2749
Telephone: 412/921-8597   Fax: 412/928-0926
E-mail: oncc@ons.org
Web site: www.oncc.org

Opthalmology

American Academy of Ophthalmology
655 Beach Street
San Francisco, CALIFORNIA 94109-1336
Telephone: 415/561-8500   Fax: 415/561-8533
E-mail: webmaster@aao.org
Web site: www.aao.org

American Association for Pediatric Ophthalmology and Strabismus
PO Box 193832
San Francisco, CALIFORNIA 94119-3832
Telephone: 415/561-5805   Fax: 415/561-8531
E-mail: aapos@aao.org
Web site: www.aapos.org

Chapter 9

American Ophthalmological Society
PO Box 193940
San Francisco, CALIFORNIA 94119-3940
Telephone: 415/561-8578   Fax: 415/561-8531
E-mail: aos@aao.org

American Osteopathic Colleges of Ophthalmology and Otolaryngology–Head and Neck Surgery
320 W. Grand Avenue
Dayton, OHIO 45405
Telephone: 800/455-9404   937/252-4958   Fax: 937/222-8840
E-mail: practicesa@aol.com
Web site: www.aocoohns.org

American Society of Cataract and Refractive Surgery
4000 Legato Road, Suite 850
Fairfax, VIRGINIA 22033
Telephone: 703/591-2220   Fax: 703/591-0614
E-mail: ascrs@ascrs.org
Web site: www.ascrs.org

American Society of Contemporary Ophthalmology
Note: Publishes journals.
820 N. Orleans, Suite 208
Chicago, ILLINOIS 60610
Telephone: 312/440-0699   Fax: 312/440-0580
E-mail: iaos@aol.com
Web site: www.ascmso.com

Association for Research in Vision and Ophthalmology
12300 Twinbrook Parkway, Suite 250
Rockville, MARYLAND 20852
Telephone: 240/221-2900   Fax: 240/221-0370
E-mail: mem@arvo.org
Web site: www.arvo.org

Canadian Ophthalmological Society
1525 Carling Avenue, Suite 610
Ottawa, ONTARIO K1Z 8R9
CANADA
Telephone: 613/729-6779   Fax: 613/729-7209
E-mail: cos@eyesite.ca
Web site: www.eyesite.ca

International Association of Ocular Surgeons
820 N. Orleans, Suite 208
Chicago, ILLINOIS 60610
Telephone: 312/440-0699   Fax: 312/440-0580
E-mail: iaos@aol.com
Web site: www.ascmso.com

Optometry

American Academy of Optometry
6110 Executive Boulevard, Suite 506
Rockville, MARYLAND 20852
Telephone: 301/984-1441   Fax: 301/984-4737
E-mail: aaoptom@aol.com
Web site: www.aaopt.org

American Optometric Foundation
6110 Executive Boulevard, Suite 506
Rockville, MARYLAND 20852
Telephone: 301/984-4734   Fax: 301/984-4737
E-mail: christine@aaoptom.org
Web site: www.ezell.org/

Oral surgery

American Cleft Palate Craniofacial Association
104 S. Estes Drive, Suite 204
Chapel Hill, NORTH CAROLINA 27514
Telephone: 919/933-9044   Fax: 919/933-9604
E-mail: cleftline@aol.com
Web site: www.cleftline.org

Orthopedic surgery

American Academy of Orthopaedic Surgeons
6300 N. River Road
Rosemont, ILLINOIS 60018-4262
Telephone: 800/346-2267   847/823-7186   Fax: 847/823-8125
E-mail: webhelp@aaos.org
Web site: www.aaos.org

American Association of Hip and Knee Surgeons
704 Florence Drive
Park Ridge, ILLINOIS 60068
Telephone: 847/698-1200   Fax: 847/825-9294
E-mail: healthdesk@aahks.org
Web site: www.aahks.org

American Osteopathic Academy of Orthopedics
PO Box 291690
Davie, FLORIDA 33329-1690
Telephone: 800/741-2626   954/262-1700   Fax: 954/262-1748
Web site: www.aoao.org

American Osteopathic Academy of Sports Medicine
7600 Terrace Avenue, Suite 203
Middleton, WISCONSIN 53562
Telephone: 608/831-4400   Fax: 608/831-5485
Web site: www.aoasm.org

American Society for Surgery of the Hand
6300 N. River Road, Suite 600
Rosemont, ILLINOIS 60018
Telephone: 847/384-8300   Fax: 847/384-1435
E-mail: info@assh.org
Web site: www.assh.org

Canadian Academy of Sport Medicine
1010 Polytek Street, Unit 14, Suite 100
Gloucester, ONTARIO K1J 9H9
CANADA
Telephone: 613/748-5851   Fax: 613/748-5792
E-mail: info@casm-acms.org
Web site: www.casm-acms.org

Canadian Orthopaedic Association
718-1440 Saint Catherine Street, W.
Montreal, QUEBEC H3G 1R8
CANADA
Telephone: 514/874-9003   Fax: 514/874-0464
E-mail: info@coa-aco.org
Web site: www.coa-aco.org

Eastern Orthopaedic Association, Inc.
2517 Eastlake Avenue E, Suite 200
Seattle, WASHINGTON 98102
Telephone: 206/860-1455   Fax: 206/860-1507
E-mail: eoa@cantrall.com
Web site: www.eoa-assn.org

The American Orthopaedic Association
American Orthopaedic Association
6300 N. River Road, Suite 505
Rosemont, ILLINOIS 60018-4263
Telephone: 847/318-7330   Fax: 847/318-7339
E-mail: info@aoassn.org
Web site: www.aoassn.org

Western Orthopaedic Association
1834 First Street, Suite 3
Napa, CALIFORNIA 94559-2353
Telephone: 707/259-9481   Fax: 707/259-9486
E-mail: info@woa-assn.org
Web site: www.woa-assn.org

Osteopathic medicine

American Academy of Osteopathy
3500 DePauw Boulevard, Suite 1080
Indianapolis, INDIANA 46268
Telephone: 317/879-1881   Fax: 317/879-0563
Web site: www.academyofosteopathy.org

American Association of Colleges of Osteopathic Medicine
Note: Association for DOs and Osteopathic Manipulative Medicine.
5550 Friendship Boulevard, Suite 310
Chevy Chase, MARYLAND 20815-7231
Telephone: 301/968-4100   Fax: 301/968-4101
Web site: www.aacom.org

American College of Osteopathic Emergency Physicians
142 E. Ontario Street, Suite 550
Chicago, ILLINOIS 60611
Telephone: 800/521-3709   312/587-3709   Fax: 312/587-3713
Web site: www.acoep.org

American College of Osteopathic Internists
3 Bethesda Metro Center, Suite 508
Bethesda, MARYLAND 20814
Telephone: 800/327-5183 (toll-free)   301/656-8877   Fax: 301/656-7133
E-mail: acoi@acoi.org
Web site: www.acoi.org

American College of Osteopathic Obstetricians and Gynecologists
900 Auburn Road
Pontiac, MICHIGAN 48342-3365
Telephone: 248/332-6360   Fax: 248/332-4607
E-mail: acoog@acoog.com
Web site: www.acoog.com

American College of Osteopathic Surgeons
123 N. Henry Street
Alexandria, VIRGINIA 22314-2903
Telephone: 703/684-0416   Fax: 703/684-3280
E-mail: info@theacos.org   Web site: www.facos.org

American Osteopathic Academy of Addiction Medicine
142 E. Ontario Street
Chicago, ILLINOIS 60611
Telephone: 312/202-8163   Fax: 312/202-8224
E-mail: aoaam@osteohdq.org

American Osteopathic Academy of Osteopathic Pain Management and Sclerotherapy, Inc.
5002 E. Woodmill Drive

Wilmington, DELAWARE 19808
Telephone: 302/996-0300   Fax: 302/996-5300

American Osteopathic Academy of Sports Medicine
7600 Terrace Avenue, Suite 203
Middleton, WISCONSIN 53562
Telephone: 608/831-4400   Fax: 608/831-5485
E-mail: info@aoasm.org
Web site: www.aoasm.org

American Osteopathic Association
Official Osteopathic Physician Profile
142 E. Ontario Street
Chicago, ILLINOIS 60611
Telephone: 800/621-1773, Ext. 8145   Fax: 312/202-8339
E-mail: info@aoa-net.org
Web site: www.aoa-net.org

American Osteopathic College of Allergy and Immunology
7025 E. McDowell Road, Suite 1B
Scottsdale, ARIZONA 85257
Telephone: 480/585-1580   Fax: 480/585-1581
Web site: www.goodnet.com/~osteo/-index.html

American Osteopathic College of Dermatology
1501 E. Illinois Street
PO Box 7525
Kirksville, MISSOURI 63501
Telephone: 660/665-2184   800/449-2623 (toll-free)   Fax: 660/627-2623
E-mail: execdirector@aocd.org

American Osteopathic College of Occupational and Preventive Medicine
PMB PMV 246
5405 Alton Parkway
Irvine, VIRGINIA 92604-3718
Telephone: 949-653-8694   Fax: 949-654-0482
E-mail: aocopm@ioc.net
Web site: www@aocopm.org

American Osteopathic College of Pathologists
12368 Northwest 13th Court
Pembroke Pines, FLORIDA 33026
Telephone: 954-432-9640   Fax: 775-587-7283
E-mail: amocpath@aol.com

American Osteopathic College of Radiology
119 E. Second Street
Milan, MISSOURI 63556-1331
Telephone: 660/265-4011   Fax: 660/265-3494
E-mail: aocr@nemr.net   Web site: www.aocr.org

Specialty Associations, Societies, Colleges, and Academies

American Osteopathic College of Rehabilitation Medicine
2214 Elmira Avenue
Des Plaines, ILLINOIS 60018
Telephone: 847/699-0048   Fax: 847/296-1366

American Osteopathic College of Rheumatology, Inc.
Attention: Dr. Robert Maurer
193 Monroe Avenue
Edison, NEW JERSEY 08820-3755
Telephone: 732/494-6688   Fax: 732/494-6689
E-mail: bmaurer107@aol.com

American Society of Bariatric Physicians
5453 E. Evans Place
Denver, COLORADO 80222
Telephone: 303/770-2526   Fax: 303/779-4834
E-mail: info@asbp.org
Web site: www.asbp.org

Canadian Osteopathic Association
575 Waterloo Street
London, ONTARIO N6B2R2
CANADA
Telephone: 519/439-5521   Fax: 519/439-2616

Community Hospital Medical Education Alliance
5550 Friendship Boulevard, Suite 300
Chevy Chase, MARYLAND 20815
Telephone: 301/968-2642   Fax: 301/968-4195
E-mail: bmerritt@chmea.org

Mississippi State Board of Medical Licensure
Note: A computerized list will be provided to hospitals and credentialing agencies for a $125 fee, to be utilized for verification purposes only. One free update may be requested within the Board's fiscal year during the months of August through April.

1867 Crane Ridge Drive, Suite 200-B
Jackson, MISSISSIPPI 39216
Telephone: 601/987-3079   Fax: 601/987-4159
E-mail: mboard@msbml.state.ms.us
Web site: www.msbml.state.ms.us

West Virginia School of Osteopathic Medicine
Office of the Registrar
400 N. Lee Street
Lewisburg, WEST VIRGINIA 24901
Telephone: 304/647-6373   Fax: 304/645-4859
E-mail: jgorby@wvsom.edu
Web site: www.wvsom.edu

Chapter 9

Otolaryngology

American Academy of Otolaryngic Allergy
1990 M Street NW, Suite 680
Washington, DISTRICT OF COLUMBIA 20036
Telephone: 202/955-5010   Fax: 202/955-5016
E-mail: aaoa@aaoaf.org
Web site: www.aaoaf.org

American Academy of Otolaryngology–Head and Neck Surgery
1 Prince Street
Alexandria, VIRGINIA 22314-3357
Telephone: 703/836-4444   Fax: 703/683-5100
E-mail: info@ent.net.org
Web site: www.entnet.org

American Bronchio-Esophagological Association
Division of Otolaryngology
University of Utah Medical Center
Room 3C120
Salt Lake City, UTAH 84132
Telephone: 801/581-7514   Fax: 801/585-5744
E-mail: r.kim.davis@hsc.utah.edu
Web site: www.abea.net

American Laryngological Association
c/o Robert Ossoff DMD,MD
Vanderbilt Medical Center
S-2100 MCN
Nashville, TENNESSEE 37232-2559
Telephone: 615/322-6326   615/343-0013 (ask for Diane)   Fax: 615/343-7604
E-mail: ossoff.assistant@vanderbilt.edu
Web site: www.ala.hns.org

American Laryngological, Rhinological, and Otological Society, Inc. (The Triological Society)
555 N. 30th Street
Omaha, NEBRASKA 68131
Telephone: 402/346-5500   Fax: 402/346-5300
E-mail: info@triological.org
Web site: www.triological.org

American Osteopathic Colleges of Ophthalmology and Otolaryngology–Head and Neck Surgery
405 W. Grand Avenue
Dayton, OHIO 45405
Telephone: 800/455-9404 937/222-8820 Fax: 937/222-8840
E-mail: info@aocoohns.org
Web site: www.aocoohns.org

Specialty Associations, Societies, Colleges, and Academies

American Rhinologic Society
Marvin P. Fried, MD
Montefiore Medical Center
Department of Otolaryngology
3400 Bainbridge Avenue, MAP Third Floor
Bronx, NEW YORK 10467
Telephone: 866/866-8656   Fax: 718/405-9014
E-mail: wperez@montefiore.org
Web site: www.american-rhinologic.org

Canadian Society of Otolaryngology–Head and Neck Surgery
Administrative Office
221 Millford Crescent, SS4
Elora, ONTARIO N0B1S0
CANADA
Telephone: 800/655-9533   519/846-0630   Fax: 519/846-9529
E-mail: cso.hns@sympatico.ca
Web site: www.csohns.com

Society of University Otolaryngologists–Head and Neck Surgeons
Department of Otolaryngology
c/o Donna Hoffman, MA
1200 N. State Street, Box 795
Los Angeles, CALIFORNIA 90033-1029
Telephone: 323/226-7315   Fax: 323/226-2780

Otology

American Otological Society, Inc.
2720 Tartan Way
Springfield, ILLINOIS 62707
Telephone: 217/785-3833   Fax: 217/524-0253
Web site: itsa.ucsf.edu/~ajo/AOS/AOS.html

Pain management

American Academy of Pain Management
13947 Mono Way #A
Sonora, CALIFORNIA 95370
Telephone: 209/533-9744   Fax: 209/533-9750
E-mail: aapm@aapainmanage.org
Web site: www.aapainmanage.org

American Academy of Pain Medicine
4700 W. Lake Avenue
Glenview, ILLINOIS 60025
Telephone: 847/375-4731   Fax: 877/734-8750
E-mail: info@amctec.com
Web site: www.painmed.org

American Chronic Pain Association
Note: Pain management support group.
c/o Penney Cowan
PO Box 850
Rocklin, CALIFORNIA 95677-0850
Telephone: 916/632-0922   Fax: 916/632-3208
E-mail: acpa@pacbell.net
Web site: www.theacpa.org

American College of Osteopathic Pain Management and Sclerotherapy, Inc.
5002 E Woodmill Drive
Wilmington, DELAWARE 19808
Telephone: 302/996-0300   800/471-6114 (toll-free)   Fax: 302/996-5300
Web site: www.acopms.com

American Pain Society
4700 W. Lake Avenue
Glenview, ILLINOIS 60025
Telephone: 847/375-4700   Fax: 847/375-6317
E-mail: info@ampainsoc.org
Web site: www.ampainsoc.org

American Society of Regional Anesthesia and Pain Medicine
2209 Dickens Road
PO Box 11086
Richmond, VIRGINIA 23230-1086
Telephone: 804/282-0010   Fax: 804/282-0090
E-mail: asra@societyhq.com
Web site: www.asra.com

International Association for the Study of Pain
909 NE 43rd Street, Suite 306
Seattle, WASHINGTON 98105
Telephone: 206/547-6409   Fax: 206/547-1703
E-mail: iaspdesk@juno.com
Web site: www.iasp-pain.org

Pathology

American Association of Neuropathologists
Office of the Secretary-Treasurer
Department of Laboratory Medicine and Pathology
Mayo Clinic
200 First Street SW
Rochester, MINNESOTA 55905
Telephone: 507/284-3394   Fax: 507/284-1599
E-mail: aanp@mayo.edu
Web site: www.aanp-jnen.com

Specialty Associations, Societies, Colleges, and Academies

American Society for Investigative Pathology
9650 Rockville Pike
Bethesda, MARYLAND 20814-3993
Telephone: 301/530-7130   Fax: 301/571-1879
E-mail: asip@pathol.faseb.org
Web site: asip.uthscsa.edu

American Society of Clinical Pathologists
2100 West Harrison Street
Chicago, ILLINOIS 60612-3798
Telephone: 312/738-7000   Fax: 312/738-1619
Web site: www.ascp.org

Canadian Association of Pathologists
774 Echo Drive
Ottawa, ONTARIO K1S 5N8
CANADA
Telephone: 613/730-6230   Fax: 613/730-1116
E-mail: cap@rcpsc.edu
Web site: www.cap.med.org

College of American Pathologists
Note: Accredits Pathology Laboratories.
325 Waukegan Road
Northfield, ILLINOIS 60093-2750
Telephone: 847/832-7000   Fax: 847/832-8000
E-mail: media@cap.org
Web site: www.cap.org

Intersociety Committee on Pathology Information
Note: Kathleen Carmody is Programming Editor.
9650 Rockville Pike
Bethesda, MARYLAND 20814
Telephone: 301/634-7932   Fax: 301/571-1879
E-mail: icpi@pathol.faseb.org
Web site: www.pathologytraining.org

Pediatrics

Ambulatory Pediatric Association
6728 Old McLean Village Drive
McLean, VIRGINIA 22101
Telephone: 703/556-9222   Fax: 703/556-8729
E-mail: info@ambpeds.org
Web site: www.ambpeds.org

Chapter 9

American Academy of Pediatric Dentistry
211 E. Chicago Avenue, Suite 700
Chicago, ILLINOIS 60611
Telephone: 312/337-2169   Fax: 312/337-6329
E-mail: aapdinfo@aapd.org
Web site: www.aapd.org

American Academy of Pediatrics
141 NW Point Boulevard
Elk Grove Village, ILLINOIS 60007
Telephone: 847/228-5005   Fax: 847/434-8000
E-mail: kidsdocs@aap.org
Web site: www.aap.org

American College of Osteopathic Pediatricians
5550 Friendship Boulevard, Suite 300
Chevy Chase, MARYLAND 20815
Telephone: 877/231-2267   Fax: 301/968-4195
E-mail: acop@osteohdq.org
Web site: www.aoha.org

American Pediatric Society
3400 Research Forest Drive, Suite B7
The Woodlands, TEXAS 77381
Telephone: 281/419-0052   Fax: 281/419-0082
E-mail: info@aps-spr.org
Web site: www.aps-spr.org

American Society of Dentistry for Children
211 E. Chicago Avenue, Suite 710
Chicago, ILLINOIS 60611-2603
Telephone: 312/943-1244   Fax: 312/943-5341
E-mail: asdckids@aol.com
Web site: www.asdckids.org

American Society of Pediatric Neuroradiology
2210 Midwest Road, Suite 207
Oak Brook, ILLINOIS 60523
Telephone: 630/574-0220   Fax: 630/574-0661
E-mail: kcammarata@asnr.org
Web site: www.asnr.org

Specialty Associations, Societies, Colleges, and Academies

Canadian Pediatric Society
100-2204 Walkley Road
Ottawa, ONTARIO K1G 4G8
CANADA
Telephone: 613/526-9397   Fax: 613/526-3332
E-mail: info@cps.ca
Web site: www.cps.ca

National Association of Pediatric Nurse Associates and Practitioners
1101 Kings Highway N, Suite 206
Cherry Hill, NEW JERSEY 08034-1912
Telephone: 877/662-7627   609/667-1773   Fax: 609/667-7187
E-mail: napnap1@aol.com
Web site: www.napnap.org

The Society for Adolescent Medicine
1916 NW Copper Oaks Circle
Blue Springs, MISSOURI 64015
Telephone: 816/224-8010   Fax: 816/224-8009
E-mail: sam@adolescenthealth.org
Web site: www.adolescenthealth.org

Pharmacology/Pharmacy

American Association of Colleges of Pharmacy
1426 Prince Street
Alexandria, VIRGINIA 22314-2841
Telephone: 703/739-2330   Fax: 703/836-8982
Web site: www.aacp.org

American College of Apothecaries
Note: Offers continuing education for pharmacists.
2830 Summer Oaks Drive
Memphis, TENNESSEE 38134
Telephone: 901/383-8119   Fax: 901/383-8882
E-mail: aca@acainfo.org
Web site: www.acainfo.org

American College of Clinical Pharmacology
3 Ellinwood Court
New Hartford, NEW YORK 13413-1105
Telephone: 315/768-6117   Fax: 315/768-6119
E-mail: accp1ssu@aol.com
Web site: www.accp1.org

American College of Clinical Pharmacy
3101 Broadway, Suite 650
Kansas City, MISSOURI 64111
Telephone: 816/531-2177   Fax: 816/531-4990
Web site: www.accp.com

Chapter 9

American Council on Pharmaceutical Education
20 N. Clark, Suite 2500
Chicago, ILLINOIS 60602
Telephone: 312/664-3575   Fax: 312/664-4652
E-mail: csinfo@acpe-accredit.org
Web site: www.acpe-accredit.org

American Pharmaceutical Association
2215 Constitution Avenue NW
Washington, DISTRICT OF COLUMBIA 20037-2985
Telephone: 202/628-4410   Fax: 202/783-2351
Web site: www.aphanet.org

American Society for Clinical Pharmacology and Therapeutics
528 N. Washington Street
Alexandria, VIRGINIA 22314
Telephone: 703/836-6981   Fax: 703/836-5223
E-mail: info@ascpt.org
Web site: www.ascpt.org

American Society for Pharmacology and Experimental Therapeutics
9650 Rockville Pike
Bethesda, MARYLAND 20814-3995
Telephone: 301/634-7060   Fax: 301/634-7061
E-mail: info@aspet.org
Web site: www.aspet.org

American Society of Health System Pharmacists
Note: Offers continuing education for pharmacists.
7272 Wisconsin Avenue
Bethesda, MARYLAND 20814
Telephone: 301/657-3000   Fax: 301/657-2747
E-mail: custserv@ashp.org
Web site: www.ashp.org

Physiatry/Rehabilitative medicine

American Orthopaedic Society for Sports Medicine
6300 N. River Road, Suite 500
Rosemont, ILLINOIS 60018
Telephone: 847/292-4900   Fax: 847/292-4905
E-mail: aossm@aossm.org
Web site: www.sportsmed.org

American Academy of Physical Medicine and Rehabilitation
1 IBM Plaza, Room 2500
Chicago, ILLINOIS 60611-3604
Telephone: 312/464-9700   Fax: 312/464-0227
E-mail: info@aapmr.org
Web site: www.aapmr.org

Specialty Associations, Societies, Colleges, and Academies

American Congress of Rehabilitation Medicine
6801 Lake Plaza Drive, Suite B205
Indianapolis, INDIANA 46220
Telephone: 317/915-2250   Fax: 317/915-2245
E-mail: acrm@acrm.org
Web site: www.acrm.org

Canadian Association of Physical Medicine and Rehabilitation
Note: Specialization in stroke, amputee, and traumatic brain injury rehabilitation.

774 Echo Drive
Ottawa, ONTARIO K1S 5N8
CANADA
Telephone: 613/730-6245   Fax: 613/730-1116
E-mail: capmr@rcpsc.edu
Web site: www.capmr.medical.org

National Rehabilitation Association
633 S. Washington Street
Alexandria, VIRGINIA 22314-4109
Telephone: 703/836-0850   Fax: 703/836-0848
E-mail: info@nationalrehab.org
Web site: www.nationalrehab.org

Physical therapy

American Board of Physical Therapy Specialties
1111 North Fairfax Street
Alexandria, VIRGINIA 22314
Telephone: 703/684-8520   Fax: 703/838-8910
Web site: www.apta.org/education/specialist

American Physical Therapy Association
1111 N. Fairfax Street
Alexandria, VIRGINIA 22314
Telephone: 703/684-2782   Fax: 703/684-7343
Web site: www.apta.org

Physician and medical assistants

American Registry of Medical Assistants
69 Southwick Road, Suite A
Westfield, MASSACHUSETTS 01085-4729
Telephone: 413/562-7336   800/527-2762 (ARMA)   Fax: 413/562-9021

National Commission on Certification of Physician Assistants
Verification of Certificate
157 Technology Parkway, Suite 800
Norcross, GEORGIA 30092-2913
Telephone: 770/734-4500   Fax: 770/734-4535
E-mail: nccpa@nccpa.net
Web site: www.nccpa.net

Plastic surgery

American Association of Plastic Surgeons
4900B S. 31st Street
Arlington, VIRGINIA 22206
Telephone: 703/820-7400   Fax: 703/931-4520
E-mail: aaps@mindspring.com
Web site: www.aaps1921.org

American Society of Plastic Surgeons
444 E. Algonquin Road
Arlington Heights, ILLINOIS 60005
Telephone: 847/228-9900   Fax: 847/228-9131
Web site: www.plasticsurgery.org

Canadian Society of Plastic Surgeons
917-30 Saint Joseph Boulevard E
Montreal, QUEBEC H2T 1G9
CANADA
Telephone: 514/843-5415   800/665-5415 (toll-free) Fax: 514/843-7005
E-mail: csps_sccp@sympatico.ca
Web site: www.plasticsurgery.ca

Podiatry

American Academy of Podiatric Sports Medicine
PO Box 723
Rockville, MARYLAND 20848-0726
Telephone: 800/438-3355   Fax: 301/962-3850
E-mail: info@aapsm.org
Web site: www.aapsm.org

American Association of Colleges of Podiatric Medicine
1350 Piccard Drive, Suite 322
Rockville, MARYLAND 20850
Telephone: 301/990-7400   Fax: 301/990-2807
Web site: www.aacpm.org

Specialty Associations, Societies, Colleges, and Academies

American College of Foot and Ankle Orthopedics and Medicine
3525 Elliott Mills Drive, Suite N
Ellicott City, MARYLAND 21043
Telephone: 800/265-8263   Fax: 410/418-4805
E-mail: acfaom@acfaom.com
Web site: www.acfaom.com

American College of Foot and Ankle Surgeons
515 Busse Highway
Park Ridge, ILLINOIS 60068
Telephone: 800/421-2237, Ext. 322   847/292-2237, Ext. 322   Fax: 847/292-2022
E-mail: bcb@acfas.org
Web site: www.acfas.org

American Podiatric Medical Association
9312 Old Georgetown Road
Bethesda, MARYLAND 20814-1621
Telephone: 301/581-9200   Fax: 301/530-2752
E-mail: askapma@apma.org
Web site: www.apma.org

Preventive medicine

American College of Preventive Medicine
1307 New York Avenue NW, Suite 200
Washington, DISTRICT OF COLUMBIA 20005
Telephone: 202/466-2044   Fax: 202/466-2662
E-mail: info@acpm.org
Web site: www.acpm.org

American Osteopathic College of Occupational and Preventive Medicine
PMB246
5405 Alton Parkway
Irvine, VIRGINIA 92604-3718
Telephone: 949-653-8694   Fax: 949-654-0482
E-mail: aocopm@ioc.net
Web site: www@aocopm.org

Psychiatry

American Academy of Addiction Psychiatry
7301 Mission Road, Suite 252
Prairie Village, KANSAS 66208
Telephone: 913/262-6161   Fax: 913/262-4311
E-mail: info@aaap.org
Web site: www.aaap.org

American Academy of Child and Adolescent Psychiatry
3615 Wisconsin Avenue NW
Washington, DISTRICT OF COLUMBIA 20016-3007
Telephone: 202/966-7300   Fax: 202/966-2891
Web site: www.aacap.org

American Academy of Clinical Psychiatrists
PO Box 458
Glastonbury, CONNECTICUT 06033
Telephone: 860/633-5045   Fax: 860/633-6023
E-mail: info-aacp@aacp.com
Web site: www.aacp.com

American Association for Geriatric Psychiatry
7910 Woodmont Avenue, Suite 1050
Bethesda, MARYLAND 20814
Telephone: 301/654-7850   Fax: 301/654-4137
E-mail: main@aagponline.org
Web site: www.aagponline.org

American Association of Psychiatric Technicians, Inc.
2000 O Street, Suite 250
Sacramento, CALIFORNIA 95814
Telephone: 800-391-7588   Fax: 916-329-9145
E-mail: npg_info@nnng.com
Web site: www.aapt.com

American Clinical Neurophysiology Society (formerly American Electroencephalographic Society)
1 Regency Drive
Bloomfield, CONNECTICUT 06002
Telephone: 860/243-3977   Fax: 860/286-0787
E-mail: acns@ssmgt.com
Web site: www.acns.org

Specialty Associations, Societies, Colleges, and Academies

American College of Neuropsychiatrists
28595 Orchard Lake Road, Suite 200
Farmington Hills, MICHIGAN 48334
Telephone: 248/553-0010, Ext. 295   Fax: 248/553-0818
E-mail: acn-aconp@msn.com

American Orthopsychiatric Association, Inc.
330 Seventh Avenue
New York, NEW YORK 10001
Telephone: 212/564-5930   Fax: 212/564-6180
E-mail: amerortho@aol.com
Web site: www.amerortho.org

American Psychiatric Association
1400 K Street NW
Washington, DISTRICT OF COLUMBIA 20005
Telephone: 202/682-6000   Fax: 202/682-6850
E-mail: apa@psych.org
Web site: www.psych.org

American Psychiatric Nurses Association
Colonial Place 3
2107 Wilson Boulevard, Suite 300A
Arlington, VIRGINIA 22201-3042
Telephone: 703/243-2443   Fax: 703/243-3390
E-mail: info@apna.org
Web site: www.apna.org

Canadian Psychiatric Association
260-441 MacLaren Street
Ottawa, ONTARIO K2P 2H3
CANADA
Telephone: 613/234-2815   Fax: 613/234-9857
E-mail: cpa@cpa-apc.org
Web site: www.cpa-apc.org

National Mental Health Association
1021 Prince Street
Alexandria, VIRGINIA 22314-2971
Telephone: 703/684-7722   800/969-6642 (toll-free) Fax: 703/684-5968
E-mail: infoctr@nmha.org
Web site: www.nmha.org

Psychology

American Group Psychotherapy Association, Inc.
25 E. 21st Street, Sixth Floor
New York, NEW YORK 10010
Telephone: 212/477-2677   Fax: 212/979-6627
E-mail: info@agpa.org

Web site: www.agpa.org

American Psychological Association College of Professional Psychology
750 First Street NE
Washington, DISTRICT OF COLUMBIA 20002-4242
Telephone: 202/336-6100   Fax: 202/336-5797
E-mail: apacollege@apa.org
Web site: www.apa.org

American Psychological Society
1010 Vermont Avenue NW, Suite 1100
Washington, DISTRICT OF COLUMBIA 20005
Telephone: 202/783-2077   Fax: 202/783-2083
E-mail: APS@aps.washington.dc.us
Web site: www.psychologicalscience.org

Association for Applied Psychophysiology and Biofeedback
10200 W. 44th Avenue, Suite 304
Wheat Ridge, COLORADO 80033-2840
Telephone: 303/422-8436   Fax: 303/422-8894
E-mail: aapb@resourcenter.com
Web site: www.aapb.org

Canadian Psychological Association
151 Slater Street, Suite 205
Ottawa, ONTARIO K1P5H3
CANADA
Telephone: 613/237-2144   Fax: 613/237-1674
E-mail: cpa@cpa.ca
Web site: www.cpa.ca

Council for the National Register of Health Service Providers in Psychology
Note: Verification type: Psychologists
1120 G Street NW, Suite 330
Washington, DISTRICT OF COLUMBIA 20005-3801
Telephone: 202/783-7663   Fax: 202/347-0550
E-mail: Available at Web site
Web site: www.nationalregister.org

Public health

American Association of Public Health Dentistry
Note: Associated with the American Board of Dental Health.
AAPHD National Office
1224 Centre W, Suite 400B
Springfield, ILLINOIS 62704
Telephone: 217/391-0218 (AAPHD Office)   Fax: 217/793-0041

E-mail: natoff@aaphd.org
Web site: www.aaphd.org

American Public Health Association
800 First Street NW
Washington, DISTRICT OF COLUMBIA 20001-3710
Telephone: 202/777-APHA   Fax: 202/777-2534
E-mail: comments@apha.org
Web site: www.apha.org

Association of Maternal and Child Health Programs
1220 19th Street NW, Suite 801
Washington, DISTRICT OF COLUMBIA 20036
Telephone: 202/775-0436   Fax: 202/775-0061
Web site: www.amchp.org

Association of Schools of Public Health, Inc.
1101 15th Street NW, Suite 910
Washington, DISTRICT OF COLUMBIA 20005
Telephone: 202/296-1099   Fax: 202/296-1252
E-mail: info@asph.org
Web site: www.asph.org

Canadian Healthcare Association
Note: Any verifications or credentialing must be done through the Canadian Medical Association.
17 York Street
Ottawa, ONTARIO K1N 9J6
CANADA
Telephone: 613/241-8005   Fax: 613/241-5055
Web site: www.cha.ca

Connecticut Department of Public Health
Note: Information packets available; packets include disk. Call for pricing information.
Data Processing Division
410 Capitol Avenue, MS 13DPR
PO Box 340308
Hartford, CONNECTICUT 06134-0308
Telephone: 860/509-7186   Fax: 860/509-8119
E-mail: lynn.carbonneau@po.state.ct.us
Web site: www.state.ct.us/dph

Radiology

American College of Radiology
1891 Preston White Drive
Reston, VIRGINIA 20191
Telephone: 703/648-8900   Fax: 703/648-9176
E-mail: info@acr.org
Web site: www.acr.org

American Healthcare Radiology Administrators
PO Box 334
Sudbury, MASSACHUSETTS 01776
Telephone: 978/443-7591   Fax: 978/443-8046
E-mail: info@ahraonline.org
Web site: www.ahraonline.org

American Osteopathic College of Radiology
119 E. Second Street
Milan, MISSOURI 63556-1331
Telephone: 660/265-4011   Fax: 660/265-3494
E-mail: aocr@nemr.net
Web site: www.aocr.org

American Society for Therapeutic Radiology and Oncology
12500 Fair Lakes Circle, Suite 375
Fairfax, VIRGINIA 22033
Telephone: 800/962-7876   Fax: 703/502-7852
E-mail: meetinga@astro.org
Web site: www.astro.org

American Society of Emergency Radiology
4550 Post Oak Place, Suite 342
Houston, TEXAS 77027
Telephone: 713/965-0566   Fax: 713/960-0488
E-mail: imm@meetingmanagers.com
Web site: www.aawr.org

American Society of Head and Neck Radiology
2210 Midwest Road, Suite 207
Oak Brook, ILLINOIS 60523-8205
Telephone: 630/574-0220, Ext. 226   Fax: 630/574-0661
E-mail: kcammarata@asnr.org or ashnr@rsna.org
Web site: www.ashnr.org

American Society of Interventional and Therapeutic Neuroradiology
Note: Also conducts verification of neuroradiology.
2210 Midwest Road, Suite 207
Oak Brook, ILLINOIS 60523-8205
Telephone: 630/574-0220   Fax: 630/574-0661
E-mail: kcammarata@asnr.org
Web site: www.asitn.org

American Society of Neuroimaging
5841 Cedar Lake Road, Suite 204
Minneapolis, MINNESOTA 55416
Telephone: 952/545-6291   Fax: 952/545-6073
E-mail: reneemolstad@msn.com
Web site: www.asnweb.org

American Society of Pediatric Neuroradiology
Note: Also verifies for neuroradiology.
2210 Midwest Road, Suite 207
Oak Brook, ILLINOIS 60523
Telephone: 630/574-0220   Fax: 630/574-0661
E-mail: kcammarata@asnr.org
Web site: www.asnr.org

American Society of Radiologic Technologists
15000 Central Avenue SE
Albuquerque, NEW MEXICO 87123-3917
Telephone: 505/298-4500   Fax: 505/298-5063
E-mail: saguilar@asrt.org
Web site: www.asrt.org

American Society of Spine Radiology
Note: Only verifies membership within society.
2210 Midwest Road, Suite 207
Oak Brook, ILLINOIS 60523-8205
Telephone: 630/574-0220, Ext. 226   Fax: 630/574-0661
E-mail: kcammarata@asnr.org/assr
Web site: www.asnr/assr.org

Radiological Society of North America
820 Jorie Boulevard
Oak Brook, ILLINOIS 60523-2215
Telephone: 630/571-2670   Fax: 630/571-7837
Web site: www.rsna.org

Society of Interventional Radiology
10201 Lee Highway, Suite 500
Fairfax, VIRGINIA 22030
Telephone: 703/691-1805   800/488-7284   Fax: 703/691-1855
E-mail: info@sirweb.org
Web site: www.sirweb.org

Respiratory care

American Association for Respiratory Care
11030 Ables Lane
Dallas, TEXAS 75229
Telephone: 972/243-2272   Fax: 972/484-2720
E-mail: info@aarc.org
Web site: www.aarc.org

Rheumatology

American College of Rheumatology
1800 Century Place, Suite 250
Atlanta, GEORGIA 30345
Telephone: 404/633-3777   Fax: 404/633-1870
E-mail: info@rheumatology.org
Web site: www.rheumatology.org

American Osteopathic College of Rheumatology, Inc.
Dr. Robert Maurer
193 Monroe Avenue
Edison, NEW JERSEY 08820
Telephone: 732/494-6688   Fax: 732/494-6689
E-mail: bmaurer107@aol.com

Canadian Rheumatology Association
43 Lundys Lane
Newmarket, ONTARIO L3Y 3R7
CANADA
Telephone: 905/478-4499   Fax: 905/478-2109
E-mail: cartho@home.com
Web site: www.cra-scr.ca

Social work

American Association for Marriage and Family Therapy
112 S. Alfred Street
Alexandria, VIRGINIA 22314
Telephone: 703/838-9808   Fax: 703/838-9805
E-mail: central@aamft.org
Web site: www.aamft.org

Council on Social Work Education
Note: Provides accreditation of colleges and universities for social work degree programs.
1725 Duke Street, Suite 500
Alexandria, VIRGINIA 22314
Telephone: 703/683-8080   Fax: 703/683-8099
E-mail: info@cswe.org
Web site: www.cswe.org

National Association of Social Workers, Inc. (NASW)
750 First Street NE, Suite 700
Washington, DISTRICT OF COLUMBIA 20002
Telephone: 202/408-8600   Fax: 202/336-8331
E-mail: cspoon@naswdc.org
Web site: www.socialworkers.org

Society for Social Work Leadership in Health Care
1 N. Franklin Street, Floor 31

Chicago, ILLINOIS 60606
Telephone: 312/422-3999   866/237-9542 (toll-free)   Fax: 312/422-4572
E-mail: zkizart@aha.org
Web site: www.sswlhc.org

Speech, language, and hearing

American Speech-Language-Hearing Association
10801 Rockville Pike
Rockville, MARYLAND 20852
Telephone: 800/498-2071   301/897-5700 (TTY)   Fax: 301/571-0457
E-mail: actioncenter@asha.org
Web site: www.asha.org

Canadian Association of Speech-Language Pathologists and Audiologists
200 Elgin Street, Suite 401
Ottawa, ONTARIO K2P 1L5
CANADA
Telephone: 613/567-9968   Fax: 613/567-2859
E-mail: caslpa@caslpa.ca
Web site: www.caslpa.ca

Surgery

American Association for Accreditation of Ambulatory Surgery Facilities, Inc. (AAAASF)
1202 Allanson Road
Mundelein, ILLINOIS 60060
Telephone: 888/545-5222 (toll-free)   847/949-6058   Fax: 847/566-4580
E-mail: aaaasf@sprynet.org
Web site: www.aaaasf.org

American Association of Hip and Knee Surgeons
704 Florence Drive
Park Ridge, ILLINOIS 60068
Telephone: 847/698-1200   Fax: 847/825-9294
E-mail: priscilla@thekneesociety.org
Web site: www.aahks.org

American Association of Surgical Physician Assistants
PO Box 867
Bernardsville, NEW JERSEY 07924
Telephone: 888/882-2772   Fax: 732/805-9582
E-mail: theaaspa@aol.com
Web site: www.aaspa.com

American College of Mohs Micrographic Surgery and Cutaneous Oncology
930 E. Woodfield Road
Schaumburg, ILLINOIS 60173

Chapter 9

Telephone: 847/330-0230   Fax: 847/330-1135
E-mail: info@mohscollege.org
Web site: www.mohscollege.org

American College of Osteopathic Surgeons
123 N. Henry Street
Alexandria, VIRGINIA 22314
Telephone: 703/684-0416   Fax: 703/684-3280
E-mail: info@theacos.org
Web site: www.facos.org

American College of Surgeons
Note: Web site will show active fellows. Although retired fellows may not appear in listings, it does not mean that they are inactive. Call for information.
633 N. Saint Clair Street
Chicago, ILLINOIS 60611-3211
Telephone: 312/202-5000   Fax: 312/202-5001
E-mail: postmaster@facs.org
Web site: www.facs.org

American Society for Dermatologic Surgery
5550 Meadowbrook Drive, Suite 120
Rolling Meadows, ILLINOIS 60008
Telephone: 847/956-0900   Fax: 847/956-0999
E-mail: info@aboutskinsurgery.com
Web site: www.aboutskinsurgery.com

American Society for Laser Medicine and Surgery, Inc.
2404 Stewart Square
Wausau, WISCONSIN 54401
Telephone: 715/845-9283   Fax: 715/848-2493
E-mail: information@aslms.org
Web site: www.aslms.org

American Society of Cataract and Refractive Surgery
4000 Legato Road, Suite 850
Fairfax, VIRGINIA 22033
Telephone: 703/591-2220   Fax: 703/591-0614
E-mail: ascrs@ascrs.org
Web site: www.ascrs.org

Canadian Association of General Surgeons
Health Sciences Center
300 Prince-Phillip Drive
St. John's, PRINCE EDWARD ISLAND A1B 3V6
CANADA
Telephone: 709/778-3611
E-mail: cags@planet.eon.net
Web site: cags.medical.org

Specialty Associations, Societies, Colleges, and Academies

International College of Surgeons, United States Section
1516 N. Lake Shore Drive
Chicago, ILLINOIS 60610-1694
Telephone: 312/787-6274   Fax: 312/787-9289
E-mail: icsus@ics-us.org
Web site: www.ics-us.org

Royal College of Physicians and Surgeons of USA
485 Allard Road
Grosse Pointe, MICHIGAN 48236-2811
Telephone: 313/882-0641   Fax: 313/882-0979
Web site: www.royalcollegeusa.com

Society for Vascular Surgery
13 Elm Street
Manchester, MASSACHUSETTS 01944-1314
Telephone: 978/526-8330   Fax: 978/526-4018
E-mail: svs@prri.com
Web site: www.vascsurg.org

Society of Thoracic Surgeons
Note: Certification performed by ABTS.
401 N. Michigan Avenue, Suite 2400
Chicago, ILLINOIS 60611-4267
Telephone: 312/321-6803   Fax: 312/527-6635
E-mail: sts@sba.com
Web site: www.sts.org

Society of University Surgeons
Attn: Barbara Beatty
1133 W. Morse Boulevard, Suite 201
Winter Park, FLORIDA 32789
Telephone: 407/644-8839   Fax: 407/629-2502
Web site: www.sus.org

The Southwestern Surgical Congress
401 N. Michigan Avenue
Chicago, ILLINOIS 60611-4267
Telephone: 312/527-6667   Fax: 312/527-6658
E-mail: swsc@sba.com
Web site: www.swscongress.org

Thoracic medicine

American Thoracic Society
61 Broadway
New York, NEW YORK 10006
Telephone: 212/315-8600   Fax: 212/315-6498
Web site: www.thoracic.org

Canadian Thoracic Society
3 Raymond Street, Suite 300
Ottawa, ONTARIO K1R 1A3
CANADA
Telephone: 613/569-6411   Fax: 613/569-8860
E-mail: info@lung.ca
Web site: www.lung.ca

Society of Thoracic Radiology
820 Jorie Boulevard
Oak Brook, ILLINOIS 60523
Telephone: 630/368-3779   Fax: 630/571-7837
E-mail: str@rsna.org
Web site: www.thoracicrad.org

Society of Thoracic Surgeons
633 N. St. Clair, Suite 2320
Chicago, ILLINOIS 60611-3658
Telephone: 312/202-5800   Fax: 312/202-5801
Web site: www.sts.org

Thyroid medicine

The American Thyroid Association, Inc.
Townhouse Office Park
55 Old Nyack Turnpike, Suite 611
Nanuet, NEW YORK 10954
Fax: 914/623-3736
E-mail: admin@thyroid.org
Web site: www.thyroid.org

Urology

American Foundation for Urologic Disease, Inc.
1128 N. Charles Street
Baltimore, MARYLAND 21201
Telephone: 410/468-1800   Fax: 410/468-1808
E-mail: admin@afud.org
Web site: www.afud.org

American Urological Association, Inc.
1120 N. Charles Street
Baltimore, MARYLAND 21201
Telephone: 410/727-1100   Fax: 410/468-1820
E-mail: aua@auanet.org
Web site: www.auanet.org

Canadian Urological Association
2D2 13 Walter MacKenzie Health Center

8440-112 Street
Edmonton, ALBERTA T6G 2B7
CANADA
Telephone: 780/407-3283   Fax: 780/407-2694
E-mail: mchetner@gpu.srv.ualberta.ca
Web site: www.cua.org

Video data transmission

National Association of Medical Examiners
1402 S. Grand Boulevard, Room C305
St. Louis, MISSOURI 63104
Telephone: 314/577-8298, Ext. 2   Fax: 314/268-5971
E-mail: settledd@slu.edu
Web site: www.thename.org

Wound care

American Academy of Wound Management
1720 Kennedy Causeway, Suite 109
North Bay Village, FLORIDA 33141
Telephone: 305/866-9592   Fax: 305/868-0905
E-mail: woundnet@aol.com
Web site: www.aawm.org

Association for the Advancement of Wound Care
Health Management Publications
83 General Warren Boulevard, Suite 100
Malvern, PENNSYLVANIA 19355
Telephone: 610/560-0500   610/237-7285   Fax: 610/688-1060
E-mail: aawchelp@voicenet.com
Web site: www.aawcone.com

The Wound Healing Society
1550 S. Coast Highway, Suite 201
Laguna Beach, CALIFORNIA 92651
Telephone: 888/434-4234   Fax: 949/376-3456
Web site: www.woundheal.org

CHAPTER 10
Credentialing and Privileging Resources

Chapter 10
Credentialing and Privileging Resources

Introduction

Many organizations provide health care professionals with credentialing and privileging resources geared toward improving their quality of service. Accreditors develop high-quality standards for organizations and publish materials designed to help the organizations meet these standards. Credentials Verification Organizations (CVOs) aid hospitals and health care organizations in the process of appointing and reappointing practitioners by verifying and reviewing their credentials. In addition, many software vendors and publishers provide credentialing and privileging resources in the form of computer software, books, periodicals, audiotapes, and videotapes.

This chapter provides a brief description of each of the above-mentioned resources, followed by a comprehensive list of contacts. As with other sections of the book, readers are encouraged to contact us with any updates or additions for the chapter. Please note that this list is provided as a resource and not as an endorsement of the listed organizations or their products.

Professional associations

Membership and participation in professional organizations can assist health care professionals in their job performance by providing access to educational materials and other resources. Most important, professional association membership offers networking opportunities with other people in the profession.

National Association of Medical Staff Services

The National Association of Medical Staff Services (NAMSS) is a national nonprofit organization for the development of individuals responsible for managing credentialing, privileging, practitioner/provider organizations, and regulatory compliance in the health care industry. It is a professional educational association of more than 4,000 members whose mission is to influence and promote quality standards for the administrative management of health care professionals. In addition to the national organization, NAMSS has associations in 46 states. Local and state meetings provide excellent networking opportunities. NAMSS offers the following two certifications:

- The Certified Medical Staff Coordinator (CMSC) certification is a comprehensive certification focusing on management expertise and expanded accreditation knowledge. The exam includes 250 questions covering a broad scope of medical staff services management issues, including hospital/health care organization management, accreditation and regulatory standards, health care law, health care definitions, and administration and management of employees.

- The Certified Provider Credentialing Specialist (CPCS) certification recognizes excellence in professionals of all health care settings whose primary function is credentialing. The job of many MSSPs, especially those in managed care, involves mainly provider credentialing and not the administrative issues involved with the medical staff. The exam contains 150 questions regarding principles of credentialing/recredentialing, accreditation standards, legal principles of credentialing, health care definitions, and information management.

NAMSS has many educational materials and resources, including an Independent Study Plan, which is available as an online study course.

The National Association for Healthcare Quality

Founded in 1976, the National Association for Healthcare Quality (NAHQ) currently comprises more than 6,000 individual members and 100 institutional members. Its goal is to promote the continuous improvement of quality in health care by providing educational and development opportunities for professionals at all management levels and within all health care settings.

Accreditors

Health care organizations seek accreditation for various reasons. Organizations accredited by some bodies are deemed to meet the Medicare *Conditions of Participation*, a set of standards with which organizations must comply in order to be reimbursed for services provided to patients under the Medicare program. Accreditation can also be a requirement for participation in managed care plans and other third-party payers, and lenders often require continuing accreditation as a condition of financing. Finally, health care organizations use voluntary accreditation as a marketing tool to enhance community confidence and to show dedication to continuous improvement of the safety and quality of the services they provide. Accrediting organizations commonly

- establish the standards of quality by which the organizations they accredit must abide
- design materials to help organizations meet these standards
- evaluate the extent to which organizations comply with these standards
- provide public recognition for those organizations that meet their standards

Accreditation or certification is almost always a voluntary, nongovernmental process where accreditors usually depend on the support of the industry they accredit. Some consumer watch groups argue that, since the health care organization is paying the accrediting body, the accrediting body is the organization's agent, thus leading to a conflict of interest. However, anyone who has been through one of these surveys can attest that this is not the case, as the survey process is very thorough and intense.

The fees for accreditation surveys vary depending on the size of the organization and the type of services to be surveyed. Costs for a single survey can be as high as $50,000, a cost that can increase if a return survey is required. Hospitals are not required to use the services of an accreditor and can request that the state agency conduct a survey at no cost to the facility. Although state and federal agencies require health care licensure and inspection, these agencies are content to leave the accreditation surveys to a private accrediting organization because governmental inspection processes are often expensive and labor-intensive.

Accreditation by a "deemed" body does not exempt an organization from additional survey by state organizations or by the Centers for Medicare & Medicaid Services (CMS). CMS routinely conducts validation of accreditation surveys based on a sample of accredited organizations or on allegations of deficiencies that could negatively affect patient health or safety.

The health care field has more than 20 accreditors, although many of them are small and offer accreditation only in highly specialized areas. The predominant standards-setting and accrediting body is the Joint Commission on Accreditation of Healthcare Organizations (JCAHO). The JCAHO evolved from the American College of Surgeons' (ACS)

Credentialing and Privileging Resources

Minimum Standard for Hospitals program, which started in 1917. After World War II, the ACS recognized that its accrediting program was becoming large and expansive and was detracting from its other objectives. As a result, the ACS assembled a group of potentially interested organizations—including the American Medical Association, the American Dental Association, the American Hospital Association, the American College of Physicians, and the Canadian Hospital Association—which together formed what is now the JCAHO.

Although the JCAHO began by accrediting hospitals only, it now accredits behavioral health, long-term care, home care, ambulatory care, clinical laboratories, assisted living facilities, critical access hospitals, office-based surgery practices, and health care networks.

The following section includes the contact information for the major health care-accrediting organizations of several health care industries. Each entry indicates the type(s) of organization(s) the accreditor evaluates.

Accreditation Association for Ambulatory Health Care, Inc.

Accredits ambulatory health care organizations, including ambulatory clinics, surgery centers, single- and multi-specialty group practices, health maintenance organization birthing centers, college and university health centers, urgent and immediate care centers, office-based surgery centers and practices, managed care organizations, diagnostic imaging centers, and networks and groups of ambulatory care organizations.

Accreditation Association for Ambulatory Health Care, Inc.
3201 Old Glenview Road, Suite 300
Wilmette, ILLINOIS 60091-2992
Telephone: 847/853-6060   Fax: 847/853-9028
E-mail: info@aaahc.org
Web site: www.aaahc.org

American Accreditation Healthcare Commission/Utilization Review Accreditation Commission/URAC

Accredits preferred provider organizations (PPOs), point of service (POS) plans, individual practice associations (IPAs), health maintenance organizations (HMOs), physician-hospital organizations (PHOs), integrated delivery networks (IDNs), physician organizations (POs), management services organizations (MSOs), and single-specialty networks (SSNs). Also accredits utilization review programs, workers' compensation utilization management programs, and workers' compensation networks.

Utilization Review Accreditation Commission, American Accreditation Healthcare Commission/URAC
1275 K Street, NW, #1100
Washington, DISTRICT OF COLUMBIA 20005
Telephone: 202/216-9010   Fax: 202/216-9006
www.urac.org

American Association for Accreditation of Ambulatory Surgery Facilities, Inc. (AAAASF)

Accredits single-specialty and multi-specialty surgery facilities.

American Association for Accreditation of Ambulatory Surgery Facilities, Inc.
1202 Allanson Road
Mundelein, ILLINOIS 60060
Telephone: 888/545-5222 (toll-free)   847/949-6058   Fax: 847/566-4580
E-mail: aaaasf@sprynet.com
Web site: www.aaaasf.org

American Association of Blood Banks
Accredits blood collection and transfusion facilities.

American Association of Blood Banks
8101 Glenbrook Road
Bethesda, MARYLAND 20814-2749
Telephone: 301/907-6977   Fax: 301/907-6895
E-mail: aabb@aabb.org
Web site: www.aabb.org

American College of Radiology
Accredits diagnostic radiology practices, radiation oncology practices, mammography practices, ultrasound facilities, and stereotactic breast biopsy facilities with specific accreditation programs for magnetic resonance imaging, computerized tomography, nuclear medicine, radiation oncology, radiography/fluoroscopy, and ultrasound.

American College of Radiology
1891 Preston White Drive
Reston, VIRGINIA 20191-4397
Telephone: 800/227-5463   Fax: 703/295-6773
Web site: www.acr.org

American College of Surgeons Commission on Cancer
Accredits hospitals, treatment centers, and cancer facilities whose goal is to decrease the morbidity and mortality caused by cancer through prevention, monitoring and reporting of care, standard setting, and education.

American College of Surgeons Commission on Cancer
633 N. Saint Clair Street
Chicago, ILLINOIS 60611-3211
Telephone: 312/202-5000   Fax: 312/202-5001
E-mail: postmaster@facs.org
Web site: www.facs.org

American Osteopathic Association
Accredits osteopathic hospitals and combination osteopathic and allopathic hospitals, osteopathic and allopathic laboratories, and ambulatory care/surgery, mental health, substance abuse, and physical rehabilitation medicine facilities.

American Osteopathic Association
142 E. Ontario Street
Chicago, ILLINOIS 60611
Telephone: 800/621-1773   Fax: 312/202-8200
Telephone: 312/202-8000
E-mail: info@aoa-net.org
Web site: www.aoa-net.org

American Society for Histocompatibility and Immunogenetics
Accredits histocompatibility laboratories.

American Society for Histocompatibility and Immunogenetics
8310 Nieman Road
Lenexa, KANSAS 66214
Telephone: 913/541-0009   Fax: 913/541-0156
E-mail: ashi.info@goAMP.com
Web site: www.ashi-hla.org

College of American Pathologists
Accredits laboratories that perform clinical drug or medical device trials and laboratories that perform tests on patients for diagnosis and treatment of disease, nonmedical tests (urine drug testing and athletic drug testing), and fertility tests.

College of American Pathologists
325 Waukegan Road
Northfield, ILLINOIS 60093-2750
Telephone: 800/323-4040   Fax: 847/832-8171
Web site: www.cap.org

Commission on Office Laboratory Accreditation
Accredits physician office laboratories, with onsite survey services, including medical and facility reviews, HEDIS reviews, ambulatory medical record reviews, and behavioral health reviews.

Commission on Office Laboratory Accreditation
9881 Broken Land Parkway, Suite 200
Columbia, MARYLAND 21046-1158
Telephone: 800/981-9883   Fax: 410/381-8611
E-mail: info@cola.org
Web site: www.cola.org

The Commission on Accreditation of Rehabilitation Facilities
Accredits facilities in the areas of adult day services, assisted living, behavioral health, employment and community services, and medical rehabilitation.

The Commission on Accreditation of Rehabilitation Facilities
4891 E. Grant Road
Tucson, ARIZONA 85712
Telephone: 520/325-1044   Fax: 520/318-1129
E-mail: info@carf.org
Web site: www.carf.org

Community Health Accreditation Program
Accredits all home and community-based health care organizations, including those specializing in nursing, social work, occupational therapy, respiratory therapy, home health aide, hospice, management services, pharmacy, home medical equipment, infusion therapy, public health nursing, community nursing center, clinics, physical therapy, speech therapy, and nutrition counseling.

Community Health Accreditation Program
61 Broadway, 33rd Floor
New York, NEW YORK 10006
Telephone: 212/480-8828   800/656-9656, Ext. 242   Fax: 212/812-0394
E-mail: chap@nln.org
Web site: www.chapinc.org

Continuing Care Accreditation Commission
Accredits continuing care retirement communities and other retirement communities and includes reviews of resident life, health, and wellness; financial resources and disclosure; and governance and administration.

Continuing Care Accreditation Commission
2519 Connecticut Avenue, NW
Washington, DISTRICT OF COLUMBIA 20008-1520
Telephone: 202/783-7286   Fax: 202/783-2255
Web site: www.ccaconline.org
Web site: www.aahsa.org

Centers for Medicare & Medicaid Services (CMS)
CMS provides health insurance for more than 74 million Americans through Medicare, Medicaid, and the State Children's Health Insurance Program. In addition to providing health insurance, CMS also performs a number of quality-focused activities, including regulation of laboratory testing (CLIA), development of coverage policies, and quality-of-care improvement.

CMS maintains oversight of the survey and certification of nursing homes and continuing care providers (including home health agencies, intermediate care facilities for the mentally retarded, and hospitals), and makes information about these activities and nursing home quality available to beneficiaries, providers, researchers, and state surveyors.

CMS has a program that allows private, national accreditation organizations to "deem" that an organization is compliant with certain Medicare requirements. To be approved for deeming authority, an accrediting organization must demonstrate that its program meets or exceeds the Medicare requirements for which it is seeking the authority to deem compliance. Health care organizations providing services under the above noted programs may opt for accreditation by one of these "deemed" organizations (e.g., the JCAHO or AOA).

CMS routinely conducts validation surveys to make sure health care facilities accredited by these agencies do, in fact, meet the Medicare Conditions of Participation for health and safety. CMS typically assigns the responsibility for these focused surveys to the state health department. Five percent of "deemed" organizations will receive a "validation" survey within 60 days of the deemed accrediting body's survey.

CMS contact information is divided among the following 10 regions:

Main Web site: www.hcfa.gov/

Region I: Boston Regional Office

John F. Kennedy Federal Building
Room 2325
Boston, Massachusetts 02203-0003
Telephone: 617/565-1232

States and territories served

Connecticut, Maine, Massachusetts, New Hampshire, Rhode Island, Vermont

Region II: New York Regional Office

26 Federal Plaza
Room 3811
New York, New York 10278-0063
Telephone: 212/264-3657

States and territories served

New Jersey, New York, Puerto Rico, Virgin Islands

Region III: Philadelphia Regional Office

Suite 216, The Public Ledger Building
150 South Independence Mall West
Philadelphia, Pennsylvania 19106
Telephone: 215/861-4140

States and territories served

Delaware, District of Columbia, Maryland, Pennsylvania, Virginia, West Virginia

Region IV: Atlanta Regional Office

Atlanta Federal Center
61 Forsyth Street SW, Suite 4T20
Atlanta, Georgia 30303-8909
Telephone: 404/562-7500

States and territories served

Alabama, Florida, Georgia, Kentucky, Mississippi, North Carolina, South Carolina, Tennessee

Region V: Chicago Regional Office

233 North Michigan Avenue, Suite 600
Chicago, Illinois 60601
Telephone: 312/886-6432

States and territories served

Illinois, Indiana, Michigan, Minnesota, Ohio, Wisconsin

Region VI: Dallas Regional Office

1301 Young Street, Eighth Floor
Dallas, Texas 75202
Telephone: 214/767-6423

States and territories served

Arkansas, Louisiana, New Mexico, Oklahoma, Texas

Region VII: Kansas City Regional Office

Richard Bolling Federal Building
601 East 12 Street, Room 235
Kansas City, MISSOURI 64106-2808
Telephone: 816/426-2866

States and territories served

Iowa, Kansas, Missouri, Nebraska

Region VIII: Denver Regional Office	States and territories served
Federal Office Building, Room 522 1961 Stout Street Denver, Colorado 80294-3538 Telephone: 303/844-4024	Colorado, Montana, North Dakota, South Dakota, Utah, Wyoming

Region IX: San Francisco Regional Office	States and territories served
75 Hawthorne Street, 4th and 5th Floors San Francisco, California 94105-3903 Telephone: 415/744-3501	American Samoa, Arizona, California, Commonwealth of Northern Marianas Islands, Guam, Hawaii, Nevada

Region X: Seattle Regional Office	States and territories served
2201 Sixth Avenue, MS/RX-40 Seattle, Washington 98121-2500 Telephone: 206/615-2354	Alaska, Idaho, Oregon, Washington

CMS—Division of Laboratories and Acute Care Centers
Laboratory certification standards required by CLIA are administered through CMS and the Centers for Disease Control and Prevention.

CMS—Division of Laboratories and Acute Care Centers
U.S. Department of Health and Human Services
7500 Security Boulevard
Baltimore, MARYLAND 21244
Telephone: 410/786-3531   Fax: 410/786-1224
Web site: www.hcfa.gov

Foundation for the Accreditation of Cellular Therapy (FACT)
[formerly the Foundation for the Accreditation of Hematopoietic Cell Therapy]
Accredits facilities that perform therapeutic cell harvest, processing, and transplants.

Foundation for the Accreditation of Cellular Therapy
FACT Accreditation Office
University of Nebraska Medical Center
986065 University Medical Center
Omaha, NEBRASKA 68198-6065, U.S.A.
Telephone: 402/561-7555   Fax: 402/561-7550
Web site: www.unmc.edu/Community/fahct/Default.htm

Credentialing and Privileging Resources

International Standards Organization
Reviews quality management and quality assurance programs in health service organizations. Organizations are not accredited by ISO but rather achieve ISO registration.

International Standards Organization
American National Standards Institute
Headquarters:
1819 L Street, NW
Washington, DISTRICT OF COLUMBIA 20036
Telephone: 202/293-8020   Fax: 202/293-9287

New York Office:
25 West 43rd Street
New York, NEW YORK 10036
Telephone: 212/642-4900   212/642-4980 (customer service)   Fax: 212/398-0023
E-mail: info@ansi.org
Web site: www.ansi.org

Joint Commission on Accreditation of Healthcare Organizations (JCAHO)
Accredits behavioral health, long-term care, home care, ambulatory care, clinical laboratories, assisted living facilities, critical access hospitals, office-based surgery practices, and health care networks. In 1995, the JCAHO launched its Cooperative Accreditation Initiative to reduce redundancy in the accreditation of health care organizations by reducing duplicative evaluation activities. The following organizations have comparative agreements with the JCAHO:
- College of American Pathologists
- Accreditation Association for Ambulatory Health Care

The following organizations have comparative agreements pending with the JCAHO:
- Commission on Office Laboratory Accreditation
- Community Health Accreditation Program

Joint Commission on Accreditation of Healthcare Organizations
1 Renaissance Boulevard
Oakbrook Terrace, ILLINOIS 60181
Telephone: 630/792-5000   Fax: 630/792-5005
Web site: www.jcaho.org

National Committee for Quality Assurance (NCQA)
Accredits preferred provider organizations (PPOs), managed care organizations (MCOs), behavioral health organizations, CVOs, and physician organizations, and new health plans with evaluations in the areas of patient safety, confidentiality, consumer protection, access, service, and continuous improvement. Also, offers certification programs for organizations that perform NCQA-specified functions but are not eligible for NCQA's accreditation programs. Certification programs include CVOs, physician organizations, credentialing and utilization review, and disease management.

National Committee for Quality Assurance
2000 L Street NW, Suite 500

Washington, DISTRICT OF COLUMBIA 20036
Telephone: 202/955-3500   Fax: 202/955-3599
E-mail: Customersupport@ncqa.org
Web site: www.ncqa.org

Credentials Verification Organizations (CVOs)

In an effort to maintain their consumers' confidence and security, health care organizations must ensure that each of their practitioners is screened and his or her credentials are verified. Because the process of screening practitioners can be a lengthy one, many hospitals and health care organizations use the services of CVOs.

A CVO is an independent contractor that performs various credentialing services on behalf of its clients, including:
- gathering evidence of practitioners' credentials
- performing primary source verification on practitioners' credentials
- conducting on-site reviews of practitioners' offices and medical records

There are hundreds of for-profit CVOs in the United States today. In addition, there are many more CVOs that provide services locally or within the organizations that sponsor them. The following section includes contact information for many national and regional CVOs.

National CVOs

Aperture Inc.
301 N. Hurstbourne Parkway, Suite 200
Louisville, KENTUCKY 40222
Telephone: 888/452-5000   Fax: 502/326-8800
Web site: www.aperture-cvo.com

Bexar Credentials Verification, Inc.
1000 Riverside Avenue, Suite 202
Jacksonville, FLORIDA 32204
Telephone: 888/663-2770   904/354-0257   Fax: 904/358-8085
Web site: www.bexarcv.com

Bexar Credentials Verification, Inc.
202 West French Place, Suite 202
San Antonio, TEXAS 78212
Telephone: 800/570-9311   Fax: 888/640-6455
E-mail: roxanna@bexarcv.com
Web site: www.bexarcv.com

The Coding Edge, Inc.
701 Central Park Drive
Sanford, FLORIDA 32771
Telephone: 800/593-0090   Fax: 407/302-0644
Web site: www.codingedge.com/pcd.html

Columbia HCA Central Credentials Services
1 Park Plaza
Nashville, TENNESSEE 37203
Telephone: 615/344-9551   Fax: 615/313-6201

Compass Resources
224 W. High Street
Bellefonte, PENNSYLVANIA 16823
Telephone: 814/237-0776   Fax: 814/237-0798
Web site: www.compassres.com

CompHealth Credentialing
4021 S. 700 E., Suite 300
Salt Lake City, UTAH 84107
Telephone: 801/264-6400   Fax: 801/284-6811 or 801/264-6464
Web site: www.comphealth.com

CreDentals
23382 Mill Creek Drive, Suite 125
Laguna Hills, CALIFORNIA 92653
Telephone: 888/273-3368   Fax: 714/470-0838
Web site: www.credentials.com

Credential America
PO Box 28478
Richmond, VIRGINIA 23228
Telephone: 888/330-7287   Fax: 877/329-7287
E-mail: Info@CredentialAmerica.com
Web site: www.CredentialAmerica.com

Credentialing Corporation of America, Inc.
20950 Center Ridge Road, Suite LL30
Rocky River, OHIO 44116
Telephone: 440/895-1900 Fax: 440/895-1901
E-mail: kbruewer@ccacredentialing.com
Web site: www.ccacredentialing.com

Credentialing Solutions
3333 Michelson Drive, #740
Irvine, CALIFORNIA 92612
Telephone: 949/260-6505 Fax: 949/833-3602
E-mail: dradu@credsolutions.com
Web site: www.credsolutions.com

Credential One
Innovative Data Solutions
5311 Northfield Road, Suite 400
Bedford Heights, OHIO 44146

Telephone: 216/587-9440   Fax: 216/587-9480
E-mail: mparianos@ids-c1.com
Web site: www.idsconnect.com

Credentials OnLine
17085 Camino San Bernardo
San Diego, CALIFORNIA 92127
Telephone: 800/733-8737   Fax: 858-673-9866
Web site: www.healthlinesystems.com

CSI Network, Inc.
480 Washington Street
Norwood, MASSACHUSETTS 02062
Telephone: 781/762-0888   Fax: 781/762-7180
E-mail: csicvs91@aol.com
Web site: www.csinetworkinc.com

First Credentialing Quality Assurance
3101 N. Central Avenue, Suite 950
Phoenix, ARIZONA 85012
Telephone: 602/279-3773 or 800/279-3773   Fax: 602/279-1635

Health Care Link, Incorp.
Notes: Managed care application preparation also.
6712 Concord Highway
Monroe, NORTH CAROLINA 28110
Telephone: 704/753-4774   Fax: 704/753-4910
E-mail: hclink@gte.net

HEALTHCHECK
3954 Youngfield Street
Wheat Ridge, COLORADO 80033
Telephone: 303/420-1006   Fax: 303/420-2461
Web site: www.healthcheck-inc.com

HealthLine Management, Inc.
9735 Landmark Parkway, Suite 110
St. Louis, MISSOURI 63103-1803
Telephone: 314/241-2345   800/443-3901   Fax: 314/206-4040
E-mail: info@hmistl.com
Web site: www.hmistl..net

Health Net Data Link, an EHDL Company
3106 Commerce Parkway
Miramar, FLORIDA 33025
Telephone: 954/331-6500   Fax: 954/331-6690
E-mail: dclaussen@healthdata.net
Web site: www.healthdata.net

Credentialing and Privileging Resources

HSP Verified, Inc.
1120 G Street NW Suite 330
Washington, DISTRICT OF COLUMBIA 20005
Telephone: 202/783-1270   Fax: 202/783-1269
Web site: www.hspverified.inc

IntegraNet Management Services, Inc.
1800 NE Loop 410, Suite 300
San Antonio, TEXAS 78217
Telephone: 210/822-3255 or 800/848-0389   Fax: 210/822-5536
E-mail: Kprimeaux@integranet-cvo.com
Web site: www.integranet-cvo.com

Mainsail Corporation
1103 Mainsail Drive
Annapolis, MARYLAND 21403
Telephone: 410/263-1932   Fax: 410/263-6806

Med Advantage, Inc.
3452 Lake Lynda Drive, Suite 250
Orlando, FLORIDA 32817
Telephone: 407/282-5131   Fax: 407/282-9240
E-mail: sales@med-advantage.com
Web site: www.med-advantage.com

Medical Society Credentials Verification Organizations of America
Academy of Medicine of Cincinnati
320 Broadway
Cincinnati, OHIO 45202
Telephone: 513/421-7010   Fax: 513/721-4378
E-mail: donnacadserv@usa.net
Web site: www.mscvoa.org

Medilert-IRIS
PO Box 14050
Scottsdale, ARIZONA 85267-4050
Telephone: 800/846-1351   Fax: 800/765-4814
Web site: www.medilert.com

National Provider Credentialing Service, Inc.
3025 Breckenridge Boulevard, Suite 150
Duluth, MINNESOTA 30096
Telephone: 800/327-5355   Fax: 678/226-5120
E-mail: info@npcs.com

National Register of Health Service Providers in Psychology
1120 G Street NW, Suite 330
Washington, DISTRICT OF COLUMBIA 20005-3801

Telephone: 202/783-7663   Fax: 202/347-0550
E-mail: info@nationalregister.org
Web site: www.nationalregister.org

Northwest Credentials Verification Service
Note: Northwest Credentials Verification Service is currently certified by NCQA for 10 of 10 verification services for both managed care and behavioral health practitioners.
PO Box 379
Bremerton, WASHINGTON 98337
Telephone: 360/405-9196 Fax: 360/405-6582
E-mail: gaild@kpshealthplans.com

Oakwood Health Care System
Corporate Medical Affairs
23400 Michigan Avenue, Suite 705
Dearborn, MICHIGAN 48124
Telephone: 313/791-1370 Fax: 313/792-7115
E-mail: bakerr@oakwood.org
Web site: www.oakwood.org

Pacific Care Credentialing, Inc.
PO Box 6006
Cypress, CALIFORNIA 90630
Telephone: 800/624-8822

Physician Credentialing and Information Service
2423 Texas Parkway
Missouri City, TEXAS 77489
Telephone: 281/403-2141 Fax: 281/261-9198
E-mail: mail@sourceverify.com
Web site: www.sourceverify.com

Precision Credentialing Services
PO Box 336
Eagleville, PENNSYLVANIA 19408-0336
Telephone: 610/454-1337
E-mail: precision.cred.serv@erols.com

Sweetwater Health Enterprises
3939 Beltline Road, Suite 600
Addison, TEXAS 75001
Telephone: 972/888-5600 Fax: 972/888-5635
Web site: www.sweetwaterhealth.com

TPI Health Systems
10300 Linn Station Road, Suite 100
Louisville, KENTUCKY 40223

Telephone: 502/425-7000 Fax: 502/423-2872
Web site: www.tpihealth.net

The Trizetto Group, Inc.
NCVO Credentialing Verification Organization
1 Columbia Circle
Albany, NEW YORK 12203
Telephone: 518/862-3400   Fax: 518/862-3480
E-mail: ncvo@trizetto.com
Web site: www.trizetto.com

Veritas Medical Services, Inc.
211 South Street, #33
Philadelphia, PENNSYLVANIA 11947
Telephone: 215/893-9772   800/895-5917   Fax: 215/893-9255
E-mail: veritasmed@aol.com
Web site: www.veritasmed.com

VeriTrac, Inc.
10700 N. Freeway Suite 900
Houston, TEXAS 77037
Telephone: 281/447-7588   Fax: 281/447-3041
Web site: www.veritrac.com

Regional CVOs

Alaska
Medical Staff Services, Inc.
PO Box 230993
Anchorage, ALASKA 99523
Telephone: 907/563-3553 Fax: 907/344-2016
E-mail: amss@alaska.net

Arizona
Credentialing/Recredentialing Unit
PO Box 42195
Alamo Building
Tucson, ARIZONA 85775-3317
Telephone: 520/324-2025 Fax: 520/324-2051
E-mail: cru.admin@tmcaz.com

Greater Arizona Central Credentialing Program
Maricopa County Medical Society
326 E. Coronado Road
Phoenix, ARIZONA 85004
Telephone: 602/256-0705 Fax: 602/256-2763
Web site: www.azcvo.com

Chapter 10

California
Checkpoint Credentials Management Services
21540 Plummer Street
Chatsworth, CALIFORNIA 91311-4103
Telephone: 800/950-2647, Ext. 8355   Fax: 818/341-1275
Web site: www.masterplan.com

Colorado
El Paso County Medical Society
730 Citader Drive E. 206
Colorado Springs, COLORADO 80917-5391
Telephone: 719/591-2424   Fax: 719/591-5649
E-mail: cwalker@epcms.org
Web site: www.epcms.org

Delaware
Credentialing Connection, Inc.
1925 Lovering Avenue
Wilmington, DELAWARE 19806-2199
Telephone: 302/571-1804   Fax: 302/571-1112
E-mail: kef@medsocdel.org
Web site: www.medsocdel.org

Georgia
GetProof.com
3050 Royal Boulevard S., Suite 100
Alpharetta, GEORGIA 30002
Telephone: 770/410-5900 or 800/366-0593   Fax: 770/410-5910
E-mail: marketing@GetProof.com
Web site: www.getproof.com

Medical Association of Atlanta
875 W. Peachtree Street
Atlanta, GEORGIA 30309
Telephone: 404/881-1714   Fax: 404/872-0601
Web site: www.maa-assn.org

Illinois
Peoria Medical Society
Suite 1006
411 Hamilton Boulevard
Peoria, ILLINOIS 61602
Telephone: 309/676-2351   Fax: 309/676-3522
Web site: www.peomedsoc.org

Winnebago County Medical Society
6991 Redansa Drive
Suite 203

Rockford, ILLINOIS 61108
Telephone: 815/395-9267   Fax: 815/484-4109
E-mail: wcms1@aol.com

Kansas
Kansas Physician Information Verification Program
1102 S. Hillside
Wichita, KANSAS 67211
Telephone: 316/683-0178   Fax: 316/683-0958
E-mail: sharonhartley@med-soc.org
Web site: www.med-soc.org

Medical Society of Sedgwick County-Kansas Physicians Information
1102 S. Hillside
Wichita, KANSAS 67211
Telephone: 316/683-0178   Fax: 316/683-0958
E-mail: sharonhartley@med-soc.org

Kentucky
Commonwealth Credentialing
Lexington Medical Society
2628 Wilhite Court, Suite 201
Lexington, KENTUCKY 40503
Telephone: 859/277-1762   Fax: 859/277-3919
E-mail: cvo@lexingtondoctors.org

Jefferson County Medical Society
101 W. Chestnut Street
Louisville, KENTUCKY 40202
Telephone: 502/589-2001   Fax: 502/581-9022
E-mail: stephemb@jcmsdocs.org
Web site: www.jcmsdocs.org

Massachusetts
Community Hospitals of Eastern Middlesex
170 Governors Avenue
Medford, MASSACHUSETTS 02155-1643
Telephone: 781/306-6500   Fax: 781/306-6896
E-mail: chemcred@yahoo.com

Minnesota
Medical Credentialing Services of Minnesota (A joint service of Hennepin and Ramsey Medical Societies)
Broadway Place E, Suite 340
3433 Broadway Street NE
Minneapolis, MINNESOTA 55413-1761
Telephone: 612/623-2887   Fax: 612/623-2842

Mississippi
The Verification Group

17 Northtown Drive
PO Box 14023
Jackson, MISSISSIPPI 39236
Telephone: 601/957-9754   Fax: 601/957-9188
E-mail: TVG14023@aol.com

Nebraska
Metropolitan Omaha Medical Society
Nebraska Credentials Verification Organization
7907 Wakeley Plaza
Omaha, NEBRASKA 68114
Telephone: 402/343-1108   Fax: 402/343-0721
E-mail: ncvo@neonramp.com
Web site: www.omahamedical.com

New York
Oneida, Madison, Herkimer, Chenango & Oswego County Medical Societies
4311 Middle Settlement Road
New Hartford, NEW YORK 13413
Telephone: 315/735-2204   Fax: 315/735-1608
E-mail: crmyers@gpoconnect.com and kdyman@gpoconnect.com

Professional Information Exchange
555 W. 57th Street, Suite 1500
New York, NEW YORK 10019
Telephone: 212/259-0790   Fax: 212/489-8820
E-mail: kim@pixny.com
Web site: www.pixcvo.com

Ohio
Academy of Medicine of Cleveland/Northern Ohio Medical Association
6000 Rockside Woods Boulevard, Suite 150
Cleveland, OHIO 44131-2352
Telephone: 216/520-1000   Fax: 216/520-0999

MedChek
320 Broadway
Cincinnati, OHIO 45202-4292
Telephone: 513/721-4377   Fax: 513/721-4378
E-mail: MedChek@fuse.net

Practitioner Credentials Verification Center
Columbus Medical Association
431 E. Broad Street, Suite 300
Columbus, OHIO 43215
Telephone: 614/240-7425   Fax: 614/240-7416

Tennessee
Tennessee Physicians Quality Verification Organization

Credentialing and Privileging Resources

6918 Shallowford Road
Suite 206
Chattanooga, TENNESSEE 37421
Telephone: 423/485-8077   Fax: 423/485-0933
E-mail: tpqvo@tpqvo.com
Web site: www.tpqvo.com

Tennessee Physicians Quality Verification Organization
422 W. Cumberland Ave.
Knoxville, TENNESSEE 37902
Telephone: 865/524-4676   Fax: 865/546-7392

Texas
Clinical Credentialing Services Bureau
Texas Medical Foundation
901 Mopac Expressway South
Building II, Suite 200
Austin, TEXAS 78746-5799
Telephone: 512/329-6610   800/725-9216   Fax: 512/327-7159
E-mail: tmanley@tmf.org
Web site: www.tmf.org/ccsb.htm

Virginia
Centralized Credentials Verification Service
1200 E. Clay Street
Richmond, VIRGINIA 23219
Telephone: 804/643-2287   Fax: 804/643-2291
E-mail: smealey@ramdocs.org
Web site: www.ramdocs.org

Credential America
PO Box 28478
Richmond, VIRGINIA 23228
Telephone: 888/330-7287   Fax: 877/329-7287
E-mail: info@CredentialAmerica.com
Web site: www.CredentialAmerica.com

Washington
Spokane County Medical Society
1101 W. College, Suite 355
Spokane, WASHINGTON 99201-2010
Telephone: 509/325-5010   Fax: 509/325-5409
E-mail: credentials@spcms.org
Web site: www.spcms.org

Wisconsin
Gundersen Lutheran Credentialing Services, Inc.
1910 S. Avenue
La Crosse, WISCONSIN 54601

Telephone: 608/791-4426   Fax: 608/791-4429
E-mail: cdholliday@gundluth.org
Web site: www.gundluth.org

United Credentials Committee
Madison Hospitals
309 W. Washington Avenue
Madison, WISCONSIN 53703
Telephone: 608/258-3229   Fax: 608/258-3265   608/258-3237

Software vendors

Applied Statistics & Management, Inc.
30520 Cabrillo Avenue
Temecula, CALIFORNIA 92592
Telephone: 800/736-7276   Fax: 909/699-4374
E-mail: info@mdstaff.com
Web site: www.mdstaff.com

Bexar Credentials Verification, Inc.
202 West French Place
San Antonio, TEXAS 78212
Telephone: 800/570-9311   Fax: 888/640-6455
E-mail: roxanna@bexarcv.com
Web site: www.bexarcb.com

CACTUS Software
7301 Mission Road, Suite 300
Prairie Village, KANSAS 66208-3005
Telephone: 913/677-0092   800/776-230   Fax: 913/677-0185
E-mail: sales@visualcactus.com
Web site: www.visualcactus.com

CBR Associates, Inc.
1018 Broad Street
Durham, NORTH CAROLINA 27705
Telephone: 919/286-1326   Fax: 919/286-1329

Clientele Solutions, Inc.
5 W. 22nd Street, Suite 355
Tulsa, OKLAHOMA 74114
Telephone: 800/797-8388   918/585-8488   Fax: 918/585-5615
E-mail: info@clientele-solutions.com
Web site: www.clientele-solutions.com

HealthLine Systems, Inc.
Notes: MedicalStaff Line™ is a software system that integrates all medical staff office functions involved in credentialing and provider management in one central database. MedicalStaff Line for the Net connects existing MedicalStaff Line

databases to your Internet Web site for electronic credentialing, physician communication, and interactive provider referral.

17085 Camino San Bernardo
San Diego, CALIFORNIA 92127
Telephone: 858/673-1700   800/733-8737   Fax: 858/673-9866

Health Planning Consultants
350 Frank H. Ogawa Plaza, Suite 701
Oakland, CALIFORNIA 94612
Telephone: 510/893-4338   Fax: 510/893-4351
E-mail: medstaff@healthplanning.com
Web site: www.medstaffmedsoftware.com

IntelliSoft Group, Inc.
23 Pondview Place
Tyngsboro, MASSACHUSETTS 01879
Telephone: 888/634-4464   Fax: 978/649-4957
E-mail: jdamelio@intellisoftgroup.com
Web site: www.credentialcentral.com

Landacorp
4151 Ashford Dunwoody Road, Suite 505
Atlanta, GEORGIA 30319
Telephone: 404/531-9956   Fax: 404/531-4826
E-mail: info@landacorp.com
Web site: www.landacorp.com

McKesson Corporations
245 First Street
Cambridge, MASSACHUSETTS 02142
Telephone: 617/679-8000   Fax: 617/679-8888
Web site: www.lmckesson.com

Medical Systems Management, Inc.
Note: Medical Systems Management, Inc. is a complete physician credentialing system that automates all documentation and reporting of your medical staff office.
200 Quannapowitt Parkway
Wakefield, MASSACHUSETTS 01880
Telephone: 781/942-1700   Fax: 781/557-3140
E-mail: info@med-sys.com
Web site: www.med-sys.com

Micro-Med
Notes: Credentialing and quality assessment software.
2640 Walnut Avenue, Suite G
Tustin, CALIFORNIA 92780

Telephone: 714/731-6803   Fax: 714/731-1635
E-mail: pkajszo@micro-med.com
Web site: www.micro-med.com

Morrisey Associates
833 W. Jackson Boulevard, Suite 500
Chicago, ILLINOIS 60607
Telephone: 312/431-0123   Fax: 312/431-0414
E-mail: jnutter@morriseyonline.com
Web site: www.morriseyonline.com

Quest Group
34 Salem Street
Wilmington, MASSACHUSETTS 01887
Telephone: 978/988-8832
E-mail: sfx88@cris.com
Web site: www.cris.com

Sweetwater Health Enterprises
3939 Beltline Road, Suite 600
Addison, TEXAS 75001
Telephone: 972/888-5600   Fax: 972/888-5635
Web site: www.sweetwaterhealth.com

Systems Group, Inc.
1018 Crestwood Lane
Stone Mountain, GEORGIA 30087
Telephone: 770/921-2128   Fax: 770/951-8963

The Trizetto Group, Inc.
1 Columbia Circle
Albany, NEW YORK 12203
Telephone: 518/862-3400   Fax: 518/862-3480
E-mail: ncvo@trizetto.com
Web site: www.ncvo.net

Vistar Technologies
12072 Old Country Road
Wellington, FLORIDA 33414
Telephone: 888/266-4532 (toll-free)   561/792-6644   Fax: 561/792-6655
E-mail: vistar@gate.net
Web site: www.vistartech.com

Wybtrak
801 S. Rancho Drive, Suite B-3
Las Vegas, NEVADA 89106
Telephone: 702/382-5858   Fax: 702/382-4116
E-mail: info@wybtrak.com

Books, periodicals, and multimedia

Many publishers produce books, periodicals, audiotapes, and multimedia geared toward credentialing and privileging. The following is a list of numerous products and contact information for the organizations that manufacture them.

Books

Acute Care Credentialing and Clinical Privilege Delineation
National Association Medical Staff Services
PO Box 140647
Austin, TEXAS 78714-0647
Telephone: 512/454-7928   Fax: 512/454-3036
E-mail: namss@namss.org
Web site: www.namss.org

Comprehensive Accreditation Manual for Hospitals
Joint Commission on Accreditation of Healthcare Organizations
1 Renaissance Boulevard
Oakbrook Terrace, ILLINOIS 60181
Telephone: 630/792-5000   Fax: 630/792-5005
Web site: www.jcaho.org

20,125 Questionable Doctors Disciplined by States or the Federal Government
(also available on CD/ROM)
Public Citizen
1600 20th Street NW
Washington, DISTRICT OF COLUMBIA 20009
Telephone: 202/588-1000   Fax: 202/588-7796
E-mail: member@citizen.org
Web site: www.citizen.org

The Official ABMS Directory of Board-Certified Medical Specialists
American Board of Medical Specialties
1007 Church Street, Suite 500
Evanston, ILLINOIS 60201-5913
Telephone: 847/491-9091   Fax: 847/328-3596
Web site: www. abms.org

AHA Guide to the Health Care Field 2001–2002
American Hospital Association, Health Forum
1 N. Franklin, 29th Floor
Chicago, ILLINOIS 60606-3421
Telephone: 312/422-3000 or 800/821-2039   Fax: 312/422-4506
Web site: www.aha.org

American Osteopathic Association Yearbook and Directory of Osteopathic Physicians
American Osteopathic Association
142 E. Ontario Street

Chicago, ILLINOIS 60611
Telephone: 312/202-8285   800/621-1773, Ext. 8285 (toll-free)   Fax: 312/202-8445
E-mail: credential@aoa-net.org
Web site: www.aoa-net.org

The NAMSS Core Curriculum
National Association Medical Staff Services
PO Box 140647
Austin, TEXAS 78714-0647
Telephone: 512/454-7928   Fax: 512/454-3036
E-mail: namss@namss.org
Web site: www.namss.org

The Compliance Guide to the Medical Staff Standards, Second Edition
Opus Communications, a division of HCPro
PO Box 1168
Marblehead, MASSACHUSETTS 01945
Telephone: 800/650-6787   Fax: 800/639-8511
E-mail: customerservice@hcpro.com
Web site: www.hcmarketplace.com

Core Privileges: A Practical Approach to Development and Implementation
Opus Communications, a division of HCPro
PO Box 1168
Marblehead, MASSACHUSETTS 01945
Telephone: 800/650-6787   Fax: 800/639-8511
E-mail: customerservice@hcpro.com
Web site: www.hcmarketplace.com

Credentialing 101 Study and Reference Guide
National Association of Medical Staff Services
PO Box 140647
Austin, TEXAS 78714-0647
Telephone: 512/454-7928   Fax: 512/454-3036
E-mail: namss@namss.org
Web site: www.namss.org

Credentialing Allied Health Professionals Study and Reference Guide
National Association of Medical Staff Services
PO Box 140647
Austin, TEXAS 78714-0647
Telephone: 512/454-7928   Fax: 512/454-3036
E-mail: namss@namss.org
Web site: www.namss.org

Credentialing and Medical Staff Law
National Association of Medical Staff Services
PO Box 140647

Austin, TEXAS 78714-0647
Telephone: 512/454-7928   Fax: 512/381-6036
E-mail: namss@namss.org
Web site: www.namss.org

The Credentialing Handbook
Aspen Publishers, Inc.
7201 McKinney Circle
Frederick, MARYLAND 21701
Telephone: 800/234-1660   Fax: 800/901-9075
Web site: www.aspenpublishers.com

The Credentialing Orientation Handbook: What Practitioners Need to Know About Credentialing
Opus Communications, a division of HCPro
PO Box 1168
Marblehead, MASSACHUSETTS 01945
Telephone: 800/650-6787   Fax: 800/639-8511
E-mail: customerservice@hcpro.com
Web site: www.hcmarketplace.com

Credentialing and Privileging Systems
American College of Physician Executives
4890 W. Kennedy Boulevard, Suite 200
Tampa, FLORIDA 33609-2575
Telephone: 800/562-8088 or 813/287-2000   Fax: 813/287-8993
Web site: www.acpe.org

Credentials Review and Privileging: Questions and Answers for Ambulatory Care
Joint Commission on Accreditation of Healthcare Organizations
1 Renaissance Boulevard
Oakbrook Terrace, ILLINOIS 60181
Telephone: 630/792-5000   Fax: 630/792-5005
Web site: www.jcaho.org

The Greeley Guide to Medical Staff Credentialing
Opus Communications, a division of HCPro
PO Box 1168
Marblehead, MASSACHUSETTS 01945
Telephone: 800/650-6787   Fax: 800/639-8511
E-mail: customerservice@hcpro.com
Web site: www.hcmarketplace.com

A Guide to AHP Credentialing: Challenges and Opportunities to Credentialing Allied Health Professionals
Opus Communications, a division of HCPro
PO Box 1168
Marblehead, MASSACHUSETTS 01945
Telephone: 800/650-6787   Fax: 800/639-8511
E-mail: customerservice@hcpro.com
Web site: www.hcmarketplace.com

Chapter 10

Hospital Phone Book
Douglas Publications, Inc.
U.S. Directory Service
2807 N. Parham Road, Suite 200
Richmond, VIRGINIA 23294
Telephone: 800/223-1797   804/762-9600   Fax: 804/217-8999
E-mail: info@douglaspublications.com
Web site: www.douglaspublications.com

Insurance Phone Book & Directory
Douglas Publications, Inc.
U.S. Directory Service
2807 N. Parham Road, Suite 200
Richmond, VIRGINIA 23294
Telephone: 800/223-1797   804/762-9600   Fax: 804/217-8999
E-mail: info@douglaspublications.com
Web site: www.douglaspublications.com

Legal Answer Book for Managed Care
Aspen Publishers, Inc.
7201 McKinney Circle
Frederick, MARYLAND 21701
Telephone: 800/234-1660   Fax: 800/901-9075
Web site: www.aspenpublishers.com

The LIP's Guide to Credentials Review and Privileging
Joint Commission on Accreditation of Healthcare Organizations
1 Renaissance Boulevard
Oakbrook Terrace, ILLINOIS 60181
Telephone: 630/792-5000   Fax: 630/792-5005
Web site: www.jcaho.org

Managed Care Credentialing Study and Reference Guide
National Association of Medical Staff Services
PO Box 140647
Austin, TEXAS 78714-0647
Telephone: 512/454-7928   Fax: 512/381-6036
E-mail: namss@namss.org
Web site: www.namss.org

Managing Medical Staff Change Through Bylaws and Other Strategies
American Hospital Association, Health Forum
1 North Franklin, 29th Floor
Chicago, ILLINOIS 60606-3421
Telephone: 312/422-3000 or 800/821-2039   Fax: 312/422-4506
Web site: www.aha.org

Medical Staff Credentialing: A Practical Guide
American Hospital Association, Health Forum

1 North Franklin, 29th Floor
Chicago, ILLINOIS 60606-3421
Telephone: 312/422-3000   800/821-2039   Fax: 312/422-4506
Web site: www.aha.org

The Medical Staff Handbook: A Guide to Joint Commission Standards
Joint Commission on Accreditation of Healthcare Organizations
1 Renaissance Boulevard
Oakbrook Terrace, ILLINOIS 60181
Telephone: 630/792-5000   Fax: 630/792-5005
Web site: www.jcaho.org

Medical Staff Leaders' Practical Guide, Fourth Edition
Opus Communications, a division of HCPro
PO Box 1168
Marblehead, MASSACHUSETTS 01945
Telephone: 800/650-6787   Fax: 800/639-8511
E-mail: customerservice@hcpro.com
Web site: www.hcmarketplace.com

Medical Staff Management: Forms, Policies, and Procedures for Health Care Providers
Aspen Publishers, Inc.
7201 McKinney Circle
Frederick, MARYLAND 21701
Telephone: 800/234-1660   Fax: 800/901-9075
Web site: www.aspenpublishers.com

The Privileging Quick Reference Guide, Second Edition
Opus Communications, a division of HCPro
PO Box 1168
Marblehead, MASSACHUSETTS 01945
Telephone: 800/650-6787   Fax: 800/639-8511
E-mail: customerservice@hcpro.com
Web site: www.hcmarketplace.com

Verify and Comply: A Quick Reference Guide to the JCAHO & NCQA Standards for Credentialing, Second Edition
Opus Communications, a division of HCPro
PO Box 1168
Marblehead, MASSACHUSETTS 01945
Telephone: 800/650-6787   Fax: 800/639-8511
E-mail: customerservice@hcpro.com
Web site: www.hcmarketplace.com

World Directory of Medical Schools
WHO Regional Office for the Americas/Pan American Health Organization
American Regional Office
525 23rd Street NW
Washington, DISTRICT OF COLUMBIA 20037
Telephone: 202/974-3000   Fax: 202/974-3663

E-mail: library@who.int
Web site: www.who.org

Periodicals

Briefings on Credentialing
Opus Communications, a division of HCPro
PO Box 1168
Marblehead, MASSACHUSETTS 01945
Telephone: 800/650-6787   Fax: 800/639-8511
E-mail: customerservice@hcpro.com
Web site: www.hcmarketplace.com

Briefings on JCAHO
Opus Communications, a division of HCPro
PO Box 1168
Marblehead, MASSACHUSETTS 01945
Telephone: 800/650-6787   Fax: 800/639-8511
E-mail: customerservice@hcpro.com
Web site: www.hcmarketplace.com

Medical Staff Briefing
Opus Communications, a division of HCPro
PO Box 1168
Marblehead, MASSACHUSETTS 01945
Telephone: 800/650-6787   Fax: 800/639-8511
E-mail: customerservice@hcpro.com
Web site: www.hcmarketplace.com

Synergy
National Association of Medical Staff Services
PO Box 140647
Austin, TEXAS 78714-0647
Telephone: 512/454-7928   Fax: 512/381-6036
E-mail: namss@namss.org
Web site: www.namss.org

Multimedia

Note: Unless otherwise indicated, the following are products of:

Opus Communications, a division of HCPro
PO Box 1168
Marblehead, MASSACHUSETTS 01945
Telephone: 800/650-6787   Fax: 800/639-8511
E-mail: customerservice@hcpro.com
Web site: www.hcmarketplace.com

Audiotapes
Conduct Effective Fair Hearings and Avoid Legal Landmines
Conducting Criminal Background Checks and Avoiding Legal Headaches
Core Privileging: A Report from the Front Lines
Credentialing and the Allied Health Professional
Credentialing Audiotape Training Series
Credentialing the Complementary & Alternative Medicine Practitioner
JCAHO's Standards on Temporary and Emergency Privileges
How to Ensure Timely Reappointments and Avoid Type I's
New Credentialing Standard: Credentialing in the Post-Swango Era
Practical Approach to Core Privileging
Quality and Peer Review for the Medical Staff

Electronic Resources
Credentialing Orientation Kit
HPCheck: Criminal and Other Background Checks of Healthcare Professionals
HCProfessor online courses in credentialing (cosponsored by NAMSS)—www.hcprofessor.com

Videos
Introduction to Credentialing for Medical Staff Leaders: The Story of Credentialing
Medical Staff Quality: How to Measure Outcomes and Improve Performance Series
Medical Executive Committee Series
Medical Staff Credentialing Interview, produced by Medical Consultants Network Inc., distributed by HCPro

Appendix

Table of Board Certification Time Limits

Board	Recertification requirements	Month/year recertification requirements instated
American Board of Medical Specialties (ABMS)		
American Board of Allergy and Immunology	Allergy: Every 10 years	January 1, 1989
	Clinical and laboratory immunology: Every 10 years	January 1, 1994
American Board of Anesthesiology	Every 10 years	2000
American Board of Colon and Rectal Surgery	Every 8 years	January 1, 1990
American Board of Dermatology	Every 10 years	
American Board of Emergency Medicine	Every 10 years	
American Board of Family Practice	General certificates: Every 7 years	
	Subspecialty certificates: Every 10 years	
American Board of Internal Medicine	Every 10 years	September 1, 1990
American Board of Medical Genetics	Every 10 years	January 1, 1993
American Board of Neurological Surgery	Lifetime certification	
American Board of Nuclear Medicine	Every 10 years	January 1, 1992
American Board of Obstetrics and Gynecology	Every 10 years	January 1, 1985
American Board of Ophthalmology	Every 10 years	January 1, 1992
American Board of Orthopaedic Surgery	Every 10 years	January 1, 1986
American Board of Otolaryngology	Every 10 years	January 1, 2002
American Board of Pathology	Every 10 years	January 1, 2006
American Board of Pediatrics	Every 7 years	May 1, 1988
American Board of Physical Medicine and Rehabilitation	Every 10 years	May 1, 1993
American Board of Plastic Surgery, Inc.	Every 10 years	November 1, 1995

Table of Board Certification Time Limits (cont.)

Board	Recertification requirements	Month/year recertification requirements instated
American Board of Medical Specialties (ABMS)		
American Board of Preventive Medicine	Every 10 years	January 1, 1997
American Board of Psychiatry and Neurology	Every 10 years	October 1, 1994
American Board of Radiology, Inc.	Every 10 years	November 1, 1995
American Board of Surgery	Voluntary	January 1, 1997
American Board of Thoracic Surgery	Every 10 years	May 1, 1976
American Board of Urology	Every 10 years	February 1, 1985
American Osteopathic Association (AOA Boards) *Effective January 1, 2004, all AOA boards will time limit their certification to 10 years or less.		
American Osteopathic Board of Anesthesiology	Every 10 years	January 1, 2000
	To be determined	January 1, 2004
American Osteopathic Board of Dermatology	General certificate: to be determined	January 1, 2004
	Certificates of added qualifications: Every 10 years	
American Osteopathic Board of Emergency Medicine	Every 10 years	January 1, 1994
American Osteopathic Board of Family Practice	Every 8 years	March 1, 1997
American Osteopathic Board of Internal Medicine	Every 10 years	January 1, 1993
American Osteopathic Board of Neurology and Psychiatry	Every 10 years	January 1, 1995
American Osteopathic Board of Neuromuskuloskeletal Medicine (formerly Special Proficiency OMM)	Every 10 years	January 1, 1995
American Osteopathic Board of Nuclear Medicine	Every 10 years	January 1, 1995
American Osteopathic Board of Obstetrics and Gynecology	To be determined	January 1, 2004

Table of Board Certification Time Limits (cont.)

Board	Recertification requirements	Month/year recertification requirements instated
American Osteopathic Association (AOA Boards) *Effective January 1, 2004, all AOA boards will time limit their certification to 10 years or less.		
American Osteopathic Board of Ophthalmology and Otorhinolaryngology	Ophthalmology: Every 10 years	January 2000
	Otorhinolaryngology: Every 10 years	January 2002
American Osteopathic Board of Orthopedic Surgery	Every 10 years	January 1, 1994
American Osteopathic Board of Pathology	Every 10 years	January 1, 1995
American Osteopathic Board of Pediatrics	Every 7 years	January 1, 1995
American Osteopathic Board of Preventive Medicine	Every 10 years	January 1, 1994
American Osteopathic Board of Proctology	To be determined	January 1, 2004
American Osteopathic Board of Radiology	To be determined	January 1, 2004
American Osteopathic Board of Rehabilitation Medicine	To be determined	January 1, 2004
American Osteopathic Board of Surgery	Every 10 years	January 1, 2004
American Dental Association (ADA Boards)		
American Board of Dental Health	Every 10 years, but must complete 10 hours of continuing education per year	January 1, 2000
American Board of Endodontics	Every 10 years	January 1, 1997
American Board of Oral and Maxillofacial Pathology	Lifetime certification (time limit in plan)	
American Board of Oral and Maxillofacial Surgery	Every 10 years	January 1, 1988
American Board of Orthodontics	15 years	January 1, 1998
American Board of Pediatric Dentistry	Every 10 years	September 6, 1991

Table of Board Certification Time Limits (cont.)

Board	Recertification requirements	Month/year recertification requirements instated
American Dental Association (ADA Boards)		
American Board of Periodontology	Lifetime certification, but must complete continuing education requirements every 3 years	February 1991
American Board of Prosthodontics	Every 8 years	January 1, 1996
American Podiatric Medical Association (APMA) Boards		
American Board of Podiatric Orthopedics & Primary Podiatric Medicine	Every 10 years	January 1, 1993
American Board of Podiatric Surgery	Every 10 years	January 1, 1991
Nursing Boards		
American Association of Nurse Anesthetists (AANA) Certification	Every 2 years	
American College of Nurse Midwives (ACNM)	Every 8 years	January 1, 1996
American Nurses Credentialing Center (ANCC)	Every 5 years	
Psychology Boards		
American Board of Professional Psychology (ABPP)	Lifetime certification	
American Psychological Association	Every 3 years	
Other Boards		
American Board of Medical Genetics	Every 10 years	January 1, 1993
American Board of Physical Therapy Specialties	Every 10 years	
Certification Board for Nutrition Specialists	Every 10 years, but must complete 75 credit hours of approved continuing education	
National Board for Certification of Orthopedic Technicians	Every 6 years	
National Commission on the Certification of Physician Assistants (NCCPA)	4 years after initial certification, and every 2 years thereafter	

Index

A

Accreditation Association for Ambulatory Health Care, Inc., 619
ACNM Certification Council, Inc. (ACC), 511
ADA, privileging and, 15
Addictionology specialty associations
    American Academy of Addiction Psychiatry, 543
    American Osteopathic Academy of Addiction Medicine, 543
    American Society of Addiction Medicine, 543
    International Society of Addiction Medicine, 543
Administration, role in credentialing and privileging, 32
Admitting privileges, 18
AHPs, credentialing, 4
Alabama Board of Examiners in Psychology, 457
Alabama Board of Nursing, 437
Alabama dental schools
    University of Alabama School of Dentistry, 161
Alabama licensing agencies
    Alabama Board of Examiners in Psychology, 457
    Alabama Board of Nursing, 437
    Alabama State Board of Chiropractic, 397
    Alabama State Board of Medical Examiners, MD and DO, 289
    Alabama State Board of Medical Examiners, Physician assistant, 289
    Alabama State Board of Podiatry, 377
    State Board of Dental Examiners of Alabama, 343
Alabama medical schools
    University of Alabama School of Medicine, 57
    University of South Alabama College of Medicine, 57
Alabama nursing schools
    University of Alabama at Birmingham, 223
    University of Alabama—Birmingham, Nurse Anesthetist program, 229
Alabama physician assistant programs
    University of Alabama at Birmingham, Surgical Physician Assistant Program, 195
Alabama residency programs
    University of Alabama School of Medicine, 57
    University of South Alabama Hospitals, 58
Alabama State Board of Chiropractic, 397
Alabama State Board of Dental Examiners, 343
Alabama State Board of Medical Examiners, MD and DO, 289
Alabama State Board of Medical Examiners, Physician assistant, 389
Alabama State Board of Podiatry, 377
Alaska licensing agencies
    Alaska Board of Nursing, 437
    Alaska Board of Psychologist and Psychological Associates, 457
Alaska State Board of Chiropractic Examiners, 397
Alaska State Medical Board, MD and DO, 290
Alaska State Medical Board, Physician assistant, 417
Alaska State Medical Board, Podiatry, 377
State of Alaska Board of Dental Examiners, 343

Index

Alaska State Medical Board, Physician assistant, 417
Alaska, State of Alaska Board of Dental Examiners, 343
Albany Hudson Valley, Physician Assistant Program, 207
Albany Medical College, 101
Albany Medical College, residencies, 101
Albert Einstein College of Medicine of Yeshiva University, 101
Alberta medical schools (Canada)
    University of Calgary Faculty of Medicine, 149
Alberta residency programs (Canada)
    University of Calgary Faculty of Medicine, 149
Alderson Broaddus College, Physician Assistant Program, 219
Allentown College of Saint Francis de Sales, Physician Assistant Program, 214
Allergy, asthma, and immunology specialty associations
    American Academy of Allergy, Asthma, and Immunology, 544
    American Academy of Otolaryngic Allergy, 544
    American Association of Immunologists, 544
    American College of Allergy, Asthma, and Immunology, 544
    American In-vitro Allergy and Immunology Society, 544
    American Osteopathic College of Allergy and Immunology, 544
    Asthma and Allergy Foundation of America, 544
    Joint Council of Allergy, Asthma, and Immunology, 545
Allied health—general specialty associations
    American Association of Bioanalysts, 545
    American Board of Electrodiagnostic Medicine, 545
    American Clinical Neurophysiology Society, 545
    American Society for Cytotechnology, 545
    American Society of Cytopathology, 545
    American Society of Neuroimaging, 545
    American Society of Radiologic Technologists, 546
    Association of Schools of Allied Health Professionals, 546
    Canadian Society for Medical Laboratory Science, 546
    National Association Medical Staff Services, 546
    National Registry of Emergency Medical Technicians, 546
American Accreditation HealthCare Commission/Utilization Review Accreditation Commission, 619
American Association for Accreditation of Ambulatory Surgery Facilities, 619
American Association for Ambulatory Health Care, Inc., 619
American Association of Blood Banks, 620
American Association of Medical Assistants, 200
American Association of Nurse Anesthetists (AANA), 511
American Board of Medical Genetics, 489
American Board of Medical Specialties (ABMS) Boards, 489
    Allergy and Immunology, 485
    Anesthesiology, 486
    Colon and Rectal Surgery, 486
    Dermatology, 487
    Emergency Medicine, 487
    Family Practice, 488
    Internal Medicine, 488
    Medical Genetics, Inc., 489

- Neurological Surgery, 490
- Nuclear Medicine, 490
- Obstetrics and Gynecology, 490
- Ophthalmology, 491
- Orthopaedic Surgery, 491
- Otolaryngology, 492
- Pathology, 492
- Pediatrics, 493
- Physical Medicine and Rehabilitation, 494
- Plastic Surgery, Inc. 494
- Preventive Medicine, 495
- Psychiatry and Neurology, 495
- Radiology, 496
- Surgery, 496
- Thoracic Surgery, 497
- Urology, 497

American Board of Professional Psychology (ABPP), 513

American Dental Association (ADA) Boards, 505
- Dental Public Health, 505
- Endodontics, 506
- Oral and Maxillofacial Pathology, 506
- Oral and Maxillofacial Surgery, 507
- Orthodontics, 507
- Pediatric Dentistry, 508
- Peridontology, 508
- Prosthodontics, 509

American Medical Association (AMA) Physician Masterfile, 530

American Nurses Credentialing Center (ANCC), 512

American Osteopathic Association (AOA) Boards, 498

American Osteopathic Association (AOA) Official Osteopathic Physician Profile Report, 498

American Osteopathic Association, 498

American Osteopathic Board of
- Anesthesiology, 499
- Dermatology, 499
- Emergency Medicine, 500
- Family Physicians, 500
- Internal Medicine (AOBIM), 501
- Neurology and Psychiatry, 501
- Neuromusculoskeletal Medicine, 502
- Nuclear Medicine, 502
- Ophthalmology and Otorhinolaryngology, 503
- Orthopedic Surgery, 503
- Preventive Medicine, 504
- Proctology, 504
- Surgery, 505

American Psychological Association, 513

American Society of Histocompatibility and Immunogenetics, 621

Anesthesiology specialty associations
- American Academy of Anesthesiologist Assistants, 547

Index

   American Association of Nurse Anesthetists, 547
   American Dental Society of Anesthesiology, Inc, 547
   American Osteopathic College of Anesthesiologists, 547
   American Society for the Advancement of Anesthesia in Dentistry, 547
   American Society of Anesthesiologists, 547
   American Society of Critical Care Anesthesiologists, 547
   American Society of Regional Anesthesia and Pain Medicine, 548
   Canadian Anesthesiologists' Society, 548
   National Board of Anesthesiology, Inc., 548
   Society for Obstetric Anesthesia and Perinatology, 548
   Society for Pediatric Anesthesia, 548
   Society of Neurological Anesthesia and Critical Care, 549

Anglo-European College of Chiropractic, 187
Applicant, role in credentialing and privileging, 32
Arizona Board of Chiropractic Examiners, 397
Arizona Board of Osteopathic Examiners in Medicine and Surgery, 290
Arizona Board of Podiatry Examiners, 377
Arizona Board of Psychologist Examiners, 457
Arizona College of Osteopathic Medicine—Midwestern University, 141
Arizona licensing agencies
   Arizona Board of Chiropractic Examiners, 397
   Arizona Board of Osteopathic Examiners in Medicine and Surgery, 290
   Arizona Board of Podiatry Examiners, 377
   Arizona Board of Psychologist Examiners, 457
   Arizona State Board of Dental Examiners, 344
   Arizona State Board of Medical Examiners, MD, 291
   Arizona State Board of Medical Examiners, Physician assistant, 417
   Arizona State Board of Nursing, 437

Arizona medical schools
   Arizona College of Osteopathic Medicine—Midwestern University, 141
   University of Arizona College of Medicine, 58

Arizona residency programs
   University of Arizona College of Medicine, 58

Arizona State Board of Dental Examiners, 344
Arizona State Board of Medical Examiners, MD, 291
Arizona State Board of Medical Examiners, Physician assistant, 417
Arizona State Board of Nursing, 437
Arkansas Board of Chiropractic, 398
Arkansas Board of Examiners in Psychology, 458
Arkansas Board of Podiatric Medicine, 378
Arkansas licensing agencies
   Arkansas Board of Chiropractic, 398
   Arkansas Board of Examiners in Psychology, 458
   Arkansas Board of Podiatric Medicine, 378
   Arkansas State Board of Dental Examiners, 345
   Arkansas State Board of Nursing, 438
   Arkansas State Medical Board, MD and DO, 291
   Arkansas State Medical Board, Physician assistant, 417

Arkansas medical schools
    University of Arkansas College of Medicine, 59
Arkansas State Board of Dental Examiners, 345
Arkansas State Board of Nursing, 438
Arkansas State Medical Board, MD and DO, 291
Arkansas State Medical Board, Physician assistant, 417
Australia chiropractic schools
    Macquarie University Department of Chiropractic, 185
    Royal Melbourne Institute of Technology, 185
Avera McKennan Hospital/University of South Dakota, School of Anesthesia for registered Nurses, 252

B

Barnes Jewish Hospital, residencies, 94
Barry University Master of Science in Anesthesia Program, 232
Barry University School of Graduate Medical Sciences, 181
Baylor College of Dentistry, 175
Baylor College of Medicine, 127
Baylor College of Medicine, Graduate Program in Nurse Anesthesia, 253
Baylor College of Medicine, Nurse-Midwifery Education Program, 270
Baylor College of Medicine, Physician Assistant Program, 215
Baylor College of Medicine, residencies, 127
Baystate Medical Center, Nurse-Midwifery Education Program, 263
Berkshire Medical Center, School of Anesthesia, 237
Board, role in credentialing and privileging, 31
Boston University School of Dental Medicine, 167
Boston University School of Public Health, Nurse-Midwifery Education Program, 263
British Columbia medical schools (Canada)
    University of British Columbia Faculty of Medicine, 59
British Columbia residency programs (Canada)
    University of British Columbia Faculty of Medicine, 59
Brooklyn Hospital Center/Long Island University, Physician Assistant Program, 210
Brown Medical School, 122
Bryan LGH Medical Center, University of Kansas, School of Nurse Anesthesia, 241

C

California Board of Registered Nursing, 438
California chiropractic schools
    Life Chiropractic College—West, 185
    Palmer College of Chiropractic—West, 186
    Southern California University of Health Sciences, Los Angeles College of Chiropractic, 186
California College of Podiatric Medicine, 181
California dental schools
    Loma Linda University School of Dentistry, 161
    University of California San Francisco School of Dentistry, 162
    University of Southern California School of Dentistry, 162
    University of the Pacific School of Dentistry, 162

Index

California Family Health Council, Inc., 259
California licensing agencies
    Board of Chiropractic Examiners, 398
    California Board of Registered Nursing, 438
    California Medical Board, Psychologist, 458
    Medical Board of California, MD, 292
    Physician Assistant Committee, 418
    State of California Board of Dental Examiners, 345
California Medical Board, Psychologist, 458
California medical schools
    Charles R. Drew University of Medicine and Science College of Medicine, 60
    Keck School of Medicine of the University of Southern California, 60
    Loma Linda University School of Medicine, 61
    Stanford University School of Medicine, 61
    Touro University College of Osteopathic Medicine, 141
    University of California at Davis School of Medicine, 61
    University of California at Irvine College of Medicine, 64
    University of California at Los Angeles School of Medicine, 62
    University of California at San Diego School of Medicine, 63
    University of California at San Francisco, School of Medicine, 64
California nursing schools
    California Family Health Council, Inc., 259
    Charles R. Drew University of medicine and Science, Nurse-Midwifery Education Program, 259
    Kaiser Permanente School of Anesthesia, 229
    UCSD Nurse-Midwifery Education Program, 259
    UCSF Interdepartmental Nurse-Midwifery Education Program, 260
    UCSF/SFGH Interdepartmental Nurse-Midwifery Education Program, 260
    University of Southern California Department of Nursing, 223
    University of Southern California Program of Nurse Anesthesia, 230
    University of Southern California, Nurse-Midwifery Education Program, 260
California Physician Assistant Committee, 418
California physician assistant programs
    Charles R. Drew University of Medicine and Science, Physician Assistant Program, 195
    Stanford University/Foothill College School of Medicine, Primary Care Associate Program, 195
    University of California—Davis Medical Center, Family Nurse Practitioner/Physician Assistant Program, 196
    University of Southern California School of Medicine, Primary Care Physician Assistant Program, 196
    Western University of Health Sciences, 196
California podiatry schools
    California College of Podiatric Medicine, 181
California residency programs
    Charles R. Drew University of Medicine and Science College of Medicine, 60
    Loma Linda University Medical Center, 60
    University of California at Davis School of Medicine, 62
    University of California at Los Angeles School of Medicine, 62
    University of California at San Diego School of Medicine, 63
    University of California Medical Center, 61
    University of California San Francisco, School of Medicine, 63
    University of California, Davis, Medical Center, 64
    University of Southern California, School of Medicine, 64

Index

California, Medical Board of California, MD, 292
California, State of California Board of Dental Examiners, 345
Canadian chiropractic schools
    Canadian Memorial Chiropractic College, 186
Canadian licensing agencies
    College des medecins du Quebec, 339
    College of Physicians and Surgeons of Alberta, 333
    College of Physicians and Surgeons of British Columbia, 333
    College of Physicians and Surgeons of Manitoba, 334
    College of Physicians and Surgeons of New Brunswick, 335
    College of Physicians and Surgeons of Nova Scotia, 337
    College of Physicians and Surgeons of Ontario, 337
    College of Physicians and Surgeons of Prince Edward Island, 338
    College of Physicians and Surgeons of Saskatchewan, 339
    Health and Social Services, Northwest Territories, 336
    Medical Profession, Health & Social Services, Northwest Territories, 336
    Newfoundland Medical Board, 335
    Yukon Medical Council, 340
Canadian medical schools
    Dalhousie University Faculty of Medicine, 152
    McGill University Faculty of Medicine, 156
    McMaster University School of Medicine, 152
    Memorial University of Newfoundland Faculty of Medicine, 151
    Queen's University Faculty of Health Sciences, 153
    Universite de Montreal Faculte de Medecine, 156
    Universite de Sherbrooke Faculte de Medecine, 156
    Universite Laval Faculte de Medecine, 157
    University of Alberta Faculty of Medicine and Dentistry, 149
    University of British Columbia Faculty of Medicine, 150
    University of Calgary Faculty of Medicine, 149
    University of Manitoba Faculty of Medicine, 150
    University of Ottawa Faculty of Medicine, 153
    University of Saskatchewan College of Medicine, 157
    University of Toronto Faculty of Medicine, 154
    University of Western Ontario Faculty of Medicine and Dentistry, 155
Canadian Memorial Chiropractic College, 186
Cardiology specialty associations
    American College of Cardiology, 549
    American College of Cardiovascular Administrators, 549
Carolinas Healthcare System/UNC—Charlotte, Nurse Anesthesia Program, 244
Case Western Reserve University School of Dentistry, 172
Case Western Reserve University School of Medicine, 111
Case Western Reserve University, Frances Payne Bolton School of Nursing, Nurse-Midwifery Program, 268
Case Western Reserve University/Mt. Sinai Medical Center/Cleveland Clinic Foundation, Frances Payne Bolton School of Nursing—School of Nurse Anesthesia, 245
Centers for Medicare and Medicaid Services, 622
CEO, role in credentialing and privileging, 32
Certification Board for Nutrition Specialists, 514

Index

Charity Hospital, School of Nurse Anesthesia, 235
Charles R. Drew University of Medicine and Science, Physician Assistant Program, 195
Charleston Area Medical Center, 255
Chatham College, Physician Assistant Program, 213
Chiropractic specialty associations
    American Chiropractic Association, 549
    Canadian Chiropractic Association, 549
    International Chiropractic Pediatric Association, 549
Clarion University School of Nursing, 225
Classifying clinical privileges, 14
Cleveland Chiropractic College, 188
Clinical data, 14
Closed organizations, 4
CMS—Division of Laboratories and Acute Care Centers, 624
COLA, 621
College of American Pathologists, 621
College of Health Sciences, Physician Assistant Program, 218
Colon and rectal surgery specialty associations
    American Society of Colon and Rectal Surgeons, 550
Colorado Board of Chiropractic Examiners, 398
Colorado Board of Medical Examiners, Physician assistants, 418
Colorado Board of Nursing, 439
Colorado Board of Psychologist Examiners, 458
Colorado dental schools
    University of Colorado School of Dentistry, 163
Colorado licensing agencies
    Board of Chiropractic Examiners, 398
    Colorado Board of Medical Examiners, Physician assistants, 418
    Colorado Board of Psychologist Examiners, 458
    Colorado Podiatry Board, 378
    Colorado State Board of Dental Examiners, 346
    Colorado State Board of Medical Examiners, MD and DO, 293
Colorado medical schools
    University of Colorado School of Medicine, 65
Colorado nursing schools
    University of Colorado, Nurse-Midwifery Program, 261
Colorado physician assistant programs
    University of Colorado Health Science Center, Child Health Associate/Physician Assistant Program, 197
Colorado Podiatry Board, 378
Colorado State Board of Dental Examiners, 346
Colorado State Board of Medical Examiners, MD and DO, 293
Columbia University College of Physicians and Surgeons, 102
Columbia University School of Dental and Oral Surgery, 171
Columbia University School of Nursing, program in Nurse Anesthesia, 242
Columbia University, Graduate Program in Nurse-Midwifery, 265
Commission on Accreditation of Rehabilitation Facilities, 621
Community College of Baltimore County, Physician Assistant Program, 204
Community Health Accreditation Program, 621
Connecticut Board of Examiners for Nursing, 439

Connecticut chiropractic schools
    University of Bridgeport, College of Chiropractic, 187
Connecticut dental schools
    University of Connecticut School of Dental Medicine, 163
Connecticut Department of Public Health, Chiropractic, 399
Connecticut Department of Public Health, Dental, 346
Connecticut Department of Public Health, 378
Connecticut Department of Public Health, MD and DO, 293
Connecticut Department of Public Health, Physician assistants, 418
Connecticut Department of Public Health, Psychologist, 459
Connecticut licensing agencies
    Connecticut Board of Examiners for Nursing, 439
    Connecticut Department of Public Health, 378
    Connecticut Department of Public Health, MD and DO, 293
    Connecticut Department of Public Health, Physician assistants, 418
    Connecticut Department of Public Health, Psychologist, 459
    Department of Public Health, Chiropractic, 399
    Department of Public Health, Dental, 346
Connecticut medical schools
    University of Connecticut School of Medicine, 65
Connecticut nursing schools
    Hospital of Saint Raphael, School of Nurse Anesthesia, 230
    New Britain School of Nurse Anesthesia, 231
    Southern Connecticut State University/Bridgeport Hospital, Nurse Anesthesia program, 231
    Yale University, Nurse-Midwifery Program, 261
Connecticut physician assistant programs
    Yale University School of Medicine, Physician Associate Program, 197
Connecticut residency programs
    University of Connecticut, 65
    Yale New Haven Hospital, 66
Continuing Care Accreditation Commission, 622
Core criteria, 4
Core privileging, 15
Credentials committee, role in credentialing and privileging, 30
Credentials verification organizations
    National, 626
    Regional, 631
Creighton University School of Dentistry, 170
Creighton University School of Medicine, 96
Creighton University School of Medicine, residencies, 96
Critical care/trauma medicine specialty associations
    American Association of Critical Care Nurses, 550
    American Burn Association, 550
    American Trauma Society, 550
    Canadian Critical Care Society, 551
CUNY/Harlem Hospital Center, Physician Assistant Program, 208
Current competence, 6
Cuyahoga Community College, Physician/Surgical Physician Assistant Program, 212

Index

D

D'Youville College, Physician Assistant Program, 208
Dartmouth Medical School, 98
Databanks, credentialing using, 5
Decatur Memorial Hospitals/Bradley University, Nurse Anesthesia Program, 232
Delaware Board of Chiropractic, 399
Delaware Board of Medical Practice, MD and DO, 294
Delaware Board of Medical Practice, Physician assistants, 419
Delaware Board of Nursing, 439
Delaware Board of Psychologists, 459
Delaware licensing agencies
    Delaware Board of Chiropractic, 399
    Delaware Board of Medical Practice, MD and DO, 294
    Delaware Board of Medical Practice, Physician assistants, 419
    Delaware Board of Nursing, 439
    Delaware Board of Psychologists, 459
    Delaware State Board of Dental Examiners, 347
Delaware State Board of Dental Examiners, 347
Delegated credentialing, 6, 39
Delineation of clinical privileges, 16
Dentistry specialty associations
    Academy of General Dentistry, 551
    Academy of Oral Dynamics, 551
    American Academy of Pediatric Dentistry, 551
    American Academy of Periodontology, 551
    American Association of Endodontists, 551
    American Association of Hospital Dentists, Inc., 551
    American College of Dentists, 552
    American College of Prosthodontists, 552
    American Dental Assistants Association, 552
    American Dental Association, 552
    American Dental Education Association, 552
    American Dental Society of Anesthesiology, Inc., 553
    American Society for the Advancement of Anesthesia Sedation in Dentistry, 553
    American Society of Dentistry for Children, 553
    Canadian Dental Association, 553
    National Association of Dental Assistants, 553
    National Dental Association, 553
Department chair, role in credentialing and privileging, 31
Department of Veterans Affairs/Drake University, Clinical Specialization in Nurse Anesthesia, 234
DePaul Medical Center, Bonsecour, Nurse anesthesia, 254
Dermatology specialty associations
    American Osteopathic College of Dermatology, 553
    American Society for Dermatologic Surgery, 554
    Canadian Dermatology Association, 554
    Dermatology Foundation, 554
Des Moines University—Osteopathic Medical Center, 142
Disclosing credentialing information, 6

District of Columbia dental schools
    Howard University College of Dentistry, 163
District of Columbia Department of Health, Chiropractic, 399
District of Columbia Department of Health, Dental, 348
District of Columbia Department of Health, MD and DO, 295
District of Columbia Department of Health, Nursing, 440
District of Columbia Department of Health, Physician assistants, 419
District of Columbia Department of Health, Psychologists, 459
District of Columbia licensing agencies
    Department of Health, Chiropractic, 399
    Department of Health, Dental, 348
    Department of Health, MD and DO, 295
    Department of Health, Physician assistants, 419
    District of Columbia Department of Health, Nursing, 440
    District of Columbia Department of Health, Psychologists, 459
District of Columbia medical schools
    George Washington University School of Medicine and Health Science, 66
    Georgetown University Medical Center, 67
    Howard University College of Medicine, 67
District of Columbia nursing schools
    Georgetown University School of Nursing and Health Sciences, 261
    Georgetown University School of Nursing, Nurse Anesthesia Program, 231
    Georgetown University, Graduate Program in Nurse-Midwifery, 261
District of Columbia physician assistant programs
    George Washington University, Physician Assistant Program, 198
    Howard University, Physician Assistant Program, 198
District of Columbia residency programs
    George Washington University School of Medicine and Health Sciences, 66
    Howard University College of Medicine, 67
Dr. William M. Scholl College of Podiatric Medicine, 181
Duke University Medical Center, Physician Assistant Program, 211
Duke University Medical School of Medicine, residencies, 108
Duke University School of Medicine, 108
Duquesne University, Physician Assistant Program, 213
Durham Regional Hospital, Watts School of Nursing, Anesthesia, 244

E

East Carolina University School of Medicine, residencies, 108
East Carolina University School of Nursing, Nurse-Midwifery Program, 267
East Tennessee State University College of Medicine, 124
East Tennessee State University College of Medicine, residencies, 124
Eastern Virginia Medical School, 132
Eastern Virginia Medical School, residencies, 133
Emergency Medicine specialty associations
    American College of Emergency Physicians, 554
    American College of Osteopathic Emergency Physicians, 554
    Canadian Association of Emergency Physicians, 554

Index

National Registry of Emergency Medical Technicians, 555
Society for Academic Emergency Medicine, 555

Emory University School of Medicine, 69
Emory University School of Medicine, Physician Assistant Program, 199
Emory University, Nell Hodgson Woodruff School of Nursing, 223
Emory University, Nell Hodgson Woodruff School of Nursing, Nurse-Midwifery Program, 262
Endocrinology specialty associations

American Association of Clinical Endocrinologists, 555
The Endocrine Society, 555
Women in Endocrinology, 555

Endoscopy specialty associations

American Society for Gastrointestinal Endoscopy, 555
Society of American Gastrointestinal Endoscopic Surgeons, 555

Environmental medicine

American Academy of Environmental Medicine, 556
American College of Occupational and Environmental Medicine, 556
National Environmental Health Association, 556
Occupational and Environmental Medical Association of Canada, 556

Erlanger Medical Center, School of Nurse Anesthesia, 252

F

Faculty of Medicine of University of Montreal, 250
Fair hearing and appeals in MCOs, 41
Family medicine specialty associations

American Academy of Family Physicians, 556
American College of Osteopathic Family Physicians, 556
College of Family Physicians of Canada, 557

Fast track credentialing, 7
Federation Credentials Verification Service, 530
The Federation Physician Data Center of the State Medical Boards (FSMB), 519
Finch University of Health Sciences/Chicago Medical School, Physician Assistant Program, 200
Finch University of the Health Sciences/Chicago Medical School, residencies, 73
Florida Board of Chiropractic, 400
Florida Board of Nursing, 440
Florida dental schools

University of Florida College of Dentistry, 164

Florida Division of Medical Quality Assurance, Dental, 348
Florida Division of Medical Quality Assurance, MD and DO, 295
Florida Division of Medical Quality Assurance, Physician assistant, 420
Florida Division of Medical Quality Assurance, Podiatric, 379
Florida licensing agencies

Board of Chiropractic, 400
Division of Medical Quality Assurance, Dental, 348
Division of Medical Quality Assurance, MD and DO, 295
Division of Medical Quality Assurance, Physician assistant, 420
Division of Medical Quality Assurance, Podiatry, 379
Florida Board of Nursing, 440

Florida medical schools
    Nova Southeastern University, College of Osteopathic Medicine, 141
    University of Florida College of Medicine, 68
    University of Miami Medical School, 69
    University of South Florida College of Medicine, 69

Florida nursing schools
    Barry University Master of Science in Anesthesia Program, 232
    Gooding Institute of Nurse Anesthesia at Bay Medical Center, 232
    University of Miami School of Nursing, 262
    University of Miami/Jackson Memorial Medical Center, Nurse-Midwifery Precertification Program, 262

Florida physician assistant programs
    Nova Southeastern University, Physician Assistant Program, 198
    University of Florida, Physician Assistant Program, 199

Florida podiatry schools
    Barry University School of Graduate Medical Sciences, 181

Florida residency programs
    Jackson Memorial Hospital, 68
    University of Florida College of Medicine, 68
    University of South Florida College of Medicine, 69

Foundation for the Accreditation of Hematopoietic Cell Therapy, 595
Franciscan Skemp Healthcare, 256
Fresno-UCSF School of Nursing, CRNA 438
Frontier School of Midwifery and Family Nursing, 263

G

Gastroenterology
    American College of Gastroenterology, 557
    American Gastroenterological Association, 557
    American Society for Gastrointestinal Endoscopy, 557
    North American Society for Pediatric Gastroenterology, Hepatology, and Nutrition, 557
    Society of American Gastrointestinal Endoscopic Surgeons, 557

General medicine specialty associations
    Accreditation Council for Graduate Medical Education, 558
    Aerospace Medical Association, 558
    American Academy of Pain Management, 558
    American Association of Physicians Specialists, Inc., 558
    American College of Medicine, 558
    American Holistic Medical Association, 558
    American Medical Association, 559
    American Physiological Society, 559
    American Society of Bariatric Physicians, 559
    American Society of Contemporary Medicine and Surgery, 559
    Association for Hospital Medical Education, 559
    Association for the Advancement of Wound Care, 559
    Association of American Medical Colleges, 559
    Association of American Physicians and Surgeons, Inc., 560
    Association of Military Surgeons of the U.S., 560
    Canadian Medical Association, 560

Index

    Committee of Interns and Residents, 560
    Council of Medical Specialty Societies, 560
    Mississippi State Board of Medical Licensure, 560
    National Health Council, Inc., 560
    National Medical Association, 561
    National Resident Matching Program, 561
    Royal College of Physicians and Surgeons of Canada, 561
    Society for Ambulatory Care Professionals, 561
    The Wound Healing Society, 561
    Tulsa County Medical Society, 561

Geriatric medicine specialty associations
    American Aging Association, 562
    American Association of Homes and Services for the Aging, 562
    American Geriatrics Society, 562
    National Council on the Aging, Inc., 562
    New England Gerontological Association, 562
    The Gerontological Society of America, 562

George Washington University School of Medicine and Health Sciences, residencies, 66
George Washington University School of Medicine and Health Sciences, 66
George Washington University, Physician Assistant Program, 198
Georgetown University School of Nursing and Health Sciences, 261
Georgetown University School of Nursing, Nurse Anesthesia Program, 231
Georgetown University, Graduate Program in Nurse-Midwifery, 261
Georgia Board of Chiropractic Examiners, 400
Georgia Board of Dentistry, 349
Georgia Board of Nursing, 440

Georgia chiropractic schools
    Life University, 187

Georgia Composite State Board of Medical Examiners, MD and DO, 296
Georgia Composite State Board of Medical Examiners, Physician assistant, 420

Georgia dental schools
    Medical College of Georgia School of Dentistry, 164

Georgia licensing agencies
    Georgia Board of Chiropractic Examiners, 400
    Georgia Board of Dentistry, 349
    Georgia Board of Nursing, 440
    Georgia Composite State Board of Medical Examiners, MD and DO, 296
    Georgia Composite State Board of Medical Examiners, Physician assistant, 420
    Georgia Psychology Board, 460
    Georgia State Board of Podiatry Examiners, 379

Georgia medical schools
    Emory University School of Medicine, 69
    Medical College of Georgia, 70
    Medical College of Georgia, Nursing Anesthesia Program, 70
    Mercer University School of Medicine, 71
    Morehouse School of Medicine, 71

Georgia nursing schools
    Emory University, Nell Hodgson Woodruff School of Nursing, 223
    Emory University, Nell Hodgson Woodruff School of Nursing, Nurse-Midwifery Program, 262

Georgia physician assistant programs

Emory University School of Medicine, Physician Assistant Program, 199
Medical College of Georgia, Physician Assistant Program, 199
Georgia Psychology Board, 460
Georgia residency programs
Medical College of Georgia, 70
Mercer University School of Medicine, 71
Morehouse School of Medicine, 72
Georgia State Board of Podiatry Examiners, 379
Gooding Institute of Nurse Anesthesia at Bay Medical Center, 232
Guam Board of Medical Examiners, MD and DO, 297
Guam licensing agencies
Guam Board of Medical Examiners, MD and DO, 297

H

Harlem Hospital, Anesthesia School for Nurses, 243
Harvard Medical School, 86
Harvard Medical School, residencies, 86
Harvard School of Dental Medicine, 167
Hawaii Board of Medical Examiners, MD and DO, 297
Hawaii Board of Nursing, 441
Hawaii Board of Psychology, 460
Hawaii Department of Commerce and Consumer Affairs Licensing Branch, Chiropractic, 400
Hawaii Department of Commerce and Consumer Affairs, Podiatry, 379
Hawaii licensing agencies
Department of Commerce and Consumer Affairs Licensing Branch, Chiropractic, 400
Department of Commerce and Consumer Affairs, Podiatry, 379
Hawaii Board of Medical Examiners, MD and DO, 297
Hawaii Board of Nursing, 441
Hawaii Board of Psychology, 460
Hawaii State Board of Dental Examiners, 349
Hawaii medical schools
University of Hawaii School of Medicine, 72
Hawaii State Board of Dental Examiners, 349
Head and neck surgery specialty associations
American Academy of Otolaryngology—Head and Neck Surgery, 562
American Head and Neck Society, 563
Healthcare Integrity and Protection Data Bank, 526
Hematology
American Society of Hematology, 563
Henry Ford Hospital, University of Detroit Mercy, Graduate Program of Nurse Anesthesia, 238
Hospice Care
American Academy of Hospice and Palliative Medicine, 563
Hospice and Palliative Nurses Association/National Board for Certification of Hospice and Palliative Nurses, 563
Hospital of Saint Raphael, School of Nurse Anesthesia, 230
Hospital-related organizations
Academy for Healthcare and Management, 564
American Academy of Hospice and Medicine, 564
American Academy of Medical Administrators, 564

Index

    American Baptist Homes and Hospitals Association, 564
    American College of Health Care Administrators, 564
    American College of Healthcare Executives, 564
    American Health Care Association, 564
    American Health Lawyers Association, 565
    American Hospital Association, 565
    American Medical Rehabilitation Providers Association, 565
    American Society of Law, Medicine and Ethics, 565
    Association of University Programs in Health Administration, 565
    Boston Medical Center, 565
    Federation of American Hospitals, 565
    Jacobi Medical Center, 566
    National Association of Psychiatric Health Systems, 566
    National Association of Public Hospitals, 566
    National Council and Association for Community Behavioral Health Care, 566
    National Rural Health Association, 566
    University of Chicago Hospitals, 566
    University of Wisconsin Hospital and Clinics, 567

Howard University College of Dentistry, 163
Howard University College of Medicine, 67
Howard University College of Medicine, residencies, 67
Howard University, Physician Assistant Program, 198
Human resources, role in credentialing and privileging, 30

I

Idaho Board of Nursing, 441
Idaho Bureau of Occupational Licenses, Chiropractic, 401
Idaho Bureau of Occupational Licensure, Podiatry, 380
Idaho licensing agencies
    Bureau of Occupational Licenses, Chiropractic, 401
    Bureau of Occupational Licensure, Podiatry, 380
    Idaho Board of Nursing, 441
    Idaho State Board of Dentistry, 350
    Idaho State Board of Medicine, MD and DO, 298
Idaho physician assistant programs
    Idaho State University, Physician Assistant Program, 200
Idaho State Board of Dentistry, 350
Idaho State Board of Medicine, MD and DO, 298
Idaho State University, Physician Assistant Program, 200
Illinois dental schools
    Southern Illinois University School of Dental Medicine, 164
    University of Illinois at Chicago College of Dentistry, 165
Illinois Department of Professional Regulation, MD and DO, 299
Illinois Department of Professional Regulation, Physician assistant, 420
Illinois Department of Professional Regulations, Nursing, 441
Illinois licensing agencies
    Illinois Department of Professional Regulation, MD and DO, 299
    Illinois Department of Professional Regulation, Physician assistant, 420

Index

Illinois Department of Professional Regulations, Nursing, 441
Licensure Maintenance Unit, Dental, 350

Illinois, Licensure Maintenance Unit, Dental, 350

Illinois medical schools
Finch University of the Health Sciences/Chicago Medical School, 72
Loyola University Chicago, Stritch School of Medicine, 73
Midwestern University, Chicago College of Osteopathic Medicine, 142
Northwestern University Medical School, 73
Pritzker School of Medicine at the University of Chicago, 74
Rush University, Rush Medical College, 75
Southern Illinois University School of Medicine, 75
University of Illinois at Chicago, 76
University of Illinois College of Medicine at Peoria, 76
University of Illinois College of Medicine at Rockford, 77
University of Illinois College of Medicine at Urbana, 78

Illinois nursing schools
Decatur Memorial Hospitals/Bradley University, Nurse Anesthesia Program, 232
Ravenswood Hospital Medical Center School of Anesthesia/DePaul University, Graduate Program in Nurse Anesthesia, 233
Rush University College of Nursing, Nurse Anesthesia Program, 233
Southern Illinois University Edwardsville, 224
Southern Illinois University—Edwardsville, School of Nursing, Nurse Anesthesia Specialization, 233

Illinois physician assistant programs
American Association of Medical Assistants, 200
Finch University of Health Sciences/Chicago Medical School, Physician Assistant Program, 200
Malcolm X College, Physician Assistant Program, 201
Midwestern University, 201
Southern Illinois University Physician Assistant Program, 201

Illinois podiatry schools
Dr. William M. Scholl College of Podiatric Medicine, 181

Illinois residency programs
Finch University of the Health Sciences/Chicago Medical School, 73
Loyola University Chicago, Stritch School of Medicine, 73
OSF Saint Francis Medical Center, 74
Rush Presbyterian St. Luke's Medical Center, 74
Southern Illinois University School of Medicine, 75
University of Illinois at Chicago College of Medicine, 76
University of Illinois College of Medicine at Peoria, 77
University of Illinois College of Medicine at Rockford, 77
University of Illinois College of Medicine at Urbana, 78

Indiana Board of Chiropractic Examiners, 402
Indiana Board of Podiatric Medicine, 380
Indiana chiropractic schools
Northwestern Health Sciences University, 188

Indiana dental schools
Indiana University School of Dentistry, 165

Indiana licensing agencies
Indiana Board of Chiropractic Examiners, 402
Indiana Board of Podiatric Medicine, 380

The 2003 Credentialing and Privileging Desk Reference

Index

    Indiana Medical Licensing Board, MD and DO, 300
    Indiana Medical Licensing Board, Physician assistant, 421
    Indiana State Board of Dental Examiners, 351
    Indiana State Nursing Board, 442
    Indiana State Psychology Board, 462

Indiana Medical Licensing Board, MD and DO, 300
Indiana Medical Licensing Board, Physician assistant, 421
Indiana medical schools
    Indiana University School of Medicine, 78
Indiana physician assistant programs
    University of Saint Francis (formerly Lutheran College of Health Professions Physician Assistant Program), 202
Indiana residency programs
    Indiana University School of Medicine, 79
Indiana State Board of Dental Examiners, 351
Indiana State Nursing Board, 442
Indiana State Psychology Board, 462
Indiana University School of Dentistry, 165
Institute of Midwifery, Women, and Health, 269
InterAmerican University of Puerto Rico, 249
Internal medicine specialty associations
    American College of Osteopathic Internists, 567
    American College of Physicians/American Society of Internal Medicine, 567
    Canadian Society of Internal Medicine, 567
    Society of General Internal Medicine, 567
International Standards Organization, 625
Interservice Physician Assistant Program, 205, 216
Iowa Board of Chiropractic Examiners, 402
Iowa Board of Dental Examiners, 351
Iowa Board of Medical Examiners, MD and DO, 301
Iowa Board of Nursing, 442
Iowa Board of Psychology Examiners, 462
Iowa chiropractic schools
    Palmer College of Chiropractic, 188
Iowa dental schools
    The University of Iowa, College of Dentistry, 165
Iowa licensing agencies
    Board of Chiropractic Examiners, 402
    Iowa Board of Dental Examiners, 351
    Iowa Board of Medical Examiners, MD and DO, 301
    Iowa Board of Nursing, 442
    Iowa Board of Psychology Examiners, 462
    Professional Licensure Division, Podiatry, 380
Iowa medical schools
    Des Moines University—Osteopathic Medical Center, 142
    University of Iowa College of Medicine, 79
Iowa nursing schools
    Department of Veterans Affairs/Drake University, Clinical Specialization in Nurse Anesthesia, 234
    University of Iowa College of Nursing, Anesthesia Nursing Program, 234

Iowa physician assistant programs
  Des Moines University—Osteopathic Medical Center, 202
  University of Iowa College of Medicine, Physician Assistant Program, 202
Iowa Professional Licensure Division, Podiatry, 380
Iowa residency programs, 79
University of Iowa Hospitals and Clinics, 79

J

Jackson Memorial Hospital, residencies, 68
Jacobi Medical Center, 566
Jefferson Medical College, 116
Johns Hopkins University School of Medicine, 84
Joint Commission on Accreditation of Healthcare Organizations, 625

K

Kaiser Permanente School of Anesthesia, 229
Kansas Board of Healing Arts, MD and DO, 301
Kansas Board of Healing Arts, Physician assistant, 421
Kansas Board of Healing Arts, Podiatry, 381
Kansas Dental Board, 352
Kansas State Board of Nursing, 442
Kansas nursing schools
  University Kansas Medical Center, Program of Nurse Anesthesia Education, 234
Kansas physician assistant programs
  Wichita State University, Physician Assistant Program, 203
Kansas residency programs
  University of Kansas Medical Center, 80
  University of Kansas School of Medicine at Wichita, 80
Kentucky Board of Chiropractic Examiners, 402
Kentucky Board of Dentistry, 353
Kentucky Board of Medical Licensure, MD and DO, 302
Kentucky Board of Medical Licensure, Physician assistant, 422
Kentucky Board of Nursing, 443
Kentucky Board of Podiatry, 381
Kentucky dental schools
  University of Kentucky College of Dentistry, 166
  University of Louisville School of Dentistry, 166
Kentucky licensing agencies
  Kentucky Board of Chiropractic Examiners, 402
  Kentucky Board of Dentistry, 353
  Kentucky Board of Medical Licensure, MD and DO, 302
  Kentucky Board of Medical Licensure, Physician assistant, 422
  Kentucky Board of Nursing, 443
  Kentucky Board of Podiatry, 381
  Kentucky State Board of Psychology, 463

Index

Kentucky medical schools
    Pikeville College, School of Osteopathic Medicine, 142
    University of Kentucky College of Medicine, 80
    University of Louisville School of Medicine, 81
Kentucky nursing schools
    Frontier School of Midwifery and Family Nursing, 263
    Trover Foundation/Murray State University Program of Anesthesia, 235
Kentucky physician assistant programs
    University of Kentucky, Physician Assistant Program, 203
Kentucky residency programs
    University of Kentucky College of Medicine, 81
    University of Louisville School of Medicine, 81
Kentucky State Board of Psychology, 463
Kettering College of Medical Arts, Physician Assistant Program, 212
King's College, Physician Assistant Program, 213
Kings County Hospital Center, School of Anesthesia for Nurses, 243

L

Lake Erie College of Osteopathic Medicine, 145
Laser medicine specialty associations
    American Society for Laser Medicine and Surgery, Inc., 568
Life Chiropractic College—West, 185
Life University, 187
Locum tenens, 7
Logan College of Chiropractic, 189
Loma Linda University Medical Center, residencies, 60
Loma Linda University School of Dentistry, 161
Louisiana dental schools
    Louisiana State University School of Dentistry, 166
Louisiana licensing agencies
    Louisiana State Board of Dentistry, 353
    Louisiana State Board of Examiners of Chiropractors, 403
    Louisiana State Board of Examiners of Psychologists, 463
    Louisiana State Board of Medical Examiners, MD and DO, 302
    Louisiana State Board of Medical Examiners, Physician assistant, 422
    Louisiana State Board of Medical Examiners, Podiatry, 381
    Louisiana State Board of Nursing, 443
Louisiana medical schools
    Louisiana State University at New Orleans School of Medicine, 82
    Louisiana State University at Shreveport School of Medicine, 82
    Tulane University School of Medicine, 83
Louisiana nursing schools
    Charity Hospital, School of Nurse Anesthesia, 235
Louisiana residency programs
    Louisiana State University at New Orleans School of Medicine, 82
    Tulane University School of Medicine, 83

Louisiana State Board of Dentistry, 353
Louisiana State Board of Examiners of Chiropractors, 403
Louisiana State Board of Examiners of Psychologists, 463
Louisiana State Board of Medical Examiners, MD and DO, 302
Louisiana State Board of Medical Examiners, Physician assistant, 422
Louisiana State Board of Medical Examiners, Podiatry, 381
Louisiana State Board of Nursing, 443
Louisiana State University at New Orleans School of Medicine, 82
Louisiana State University at New Orleans School of Medicine, residencies, 82
Louisiana State University at Shreveport School of Medicine, 82
Louisiana State University School of Dentistry, 166
Loyola University Chicago, Stritch School of Medicine, residencies, 73

M

Macquarie University Department of Chiropractic, 185
Maine Board of Chiropractic Licensure, 403
Maine Board of Dental Examiners, 354
Maine Board of Examiners of Psychologists, 463
Maine Board of Licensure in Medicine, MD, 303
Maine Board of Licensure in Medicine, Physician assistant, 422
Maine Board of Licensure of Podiatric Medicine, 382
Maine licensing agencies
    Board of Chiropractic Licensure, 403
    Board of Licensure of Podiatric Medicine, 382
    Maine Board of Dental Examiners, 354
    Maine Board of Examiners of Psychologists, 463
    Maine Board of Licensure in Medicine, MD, 303
    Maine Board of Licensure in Medicine, Physician assistant, 422
    Maine State Board of Nursing, 444
Maine medical schools
    University of New England, College of Osteopathic Medicine, 143
Maine nursing schools
    University of New England, School of Nurse Anesthesia, 235
Maine State Board of Nursing, 444
Malcolm X College, Physician Assistant Program, 201
Managed care
    Accreditation, 35
    Credentialing requirements, 36
    Credentialing, 37
    LIPs, 37
    MCO-owned hospitals, credentialing in, 41
    Physicians, 37
    Practitioner office audits, 42
    Unique challenges, 44
Managed Care specialty associations
    Academy for Healthcare and Management, 568
    American Association of Managed Care Nurses, 568
    American College of Managed Care Medicine, 568

Index

National Association of Managed Care Physicians, Inc., 568
Manitoba medical schools (Canada)
University of Manitoba Faculty of Medicine, 150
Manitoba residency programs (Canada)
University of Manitoba Faculty of Medicine, 151
Marquette University College of Nursing, Nurse-Midwifery Program, 273
Marquette University School of Dentistry, 177
Marquette University, 219
Marshall University, Joan C. Edwards School of Medicine, 135
Maryland Board of Chiropractic Examiners, 403
Maryland Board of Examiners of Psychologists, 464
Maryland Board of Nursing, 444
Maryland Board of Physician Quality Assurance, MD and DO, 304
Maryland Board of Podiatry, 382
Maryland dental schools
University of Maryland Dental School, 167
Maryland licensing agencies
Board of Chiropractic Examiners, 403
Maryland Board of Examiners of Psychologists, 464
Maryland Board of Nursing, 444
Maryland Board of Physician Quality Assurance, MD and DO, 304
Maryland Board of Podiatry, 382
Maryland State Board of Dental Examiners, 354
Maryland medical schools
Johns Hopkins University School of Medicine, 84
Naval School of Health Sciences, 84
Uniformed Services University of the Health Sciences School of Medicine, 84
University of Maryland Baltimore, 85
Maryland nursing schools
Durham Regional Hospital, School of Anesthesia for Nurses, 236
Maryland physician assistant programs
The Community College of Baltimore County, Physician Assistant Program, 204
Maryland residency programs
Uniformed Services University of the Health Sciences School of Medicine, 85
University of Maryland Medical Systems, 85
Maryland State Board of Dental Examiners, 354
Marshall University, Medicine, 135
Massachusetts Board of Podiatry, 382
Massachusetts Board of Registration in Dentistry, 355
Massachusetts Board of Registration in Medicine, MD and DO, 304
Massachusetts Board of Registration in Nursing, 444
Massachusetts Board of Registration of Chiropractors, 404
Massachusetts Board of Registration of Physician Assistants, 423
Massachusetts dental schools
Boston University School of Dental Medicine, 167
Harvard School of Dental Medicine, 167
Tufts University School of Dental Medicine, 168
Massachusetts Division of Professional Licensure, 464
Massachusetts licensing agencies

    Board of Registration of Chiropractors, 404
    Massachusetts Board of Podiatry, 382
    Massachusetts Board of Registration in Dentistry, 355
    Massachusetts Board of Registration in Medicine, MD and DO, 304
    Massachusetts Board of Registration in Nursing, 444
    Massachusetts Board of Registration of Physician Assistants, 423
    Massachusetts Division of Professional Licensure, 464

Massachusetts medical schools
    Boston University School of Medicine, 86
    Harvard Medical School, 86
    Tufts University School of Medicine, 86
    University of Massachusetts Medical School, 87

Massachusetts nursing schools
    Baystate Medical Center, Nurse-Midwifery Education Program, 263
    Berkshire Medical Center, School of Anesthesia, 237
    Boston University School of Public Health, Nurse-Midwifery Education Program, 263
    Northeastern University Graduate School of Nursing, Nurse Anesthesia Program, 237

Massachusetts physician assistant programs
    Northeastern University, Physician Assistant Program, 204

Massachusetts residency programs
    Harvard Medical School, 86
    University of Massachusetts Medical School, 87

Maxillofacial surgery specialty associations
    American Association of Oral and Maxillofacial Surgeons, 568
    American Cleft Palate—Craniofacial Association, 569

Mayo Graduate School of Medicine, residencies, 91
Mayo Medical School, 91
Mayo School of Health-Related Sciences, Nurse Anesthesia Program, 239
McGill University Faculty of Medicine, 156
McMaster University School of Medicine, 152
MCO-owned hospitals, credentialing in, 35
MCP Hahnemann University School of Medicine, residencies, 117
MCP Hahnemann University, 117
MCP Hahnemann University, Physician Assistant Program, 214
Medical College of Georgia School of Dentistry, 164
Medical College of Georgia, 70
Medical College of Georgia, Physician Assistant Program, 199
Medical College of Georgia, residencies, 70
Medical College of Ohio at Toledo, residencies, 111
Medical College of Ohio, 111
Medical College of Virginia Hospitals, residencies, 133
Medical College of Wisconsin, 136
Medical College of Wisconsin, residencies, 136
Medical executive committee, role in credentialing and privileging, 30
Medical staff services professional, role in credentialing and privileging, 30
Medical staff, role in credentialing and privileging, 30
Medical University of South Carolina College of Dental Medicine, 174
Medical University of South Carolina College of Medicine, 122
Medical University of South Carolina College of Medicine, residencies, 123

Index

Medical University of South Carolina, Anesthesia for Nurses Program, 251
Medical University of South Carolina, Nurse-Midwifery Program, 270
Meharry Medical College School of Dentistry, 175
Meharry Medical College School of Medicine, residencies, 125
Meharry Medical College, 125
Memorial Hospital of Rhode Island, School of Nurse Anesthesia, 250
Memorial University of Newfoundland Faculty of Medicine, 151
Mercer University School of Medicine, 71
Mercer University School of Medicine, residencies, 71
Michigan Board of Nursing, 445
Michigan Bureau of Occupational and Professional Regulation, Dental, 356
Michigan Bureau of Occupational and Professional Regulation, Podiatry, 383
Michigan dental schools
    University of Detroit Mercy School of Dentistry, 168
    University of Michigan School of Dentistry, 168
Michigan Department of Consumer and Industry Services, Chiropractic, 404
Michigan Department of Consumer and Industry Services, Physician assistant, 423
Michigan licensing agencies
    Bureau of Occupational and Professional Regulation, Podiatry, 383
    Department of Consumer and Industry Services, Chiropractic, 404
    Department of Consumer and Industry Services, MD and DO, 305
    Michigan Board of Nursing, 445
    Michigan Bureau of Occupational and Professional Regulation, Dental, 356
    Michigan Department of Consumer and Industry Services, Physician assistant, 423
Michigan medical schools
    Michigan State University College of Human Medicine, 88
    Michigan State University, College of Osteopathic Medicine, 143
    University of Michigan Medical School, 90
    Wayne State University School of Medicine, 90
Michigan nursing schools
    Henry Ford Hospital, University of Detroit Mercy, Graduate Program of Nurse Anesthesia, 238
    Oakland University/William Beaumont Hospital, Education Program in Nurse Anesthesia, 238
    St. Joseph Mercy/University of Detroit Mercy, Graduate Program of Nurse Anesthesiology, 238
    University of Michigan School of Nursing, Nurse-Midwifery Program, 264
    University of Michigan—Flint/Hurley Medical Center, Anesthesia Program, 239
    Wayne State University College of Pharmacy and Allied Health Professions/Detroit Receiving Hospital, Department of Nurse Anesthesia, 239
Michigan physician assistant programs
    University of Detroit Mercy, Physician Assistant Program, 204
    Western Michigan University, Physician Assistant Program, 205
Michigan residency programs
    Michigan State University College of Human Medicine, 88
    University of Michigan Health Systems, 90
    Wayne State University School of Medicine, 90
Michigan State University College of Human Medicine, 88
Michigan State University College of Human Medicine, residencies, 88
Michigan State University, 88
Middle Tennessee School of Anesthesia, nursing, 253
Midwestern University, 201
Midwestern University, Chicago College of Osteopathic Medicine, 142

Index

Minneapolis School of Anesthesia, 240
Minneapolis VA School of Anesthesia, 240
Minnesota Board of Chiropractic Examiners, 405
Minnesota Board of Dentistry, 356
Minnesota Board of Medical Practice, MD and DO, 306
Minnesota Board of Medical Practice, Physician assistant, 423
Minnesota Board of Nursing, 445
Minnesota Board of Podiatric Medicine, 383
Minnesota Board of Psychology, 465
Minnesota dental schools
    University of Minnesota Dental School, 169
Minnesota licensing agencies
    Minnesota Board of Chiropractic Examiners, 405
    Minnesota Board of Dentistry, 356
    Minnesota Board of Medical Practice, MD and DO, 306
    Minnesota Board of Medical Practice, Physician assistant, 423
    Minnesota Board of Nursing, 445
    Minnesota Board of Podiatric Medicine, 383
    Minnesota Board of Psychology, 465
Minnesota medical schools
    Mayo Medical School, 91
    University of Minnesota at Duluth School of Medicine, 92
    University of Minnesota at Minneapolis Medical School, 92
Minnesota nursing schools
    Mayo School of Health-Related Sciences, Nurse Anesthesia Program, 239
    Minneapolis School of Anesthesia, 240
    Minneapolis VA School of Anesthesia, 240
    St. Mary's University Graduate Program in Nurse Anesthesia, 240
    University of Minnesota School of Nursing, Nurse-Midwifery Program, 264
Minnesota residency programs
    Mayo Graduate School of Medicine, 91
    University of Minnesota Medical School, 92
Mississippi Board of Nursing, 445
Mississippi Board of Psychology, 465
Mississippi dental schools
    University of Mississippi School of Dentistry, 169
Mississippi licensing agencies
    Mississippi Board of Nursing, 445
    Mississippi Board of Psychology, 465
    Mississippi State Board of Dental Examiners, 357
    Mississippi State Board of Medical Licensure, MD and DO, 306
    Mississippi State Board of Medical Licensure, Podiatry, 384
Mississippi medical schools
    University of Mississippi Medical Center School of Medicine, 93
Mississippi nursing schools
    University of Southern Mississippi College of Nursing, 224
Mississippi State Board of Dental Examiners, 357
Mississippi State Board of Medical Licensure, MD and DO, 306
Mississippi State Board of Medical Licensure, Podiatry, 384

Index

Missouri chiropractic schools
    Cleveland Chiropractic College, 188
    Logan College of Chiropractic, 189

Missouri dental schools
    University of Missouri—Kansas City School of Dentistry, 169

Missouri Department of Health, 307

Missouri licensing agencies
    Missouri Dental Board, 357
    Missouri Department of Health, 307
    Missouri State Board of Nursing, 446
    Missouri State Board of Registration of Healing Arts, Physician assistant, 424
    Missouri State Board of Registration of the Healing Arts, MD and DO, 307
    Missouri State Committee of Psychologists, 465
    State Board of Chiropractic Examiners, 405

Missouri medical schools
    St. Louis University School of Medicine, 94
    The University of Health Sciences, College of Osteopathic Medicine, 143
    University of Missouri at Columbia School of Medicine, 94
    University of Missouri at Kansas City School of Medicine, 95
    Washington University School of Medicine, 96

Missouri nursing schools
    Southwest Missouri School of Anesthesia, 241
    Truman Medical Center, School of Nurse Anesthesia, 241

Missouri physician assistant programs
    St. Louis University, Physician Assistant Program, 205

Missouri residency programs
    Barnes Jewish Hospital, 94
    University of Missouri at Kansas City School of Medicine, 95
    University of Missouri—Columbia School of Medicine, 95

Missouri State Board of Chiropractic Examiners, 405
Missouri State Board of Nursing, 446
Missouri State Board of Registration of Healing Arts, Physician assistant, 424
Missouri State Board of Registration of the Healing Arts, MD and DO, 307
Missouri State Committee of Psychologists, 465
Montana Board of Chiropractors, 405
Montana Board of Dentistry, 358
Montana Board of Medical Examiners, MD and DO, 308
Montana Board of Medical Examiners, Physician assistant, 424
Montana Board of Medical Examiners, Podiatry, 384
Montana Board of Psychologists, 466

Montana licensing agencies
    Board of Chiropractors, 405
    Montana Board of Dentistry, 358
    Montana Board of Medical Examiners, MD and DO, 308
    Montana Board of Medical Examiners, Physician assistant, 424
    Montana Board of Medical Examiners, Podiatry, 384
    Montana Board of Psychologists, 466
    Montana State Board of Nursing, 446

Montana State Board of Nursing, 446
Morehouse School of Medicine, 71
Morehouse School of Medicine, residencies, 72
Mount Marty College, Graduate Program in Nurse Anesthesia, 252
Mount Sinai Hospital, 103
Mount Sinai Hospital, residencies, 102

N

National Association for Healthcare Quality, 618
National Association of Medical Staff Services, 617
National Board for Certification of Orthopedic Technicians, 515
National Commission on Certification of Physician Assistants (NCCPA), 514
National Committee for Quality Assurance, 625
National Practitioner Data Bank (NPDB), 519
National Register of Health Service Providers in Psychology, 629
Naval School of Health Sciences, Physician Assistant Program, 203
Nebraska dental schools
    Creighton University School of Dentistry, 170
Nebraska Department of Health and Human Services, Dental, 358
Nebraska Department of Health and Human Services, MD and DO, 308
Nebraska Department of Health and Human Services, Physician assistant, 425
Nebraska Department of Health and Human Services, Podiatry, 384
Nebraska Department of Regulation and Licensure, Nursing, 446
Nebraska Department of Regulation and Licensure—Credentials, Psychologist, 466
Nebraska licensing agencies
    Nebraska Department of Health and Human Services, Dental, 358
    Nebraska Department of Health and Human Services, MD and DO, 308
    Nebraska Department of Health and Human Services, Physician assistant, 425
    Nebraska Department of Health and Human Services, Podiatry, 384
    Nebraska Department of Regulation and Licensure, Nursing, 446
    Nebraska Department of Regulation and Licensure—Credentials, Psychologist, 466
    Regulations and Licensure Credentials Division, Chiropractic, 406
Nebraska medical schools
    Creighton University School of Medicine, 96
    University of Nebraska Medical Center, 97
Nebraska nursing schools
    Bryan LGH Medical Center, University of Kansas, School of Nurse Anesthesia, 241
Nebraska physician assistant programs
    University of Nebraska Medical Center, Physician Assistant Program, 205
Nebraska Regulations and Licensure Credentials Division, Chiropractic, 406
Nebraska residency programs
    Creighton University School of Medicine, 96
    University of Nebraska College of Medicine, 97
Nephrology specialty associations
    Renal Physicians Association, 569
Neurological surgery specialty associations
    American Association of Neurological Surgeons, 569

Index

The Society of Neurological Surgeons University of Michigan Hospital, 569
UCLA Medical Center Division of Neurosurgery, 569

Neurology specialty associations
American Academy of Neurology, 570
American Association of Neuroscience Nurses, 570
American College of Neuropsychiatrists, 570
American Society of Electroneurodiagnostic Technologists, Inc., 570
American Society of Pediatric Neuroradiology, 570

Nevada licensing agencies
Nevada State Board of Dental Examiners, 359
Nevada State Board of Medical Examiners, MD, 309
Nevada State Board of Medical Examiners, Physician assistant, 425
Nevada State Board of Nursing, 447
Nevada State Board of Osteopathic Medicine, DO, 310
Nevada State Board of Podiatry, 385
Nevada, State of, Board of Psychological Examiners, 467

Nevada medical schools
University of Nevada School of Medicine, 97

Nevada residency programs
University of Nevada School of Medicine, 95

Nevada State Board of Dental Examiners, 359
Nevada State Board of Medical Examiners, MD, 309
Nevada State Board of Medical Examiners, Physician assistant, 425
Nevada State Board of Nursing, 447
Nevada State Board of Osteopathic Medicine, DO, 310
Nevada State Board of Podiatry, 385
Nevada, State of, Board of Psychological Examiners, 467
New Britain School of Nurse Anesthesia, 231
New Hampshire Board of Chiropractic Examiners, 406
New Hampshire Board of Dental Examiners, 360
New Hampshire Board of Medicine, MD and DO, 310
New Hampshire Board of Medicine, Physician assistant, 425
New Hampshire Board of Medicine, Podiatry, 385
New Hampshire Board of Mental Practice, 467
New Hampshire Board of Nursing, 447

New Hampshire licensing agencies
New Hampshire Board of Chiropractic Examiners, 406
New Hampshire Board of Dental Examiners, 360
New Hampshire Board of Medicine, MD and DO, 310
New Hampshire Board of Medicine, Physician assistant, 425
New Hampshire Board of Medicine, Podiatry, 385
New Hampshire Board of Mental Practice, 467
New Hampshire Board of Nursing, 447

New Hampshire medical schools
Dartmouth Medical School, 98

Newfoundland medical schools (Canada)
Memorial University of Newfoundland Faculty of Medicine, 151

Newfoundland residency programs (Canada)
Memorial University of Newfoundland Faculty of Medicine, 151

New Jersey Board of Nursing, 447
New Jersey dental schools
> University of Medicine and Dentistry of New Jersey, New Jersey Dental School, 170

New Jersey licensing agencies
> New Jersey Board of Nursing, 447
> New Jersey State Board of Dentistry, 360
> New Jersey State Board of Medical Examiners, Podiatry, 385
> New Jersey State Board of Psychological Examiners, 467
> New Jersey State Medical Board, MD and DO, 311
> New Jersey State Medical Board, Physician assistant, 426
> State Board of Chiropractic Examiners, 407

New Jersey medical schools
> New Jersey Medical School at the University of Medicine and Dentistry of New Jersey, 99
> Robert Wood Johnson Medical School at the University of Medicine and Dentistry of New Jersey at Piscataway, 100
> University of Medicine and Dentistry of New Jersey, School of Osteopathic Medicine, 144

New Jersey nursing schools
> University of Medicine and Dentistry of New Jersey—Newark School of Health-Related Professions, Nurse-Midwifery Program, 265

New Jersey Medical School at the University of Medicine and Dentistry of New Jersey at Newark, residencies, 99
New Jersey Medical School at the University of Medicine and Dentistry of New Jersey, 99
New Jersey physician assistant programs
> Rutgers University/University of Medicine and Dentistry of New Jersey at Piscataway Physician Assistant Program, 206

New Jersey residency programs
> New Jersey Medical School at the University of Medicine and Dentistry of New Jersey at Newark, 99
> Robert Wood Johnson Medical School at the University of Medicine and Dentistry of New Jersey at Piscataway, 100

New Jersey State Board of Chiropractic Examiners, 407
New Jersey State Board of Dentistry, 360
New Jersey State Board of Medical Examiners, Podiatry, 385
New Jersey State Board of Psychological Examiners, 467
New Jersey State Medical Board, MD and DO, 311
New Jersey State Medical Board, Physician assistant, 426
New Mexico Board of Chiropractic Examiners, 407
New Mexico Board of Dental Health Care, 361
New Mexico Board of Medical Examiners, MD, 312
New Mexico Board of Nursing, 448
New Mexico Board of Osteopathic Medical Examiners, DO, 312
New Mexico Board of Podiatry, 386
New Mexico Board of Psychologist Examiners, 468
New Mexico licensing agencies
> New Mexico Board of Chiropractic Examiners, 407
> New Mexico Board of Dental Health Care, 361
> New Mexico Board of Medical Examiners, MD, 312
> New Mexico Board of Nursing, 448
> New Mexico Board of Osteopathic Medical Examiners, DO, 312

Index

New Mexico Board of Podiatry, 386
New Mexico Board of Psychologist Examiners, 468

New Mexico medical schools
University of New Mexico Health Sciences Center School of Medicine, 100

New Mexico nursing schools
University of New Mexico College of Nursing, Nurse-Midwifery Program, 265

New Mexico physician assistant programs
The University of New Mexico School of Medicine, Physician Assistant Program, 207

New Mexico residency program
University of New Mexico Medical School, 100

New York Chiropractic College, 189

New York chiropractic schools
New York Chiropractic College, 189

New York College of Osteopathic Medicine of the New York Institute of Technology, 144

New York dental schools
Columbia University School of Dental and Oral Surgery, 171
New York University College of Dentistry, 171
State University of New York at Buffalo School of Dental Medicine, 171

New York licensing agencies
New York Office of the Professions, Physician assistant, 426
New York Office of the Professions—Psychology Licensing, 468
Office of Professions, Medical Licensing, MD and DO, 313
Office of the Professions, Chiropractic Licensing Agency, 407
Office of the Professions, Dental Licensing, 362
Office of the Professions, Podiatric Licensing Agency, 386

New York Medical College, 103

New York medical schools
Albany Medical College, 101
Albert Einstein College of Medicine of Yeshiva University, 101
Columbia University College of Physicians and Surgeons, 102
Mount Sinai Hospital, 103
New York College of Osteopathic Medicine of the New York Institute of Technology, 144
New York Medical College, 103
New York University School of Medicine, 104
State University of New York at Buffalo School of Medicine, 104
State University of New York at Stony Brook School of Medicine, 106
State University of New York Downstate Medical Center, 105
State University of New York Upstate Medical University, 106
University of Rochester School of Medicine and Dentistry, 107
Weill Medical College of Cornell University, 107

New York nursing schools
Albany Medical College, Nurse Anesthesiology Program, 242
Columbia University School of Nursing, Program in Nurse Anesthesia, 242
Columbia University, Graduate Program in Nurse-Midwifery, 265
Harlem Hospital, Anesthesia School for Nurses, 243
King's County Hospital Center, School of Anesthesia for Nurses, 243
New York University, Nurse-Midwifery Education Program, 266
North Central Bronx Hospital, Nurse-Midwifery Precertification Program, 266
State University of New York at Stony Brook School of Nursing, Pathways to Midwifery Program, 266

Index

State University of New York Downstate Medical Center Midwifery Education program, 267
State University of New York Downstate Medical Center, 243
University at Buffalo School of Nursing, Advanced Certificate, 224
University at Buffalo School of Nursing, Nurse Anesthesia Program, 244
University of Rochester School of Nursing, nurse-midwifery, 267

New York Office of the Professions, Chiropractic Licensing Agency, 407
New York Office of the Professions, Dental Licensing, 362
New York Office of Professions, Medical Licensing, MD and DO, 313
New York Office of the Professions, Physician assistant, 426
New York Office of the Professions, Podiatric Licensing Agency, 386
New York Office of the Professions—Psychology Licensing, 468
New York physician assistant programs

Albany Hudson Valley, Physician Assistant Program, 207
CUNY/Harlem Hospital Center, Physician Assistant Program, 208
D'Youville College, Physician Assistant Program, 208
Physician Assistant Program, Sisters of Charity Medical Center, 209
Rochester Institute of Technology, Physician Assistant Program, 208
State University of New York at Stony Brook, School of Health Technology & Management,
   Physician Assistant Program, 209
SUNY—Health Science Center at Brooklyn (Downstate), Physician Assistant Program, 209
The Brooklyn Hospital Center/Long Island University, Physician Assistant Program, 210
Touro College, Physician Assistant Program, 210
Weill Cornell Medical College, Physician Assistant Program, 210

New York Presbyterian Hospital, Columbia Presbyterian Campus, residencies, 104
New York Presbyterian Hospital, residencies, 103
New York residency programs

Albany Medical College, 101
King's County Hospital, State University of New York at Brooklyn College of Medicine, 102
Mount Sinai Hospital, 102
New York Presbyterian Hospital, 103
New York Presbyterian Hospital, Columbia Presbyterian Campus, 104
New York University School of Medicine, 104
State University of New York at Buffalo School of Medicine, 105
State University of New York at Syracuse College of Medicine, 105
University Hospital, State University of New York at Stony Brook, 106
University of Rochester Strong Memorial Hospital, 107
Westchester Medical Center, 108

New York University College of Dentistry, 171
New York University School of Medicine, 104
New York University School of Medicine, residencies, 104
New York University, Nurse-Midwifery Education Program, 266
North Carolina Board of Chiropractic, 408
North Carolina Board of Medical Examiners, MD and DO, 313
North Carolina Board of Medical Examiners, Physician assistant, 427
North Carolina Board of Nursing, 448
North Carolina Board of Podiatry Examiners, 386
North Carolina dental schools

University of North Carolina School of Dentistry, 172

North Carolina licensing agencies

Index

North Carolina Board of Chiropractic, 408
North Carolina Board of Medical Examiners, MD and DO, 313
North Carolina Board of Medical Examiners, Physician assistant, 427
North Carolina Board of Nursing, 448
North Carolina Board of Podiatry Examiners, 386
North Carolina Psychology Board, 468
North Carolina State Board of Dental Examiners, 362

North Carolina medical schools
Duke University School of Medicine, 108
The Brody School of Medicine at East Carolina University, 109
University of North Carolina at Chapel Hill School of Medicine, 109
Wake Forest University School of Medicine, 110

North Carolina nursing schools
Carolinas Healthcare System/UNC—Charlotte, Nurse Anesthesia Program, 244
Durham Regional Hospital, Watts School of Nursing, 244
East Carolina University School of Nursing, Nurse-Midwifery Program, 267

North Carolina physician assistant programs
Duke University Medical Center, Physician Assistant Program, 211
Wake Forest University School of Medicine, Physician Assistant Program, 211

North Carolina Psychology Board, 468

North Carolina residency programs
Duke University Medical School of Medicine, 108
East Carolina University School of Medicine, 108
University of North Carolina at Chapel Hill School of Medicine, 110

North Carolina State Board of Dental Examiners, 362
North Central Bronx Hospital, Nurse-Midwifery Precertification Program, 266
North Dakota Board of Dentistry, 363
North Dakota Board of Nursing, 449
North Dakota Board of Podiatric Medicine, 387
North Dakota licensing agencies
North Dakota Board of Dentistry, 363
North Dakota Board of Nursing, 449
North Dakota Board of Podiatric Medicine, 387
North Dakota Medical Association, 314
North Dakota State Board of Medical Examiners, MD and DO, 314
North Dakota State Board of Medical Examiners, Physician assistant, 427
North Dakota State Board of Psychologist Examiners, 469

North Dakota medical schools
University of North Dakota School of Medicine and Health Sciences, 110

North Dakota nursing schools
University of North Dakota, Anesthesia Nursing Specialization, 245

North Dakota physician assistant programs
University of North Dakota School of Medicine, Physician Assistant Program, 211

North Dakota State Board of Medical Examiners, MD and DO, 314
North Dakota State Board of Medical Examiners, Physician assistant, 427
North Dakota State Board of Psychologist Examiners, 469
Northeastern Ohio Universities College of Medicine, residencies, 112
Northeastern Ohio Universities College of Medicine, 112
Northeastern University Graduate School of Nursing, Nurse Anesthesia Program, 237

Northeastern University, Physician Assistant Program, 204
Northwestern Health Sciences University, 188
Nova Scotia medical schools (Canada)
    Dalhousie University Faculty of Medicine, 152
Nova Scotia residency programs (Canada)
    Dalhousie University Faculty of Medicine, 152
Nova Southeastern University, College of Osteopathic Medicine, 141
Nova Southeastern University, Physician Assistant Program, 198
Nuclear Medicine specialty associations
    Canadian Association of Nuclear Medicine, 570
    Society of Nuclear Medicine, 570
    Washington Hospital School of Radiography, 571
Nursing Boards, 511
    ACNM Certification Council, Inc. (ACC), 511
    American Association of Nurse Anesthetists (AANA), 511
    American Nurses Credentialing Center (ANCC), 512
Nursing specialty associations
    Air & Surface Transport Nurses Association (formerly National Flight Nurses Association), 571
    American Academy of Ambulatory Care Nursing, 571
    American Academy of Nurse Practitioners, 571
    American Academy of Nursing, 571
    American Association of Colleges of Nursing, 571
    American Association of Critical Care Nurses, Certification Corporation, 572
    American Association of Legal Nurse Consultants, 572
    American Association of Managed Care Nurses, 572
    American Association of Neuroscience Nurses, 572
    American Association of Nurse Anesthetists, 572
    American Association of Nurse Attorneys, 572
    American Association of Occupational Health Nurses, 572
    American Association of Spinal Cord Injury Nurses, 573
    American College of Nurse-Midwives, 573
    American Holistic Nurses' Association, 573
    American Nephrology Nurses' Association, 573
    American Nurses Credentialing Center, 573
    American Nurses Foundation, 573
    American Organization of Nurse Executives, 574
    Association of Operating Room Nurses, Inc., 574
    Association of Pediatric Oncology Nurses, 574
    Association of Peri Operative Registered Nurses, Inc., 574
    Association of Rehabilitation Nurses, 574
    Baromedical Nurses Association, 574
    Canadian Nurses Association, 575
    Emergency Nurses Association, 575
    Hospice and Palliative Nurses Association/National Board for Certification of Hospice and Palliative Nurses, 576
    Infusion Nurses Society, Inc., 577
    National Association for Practical Nurse Education and Service, 577
    National Association of Hispanic Nurses, 578
    National Association of Pediatric Nurse Practitioners, 578
    National Association of Physician Nurses, 578

Index

National Association of Registered Nurses, 578
National Black Nurses Association, 578
National Federation of Licensed Practical Nurses, 578
National League for Nursing, 578
National Student Nurses' Association, Inc., 578
Oncology Nursing Certification Corporation, 578
Society of Otorhinolaryngology and Head-Neck Nurses, 579
The Association of Women's Health, Obstetric, and Neonatal Nurses, 579

O

Oakland University/William Beaumont Hospital, Education Program in Nurse Anesthesia, 238
Obstetrics and gynecology specialty associations
American College of Nurse-Midwives, 583
American College of Obstetricians and Gynecologists, 583
American College of Osteopathic Obstetricians and Gynecologists, 583
Association of Reproductive Health Professionals, 583
International Childbirth Education Association, Inc., 583
National Perinatal Association, 583
Society of Obstetricians and Gynecologists of Canada, 584
The Association of Women's Health, Obstetric, and Neonatal Nurses, 584
Occupational medicine specialty associations
American Association of Occupational Health Nurses, Inc., 584
American Osteopathic College of Occupational and Preventive Medicine, 584
Occupational and Environmental Medical Association of Canada, 584
Occupational therapy specialty associations
American Occupational Therapy Association, Inc., 584
Ohio Board of Nursing, 449
Ohio College of Podiatric Medicine, 182
Ohio dental schools
Case Western Reserve University School of Dentistry, 172
Ohio State University College of Dentistry, 172
Ohio licensing agencies
Ohio Board of Nursing, 449
Ohio State Board of Psychology, 469
Ohio State Chiropractic Board, 386
Ohio State Dental Board, 363
Ohio State Medical Board, MD and DO, 315
Ohio State Medical Board, Physician assistant, 427
State Medical Board of Ohio, Podiatry, 387
Ohio medical schools
Case Western Reserve University School of Medicine, 111
Medical College of Ohio, 111
Northeastern Ohio Universities College of Medicine, 112
Ohio State University College of Medicine, 112
Ohio University, College of Osteopathic Medicine, 144
University of Cincinnati College of Medicine, 114
Wright State University School of Medicine, 114
Ohio nursing schools
Case Western Reserve University, Frances Payne Bolton School of Nursing, Nurse-Midwifery Program, 268

Index

Case Western Reserve University/Mt. Sinai Medical Center/Cleveland Clinic Foundation, Frances Payne Bolton School of Nursing—School of Nurse Anesthesia, 245
Ohio State University College of Nursing, Nurse-Midwifery Education Program, 268
St. Elizabeth Health Center School for Nurse Anesthetists, Inc., 245
The University of Akron College of Nursing, Anesthesia Track, 246
University of Cincinnati Nurse Midwifery Education Program, 268
University of Cincinnati, Nurse Anesthesia, 246

Ohio physician assistant programs
Cuyahoga Community College, Physician/Surgical Physician Assistant Program, 212
Kettering College of Medical Arts, Physician Assistant Program, 212

Ohio podiatry schools
Ohio College of Podiatric Medicine, 182

Ohio residency programs
Medical College of Ohio at Toledo, 111
Ohio State University Medical Center, 113
University Hospital/University of Cincinnati College of Medicine, 113
Wright State University School of Medicine, 114

Ohio State Board of Psychology, 469
Ohio State Dental Board, 363
Ohio State Medical Board, MD and DO, 315
Ohio State Medical Board, Podiatry, 387
Ohio State University College of Dentistry, 172
Ohio State University College of Medicine, 112
Ohio State University College of Nursing, Nurse-Midwifery Education Program, 268
Ohio State University Medical Center, residencies, 111
Ohio University, College of Osteopathic Medicine, 144
Oklahoma Board of Dentistry, 364
Oklahoma Board of Nursing, 449

Oklahoma dental schools
University of Oklahoma Health Sciences Center College of Dentistry, 173

Oklahoma licensing agencies
Board of Dentistry, 364
Oklahoma Board of Nursing, 449
Oklahoma State Board of Examiners of Psychologists, 469
Oklahoma State Board of Medical Licensure and Supervision, MD, 316
Oklahoma State Board of Osteopathic Examiners, DO, 316
Oklahoma State Board of Podiatry, 387

Oklahoma medical schools
Oklahoma State University, Center of Health Sciences, 145
University of Oklahoma at Tulsa College of Medicine, 115

Oklahoma physician assistant programs
University of Oklahoma at Oklahoma City, Physician Assistant Program, 212

Oklahoma residency program
University of Oklahoma Health Sciences Center at Oklahoma City, 115

Oklahoma State Board of Examiners of Psychologists, 469
Oklahoma State Board of Medical Licensure and Supervision, MD, 316
Oklahoma State Board of Osteopathic Examiners, DO, 316
Oklahoma State Board of Podiatry, 387
Oklahoma State University, Center of Health Sciences, 145

Index

Old Dominion University School of Nursing, Nurse Anesthesia Program, 255
Oncology specialty associations
- American College of Mohs Micrographic Surgery and Cutaneous Oncology, 585
- American Society for Therapeutic Radiology and Oncology, 585
- American Society of Clinical Oncology, 585
- Oncology Nursing Certification Corporation, 585

Ontario medical schools (Canada)
- McMaster University School of Medicine, 152
- Queen's University Faculty of Health Sciences, 153
- University of Ottawa Faculty of Medicine, 153
- University of Toronto Faculty of Medicine, 154
- University of Western Ontario Faculty of Medicine and Dentistry, 155

Ontario residency programs (Canada)
- McMaster University School of Medicine, 153
- University of Ottawa Faculty of Medicine, 154
- University of Toronto Faculty of Medicine, 154
- University of Western Ontario Faculty of Medicine and Dentistry, 155

Ophthalmology specialty associations
- American Academy of Ophthalmology, 585
- American Association for Pediatric Ophthalmology and Strabismus, 585
- American Ophthalmologic Society, 586
- American Osteopathic Colleges of Ophthalmology and Otolaryngology-Head and Neck Surgery, 586
- American Society of Cataract and Refractive Surgery, 586
- American Society of Contemporary Ophthalmology, 586
- Association for Research in Vision and Ophthalmology, 586
- Canadian Ophthalmological Society, 586
- International Association of Ocular Surgeons, 586

Optometry specialty associations
- American Academy of Optometry, 586
- American Optometric Foundation, 586

Oral Surgery specialty associations
- American Cleft Palate-Craniofacial Association, 586

Oregon Board of Chiropractic Examiners, 408
Oregon Board of Dentistry, 364
Oregon Board of Psychologist Examiners, 470
Oregon chiropractic schools
- Western States Chiropractic College, 189

Oregon dental schools
- Oregon Health Science University School of Dentistry, 173

Oregon Health Sciences University School of Medicine, 116
Oregon Health Sciences University School of Medicine, residencies, 116
Oregon licensing agencies
- Oregon Board of Chiropractic Examiners, 408
- Oregon Board of Dentistry, 364
- Oregon Board of Psychologist Examiners, 470
- Oregon State Board of Medical Examiners, MD and DO, 317
- Oregon State Board of Medical Examiners, Physician assistant, 428
- Oregon State Board of Medical Examiners, Podiatry, 388

Index

Oregon State Board of Nursing, 450
Oregon medical schools
Oregon Health Sciences University School of Medicine, 116
Oregon nursing schools
Oregon Health Sciences University School of Nursing, Nurse-Midwifery Program, 269
Oregon residency program
Oregon Health Sciences University School of Medicine, 116
Oregon State Board of Medical Examiners, MD and DO, 317
Oregon State Board of Medical Examiners, Physician assistant, 428
Oregon State Board of Medical Examiners, Podiatry, 388
Oregon State Board of Nursing, 450
Orthopedic surgery specialty associations
American Academy of Orthopedic Surgeons, 587
American Association of Hip and Knee Surgeons, 587
American Osteopathic Academy of Orthopedics, 587
American Society for Surgery of the Hand, 588
Canadian Academy of Sport Medicine, 588
Canadian Orthopaedic Association, 588
Eastern Orthopaedic Association, Inc., 588
The American Orthopaedic Association, Inc., 588
Western Orthopaedic Association, 588
OSF Saint Francis Medical Center, residencies, 74
Osteopathic medicine specialty associations
American Academy of Osteopathy, 589
American Association of Colleges of Osteopathic Medicine, 589
American College of Osteopathic Emergency Physicians, 589
American College of Osteopathic Internists, 589
American College of Osteopathic Obstetricians and Gynecologists, 589
American College of Osteopathic Surgeons, 589
American Osteopathic Academy of Addiction Medicine, 589
American Osteopathic Academy of Osteopathic Pain Management and Sclerotherapy, Inc., 589
American Osteopathic Academy of Sports Medicine, 590
American Osteopathic Association, 590
American Osteopathic College of Allergy and Immunology, 590
American Osteopathic College of Dermatology, 590
American Osteopathic College of Occupational and Preventive Medicine, 590
American Osteopathic College of Pathologists, 590
American Osteopathic College of Radiology, 590
American Osteopathic College of Rehabilitation Medicine, 591
American Osteopathic College of Rheumatology, Inc., 591
American Society of Bariatric Physicians, 591
Canadian Osteopathic Association, 591
Community Hospital Medical Education Alliance, 591
Otolaryngology specialty associations
American Academy of Otolaryngic Allergy, 592
American Academy of Otolaryngology—Head and Neck Surgery, Inc., 592
American Bronchoesophagological Association, 592
American Laryngological Association, 592

Index

American Laryngological, Rhinological, and Otological Society, Inc. (The Triological Society), 592
American Osteopathic Colleges of Ophthalmology and Otolaryngology—Head and Neck Surgery, 592
American Rhinologic Society, 593
Canadian Society of Otolaryngology—Head and Neck Surgery, 593
Society of American Otolaryngologists—Head and Neck Surgeons, 593

Otology specialty associations
American Otological Society, Inc., 593

Our Lady of Lourdes Medical Center, Nurse Anesthesia Program, 242

P

Pain management specialty associations
American Academy of Pain Management, 593
American Academy of Pain Medicine, 593
American Chronic Pain Association, 594
American College of Osteopathic Pain Management and Sclerotherapy, Inc., 594
American Pain Society, 594
American Society of Regional Anesthesia and Pain Medicine, 594
International Association for the Study of Pain, 594

Palmer College of Chiropractic, 188
Palmer College of Chiropractic—West, 186
Palmetto Richland Memorial Hospital/USC/PRMH Graduate Program in Nurse Anesthesia, 251
Parker College of Chiropractic, 190
Parkland School of Nurse-Midwifery, 271
Pathology specialty associations
American Association of Neuropathologists, 594
American Society for Investigative Pathology, 595
American Society of Clinical Pathologists, 595
Canadian Association of Pathologists, 595
College of American Pathologists, 595
Intersociety Committee on Pathology Information, 595

Pediatrics specialty associations
Ambulatory Pediatric Association, 596
American Academy of Pediatric Dentistry, 596
American Academy of Pediatrics, 596
American College of Osteopathic Pediatricians, 596
American Pediatric Society, 596
American Society of Dentistry for Children, 596
American Society of Pediatric Neuroradiology, 596
Canadian Pediatric Society, 597
National Association of Pediatric Nurse Associations and Practitioners, 597
Society for Adolescent Medicine, Inc., 597

Peer recommendation, 7, 17
Peer review, 7, 18
Pennsylvania Bureau of Professional and Occupational Affairs, 317
Pennsylvania dental schools
Temple University School of Dentistry, 173

Index

University of Pennsylvania School of Dental Medicine, 174
University of Pittsburgh School of Dental Medicine, 174

Pennsylvania licensing agencies
Bureau of Professional and Occupational Affairs, 317
Chiropractic Licensing Agency, 409
Pennsylvania State Board of Dentistry, 365
Pennsylvania State Board of Medicine, MD, 318
Pennsylvania State Board of Medicine, Physician assistant, 428
Pennsylvania State Board of Nursing, 450
Pennsylvania State Board of Osteopathic Medicine, DO, 318
Pennsylvania State Board of Psychology, 470
State Board of Podiatry, 388

Pennsylvania medical schools
Jefferson Medical College, 116
Lake Erie College of Osteopathic Medicine, 145
MCP Hahnemann University, 117
Pennsylvania State University College of Medicine, 118
Philadelphia College of Osteopathic Medicine, 145
Temple University School of Medicine, 118
University of Pennsylvania School of Medicine, 120
University of Pittsburgh School of Medicine, 120

Pennsylvania nursing schools
Clarion University School of Nursing, 225
Hamot Medical Center, School of Anesthesia, 246
Institute of Midwifery, Women, and Health, 269
Lankenau Hospital, School of Nurse Anesthesia, 247
MCP Hahnemann University, Graduate Program of Nurse Anesthesia, 247
Montgomery Hospital, School of Anesthesia, 247
Nazareth Hospital, School of Nurse Anesthesiology, 248
Pennsylvania Hospital, School of Nurse Anesthesia, 248
St. Francis Medical Center/LaRoche College, School of Anesthesia, nursing, 248
University of Pennsylvania School of Nursing, Nurse-Midwifery Program, 269
University of Pittsburgh School of Nursing, Nurse Anesthesia, 249
Westmoreland-LaTrobe Hospitals/LaRoche College, School of Anesthesia, 249

Pennsylvania physician assistant programs
Allentown College of Saint Francis de Sales, Physician Assistant Program, 214
Chatham College, Physician Assistant Program, 213
Duquesne University, Physician Assistant Program, 213
King's College, Physician Assistant Program, 213
MCP Hahnemann University, Physician Assistant Program, 214
St. Francis University of Pennsylvania, Physician Assistant Program, 214

Pennsylvania podiatry schools
Temple University School of Podiatric Medicine, 182

Pennsylvania residency programs
MCP Hahnemann University School of Medicine, 117
Pennsylvania State University College of Medicine, 118
Temple University Hospital, 118
Thomas Jefferson University Hospital, 119
University Health Center of Pittsburgh, 119

Index

University of Pennsylvania Health System, 119
Pennsylvania State Board of Chiropractic, 409
Pennsylvania State Board of Dentistry, 365
Pennsylvania State Board of Medicine, MD, 318
Pennsylvania State Board of Medicine, Physician assistant, 428
Pennsylvania State Board of Nursing, 450
Pennsylvania State Board of Osteopathic Medicine, DO, 318
Pennsylvania State Board of Psychology, 470
Personnel, role in credentialing and privileging, 30
Pharmacology/Pharmacy specialty associations
    American Association of Colleges of Pharmacy, 597
    American College of Apothecaries, 597
    American College of Clinical Pharmacology, 597
    American College of Clinical Pharmacy, 597
    American College on Pharmaceutical Education, 598
    American Pharmaceutical Association, 598
    American Society for Clinical Pharmacology and Therapeutics, 598
    American Society for Pharmacology and Experimental Therapeutics, 598
    American Society of Health-System Pharmacists, 598
Philadelphia College of Osteopathic Medicine, 145
Photographs, use in credentialing, 8
Physiatry/Rehabilitative medicine specialty associations
    American Academy of Physical Medicine and Rehabilitation, 598
    American Congress of Rehabilitation Medicine, 598
    American Orthopaedic Society for Sports Medicine, 598
    Canadian Association of Physical Medicine and Rehabilitation, 599
    National Rehabilitation Association, 599
Physical therapy specialty associations
    American Board of Physical Therapy Specialties, 599
    American Physical Therapy Association, 599
Physician Assistant Program, Sisters of Charity Medical Center, 209
Physician and medical assistants specialty associations
    American Registry of Medical Assistants, 599
    National Commission on Certification of Physician Assistants, 600
Pikeville College, School of Osteopathic Medicine, 142
Plastic surgery specialty associations
    American Association of Plastic Surgeons, 600
    American Society of Plastic Surgeons, 600
    Canadian Society of Plastic Surgeons, 600
Podiatry specialty associations
    American Academy of Podiatric Sports Medicine, 600
    American Association of Podiatric Medicine, 600
    American College of Foot and Ankle Orthopedics and Medicine, 601
    American College of Foot and Ankle Surgeons, 601
    American Podiatric Medical Association, 601
Preventive medicine specialty associations
    American College of Preventive Medicine, 601
    American Osteopathic College of Occupational and Preventive Medicine, 601
Primary source verification, 8
Pritzker School of Medicine at the University of Chicago, 74

Index

Privileging
- Admitting, 18
- AHPs, 19
- Clinics, 21
- House staff, 22
- LIPs, 22
- Mergers and acquisitions, 21
- Outpatient services, 20
- Physician offices, 21
- Trainees, 22

Psychiatry specialty associations
- American Academy of Addiction Psychiatry, 602
- American Academy of Child and Adolescent Psychiatry, 602
- American Academy of Clinical Psychiatrists, 602
- American Association for Geriatric Psychiatry, 602
- American Association of Psychiatric Technicians, Inc., 602
- American Clinical Neurophysiology Society (formerly American Electroencephalographic Society), 602
- American College of Neuropsychiatrists, 603
- American Orthopsychiatric Association, Inc., 603
- American Psychiatric Association, 603
- American Psychiatric Nurses Association, 603
- Canadian Psychiatric Association, 603
- National Mental Health Association, Inc., 603

Psychology Boards, 513
- American Board of Professional Psychology (ABPP), 513
- American Psychological Association, 513

Psychology specialty associations
- American Group Psychotherapy Association, Inc., 603
- American Psychological Association, College of Professional Psychology, 604
- American Psychological Society, 604
- Association for Applied Psychophysiology and Biofeedback, 604
- Canadian Psychological Association, 604
- Council for the National Register of Health Service Providers in Psychology, 604

Public health specialty associations
- American Association of Public Health Dentistry, 604
- American Public Health Association, 605
- Association of Maternal and Child Health Programs, 605
- Association of Schools of Public Health, Inc., 605
- Canadian Healthcare Association, 605
- Connecticut Department of Public Health, 605

Puerto Rico Board of Dental Examiners, 366
Puerto Rico Board of Medical Examiners, MD and DO, 319
Puerto Rico Chiropractic Licensing Agency, 409
Puerto Rico dental schools
- University of Puerto Rico School of Dentistry, 174

Puerto Rico licensing agencies
- Office of Regulation and Certification of Health Care Professionals, Podiatry, 388
- Puerto Rico Board of Dental Examiners, 366
- Puerto Rico Board of Medical Examiners, MD and DO, 319

Index

Puerto Rico Office of Regulation and Certification of Health Care Professionals, Nursing, 450
Puerto Rico Office of Regulation and Certification of Health Care Professionals, 470

Puerto Rico medical schools
Ponce School of Medicine, 120
Universidad Central del Caribe School of Medicine, 121
University of Puerto Rico, 121

Puerto Rico nursing schools
InterAmerican University of Puerto Rico, 249
University of Puerto Rico, 249

Puerto Rico Office of Regulation and Certification of Health Care Professionals, Dental, 366
Puerto Rico Office of Regulation and Certification of Health Care Professionals, Nursing, 450
Puerto Rico Office of Regulation and Certification of Health Care Professionals, Podiatry, 388
Puerto Rico Office of Regulation and Certification of Health Care Professionals, Psychology, 470

Q

Quebec medical schools (Canada)
McGill University Faculty of Medicine, 156
University de Montreal Faculte de Medecine, 121
University de Sherbrooke Faculte de Medecine, 156
University Laval Faculte de Medecine, 157

Quebec residency programs (Canada)
McGill University Faculty of Medicine, 156
University de Montreal Faculte de Medecine, 121
University Laval Faculte de Medecine, 157

Queen's University Faculty of Health Sciences, 153

R

Radiology specialty associations
American College of Radiology, 605
American Healthcare Radiology Administrators, 606
American Osteopathic College of Radiology, 606
American Society for Therapeutic Radiology and Oncology, 606
American Society of Emergency Radiology, 606
American Society of Head and Neck Radiology, 606
American Society of Interventional and Therapeutic Neuroradiology, 606
American Society of Neuroimaging, 606
American Society of Pediatric Neuroradiology, 607
American Society of Radiologic Technologists, 607
American Society of Spine Radiology, 607
Radiological Society of North America, 607
Society of Cardiovascular & Interventional Radiology, 607

Ramsey Clinic, Nurse-Midwifery Precertification program, 273
Ravenswood Hospital Medical Center School of Anesthesia/DePaul University, Graduate Program in Nurse Anesthesia, 233

Index

Respiratory care specialty associations
    American Association for Respiratory Care, 607
Rheumatology specialty associations
    American College of Rheumatology, 608
    American Osteopathic College of Rheumatology, Inc., 608
    Canadian Rheumatology Association, 608
Rhode Island Board of Medical Licensure and Discipline, MD and DO, 319
Rhode Island Board of Medical Licensure and Discipline, Physician assistant, 428
Rhode Island Board of Nurse Registration and Nursing Education, 451
Rhode Island Division of Professional Regulation, 409
Rhode Island Division of Professional Regulation, Psychologist, 471
Rhode Island licensing agencies
    Division of Professional Regulation, 409
    Rhode Island Board of Medical Licensure and Discipline, MD and DO, 428
    Rhode Island Board of Medical Licensure and Discipline, Physician assistant, 428
    Rhode Island Board of Nurse Registration and Nursing Education, 451
    Rhode Island Division of Professional Regulation, Psychologist, 471
    Rhode Island State Board of Examiners in Dentistry, 367
Rhode Island medical schools
    Brown Medical School, 122
Rhode Island nursing schools
    Memorial Hospital of Rhode Island, School of Nurse Anesthesia, 250
    St. Joseph Hospital, School of Anesthesia for Nurses, 251
    University of Rhode Island College of Nursing, Nurse-Midwife Program, 270
Rhode Island State Board of Examiners in Dentistry, 367
Robert Wood Johnson Medical School at the University of Medicine and Dentistry of New Jersey at Piscataway, residencies, 100
Robert Wood Johnson Medical School at the University of Medicine and Dentistry of New Jersey at Piscataway, 100
Rochester Institute of Technology, Physician Assistant Program, 208
Roles in credentialing and privileging
    Administration, 32
    Applicant, 32
    Board, 31
    CEO, 32
    Credentials committee, 30
    Department chair, 31
    Human resources, 30
    Medical executive committee, 30
    Medical staff services professional, 30
    Medical staff, 30
Royal Melbourne Institute of Technology, 185
Rush Presbyterian St. Luke's Medical Center, residencies, 74
Rush University College of Nursing, Nurse Anesthesia Program, 233
Rush University, Rush Medical College, 75
Rutgers University/University of Medicine and Dentistry of New Jersey at Piscataway Physician Assistant Program, 206

Index

S

Samuel Merritt College, Graduate Program of Nurse Anesthesia, 230
Saskatchewan medical schools (Canada)
    University of Saskatchewan College of Medicine, 157
Saskatchewan residency programs (Canada)
    University of Saskatchewan College of Medicine, 157
Sedation and anesthesia, 22
Sherman College of Straight Chiropractic, 190
Social work specialty associations
    American Association for Marriage and Family Therapy, 608
    Council on Social Work Education, 608
    National Association of Social Workers, Inc. (NASW), 608
    Society for Social Work Leadership in Healthcare, 609
Software vendors, 636
South Carolina Board of Chiropractic Examiners, 410
South Carolina Board of Examiners in Psychology, 471
South Carolina Board of Medical Examiners, MD and DO, 320
South Carolina Board of Podiatry Examiners, 389
South Carolina chiropractic schools
    Sherman College of Straight Chiropractic, 190
South Carolina dental schools
    Medical University of South Carolina College of Dental Medicine, 174
South Carolina licensing agencies
    South Carolina Board of Chiropractic Examiners, 410
    South Carolina Board of Examiners in Psychology, 471
    South Carolina Board of Medical Examiners, MD and DO, 320
    South Carolina Board of Podiatry Examiners, 389
    South Carolina State Board of Dentistry, 367
    South Carolina State Board of Medical Examiners, Physician assistant, 429
    South Carolina State Board of Nursing, 451
South Carolina medical schools
    Medical University of South Carolina College of Medicine, 122
    University of South Carolina School of Medicine, 123
South Carolina nursing schools
    Medical University of South Carolina, Anesthesia for Nurses Program, 251
    Medical University of South Carolina, Nurse-Midwifery Program, 270
    Palmetto Richland Memorial Hospital/USC/PRMH Graduate Program in Nurse Anesthesia, 251
    University of South Carolina College of Nursing, 582
South Carolina residency program
    Medical University of South Carolina College of Medicine, 122
South Carolina State Board of Dentistry, 367
South Carolina State Board of Medical Examiners, Physician assistant, 429
South Carolina State Board of Nursing, 451
South Dakota Board of Chiropractic Examiners, 410
South Dakota Board of Examiners of Psychologists, 471
South Dakota Board of Nursing, 451

Index

South Dakota Board of Podiatry Examiners, 389
South Dakota licensing agencies
    Board of Chiropractic Examiners, 410
    South Dakota Board of Examiners of Psychologists, 471
    South Dakota Board of Nursing, 451
    South Dakota Board of Podiatry Examiners, 389
    South Dakota State Board of Dentistry, 368
    South Dakota State Board of Medical and Osteopathic Examiners, MD and DO, 321
    South Dakota State Board of Medical and Osteopathic Examiners, Physician assistant, 429
South Dakota medical schools
    University of South Dakota School of Medicine, 123
South Dakota nursing schools
    Avera McKennan Hospital/University of South Dakota, School of Anesthesia for registered Nurses, 252
    Mount Marty College, Graduate Program in Nurse Anesthesia, 252
South Dakota physician assistant programs
    University of South Dakota School of Medicine, Physician Assistant Program, 215
South Dakota residency program
    University of South Dakota School of Medicine, 124
South Dakota State Board of Dentistry, 368
South Dakota State Board of Medical and Osteopathic Examiners, MD and DO, 321
South Dakota State Board of Medical and Osteopathic Examiners, Physician assistant, 429
Southern California University of Health Sciences, Los Angeles College of Chiropractic, 186
Southern Connecticut State University/Bridgeport Hospital, Nurse Anesthesia program, 231
Southern Illinois University Edwardsville, nursing, 224
Southern Illinois University Physician Assistant Program, 201
Southern Illinois University School of Dental Medicine, 164
Southern Illinois University School of Medicine, 75
Southern Illinois University School of Medicine, residencies, 75
Southern Illinois University—Edwardsville, School of Nursing, Nurse Anesthesia Specialization, 233
Southwest Missouri School of Anesthesia, 241
Speech, language, hearing specialty associations
    American Speech-Language-Hearing Association, 609
    Canadian Association of Speech-Language Pathologists and Audiologists, 609
St. Elizabeth Health Center School for Nurse Anesthetists, Inc., 245
St. Francis University of Pennsylvania, Physician Assistant Program, 214
St. Joseph Hospital, School of Anesthesia for Nurses, 238
St. Louis University, Physician Assistant Program, 205
St. Mary's University Graduate Program in Nurse Anesthesia, 240
Stanford University/Foothill College School of Medicine, Primary Care Associate Program, 195
State University of New York at Buffalo School of Dental Medicine, 171
State University of New York at Buffalo School of Medicine, 104
State University of New York at Buffalo School of Medicine, residencies, 105
State University of New York at Stony Brook School of Medicine, 106
State University of New York at Stony Brook School of Nursing, Pathways to Midwifery Program, 266
State University of New York at Stony Brook, School of Health Technology & Management, Physician Assistant Program, 209
State University of New York at Syracuse College of Medicine, residencies, 105
State University of New York Downstate Medical Center Midwifery Education program, 266

Index

State University of New York Downstate Medical Center, medical school, 105
State University of New York Downstate Medical Center, nurse anesthesia program, 243
State University of New York Upstate Medical University, 106
Stritch School of Medicine, see Loyola University Chicago, residencies, 73
SUNY—Health Science Center at Brooklyn (Downstate), Physician Assistant Program, 209
Supplemental credentialing criteria, 8
Surgery specialty associations
    American Association for Accreditation of Ambulatory Surgery Facilities, Inc., 609
    American Association of Hip and Knee Surgeons, 609
    American Association of Surgical Physician Assistants, 609
    American College of Mohs Micrographic Surgery and Cutaneous Oncology, 609
    American College of Osteopathic Surgeons, 610
    American College of Surgeons, 610
    American Society for Dermatologic Surgery, 610
    American Society for Laser Medicine and Surgery, Inc., 610
    American Society of Cataract and Refractive Surgery, 610
    Canadian Association of General Surgeons, 610
    International College of Surgeons/United States Section, 611
    Royal College of Physicians and Surgeons of USA, 611
    Society for Vascular Surgery, 611
    Society of Thoracic Surgeons, 611
    Society of University Surgeons, 611
    The Southwestern Surgical Congress, 611

T

Telemedicine, 23
Temple University Hospital, residencies, 118
Temple University School of Dentistry, 173
Temple University School of Medicine, 118
Temple University School of Podiatric Medicine, 182
Tennessee Board in Psychology, 472
Tennessee Board of Dentistry, 369
Tennessee Board of Nursing, 452
Tennessee Board of Registration in Podiatry, 390
Tennessee Bureau of Health, Licensure & Regulations, Chiropractic, 411
Tennessee Committee for Physicians Assistants, 429
Tennessee dental schools
    Meharry Medical College School of Dentistry, 175
    University of Tennessee College of Dentistry, 175
Tennessee Department of Health, MD, 322
Tennessee licensing agencies
    Bureau of Health, Licensure & Regulations, Chiropractic, 411
    Tennessee Board in Psychology, 472
    Tennessee Board of Dentistry, 369
    Tennessee Board of Nursing, 452
    Tennessee Board of Registration in Podiatry, 390

Tennessee Committee for Physicians Assistants, 429
Tennessee Department of Health, MD, 322
Tennessee medical schools
East Tennessee State University College of Medicine, 124
Meharry Medical College, 125
University of Tennessee Health Science Center, 125
Vanderbilt University Office of the University Registrar, 126
Tennessee nursing schools
Erlanger Medical Center, School of Nurse Anesthesia, 252
Middle Tennessee School of Anesthesia, nursing, 253
University of Tennessee Medical Center, School of Nurse Anesthesia, 253
Tennessee physician assistant programs
Trevecca Nazarene University, Physician Assistant Program, 215
Tennessee residency programs
East Tennessee State University College of Medicine, 124
Meharry Medical College School of Medicine, 125
University of Tennessee College of Medicine, 126
Vanderbilt University Medical Center, 126
Texas A&M University System Health Science Center College of Medicine, 127
Texas Board of Chiropractic Examiners, 411
Texas Board of Medical Examiners, Nursing, 452
Texas Chiropractic College, 190
Texas chiropractic schools
Parker College of Chiropractic, 190
Texas Chiropractic College, 190
Texas dental schools
Baylor College of Dentistry, 175
University of Texas Health Science Center at San Antonio Dental School, 176
University of Texas Houston Health Science Center Dental School, 176
Texas licensing agencies
Texas Board of Chiropractic Examiners, 411
Texas Board of Medical Examiners, Nursing, 452
Texas State Board of Dental Examiners, 369
Texas State Board of Examiners of Psychologists, 472
Texas State Board of Medical Examiners, Acupuncture and Physician Assistant, 323
Texas State Board of Medical Examiners, Acupuncture Examiners and Physician Assistant Examiners, Physician assistant, 430
Texas State Board of Podiatric Medical Examiners, 390
Texas medical schools
Baylor College of Medicine, 127
Texas A&M University System Health Science Center College of Medicine, 127
Texas Tech University School of medicine, 128
University of Texas Health Science Center at San Antonio, 129
University of Texas Health Science Center Houston, 128
University of Texas Medical Branch at Galveston, 129
University of Texas Southwestern Medical Center at Dallas School of Medicine, 130
Texas nursing schools
Baylor College of Medicine, Graduate Program in Nurse Anesthesia, 253
Baylor College of Medicine, Nurse-Midwifery Education Program, 270
Parkland School of Nurse-Midwifery, 271

Index

University of Texas Health Sciences Center—Houston School of Nursing, anesthesia, 254
University of Texas Medical Branch—Galveston, Nurse-Midwifery Program, 271
University of Texas—El Paso/Texas Tech University, Collaborative Nurse-Midwifery Program at Texas Tech University Health Science Center, 271

Texas physician assistant programs
Baylor College of Medicine, Physician Assistant Program, 215
Interservice Physician Assistant Program, 216
University of North Texas Health Science Center at Fort Worth, Physician Assistant Program, 216
University of Texas Medical Branch at Galveston, Physician Assistant Program, 216
University of Texas Southwestern Medical Center, Physician Assistant Program, 217

Texas residency programs
Baylor College of Medicine, 127
Texas Tech University School of Medicine, 128
University of Texas Medical Branch at Galveston, 130
University of Texas Medical School at Houston, 128
University of Texas Southwestern Medical Center at Dallas School of Medicine, 130

Texas State Board of Dental Examiners, 369
Texas State Board of Examiners of Psychologists, 472
Texas State Board of Medical Examiners, Acupuncture Examiners and Physician Assistant Examiners, MD, 323
Texas State Board of Medical Examiners, Acupuncture Examiners and Physician Assistant Examiners, Physician assistant, 430
Texas State Board of Podiatric Medical Examiners, 390
Texas Tech University School of medicine, 128
Texas Tech University School of Medicine, residencies, 128
The Brody School of Medicine at East Carolina University, 109
The Naval School of Health Sciences, Navy Nurse Corps Anesthesia Program, 236
The University of Akron College of Nursing, Anesthesia Track, 246
The University of New Mexico School of Medicine, Physician Assistant Program, 207
Thoracic medicine specialty associations
American Thoracic Society, 611
Canadian Thoracic Society, 612
Society of Thoracic Radiology, 612
Society of Thoracic Surgeons, 612

Touro College, Physician Assistant Program, 210
Touro University College of Osteopathic Medicine, 141
Trevecca Nazarene University, Physician Assistant Program, 215
Trover Foundation/Murray State University Program of Anesthesia, 235
Truman Medical Center, School of Nurse Anesthesia, 241
Tufts University School of Dental Medicine, 168
Tufts University School of Medicine, 87
Tulane University School of Medicine, 83
Tulane University School of Medicine, residencies, 83

U

UCSD Nurse-Midwifery Education Program, 259
UCSF Interdepartmental Nurse-Midwifery Education Program, 259
UCSF/SFGH Interdepartmental Nurse-Midwifery Education Program, 260
Uniformed Services nursing schools

Index

    The Naval School of Health Sciences, Navy Nurse Corps Anesthesia Program, 236
    Uniformed Services University of the health Sciences, Graduate School of Nursing,
        Nurse Anesthesia Program, 236
    United States Air Force Graduate Program of Nurse Anesthesia, 237
    United States Army Graduate Program in Anesthesia Nursing, 254

Uniformed Services physician assistant programs
    Naval School of Health Sciences, Physician Assistant Program, 203

Uniformed Services University of the Health Sciences School of Medicine, residencies, 85
Uniformed Services University of the Health Sciences School of Medicine, 84
Uniformed Services University of the health Sciences, Graduate School of Nursing, Nurse Anesthesia Program, 236
United Hospital Center/LaRoche College, Nurse Anesthesia Program, 256
United Kingdom chiropractic schools
    Anglo-European College of Chiropractic, 187

United States Air Force Graduate Program of Nurse Anesthesia, 237
United States Army Graduate Program in Anesthesia Nursing, 254
University at Buffalo, School of Nursing, Nurse Anesthesia Program, 244
University Health Center of Pittsburgh, residencies, 119
University Hospital/University of Cincinnati College of Medicine, residencies, 113
University Hospitals of Cleveland, residencies, 113
University of Alabama at Birmingham, Nurse Anesthetist program, 229
University of Alabama at Birmingham, nursing, 223
University of Alabama at Birmingham, Surgical Physician Assistant Program, 195
University of Alabama School of Dentistry, 161
University of Alabama School of Medicine, 57
University of Alabama School of Medicine, residencies, 57
University of Arizona College of Medicine, 58
University of Arizona College of Medicine, residencies, 58
University of Arkansas College of Medicine, 59
University of Bridgeport, College of Chiropractic, 187
University of British Columbia Faculty of Medicine, 59
University of California, Davis, Medical Center, residencies, 62
University of California—Davis Medical Center, Family Nurse Practitioner/Physician Assistant Program, 196
University of California at Davis School of Medicine, 61
University of California at Davis School of Medicine, residencies, 64
University of California at Irvine College of Medicine, 64
University of California at Los Angeles (UCLA) School of Dentistry, 161
University of California at Los Angeles School of Medicine, 62
University of California at Los Angeles School of Medicine, residencies, 62
University of California at San Diego School of Medicine, 63
University of California at San Diego School of Medicine, residencies, 63
University of California at San Francisco, School of Medicine, 63
University of California Medical Center, residencies, 61
University of California San Francisco School of Dentistry, 162
University of California San Francisco, School of Medicine, residencies, 64
University of Cincinnati College of Medicine, 114
University of Cincinnati Nurse Midwifery Education Program, 268
University of Cincinnati, Nurse Anesthesia, 246
University of Colorado Health Science Center, Child Health Associate/Physician Assistant Program, 197
University of Colorado, Nurse-Midwifery Program, 261
University of Colorado School of Dentistry, 163

Index

University of Connecticut School of Dental Medicine, 163
University of Connecticut School of Medicine, 65
University of Connecticut School of Medicine, residencies, 65
University of Detroit Mercy School of Dentistry, 168
University of Detroit Mercy, Physician Assistant Program, 204
University of Florida College of Dentistry, 164
University of Florida College of Medicine, 68
University of Florida College of Medicine, residencies, 68
University of Florida, Physician Assistant Program, 199
University of Hawaii School of Medicine, 72
University of Health Sciences, College of Osteopathic Medicine, 143
University of Illinois at Chicago College of Dentistry, 165
University of Illinois at Chicago College of Medicine, residencies, 76
University of Illinois at Chicago, 76
University of Illinois College of Medicine at Peoria, 76
University of Illinois College of Medicine at Peoria, residencies, 77
University of Illinois College of Medicine at Rockford, 77
University of Illinois College of Medicine at Rockford, residencies, 77
University of Illinois College of Medicine at Urbana, 78
University of Illinois College of Medicine at Urbana, residencies, 78
University of Iowa College of Dentistry, 165
University of Iowa College of Medicine, 79
University of Iowa College of Medicine, Physician Assistant Program, 202
University of Iowa College of Nursing, Anesthesia Nursing Program, 234
University of Iowa Hospitals and Clinics, residencies, 79
University of Kansas Medical Center, 80
University of Kansas School of Medicine at Wichita, residencies, 80
University of Kentucky College of Dentistry, 166
University of Kentucky College of Medicine, 80
University of Kentucky College of Medicine, residencies, 81
University of Kentucky, Physician Assistant Program, 203
University of Louisville School of Dentistry, 166
University of Louisville School of Medicine, 81
University of Louisville School of Medicine, residencies, 81
University of Manitoba Faculty of Medicine, 150
University of Maryland Baltimore, 85
University of Maryland Dental School, 167
University of Maryland Medical Systems, residencies, 85
University of Massachusetts Medical School, 87
University of Massachusetts Medical School, residencies, 87
University of Medicine and Dentistry of New Jersey, New Jersey Dental School, 170
University of Medicine and Dentistry of New Jersey, School of Osteopathic Medicine, 144
University of Medicine and Dentistry of New Jersey—Newark School of Health-Related Professions, Nurse-Midwifery Program, 265
University of Miami Medical School, 69
University of Miami School of Nursing, 262
University of Miami/Jackson Memorial Medical Center, Nurse-Midwifery Precertification Program, 262
University of Michigan—Flint/Hurley Medical Center, Anesthesia Program, 239
University of Michigan Health Systems, residencies, 90
University of Michigan Medical School, 90

University of Michigan School of Dentistry, 168
University of Michigan School of Nursing, Nurse-Midwifery Program, 264
University of Minnesota at Duluth School of Medicine, 92
University of Minnesota at Minneapolis Medical School, 92
University of Minnesota Dental School, 169
University of Minnesota Medical School, residencies, 92
University of Minnesota School of Nursing, Nurse-Midwifery Program, 264
University of Mississippi Medical Center School of Medicine, 93
University of Mississippi School of Dentistry, 169
University of Missouri at Columbia School of Medicine, 94
University of Missouri—Columbia School of Medicine, residencies, 94
University of Missouri—Kansas City School of Dentistry, 169
University of Missouri at Kansas City School of Medicine, 95
University of Missouri at Kansas City School of Medicine, residencies, 95
University of Nebraska College of Medicine, residencies, 97
University of Nebraska Medical Center, 97
University of Nebraska Medical Center, Physician Assistant Program, 205
University of Nevada School of Medicine, 97
University of Nevada school of Medicine, residencies, 98
University of New England, College of Osteopathic Medicine, 143
University of New England, School of Nurse Anesthesia, 235
University of New Hampshire Department of Nursing, 582
University of New Mexico College of Nursing, Nurse-Midwifery Program, 265
University of New Mexico Health Sciences Center School of Medicine, 100
University of New Mexico Medical School, residencies, 100
University of North Carolina at Chapel Hill School of Medicine, 109
University of North Carolina at Chapel Hill School of Medicine, residencies, 110
University of North Carolina School of Dentistry, 172
University of North Dakota School of Medicine and Health Sciences, 110
University of North Dakota School of Medicine, Physician Assistant Program, 211
University of North Dakota, Anesthesia Nursing Specialization, 245
University of North Texas Health Science Center at Fort Worth, Physician Assistant Program, 216
University of North Texas Health Science Center at Fort Worth, Texas College of Osteopathic Medicine, 146
University of Oklahoma at Oklahoma City, Physician Assistant Program, 212
University of Oklahoma at Tulsa College of Medicine, 115
University of Oklahoma Health Sciences Center at Oklahoma City, 115
University of Oklahoma Health Sciences Center at Oklahoma City, residencies, 115
University of Oklahoma Health Sciences Center College of Dentistry, 173
University of Pennsylvania Health System, residencies, 119
University of Pennsylvania School of Dental Medicine, 174
University of Pennsylvania School of Medicine, 120
University of Pennsylvania School of Nursing, Nurse-Midwifery Program, 269
University of Pittsburgh School of Dental Medicine, 174
University of Pittsburgh School of Medicine, 120
University of Puerto Rico, medical school, 121
University of Puerto Rico Nurse Anesthesia Program, 249
University of Puerto Rico School of Dentistry, 174
University of Rhode Island College of Nursing, Nurse-Midwife Program, 270
University of Rochester School of Medicine and Dentistry, 107

Index

University of Rochester School of Nursing, nurse-midwifery, 267
University of Rochester Strong Memorial Hospital, residencies, 107
University of Saint Francis (formerly Lutheran College of Health Professions Physician Assistant Program), 202
University of Saskatchewan College of Medicine, 157
University of South Carolina School of Medicine, 123
University of South Dakota School of Medicine, 123
University of South Dakota School of Medicine, Physician Assistant Program, 215
University of South Dakota School of Medicine, residencies, 124
University of South Florida College of Medicine, 69
University of South Florida College of Medicine, residencies, 69
University of Southern California Department of Nursing, 223
University of Southern California Nurse-Midwifery Education Program, 260
University of Southern California Program of Nurse Anesthesia, 230
University of Southern California School of Dentistry, 162
University of Southern California School of Medicine, Primary Care Physician Assistant Program, 196
University of Southern California School of Medicine, residencies, 64
University of Southern Mississippi College of Nursing, 224
University of Tennessee College of Dentistry, 175
University of Tennessee College of Medicine, residencies, 126
University of Tennessee Health Science Center, 125
University of Tennessee Medical Center, School of Nurse Anesthesia, 253
University of Texas Health Science Center at San Antonio Dental School, 175
University of Texas Health Science Center at San Antonio, 129
University of Texas Health Science Center Houston, 128
University of Texas Health Sciences Center—Houston School of Nursing, anesthesia, 254
University of Texas Houston Health Science Center Dental School, 176
University of Texas Medical Branch at Galveston, 129
University of Texas Medical Branch—Galveston, Nurse-Midwifery Program, 271
University of Texas Medical Branch at Galveston, Physician Assistant Program, 216
University of Texas Medical Branch at Galveston, residencies, 130
University of Texas Medical School at Houston, residencies, 128
University of Texas Southwestern Medical Center at Dallas School of Medicine, 130
University of Texas Southwestern Medical Center at Dallas School of Medicine, residencies, 130
University of Texas Southwestern Medical Center, Physician Assistant Program, 217
University of Texas—El Paso/Texas Tech University, Collaborative Nurse-Midwifery Program at Texas Tech University Health Science Center, 271
University of the Pacific School of Dentistry, 162
University of Utah College of Nursing, Graduate Program in Nurse-Midwifery, 272
University of Utah School of Medicine, 131
University of Utah School of Medicine, Physician Assistant Program, 217
University of Utah School of Medicine, residencies, 131
University of Vermont College of Medicine, 131
University of Vermont College of Medicine, residencies, 132
University of Virginia School of Medicine, 133
University of Virginia School of medicine, residencies, 134
University of Washington School of Dentistry, 177
University of Washington School of Medicine, 134
University of Washington School of Medicine, residencies, 135
University of Washington School of Nursing, Nurse-Midwifery Program, 272

University of Washington/MEDEX Northwest, Physician Assistant Program, 218
University of Wisconsin Medical School, 137
University of Wisconsin—Madison Medical Sciences Center, Physician Assistant Program, 219
Utah Board of Dentists and Dental Hygienists, 370
Utah Division of Occupational and Professional Licensing, Chiropractic, 411
Utah Division of Occupational and Professional Licensing, Psychologists, 473
Utah Division of Occupational and Professional Licensure, MD and DO, 323
Utah Division of Occupational and Professional Licensure, Physician assistant, 430
Utah Division of Occupational and Professional Licensure, Podiatry, 391
Utah licensing agencies
> Utah Board of Dentists and Dental Hygienists, 370
> Utah Division of Occupational and Professional Licensing, Chiropractic, 411
> Utah Division of Occupational and Professional Licensing, Psychologists, 473
> Utah Division of Occupational and Professional Licensure, MD and DO, 323
> Utah Division of Occupational and Professional Licensure, Physician assistant, 430
> Utah Division of Occupational and Professional Licensure, Podiatry, 391

Utah medical schools
> University of Utah School of Medicine, 131

Utah nursing schools
> University of Utah College of Nursing, Graduate Program in Nurse-Midwifery, 272

Utah physician assistant programs
> University of Utah School of Medicine, Physician Assistant Program, 217

Utah residency program
> University of Utah School of Medicine, 131

Utilization Review Accreditation Commission, American Accreditation HealthCare Commission, 619

V

Vanderbilt University Medical Center, residencies, 126
Vanderbilt University Office of the University Registrar, 126
Vermont Board of Dental Examiners, 370
Vermont Board of Medical Practice, MD, 324
Vermont Board of Medical Practice, Physician assistant, 430
Vermont Board of Medical Practice, Podiatry, 391
Vermont Board of Osteopathic Physicians and Surgeons, DO, 324
Vermont Board of Psychological Examiners, 473
Vermont licensing agencies
> Office of the Secretary of State, License Verification Unit, Chiropractic, 412
> Vermont Board of Dental Examiners, 370
> Vermont Board of Medical Practice, MD, 324
> Vermont Board of Medical Practice, Physician assistant, 430
> Vermont Board of Medical Practice, Podiatry, 391
> Vermont Board of Osteopathic Physicians and Surgeons, DO, 324
> Vermont Board of Psychological Examiners, 473
> Vermont State Board of Nursing, 452

Vermont medical schools
> University of Vermont College of Medicine, 131

Vermont Office of the Secretary of State, License Verification Unit, Chiropractic, 412

Vermont residency program
    University of Vermont College of Medicine, 132
Vermont State Board of Nursing, 452
Video Data Transmission specialty associations
    National Association of Medical Examiners, 613
Virgin Islands licensing agencies
    Virgin Islands Board of Medical Examiners, MD and DO, 325
Virginia Board of Dentistry, 371
Virginia Board of Medicine, MD and DO, 325
Virginia Board of Medicine, Physician assistant, 431
Virginia Board of Medicine, Podiatry, 391
Virginia Board of Nursing, 453
Virginia Board of Psychology, 473
Virginia Commonwealth University School of Dentistry, 173
Virginia Commonwealth University, Department of Nurse Anesthesia, 255
Virginia Commonwealth University, School of Medicine, Medical College of Virginia Campus, 134
Virginia dental schools
    Virginia Commonwealth University School of Dentistry, 173
Virginia licensing agencies
    State Board of Medicine, Chiropractic, 412
    Virginia Board of Dentistry, 371
    Virginia Board of Medicine, MD and DO, 325
    Virginia Board of Medicine, Physician assistant, 431
    Virginia Board of Medicine, Podiatry, 391
    Virginia Board of Nursing, 453
    Virginia Board of Psychology, 473
Virginia medical schools
    Eastern Virginia Medical School, 132
    University of Virginia School of Medicine, 133
    Virginia Commonwealth University, School of Medicine, Medical College of Virginia Campus, 134
Virginia nursing schools
    DePaul Medical Center, Bonsecour, nurse anesthesia, 254
    Old Dominion University School of Nursing, Nurse Anesthesia Program, 255
    Virginia Commonwealth University, Department of Nurse Anesthesia, 255
Virginia physician assistant program
    American Academy of Physicians Assistants, 217
    Association of Physician Assistant Programs, 218
    College of Health Sciences, Physician Assistant Program, 218
Virginia residency programs
    Eastern Virginia Medical School, 132
    Medical College of Virginia Hospitals, 133
    University of Virginia School of Medicine, 134
Virginia State Board of Medicine, Chiropractic, 412

W

Wake Forest University School of Medicine, 110
Wake Forest University School of Medicine, Physician Assistant Program, 211

Index

Washington dental schools
    University of Washington School of Dentistry, 177
Washington Department of Health Dental Quality Assurance Commission, 372
Washington Division of Professional Licensing, MD, 326
Washington Examining Board of Psychology, 474
Washington Health Professions Quality Assurance Division, Physician assistant, 431
Washington Health Professions Quality Assurance, Chiropractic, 412
Washington licensing agencies
    Department of Health Dental Quality Assurance Commission, 372
    Health Professions Quality Assurance, Chiropractic, 412
    Washington Division of Professional Licensing, MD, 326
    Washington Examining Board of Psychology, 474
    Washington Health Professions Quality Assurance Division, Physician assistant, 431
    Washington State Board of Osteopathic Medicine and Surgery, DO, 326
    Washington State Nursing Care Quality Assurance Commission, 453
    Washington State Podiatric Medical Board, 392
Washington medical schools
    University of Washington School of Medicine, 134
Washington nursing schools
    University of Washington School of Nursing, Nurse-Midwifery Program, 272
Washington physician assistant programs
    University of Washington/MEDEX Northwest, Physician Assistant Program, 218
Washington residency program
    University of Washington School of Medicine, 135
Washington State Board of Osteopathic Medicine and Surgery, DO, 326
Washington State Nursing Care Quality Assurance Commission, 453
Washington State Podiatric Medical Board, 392
Washington University School of Medicine, 96
Wayne State University College of Pharmacy and Allied Health Professions/Detroit Receiving Hospital, Department of Nurse Anesthesia, 239
Wayne State University School of Medicine, 90
Wayne State University School of Medicine, residencies, 90
Weill Cornell Medical College, Physician Assistant Program, 210
Weill Medical College of Cornell University, 107
West Virginia Board of Dental Examiners, 372
West Virginia Board of Examiners of Psychologists, 474
West Virginia Board of Medical Examiners for Registered Professional Nurses, 453
West Virginia Board of Medicine, MD, 327
West Virginia Board of Medicine, Physician assistant, 432
West Virginia Board of Osteopathy, DO, 328
West Virginia dental schools
    West Virginia University School of Dentistry, 177
West Virginia licensing agencies
    West Virginia Board of Dental Examiners, 372
    West Virginia Board of Examiners of Psychologists, 474
    West Virginia Board of Medical Examiners for Registered Professional Nurses, 453
    West Virginia Board of Medicine, MD, 327
    West Virginia Board of Medicine, Physician assistant, 432
    West Virginia Board of Osteopathy, DO, 328

Index

West Virginia medical schools
    Marshall University, Joan C. Edwards School of Medicine, 135
    West Virginia University School of Medicine, 136
West Virginia nursing schools
    Charleston Area Medical Center, 255
    United Hospital Center/LaRoche College, Nurse Anesthesia Program, 256
West Virginia physician assistant programs
    Alderson Broaddus College, Physician Assistant Program, 219
West Virginia residency program
    West Virginia University Hospitals Inc., 135
West Virginia University School of Dentistry, 177
Westchester Medical Center, 108
Western Michigan University, Physician Assistant Program, 205
Western States Chiropractic College, 189
Western Univers.ity of Health Sciences, Physician Assistant Program, 196
Wichita State University, Physician Assistant Program, 203
Wisconsin dental schools
    Marquette University, 177
Wisconsin Dentistry Examining Board, 373
Wisconsin Department of Regulation and Licensing, Chiropractic, 413
Wisconsin licensing agencies
    Department of Regulation and Licensing, Chiropractic, 413
    Wisconsin Dentistry Examining Board, 373
    Wisconsin Medical Examining Board, MD and DO, 328
    Wisconsin Medical Examining Board, Physician assistant, 432
    Wisconsin Medical Examining Board, Podiatry, 392
    Wisconsin Psychology Examining Board, 474
    Wisconsin, State of, Department of Regulation and Licensing, Board of Nursing, 454
Wisconsin Medical Examining Board, MD and DO, 328
Wisconsin Medical Examining Board, Physician assistant, 432
Wisconsin Medical Examining Board, Podiatry, 392
Wisconsin medical schools
    Medical College of Wisconsin, 136
    University of Wisconsin Medical School, 137
Wisconsin nursing schools
    Franciscan Skemp Healthcare, 256
    Marquette University College of Nursing, Nurse-Midwifery Program, 273
Wisconsin physician assistant programs
    Marquette University, Physician Assistant Program, 219
    University of Wisconsin—Madison Medical Sciences Center, Physician Assistant Program, 219
    UW—La Crosse-Gundersen-Mayo, Physician Assistant Program, 220
Wisconsin Psychology Examining Board, 474
Wisconsin residency programs
    Medical College of Wisconsin, 136
Wisconsin, State of, Department of Regulation and Licensing, Board of Nursing, 454
Wound care specialty associations
    American Academy of Wound Management, 613
    Association for the Advancement of Wound Care, 613
    The Wound Healing Society, 613

Wright State University School of Medicine, 114
Wright State University School of Medicine, residencies, 114
UW—La Crosse-Gundersen-Mayo, Physician Assistant Program, 220
Wyoming Board of Dental Examiners, 374
Wyoming Board of Medicine, MD and DO, 329
Wyoming Board of Medicine, Physician assistant, 432
Wyoming Board of Registration in Podiatry, 392
Wyoming licensing agencies
    Professional Licensing Boards, Chiropractic, 413
    Wyoming Board of Dental Examiners, 374
    Wyoming Board of Medicine, MD and DO, 329
    Wyoming Board of Medicine, Physician assistant, 432
    Wyoming Board of Registration in Podiatry, 392
    Wyoming Professional Licensing Board, Psychologist, 475
    Wyoming State Board of Nursing, 454
Wyoming Professional Licensing Board, Psychologist, 475
Wyoming Professional Licensing Boards, Chiropractic, 413
Wyoming State Board of Nursing, 454

Y

Yale New Haven Hospital, residencies, 66
Yale University, Nurse-Midwifery Program, 261
Yale University School of Medicine, Physician Associate Program, 197